SURGICAL CARE
FOR THE ELDERLY

SURGICAL CARE FOR THE ELDERLY

Edited by

R. BENTON ADKINS, JR., M.D.

Professor of Surgery and Anatomy
Vanderbilt University Medical Center

Surgeon-in-Chief
Metropolitan Nashville General Hospital
Nashville, Tennessee

H. WILLIAM SCOTT, JR., M.D.

Professor of Surgery Emeritus
Director, Section of Surgical Sciences, Emeritus
Vanderbilt University Medical Center
Nashville, Tennessee

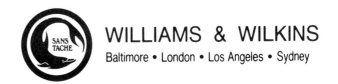

WILLIAMS & WILKINS

Baltimore • London • Los Angeles • Sydney

Editor: Kimberly Kist
Associate Editor: Victoria M. Vaughn
Copy Editor: Gail Naron Chalew
Design: Norman W. Och
Illustration Planning: Wayne Hubbel
Production: Anne G. Seitz

Copyright © 1988
Williams & Wilkins
428 East Preston Street
Baltimore, MD 21202, U.S.A.

Accurate indications, adverse reactions, and dosage schedules for drugs are provided in this book, but it is possible that they may change. The reader is urged to review the package information data of the manufacturers of the medications mentioned.

Printed in the United States of America

Library of Congress Cataloging-in-Publication Data

Surgical care for the elderly.

Includes index.
1. Aged—Surgery. I. Adkins, R. Benton. II. Scott,
H. William (Henry William), 1916–   [DNLM:
1. Surgery, Operative—in old age. W0 950 S959]
RD145.S92 1986   617'.97   87-10579
ISBN 0-683-00054-3

88 89 90 91 92
10 9 8 7 6 5 4 3 2 1

To Our Parents and Grandparents

Preface

The intention of this book is to provide an overview of the challenges, risks, and rewards involved in providing surgical care to the elderly Older persons constitute a rapidly growing segment of our society, and they are beginning to receive more and more of the medical resources of this country. They will, by necessity, require a larger share of the health care dollar, occupy more space in hospitals and other health facilities, and claim more professional attention for the solutions to their special needs.

Because of the growing realization that there are increasing numbers of Americans who are age 65 and older, because of the cost involved in their health care, and because of the volatile ethical questions that arise in the course of their medical and surgical management, media and political interest in this subject has been intense. Simultaneous with the growth in numbers of the elderly segment of the population, an attitude of increased government surveillance and cost-saving measures has been instituted in the Medicare program. The current effects of this trend of accountability are discussed briefly in this book and will likely be an issue of importance for many years to come. The circumstances now demand that health care providers be aware of these issues.

The subjects of these chapters were selected and designed to allow the reader to use this book as a reference source for his or her specific areas of interest. A few chapters address the general problems distinctive to the care of the elderly. Most chapters are devoted to specific organ systems with special emphasis on the particular problems of each of these systems where the surgical care of the elderly is involved. Other chapters deal with the issues of interest to allied health professionals. Bibliographies are selected to serve as a ready source of reference for nurses, dieticians, social service personnel, physical therapists, respiratory therapists, occupational therapists, home health care providers, nursing home personnel, psychology specialists, and those interested in gerontology in general.

Our intention is that this book would allow the practicing physician, house officer, medical student, and allied health professional easy access to advice and counsel for the specific problems that arise in the day-to-day care of the surgical diseases of the older patient. It is our hope that this text will serve as an especially valuable source of information and advice for the practitioners of all of the surgical specialties involved in the care of the elderly.

In virtually every chapter, examples are given of common disease processes that require special attention when they occur in the elderly. Whatever the disease process, the elderly patient's symptoms are often subtle. Complaints of the aged patient sometimes border on those of functional disorders and they may mimic many "normal" age-related problems. It is when these early signs and symptoms of a subtle nature are thoroughly investigated that many disease processes are detected at a time when they are curable and when life-threatening complications can be avoided. In an older patient, failure to investigate subtle symptoms, some of which will *not* lead to a firm diagnosis of organic disease, may result in the neglect of conditions until they have progressed to the point of an irretrievable pathologic state.

The theme of this book has developed into a surprisingly optimistic message for those involved with the surgical care of the elderly. This encouraging theme appears repeatedly where contributors report results of surgical treatment for many of the life-threatening and debilitating diseases in the elderly that are shown to be amazingly good. This is especially true of elective surgical treatment for most conditions.

It is our hope that this effort will stimulate further interest in research and study for the solution of those special problems that are encountered when the treatment of the elderly is undertaken. If the elderly patient needing surgical care can be treated in the appropriate manner and can be afforded the proper care, and if readers of this book can find information that might acquaint them with the many problems that are peculiar to the care of the elderly, and if those providing medical and supportive care for the elderly can find here a ready reference for many of the medical needs for these special individuals—our efforts will have been well rewarded.

Acknowledgments

We wish to express our sincere gratitude to each contributor and his or her assistants for making this text a comprehensive review. We are also indebted to Ms. Candy Hart, Ms. Julia Lacy, Ms. Jerri Smith, and Ms. Mary Lou Vantrease for their assistance in manuscript preparation. The assistance and encouragement given by Ms. Kim Kist, Ms. Vicki Vaughn, and Ms. Theda Harris at Williams & Wilkins are also greatly appreciated. Most of the difficult and time-consuming work on this book was done by our Editorial Associate, Ms. Wanda McKnight, to whom we owe special thanks.

Contributors

Bess A. Adkins, M.D., Research Associate, Department of Molecular Physiology and Biophysics, Nashville, Tennessee

R. Benton Adkins, Jr., M.D., F.A.C.S., Surgeon-in-Chief, Metropolitan Nashville General Hospital, Professor of Surgery and Anatomy, Vanderbilt University Medical Center, Nashville, Tennessee

Perry Aievoli, M.S.N., R.N.C., Mercerville, New Jersey

George R. Avant, M.D., Associate Professor of Medicine, Vanderbilt University Medical Center, Nashville, Tennessee

Brian A. Bacon, R.R.A., President, Medical Home Health Care, Tullahoma, Tennessee

Oliver H. Beahrs, M.D., F.A.C.S., Professor of Surgery, Emeritus, Mayo Medical School, Rochester, Minnesota

F. Tremaine Billings, M.D., F.A.C.P., Clinical Professor of Medicine, Emeritus, Vanderbilt University Medical Center, Nashville, Tennessee

Lonnie S. Burnett, M.D., F.A.C.O.G., Professor and Chairman, Department of Obstetrics and Gynecology, Vanderbilt University Medical Center, Nashville, Tennessee

John L. Cameron, M.D., F.A.C.S., The Warfield M. Firor Professor and Director, Section of Surgical Sciences, Surgeon-in-Chief, The Johns Hopkins Hospital, Baltimore, Maryland

Anh H. Dao, M.D., Assistant Professor of Pathology, Vanderbilt University Medical Center, Chief of Pathology, Metropolitan Nashville General Hospital, Nashville, Tennessee

Jack Davies, M.D., Professor of Anatomy and Surgery, Vanderbilt University Medical Center, Nashville, Tennessee

Gerald B. Demarest, M.D., F.A.C.S., Associate Professor of Surgery, Director, Division of Burn and Trauma, The University of New Mexico School of Medicine, Albuquerque, New Mexico

Eva A. Dimitrov, M.D., Fellow, Otolaryngology, The Otology Group, Nashville, Tennessee

James H. Elliott, M.D., F.A.C.S., George Weeks Hale Professor and Chairman, Department of Ophthalmology, Vanderbilt University Medical Center, Nashville, Tennessee

Stephen S. Feman, M.D., F.A.C.S., Associate Professor of Ophthalmology, Director of Retinal Services, Vanderbilt University Medical Center, Nashville, Tennessee

Mark K. Ferguson, M.D., Assistant Professor of Surgery, The University of Chicago, Chicago, Illinois

Michael H. Fritsch, M.D., Assistant Professor of Otology and Neurotology, Indiana University School of Medicine, Indianapolis, Indiana

R. Neal Garrison, M.D., F.A.C.S., Associate Professor of Surgery, University of Louisville School of Medicine, Surgical Service, Veterans Administration Medical Center, Louisville, Kentucky

Michael E. Glasscock, III, M.D., F.A.C.S., Clinical Professor of Otology and Neurotology, Vanderbilt University Medical Center, The Otology Group, Nashville, Tennessee

Clive S. Grant, M.D., F.A.C.S., Assistant Professor of Surgery, Section Head, Gastro-enterologic and General Surgery, Mayo Clinic, Rochester, Minnesota

John D. Hainsworth, M.D., Assistant Professor of Medicine, Division of Medical Oncology, Vanderbilt University Medical Center, Nashville, Tennessee

Phil J. Harbrecht, M.D., F.A.C.S., Chief of Surgery, Veterans Administration Medical Center, Professor of Surgery, University of Louisville School of Medicine, Louisville, Kentucky

Howard W. Jones, III, M.D., F.A.C.O.G., Associate Professor of Obstetrics and Gynecology, Director of Gynecologic Oncology, Vanderbilt University Medical Center, Nashville, Tennessee

Anne Keane, Ed.D., R.N., Associate Professor of Nursing, Director of Graduate Programs in Adult Health and Illness, University of Pennsylvania, Philadelphia, Pennsylvania

Duncan A. Killen, M.D., F.A.C.S., Clinical Professor of Surgery, University of Missouri, Kansas City School of Medicine, Staff Surgeon, Mid-America Heart Institute of St. Luke's Hospital, Kansas City, Missouri

Fred K. Kirchner, Jr., M.D., F.A.C.S., Chief of Urology, Metropolitan Nashville General Hospital, Associate Professor of Urology, Vanderbilt University Medical Center, Nashville, Tennessee

Michael O. Koch, M.D., Assistant Professor of Urology, Vanderbilt University Medical Center, Nashville, Tennessee

Michael Lichtenstein, M.D., M.Sc., Assistant Professor of Medicine, Vanderbilt University Medical Center, Nashville, Tennessee

Keith D. Lillemoe, M.D., Assistant Professor of Surgery, The Johns Hopkins Hospital, Baltimore, Maryland

John B. Lynch, M.D., F.A.C.S., Professor and Chairman, Department of Plastic Surgery, Vanderbilt University Medical Center, Nashville, Tennessee

Richard A. Margolin, M.D., Assistant Professor of Psychiatry and Radiology, Vanderbilt University Medical Center, Nashville, Tennessee

Kenneth L. Mattox, M.D., F.A.C.S., Professor of Surgery, Baylor College of Medicine, Deputy Surgeon-in-Chief, Ben Taub General Hospital, Houston, Texas

Wanda G. McKnight, A.R.T., Editorial Associate, Department of Surgery, Vanderbilt University Medical Center, Nashville, Tennessee

Patrick W. Meacham, M.D., Assistant Professor of Surgery, Vascular Division, Vanderbilt University Medical Center, Nashville, Tennessee

William F. Meacham, M.D., F.A.C.S., Clinical Professor of Neurosurgery, Emeritus, Vanderbilt University Medical Center, Nashville, Tennessee

W. Jerry Merrell, M.D., Assistant Professor of Anesthesiology and Pharmacology, University of Florida College of Medicine, Gainesville, Florida

Anne E. Missavage, M.D., Major MC, Chief, Burn Study Branch, US Army Institute of Surgical Research, Fort Sam Houston, San Antonio, Texas

James L. Netterville, M.D., Assistant Professor of Otolaryngology, Vanderbilt University Medical Center, Nashville, Tennessee

Lloyd M. Nyhus, M.D., F.A.C.S., F.R.C.S. (Eng)(Hon), F.R.C.S.I. (Hon), Professor and Head, Department of Surgery, The University of Illinois College of Medicine at Chicago, Chicago, Illinois

Robert H. Ossoff, M.D., D.M.D., F.A.C.S., Guy M. Maness Professor and Chairman, Department of Otolaryngology, Vanderbilt University Medical Center, Nashville, Tennessee

Richard M. Peters, M.D., F.A.C.S., Professor of Surgery and Bioengineering, Director of Surgery, Research, and Education, Co-Head, Cardiothoracic Training Program, University of California Medical Center, San Diego, California

Raymond Pollak, M.B., F.R.C.S. (Edin.), Assistant Professor of Surgery, The University of Illinois Hospital, Chicago, Illinois

Raymond W. Postlethwait, M.D., F.A.C.S., Professor of Surgery, Emeritus, Duke University, Durham, North Carolina

Basil A. Pruitt, Jr., M.D., F.A.C.S., Colonel MC, Commander and Director, US Army Institute of Surgical Research, Fort Sam Houston, San Antonio, Texas

Riley S. Rees, M.D., F.A.C.S., Chief of Plastic Surgery, Veterans Administration Medical Center, Associate Professor of Plastic Surgery, Vanderbilt University Medical Center, Nashville, Tennessee

Louis Rosenfeld, M.D., F.A.C.S., Clinical Professor of Surgery, Emeritus, Vanderbilt University Medical Center, Nashville, Tennessee

Ronald E. Rosenthal, M.D., F.A.C.S., Associate Professor of Clinical Orthopaedic Surgery, State University of New York at Stony Brook, Chief, Division of Trauma, Department of Orthopaedic Surgery, Long Island Jewish Medical Center, New Hyde Park, New York

Joel J. Roslyn, M.D., F.A.C.S., Assistant Professor of Surgery, University of California, Los Angeles Medical Center, Los Angeles, California

John L. Sawyers, M.D., F.A.C.S., John Clinton Foshee Distinguished Professor and Chairman, Department of Surgery, Director, Section of Surgical Sciences, Vanderbilt University Medical Center, Nashville, Tennessee

H. William Scott, Jr., M.D., D.Sc. (Hon), F.A.C.S., F.R.A.C.S., Professor of Surgery, Emeritus, Vanderbilt University Medical Center, Nashville, Tennessee

R. Bruce Shack, M.D., F.A.C.S., Associate Professor of Plastic Surgery, Vanderbilt University Medical Center, Nashville, Tennessee

David B. Skinner, M.D., F.A.C.S., Dallas B. Phemister Professor and Chairman, Department of Surgery, The University of Chicago, Chicago, Illinois

Bradley E. Smith, M.D., Professor of Anesthesiology, Chairman, Department of Anesthesiology, Vanderbilt University Medical Center, Nashville, Tennessee

Ronald K. Tompkins, M.D., F.A.C.S., Professor and Chief, General Surgery, University of California, Los Angeles Medical Center, Los Angeles, California

Jon A. van Heerden, M.B., F.R.C.S.(C), F.A.C.S., Professor of Surgery, Mayo Clinic, Rochester, Minnesota

Mary G. Wallace, R.R.A., Director, Medical Information Services, Vanderbilt University Medical Center, Nashville, Tennessee

Charles E. Wells, M.D., Clinical Professor of Psychiatry and Neurology, Vanderbilt University Medical Center, Nashville, Tennessee

Contents

Chapter 1

History and Philosophy

R. Benton Adkins, Jr., M.D., F.A.C.S., Wanda G. McKnight, A.R.T.

Recently there has been an increasing acceptance among internists and general practitioners of the concept of elective surgical care in the elderly. Biliary tract disease, peptic ulcer disease, herniae, and vascular diseases are excellent examples of disorders for which surgical consultations are being requested earlier in the disease process (1). Correctable conditions that require relatively major surgical procedures are being successfully managed in older and older people. When done under well controlled elective conditions, the results are fantastically good (2, 3). Even in urgent and emergency settings, the situation is not always hopeless. In this book, we have undertaken the task of documenting the current status of and recommendations for surgical treatment of the elderly.

The surgical care of older persons is not a new concept facing the medical profession. Physicians have always devoted what sometimes appears to be a disproportionate share of their time to the care of the elderly. The number of elderly persons in our society is steadily increasing, to the point that many medical doctors are now choosing to devote their entire practice to the care of older patients. It has been estimated that 40%–50% of the time of most non-pediatric physicians and more than 30% of all health care dollars are currently devoted to the diagnosis, treatment, and long-term care of older persons (4). The population of elderly persons is growing steadily in numbers and in age level, and their medical needs are gradually changing. The special problem of the surgical care for these older, more active, generally healthy members of American society is now of great interest to most political, business, industrial, medical, and social groups.

The medical advances of the 19th century have enabled people in our society to live longer and to remain healthy longer. The discovery of anesthesia, the understanding of the relationship between microorganisms and disease, the concept of antisepsis, the inadvertent discovery of antimicrobials, and the better understanding of the physiologic basis of many metabolic diseases have led to a more effective life-saving and life-prolonging medical care environment (5). The 20th century has brought with it an extension, refinement, and an elaboration of the discoveries of the previous 100 years. In recent years, epidemics have been rare. Infections, which were lethal only a few years ago, are now either nonexistent or readily treated by the use of the appropriate antibiotic. Surgical techniques are continually being refined, and the recent use of surgical mechanical devices, grafts, and organ transplantation has allowed persons who would have died of their diseases just a few years ago to return to healthy, productive lives. The electron microscope, invented in the late 1930s, has led to medical advances in the fields of oncology and virology. The culture and study of viruses resulted in control of poliomyelitis and other viral diseases. Public health and sanitation have continued to improve (5). Appendicitis was first recognized as a surgical entity only 100 years ago. Consider that a person born in 1900 (who at the time of this writing is 87 years old) has seen during his or her adult years the discovery of major red blood cell types, the discovery of penicillin, the advances of roentgenography, the discovery of insulin, internal fixation of fractures, the evolution of kidney dialysis and organ transplantation, and major advances in cardiovascular procedures. Advances in the care of trauma and cancer victims in the last 50 years have resulted in the saving and the prolonging of many additional lives. The rapidly developing fields of computerized body scanning, immunologic typing, and cancer chemotherapy are having an incalculable influence on longevity at this time. The benefactors of these scientific and medical phenomena are now adding to the population pool of elderly Americans at the most dramatic rate in the history of our country.

IMPACTS OF AGING AND THE AGED: DEMOGRAPHIC TRENDS

Population

We are now living in what has been called "the century of old age" (4). The increase in average life expectancy realized in this century almost equals the total increase of the previous 5000 years. Even at age 100, one is expected to live almost 3 more years. (See Table 1.1) It has been estimated that by the year 2030 there will be 55 million people in the United States who are 65 years of age or older as compared to only 9 million in 1940 (4). This steady increase in the proportion of older people in this country is due in part to the relatively stable fertility, mortality, and immigration rates seen now in the United States. Persons born in the 1980s can expect to see the proportion of elderly persons *double* in their lifetimes. Seven of ten newborns today can

Table 1.1 Life Expectancy

Age	Years Expected
65	16.6
70	13.4
75	10.6
80	8.4
85	6.7[a]
90	4.4
95	3.3
100	2.7
105	2.4
110	2.2[b]

[a]From Expectation of Life at Single Years of Age, by Race and Sex, United States, 1979, *Vital Statistics of the United States*. Washington, DC, US Department of Health and Human Services, Public Health Service, National Center for Health Statistics, 1979.
[b]From United States Life Tables: 1969–1971. Washington, DC, DHEW Publication No. HRA 75-1150, Public Health Service, National Center for Health Statistics, 1975.

expect to reach age 65 (4). Over the course of a decade, 60% of the older population is replaced by other individuals who become 65 years of age and older (4). This rapid turnover of membership in the elite club of elderly may become less rapid as our medical successes complicate the equation. Some authors have subdivided the population of older persons into two groups: young-old (55–75 years) and old-old (over 75 years). Surprisingly, the over 75 year group is now growing proportionally faster than the elderly population as a whole. It is estimated that by the year 2040, there will be 8 million persons over age 85 (14.5% of all elderly persons) (4). We can expect females to continue to outnumber males. The percentage of older persons will continue to be greater in the white population than it is among blacks.

Socioeconomic Trends

Increased incidence and prevalence of disease and disability in older persons obviously result in an increased need for medical care. The current financial impact of health care for increasing numbers of older persons is substantial, and the future impact can be anticipated based on current statistics. Even now, 30% of all health costs are associated with persons over 65 years of age. In 1982, 10% of the gross national product (approximately $320 billion) was spent on health care—$83 billion for Medicare and Medicaid (largely consumed by older Americans) (4). Forty percent of our Medicaid dollars are now being spent for nursing home care. There are some 20,000 long-term care facilities in this country housing approximately 1.4 million older Americans or only 5% of our elderly population at any given time. However, in the group of persons 85 years of age and older, a greater percentage (22%) are living in nursing homes (4). The demands for the medical community to respond more effectively and efficiently to older patients' medical needs will increase dramatically in the next few years.

As greater demands are being placed on the medical community, there is a simultaneous demand to lower the cost of health care. The federally supported and the private insurers have initiated programs designed to encourage physicians and hospitals to hospitalize fewer patients for shorter periods of time and use the absolute minimum of resources for each patient. These efforts could potentially lower the quality of care for all patients, especially for the most costly—the elderly. Immediate, expedient treatment is obviously less costly than long-term treatment for a condition that could be corrected. This issue will receive more attention in later chapters.

Although they use a substantial percentage of health care dollars, many elderly citizens are not financially secure. However, the economic disadvantage that has generally been associated with the elderly population has lessened in recent years. In 1959, 35.2% of elderly persons lived below the poverty level; in 1974 the percentage had decreased to only 14.6% (4). Of those elderly persons living alone, however, 27% were poor in 1977. Only 8% of those living with their own families were classified as poor (4).

Social and Cultural Trends

In addition to the ever-increasing numbers of older Americans, the characteristics of the population of older people are constantly changing as well. As new individuals enter the older age group each year, they bring with them slightly different values, ideals, expectations, and life experiences. They are becoming a group of well-informed, "modern" individuals.

In the past, there has been a considerable educational disadvantage among the elderly. Today, slightly more than 40% of our elderly have only an elementary school education. This percentage will decrease to 20% in the next few years (4). Before many years, a substantial percentage will be college graduates.

Other social and cultural aspects of aging have also changed dramatically in the last century. In 18th-century America, older citizens were highly respected and venerated. In that mostly agrarian culture, they controlled most of the wealth and the land, served as role models, and were the keepers of traditions and history within the society. Most historians suggest that the bias began to shift toward the young in the mid-19th century with gradually increasing urbanization and industrialization. Many young adults broke the bonds of clan and family dependence and became self-reliant in the industrial arena. This bias in favor of the young is consistent with the findings of many cross-cultural researchers who maintain that the status of elderly persons varies

directly with the control that they have over the valued resources of the family (6). The mid-20th century brought with it forced retirement, a degree of family abandonment, increased poverty among the elderly, and a correspondingly diminished social status of some of the aged members of society.

Nevertheless, the financial and social status of most older persons has significantly improved since World War II, due in part to government social programs, which resulted from widespread revival of a sensitivity within our society to the plight of the elderly. Evidence of increased sensitivity to the needs of the elderly can be found in the large number of social programs now in existence. Many of the first gerontologic researchers had assumed that the public's view of the elderly was basically negative, but the opposite was actually found to be true. In fact, elderly persons in this country are not generally the victims of social prejudice. Due in part to widespread news media coverage, Americans are taught to overestimate the dismal plight of the elderly today. We tend to have an inflated perception of the percentage of older persons living in institutions and/or below the poverty line. There is no statistical evidence to support the notion that a large percentage of older persons are neglected by their children or are left alone to die in nursing homes. Conversely, 81% of older Americans have caring, loving, living children, and in one study, more than 80% of the older persons surveyed had seen at least one of their children in the preceding week (6). In a similar study, 55% of those surveyed had seen at least one of their children within the past 24 hours (6). This is not to belittle or underestimate the serious disadvantage that a few elderly people do experience even today both financially and socially when little or no family support is available.

We can realistically expect that the social status of America's elderly will continue to improve in the coming years. Evidence of our increased awareness of the importance of the elderly is growing in this country. For instance, the highly influential advertising agencies are now recognizing the over-50 as group as a very large and desirable segment of consumers (7). This is a radical change from the youth-oriented attitude of advertising in the recent past. In movies and television shows, more and more older Americans are being featured in positive, attractive roles. The list of much older Americans in politics, business, and the entertainment industry continues to grow and, in fact, has become lengthy and impressive. These Americans are setting the pace for the average older American and are helping to change the attitudes of all Americans toward older people. The elderly are now also in the position to know what is available medically, will expect to benefit from it, and will continue to demand consideration for more and more aggressive medical and surgical treatment.

Health Status and Medical Care

The general public tends to underestimate the good health status of most older Americans. Although only about one-half of America's elderly are limited at all in their daily living activities, it is true that over 80% of older persons report having one or more chronic medical conditions (8). The incidence of acute disease in the elderly is relatively low; the treatment of chronic illness therefore constitutes the major health care problem and cost for older Americans. Despite this high incidence of a variety of chronic medical conditions, most older persons do not actually consider themselves to be seriously handicapped by their age or by these conditions. The overwhelming majority of older persons when questioned will rate their health as "good" or "excellent" and, when asked to compare their health status to that of others in their own age group, will rate it as better (8).

The major causes of death in persons 65 years of age and older are heart disease, malignant tumors, and cerebrovascular disease. As mentioned earlier, this older group of our population now accounts for almost one-third of the nation's health care expenditures, generally require more frequent hospital visits and more physician time, and consume about one-fourth of all legal drugs purchased in the United States (8).

In spite of the few well-publicized and dramatic instances of fraud and abuse, there are actually very few inadequacies in the vast health care system in this country. It is true that the few "service gaps" that do exist generally tend to affect older patients, especially those with lower incomes, more than younger patients. Delivery systems for home health care, long-term care, rehabilitation, and preventive services are not as efficient, well-defined, or as intensely monitored as are other more traditional health care delivery systems. Attention to these areas is increasing at the time of this writing. This will be addressed in subsequent chapters. The special health needs of the elderly are becoming a top priority for health care planners.

In addition to improving the health care system for all of those who need medical care in this country, attention is now being focused on promoting healthy lifestyles. This will undoubtedly have a positive effect on the health status of the future elderly and also upon longevity itself. Decreased pollution exposure, better exercise habits, improved nutrition, elimination of smoking, and modification of drinking habits will significantly affect the health status of all age groups. The beneficial effect of these efforts is already being reflected in the numbers of healthy, well-educated Americans reaching more advanced age groups each year. They will expect and demand the same health care offered to their younger countrymen.

THE IMPACT OF CHRONIC DISEASE IN THE AGED

Chronic disease is the major health factor among the elderly. In the population age group 45–64, approximately 72% have one or more chronic illnesses. The percentage increases to 86% for persons 65 years of age and older. Additionally, the incidence of *multiple* chronic conditions also increases. The most common of these are reported to be arthritis (38%), hearing impairments (29%), vision impairments (20%), hypertension (20%), and heart conditions (20%) (8). The incidence of arthritis and hypertension is higher among older females, but they demonstrate a lower incidence of hearing impairments. Heart conditions occur with similar frequency in men and women. All chronic conditions except for peptic ulcer disease are found to occur more frequently among those elderly who are classified as "poor" (8).

The impact of chronic disease on the daily living activities of the elderly is statistically substantial in spite of the fact that most individuals in this age group do not consider themselves to be seriously handicapped by their condition.

Most older persons do not experience *serious* activity limitations, but almost half of all elderly persons are limited to some degree in carrying out the activities of daily living. The conditions that are most limiting are heart conditions (52%), diabetes (34%), asthma (27%), and arthritis (23%) (8).

In terms of general mobility, most elderly persons (approximately 82%) are not seriously restricted. Females are more likely to have some degree of mobility limitation than males. The major causes of mobility limitation are arthritis, rheumatism, lower extremity disorders, heart conditions, and cerebrovascular disease. It is interesting to note that if the major cardiovascular-renal diseases (i.e., heart disease, stroke, hypertension, etc.) were eliminated, we would realize an extra 11.4 years in life expectancy after age 65. These are the illnesses that are and should be receiving major research emphasis at this time (8). As mentioned earlier, most of the health care costs for the elderly are attributed to these chronic conditions. They also consume the largest part of the time and support given by family members and health care providers to elderly patients. Surprisingly, the chronic illnesses do not affect results of surgical care of older patients to the degree that one might expect.

THE IMPACT OF DELAYED TREATMENT IN THE ELDERLY

In spite of the prevalence of chronic disease among the elderly, America's elderly are amazingly resilient. Several investigators have found little correlation between the presence of chronic disease and operative mortality when surgical conditions arise. In many studies, urgent and emergency operations rather than chronic disease have proved to be the greatest risk factor in operative mortality of elderly patients who require surgical treatment (2, 3, 9–11). Emergency procedures have been shown to increase the risk of operative mortality two to threefold (12, 13). The operative mortality rate in the elderly varies from a low of 0.85% (9) for elective procedures to a high of 45% (3) for emergency operations. When surgical disease states are recognized and corrected in a timely manner under careful, controlled, elective conditions, older patients have been found to tolerate even the most major surgical procedures and to recover remarkably well. However, the elderly patient's tolerance for delay, technical mistakes, or errors in judgement is lower than seen in younger patients. Accurate preoperative appraisal of the elderly patient and *early,* careful attention to the surgical needs of the patient are essential in producing a good outcome for the patient. The use of the American Society of Anesthesiologists Physical Status Scale with the addition of invasive evaluation in very high-risk patients has been suggested (14). This type of aggressive evaluation will allow us to chose more intelligently the proper surgical candidates from all age groups.

As patients are living longer, most physicians are seeing that, when surgical problems are left unattended, an emergency situation is likely to arise. In a recent review of 75 patients aged 90 or more who had 85 major surgical procedures, we found strong evidence to support the notion that elective operations are tolerated well in the elderly. In 42 elective cases, postoperative mortality was only 2.3% compared to 45% in the group of patients whose situations had progressed to the point of requiring emergency procedures. (See Figure 1.1) Even under urgent and emergency conditions, the results were not overwhelmingly disasterous in these very old patients.

SPECIAL SURGICAL CONSIDERATIONS FOR THE ELDERLY

The special needs and problems of elderly patients should receive personalized attention before any significant operation is considered. This, of course, is not always possible in some urgent and most true emergency situations. In cases of planned, elective procedures, however, the surgeon will do well to consider all of the special needs of his elderly patient. (See Chapter 3)

The patient's home or extended care environment should also be evaluated. Will the patient be returning to a safe atmosphere for recovery after the operation? If it seems unlikely that the patient will be able to return home, efforts must be initiated early to find placement in an extended care facility where rehabilitation, return to independence, and return to a home environment can be pursued. A close relationship with the pa-

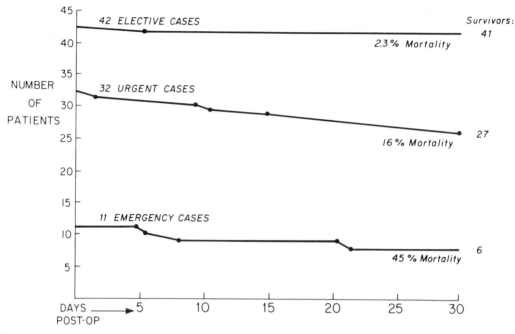

Figure 1.1 Postoperative deaths related to original exigency of operative procedure. Elective operations were those for which indications allowed ample time for preparation of patient. Urgent operations were done after short planning and preparation time for potentially life-threatening conditions. Emergency procedures were those done for progressive, life-threatening conditions. (Reprinted by permission from the *South Med J* 77:1357–1364, 1984.)

tient's family and the Social Services Department of the hospital can expedite these procedures. The economic impact of the operative procedure and recovery period upon the patient, the family, the community, and the public resources that will be required should be considered, but these factors should not outweigh the purely medical and surgical needs of the patient in the decision-making process. Elderly patients themselves may be able to assist in these deliberations, and their wishes must always be considered.

Another special concern that must be remembered in the surgical care of the elderly is the patient's concept of hospitals and attitude toward doctors in general. Consider that many of an elderly person's peers have died in hospitals and that some of them may fear the same fate. Although most older people continue to have a great reverence for doctors in general, their previous experience with hospitals may have been before many of the new technological advances were available. Moreover, because older persons have probably seen some of their counterparts become disabled and helpless over the

years, their fear of disability and dependency is usually greater than in the young. Other authors have described this situation (13).

An honest appraisal of the elderly patient's prognosis and expectations should be communicated to him or her and the family. The surgeon and the referring doctor must do this in a straight-forward manner. The fact that patients are older is not necessarily an indication that they cannot understand their disorder and make their own intelligent decisions about their future. As in dealing with any surgical patient, the necessary emotional support should be provided, utilizing all available and necessary resources. Geriatric nurses are specially trained to meet the needs of older patients. (See Chapter 7)

More than any other group of physicians, American doctors must be aware of the special cultural characteristics of our many ethnic groups. Such characteristics as those seen in some ethnic groups with a strong matriarchal structure and in many Eastern cultures where there is an adoration of the parents, the fatalistic approach of some religious groups, and the stoicism of such groups as the American Indian all become very important factors to consider when doctors and families plan operative, postoperative, and rehabilitative care for the elderly patient.

Problems that are known to be more common in the postoperative period for the older patient should be anticipated and avoided by appropriate measures taken in the preoperative preparation period. Pulmonary function, renal function, and nutritional status should be carefully evaluated preoperatively, and corrective steps should be taken whenever possible in an attempt to avoid postoperative complications. The widespread use of steroids and antihypertensives in the elderly should be remembered and documented. Their effect should be recognized and their continued use monitored. If possible, steroids should be tapered and discontinued during the preoperative period (13). Special attention to these and other specific medical conditions will be addressed in subsequent chapters.

WHEN ENOUGH IS ENOUGH

In the course of events that are associated with any terminal disease or condition, there arrives a time, regardless of the patient's age, when the hope of reasonable success is unlikely. To press forward with heroic measures beyond this point becomes an exercise in prolonging death, rather than prolonging life. Before this point is reached, we, like Wagner (15) and others, would suggest that some understanding of the patient's wishes be discussed. This must always be considered when the propriety of withholding or offering cardiopulmonary resuscitation in the elderly is at issue. As Levinson (16) has so eloquently stated, there comes a time when "death is the best life has to offer." Obviously, advanced age alone must not be equated arbitrarily with universally hopeless situations (17, 18). It is to be our office to distinguish that which is appropriate, advise that which should be done, and administer the correct decision in these circumstances.

TROUBLING TRENDS

Since there has been a progressive increase in the numbers of elderly individuals living for longer periods of time and needing more medical, surgical, and long term care, the cost of keeping the elderly alive and healthy has become an issue of great social importance. The Health Care Financing Administration (HCFA) has placed a priority on cutting Medicare costs. In 1982, the Tax Equity Fiscal Responsibility Act (TEFRA—PL 97.248) was passed that established a Prospective Payment System (PPS) and Professional Review Organizations (PROs) to reduce the federal expenditures in the Medicare program.

The Inspector General of HCFA has vowed to seek out the "criminal element" in the medical profession that is perceived as the culprit (19). PROs have been given specific guidelines regarding the amount of money to recover each year by denying hospital payment for medical care. Immediate review of cases and eventually sanctions against physicians and hospitals for perceived inappropriate care are being determined based upon a generic screening process. These so-called quality screens include situations that often occur in the course of treatment through the fault of no one but as the result of uncontrollable circumstances. The generic screens currently in use are outlined in Table 1.2. Although they are modified frequently, the authors feel that the screens warrant mention because of the impact of the screening process on surgical care. They are generally effective retroactively.

When the PRO determines that a provider or practitioner has violated Medicare guidelines, notice is given to the affected party. An opportunity for informal discussion and formal appeal follows. The final PRO determination is reported to the Office of the Inspector General who then reviews the PRO recommendation. If the final determination is that a violation of the guidelines did occur, notice of such determination is given to the practitioner or provider; the local and regional PROs; state licensing bodies; state Medicaid agencies; hospitals, skilled nursing facilities, and Health Maintenance Organizations where the practitioner has privileges; medical societies and other professional organizations; fiscal intermediaries; and often local newspapers. The effect of the sanction is in financial assessment or invalidation of Medicare assignments. The affected practitioner or provider has the right to judicial review *after* the sanction has been im-

Table 1.2 Generic Quality Screens[a]

1. Admission following inadequate outpatient management and/or complication of outpatient procedure.
2. Unplanned transfer from general care unit to special care unit (ICU/CCU).
3. *Inappropriate* transfer to another acute care facility.
4. *Unapproved* transfer to another acute care facility.
5. Blood administration incident/error (NOT life-threatening complications).
6. Operation for perforation, laceration, tear, or injury of an organ incurred during an invasive procedure.
7. *Unnecessary* invasive procedure.
8. *Inappropriate* invasive procedure.
9. Cancellation of or repeat diagnostic procedure due to improper preparation of patient, technician error, or equipment failure.
10. Myocardial infarction during or within 48 hours of a surgical procedure on this admission.
11. Neurological deficit or footdrop present at discharge which was not present upon admission.
12. Cardiac or respiratory arrest (not resulting in death).
13. Adverse reaction and/or complication resulting from respiratory therapy.
14. Delay in administration of services.
15. Repeated laboratory test due to error in obtaining, handling, or storage of lab samples.
16. History and physical, discharge summary, operative reports, etc. not dictated on a timely basis as defined.
17. No chest x-ray to validate primary diagnosis of pneumonia.
18. No smear and culture of sputum and/or bronchial secretions to validate primary diagnosis of pneumonia.
19. No culture and sensitivity and/or appropriate bacterial investigation prior to initiating antibiotic for pneumonia.
20. Pathology report does not match pre-operative diagnosis.
21. Unexpected specimen received by pathology department.
22. Patient ordered NPO, but received diet despite the order.
23. Diet not given to the patient as ordered.
24. Reaction to x-ray dye during cardiac cath or x-ray procedures (*not* life-threatening complications).
25. Attempted or unsuccessful radiological or angiographic procedures.
26. Attempted or unsuccessful cardiac catheterization.
27. Attempted or unsuccessful PTCA procedure.
28. Hematoma as a result of an invasive procedure (*no* major treatment necessary).
29. Surgical back-up not documented prior to PTCA procedure.
30. Barium administered without physician's orders.
31. Other complications *or* quality of care concerns not classifiable in any of the above mentioned elements.

[a]From the Mid-South Foundation for Medical Care, Inc., Memphis, TN)

posed and publicized.

The PROs have been charged with reducing the number of hospital admissions and thereby saving federal dollars spent through the Medicare program. In actuality, the great reduction has been in *reimbursed* hospitalizations; most physicians and hospitals have continued to admit and treat the elderly sick as indicated regardless of the patient's financial status or the threat of sanction.

It seems inevitable that most of the physician contributors to this text, because of their love for and interest in the medical and surgical care of elderly citizens in this country, will have their names listed among those against whom sanctions have been levied by HCFA. It is ironic that those of us who have the strongest interest in the elderly and indeed who love them most are liable to be excluded from participating in their care by these punitive and arbitrary rules. We have, it seems, returned to the Code of Hammurabi (5), wherein failure to cure, a perception of inefficient care, or the unavoidable trap of a "Catch-22" situation imposed by the sanctioning process will result in the "cutting off" of the hand that cares for the aged. Examples that horrify and frustrate the medical profession are already abundant. In a few instances, the medical care in rural communities has been seriously hampered by sanctions against all of the few available providers and practitioners in that area. (*American Medical News*, April 10, 1987, p 1; 53.)

PROSPECTS FOR THE FUTURE

The emergence of geriatric medicine as a viable treatment and research specialty is evidence of the growing concern of the profession for the medical care of the elderly in our country. The premise of geriatric medicine is that aging itself is a clinical phenomenon that is worthy of a group of clinicians' full attention. This is not to say that only gerontologists are qualified to care for older patients. As noted earlier, America's physicians have always spent a large percentage of their time caring for the elderly. As is appropriate with all special patient populations, the medical community must commit itself to providing the best possible care for and meeting the health needs of the older patient. We must work toward developing improved attitudes, efficient and effective service organizations, sufficient monetary funds, and an accurate appreciation of the importance of the elderly person's role in our society and within our professions. It is obvious to all of us that each year a larger percentage of our population is living to enter the older decades of life. It behooves the medical profession, which is at least partially responsible for creating this predicament, to prepare for the challenge of dealing with the medical and surgical care of more and more of these not-so-fragile survivors of the game of life.

REFERENCES

1. Glenn F: Surgical principles for the aged patient. In Reichel W (ed): *Clinical Aspects of Aging.* Baltimore, Williams & Wilkins, 1983, pp 453–468.

2. Harbrecht PH, Garrison RN, Fry DE: Surgery in elderly patients. *South Med J* 74:594–598, 1981.

3. Adkins RB, Scott HW: Surgical procedures in patients aged 90 years and older. *South Med J* 77:1357–1364, 1984.

4. Watts D, McCally M: Demographic perspectives. In Cassel DK, Walsh JR (eds): *Geriatric Medicine.* New York, Springer-Verlag, 1984, pp 3–15.

5. Lyons AS, Petrucelli RJ: *Medicine, An Illustrated History.* New York, Harry N. Abrams, Inc, 1978.

6. Schulz R, Manson S: Social perspectives. In Cassel DK, Walsh JR (eds): *Geriatric Medicine.* New York, Springer-Verlag, 1984, pp 16–27.

7. Hoyt MF: The new prime time. *USA Weekend* December 13–15, 1985.

8. *Fact Book on Aging.* Washington, DC, The National Council on the Aging, Inc., Washington, 1978.

9. Greenburg AF, Saik RP, Farris JM, Peskin GW: Operative mortality in general surgery. *Am J Surg* 144:22–28, 1982. 10. Linn BS, Linn MW, Wallen N: Evaluation of results of surgical procedures in the elderly. *Ann Surg* 195:90–96, 1982.

11. Kohn P, Zekert F, Vormittag E, Grabner H: Risks of operation in patients over 80. *Geriatrics* 28:100–105, 1973.

12. Greenburg AG, Saik RP, Coyle JJ, Peskin GW: Mortality and gastrointestinal surgery in the aged. *Arch Surg* 116:788–791, 1981.

13. Robins RE, Budden MK: Major abdominal surgery in patients over 70 years of age, results during 1962 to 1966 compared with those during 1950 to 1959. *Can J Surg* 15:1–6, 1972.

14. Mohr DN: Estimation of surgical risk in the elderly, a correlative review. *J Am Geriatr Soc* 31:99–102, 1983.

15. Wagner A: Cardiopulmonary resuscitation in the aged. *N Engl J Med* 310:1129–1130, 1984.

16. Levinson AJR: Termination of life support systems in the elderly: ethical issues. *J Geriatr Psych* 14:71–85, 1981.

17. DeBard ML: Cardiopulmonary resuscitation: analysis of six years' experience and review of the literature. *Ann Emerg Med* 10:408–416, 1981.

18. Gulati RS, Bhan GL, Horan MA: Cardiopulmonary resuscitation of old people. *Lancet* 2:267–269, 1983.

19. Hostetler D: AHA meeting focuses on federal budget: "The only game in town." *JAMRA* 58(3):42–44, 1987.

Chapter 2

The Anatomic and Physiologic Aspects of Aging

Bess A. Adkins, M.D., Jack Davies, M.D., R. Benton Adkins, Jr., M.D., F.A.C.S.

All organ systems are affected by the aging process. Some tissues and organ systems respond to the wear and tear of daily existence at a different rate from that of others. The most important effects of aging, which alter the physician's approach to aggressive medical and surgical care, are those that materially diminish the quality of life or those that would by their changes exert undue risk if surgical procedures were needed. Some of these changes are irreversible by any medical or surgical intervention. It is the purpose of this chapter to address those issues of aging existing within each organ system that significantly alter the physician's approach to the care of the elderly and the methods of care that may be necessary for success in their management.

The process of aging has been attributed to an incredible variety of factors, including the existence of a finite and immutable maximum number of doublings for a given cell population (the Hayflick principle) (1), cumulative cellular damage from free radicals and radiations (2), errors in protein synthesis (3), alterations in the immune system (4), deleterious effects of endogenous steroid hormones (5), and the cross-linkage theory (6). (See Chapter 37)

The Hayflick principle deserves special consideration because it is backed by solid laboratory observations to support its point of view that aging is based upon a genetic clock and that species-specific numbers of cell doublings can occur before all the cells from that parent organism die and will not divide further (7). If true, the known life span, like that of all species, is genetically fixed at a finite maximum length. For humans senescence is reached after approximately 50 population doublings (8).

The immune-autoimmune theory proposes that the cells of successive generations of divisions begin to produce "defective proteins" within the DNA and RNA phases of replication during cellular growth. These proteins then act as antigens to the immune system, which then begins to attack and damage all the tissues that have developed this histo-incompatible state. As the organism ages, more antigens are formed and more tissues are affected and eliminated by the immune response.

The cross-linkage theory of aging assumes that the constant bonding of two or more molecules in a side to side arrangement is taking place within all cells. Age-dependent changes result in damage to the tissues, such as loss of elasticity in the connective tissue, reduced "swelling" capacity of all cells, increased molecular weight of critical nuclear molecules, and a "brittleness" of the tissues. Bjorksten has published an excellent discussion of this concept of aging (6).

Only severe caloric restriction in certain rats and mice has been found consistently to prolong the life span (9), although exercise begun early in life may also extend the life span of mice (10). The claims of persons living to be as old as 170 years in the Georgia Republic of the Soviet Union, the village of Vilcabamba in the Ecuador Andes, and in the Hunza region in Pakistan have been found to be greatly exaggerated. The uncertainty of the true age of these people is due to the illiteracy of those involved and due to the desire for political gain for the leaders of the region and for other economic reasons (11–13). As yet, no data exist to confirm or refute the effectiveness of any intervention aimed at extending the human life span (14). Thus, although eliminating various diseases has increased our life expectancy, allowing a greater proportion of the population to approach the maximum life span, nothing has been shown to alter that maximum age to which one individual may aspire, which is, presumably, determined by normal physiologic aging (11).

It is sometimes confusing to the laity and even to some members of the medical profession when an overlap of the normal processes of aging and some unrelated true pathologic processes begin to blend into the same circumstance. We have tried to separate those true pathologic situations that are apt to occur in the elderly from those processes that are most likely due to the "normal" processes of aging. This chapter deals with the latter, whereas the former is covered in many of the subsequent chapters on specific diseases of each organ system in the elderly.

CARDIOVASCULAR SYSTEM

A major consideration that is necessary to remember when discussing the aging cardiovascular system is the issue of atherosclerosis, which is felt by most to be a pathologic condition, rather than a normal process of aging. In this country, it is nonetheless so prevalent and so parallel to aging that it confuses many human studies aimed at examining the normal changes of aging. This discussion will deal primarily with the anatomic and physiologic changes associated with aging that are expected to occur regardless of the presence or absence of atherosclerosis.

Vasculature

Histologic studies reveal intimal hyperplasia and thickening that progress with age, beginning early in life (15) with fragmentation of the internal elastic lamina in the arteries, especially those of the lower extremities. Medial sclerosis with calcification is seen in the lower extremity arteries in most persons greater than 50 years old (15). Upper extremity arteries will show these changes in much milder forms with progressing age, suggesting that the greater hydrostatic pressure present in the legs contributes to these changes. In the same study, intimal hyperplasia was found in the aorta of all ages (15).

Pulmonary vessels demonstrate a decrease in medial collagen content of about 1% per decade, and the wall of pulmonary arteries shows a fall in elastin content and a rise in muscle content with progressive age. The total wall thickness of the arteries and veins changes little with age, but the intima thickens with age in the arteries (16) and may demonstrate fibrosis after the fourth decade (17).

Physiologically, age changes of the vasculature include increased stiffness and decreased compliance of the pulmonary arteries but not of the veins (18) and decreased distensibility and increased stiffness of the systemic arteries (19, 20). Presumably, as a result of these changes, the maximum systolic blood pressure increases significantly with age with no increase in mean blood pressure (21).

The elderly vascular system responds to and recovers as well as the young when a sudden "tilt" from supine to erect position is made although the older person apparently requires a larger rise in vasopressin and possibly also in sympathetic drive to effect a similar response (22). (See Chapter 29)

Heart

Anatomically, there are few changes in the heart that are specifically associated with normal aging, and according to Pomerance, "Its appearance in an octerarian may be indistinguishable from that in a patient half a century younger," (23). The size and weight of the heart in a population without ischemic heart disease or hypertension are proportional to body weight (24). Microscopically, the old myocardium shows a decrease in muscle mass and an increase in collagen, elastic tissue, and fat (23). The endocardium of the atrium and the valve edges continue to thicken until about age 60 (25), with changes similar to the intimal thickening seen in systemic arteries. Echocardiographic studies demonstrate a decrease in the "EF slope" of the anterior mitral valve leaflet of older subjects (26). This parameter is usually considered to be proportional to early diastolic left ventricular filling. The age-related decrease in the slope could indicate a decrease in left ventricular filling due, for example, to delayed ventricular relaxation, which has been reported (27), or is perhaps due to increased myocardial "stiffness." The change in the slope could also reflect age-related changes in the valve (26). The echocardiogram also shows an increase with age in the left ventricular wall thickness. This change is proportional to the square meters of body surface area, but bears no apparent change or relationship to left ventricular cavity size (26). The aortic root's diastolic diameter increases with age, which, Gerstenblith suggests, occurs to compensate for the aorta's increased stiffness. The larger volume of blood in the aorta during diastole would present the heart with a greater inertial load against which to pump and thus would be expected to cause the observed thickening of the left ventricular wall (26).

The physiologic alterations in cardiac function found to be associated with aging are, like the anatomic changes, difficult to separate from the alterations associated with atherosclerotic changes and from other diseases. The apparently healthy elderly myocardium has a prolonged relaxation time, which means the old heart will not function as well as a young heart during periods of tachycardia (27). Perhaps because of this change, the heart rate of patients over 50 years old is not significantly different from younger patients at rest, but increases significantly less than that of younger patients in response to equivalent exercise (28). Similarly, there is a decreased response of heart rate to a rise in blood pressure. This may not be due to the heart itself but possibly to the decreased distensibility of the arteries, which would then obviously prevent an accurate stimulation of the baroreceptor mechanism (29). Reports on changes in stroke volume with age do not give consistent results, but at least one reliable source says that there is a decline of about 1% per year in cardiac output, which Landowne attributes almost entirely to a rise of similar degree in peripheral vascular resistance (21).

Studies of the heart's rhythm in the apparently health elderly (65 + years old) allow us to conclude that supraventricular ectopic contractions, premature ventricular contractions, and sinus tachycardia or other types of tachycardias due to atrial arrhythmia are not uncommon, but sinus pauses, atrioventricular block, and bradycardias are extremely uncommon (30, 31).

In summary, the major changes with aging in the cardiovascular system are related to a stiffening and decreased distensibility of the pulmonary and systemic arteries and of the heart wall itself.

This change is due to changes in collagen and elastic tissue. Under normal conditions, these changes do not adversely affect the functioning of the system, but when the aged cardiovascular system is over-stressed, the old heart may not perform as well as the young heart due to slowed filling in diastole. The reduced distensibility of the aorta and systemic arteries contributes to a higher systolic blood pressure in the aged despite a normal mean pressure, and if extrapolated to a stressed heart this could impair coronary perfusion to the myocardium and lead to myocardial ischemia and damage.

RESPIRATORY SYSTEM

There are three major effects of aging upon the respiratory system that account for changes in pulmonary function. They are loss of elastic recoil of lung tissue, fixation and stiffening of the chest wall, and atrophy and weakening of respiratory muscles (32, 33).

The alveolar ducts and bronchioles are supported by a helical arrangement of elastin and collagen fibers. The elastic behavior and recoil of the lung result from an enfolding of this complex structure, rather than the lengthening of each individual fiber. This recoil ability is lost, elastic recoil fails, and lung compliance decreases when the lung's elastic quality changes. There is evidence that with age the size of the alveolar ducts increases, the resting size of the lung's elastic components increases, and airway conductants may remain static or become increased (34). This results in the so-called senile emphysema that is common in the elderly. The loss of elastic recoil is responsible for an increase in residual volume, a decrease in compliance, and an increase in closing volume (32). *Closing volume* is the lung volume at which small airways start to close and increasing intrapleural pressure is unable to reopen the small airways. This results in air trapping and in uneven distribution of ventilation and perfusion (33).

The anteroposterior (AP) diameter of the chest increases and the chest wall stiffens as a result of calcification of the costal cartilages. The intervertebral disc spaces decrease, kypho-scoliosis develops, and a ''barrel-chest'' deformity becomes the hallmark of old age. The physiologic results of these changes are increased lung volume, reduced rib cage excursion, shortening of diaphragmatic excursion, and increasing abdominal wall involvement with respiratory movement (35). Total lung capacity is not appreciably changed.

A perceived effect of decreased respiratory muscle strength that occurs with aging might very well be due to the reduced compliance of the chest wall. For forced expiration, limitation of movement results from a rounded, stiffened, fixed rib cage and vertebral mechanism covering an inelastic lung with altered closing pressures. These factors would pose formidable obstacles even for young, healthy muscles to overcome.

The increased AP diameter and flaring of the lateral margins of the "barrel-chest" increase the span of peripheral attachments of the diaphragm and contribute to the flattening of the dome effect of that fibromuscular structure. This increased circumference has the added effect of shortening the effective excursion length of the diaphragmatic muscle. This compounds the effects of increased lung volume, which occurs secondary to the "senile emphysema" (35, 36). Deep inspiration is affected most by these changes, which also decrease the excursion distance of the diaphragm in its ascent and descent, thereby requiring more assistance by the abdominal muscles for this respiratory activity.

Age-related changes in the pulmonary blood vessels are mostly due to intimal fibrosis and loss of elasticity of both pulmonary arteries and veins. These changes are less pronounced than the changes of aging usually seen in peripheral vessels (37). The actual pulmonary function appears to be unaffected by these pulmonary vascular changes. However, when combined with several pathologic states, such as cor pulmonale and other forms of pulmonary hypertension, they may become quite important.

GASTROINTESTINAL TRACT

The aging gastrointestinal tract has changes that decrease its motility, secretions, and perhaps its absorptive ability. There is altered distensibility and thinning of perivascular channels due to muscular and collagen weakness.

Esophagus

Deglutition is the result of a complex coordination of reflexes that is dependent upon neuromuscular interplay and that is easily affected by any changes in the neuromuscular pathways. Muscular weakness in specific sites may lead to abnormal contraction patterns. This may result in diverticular formation, diffuse spasm, chalasia, achalasia, and gastroesophageal reflux.

The changes in swallowing patterns in the elderly usually indicate a degree of neuromuscular degeneration that can mimic true disorders of the esophagus, such as those caused by diffuse spasm and gastroesophageal reflux. The subtle differences between the effects of the normal process of aging and the true pathologic situation related to spasm and reflux must be recognized when interpreting esophageal motility patterns in the elderly (38).

Motility pattern changes that are normal in the aging esophagus are similar to those seen in true neuromuscular disorders of the esophagus. Presbyesophagus may be associated with a mild form of spasm due to age-related changes that, when advanced to a severe degree, will represent a pathologic situation. Motility disorders of the pharyngoesophageal region at the level of the cricopharyngeus muscle and the upper esophageal sphincter are not uncommon in the elderly. Disturbances of contraction in this area may produce a misdirection of food and liquids during swallowing and lead to aspiration, Zenker's diverticulum, and dysphagia (39).

It may be difficult to separate problems related to primary esophageal disorders from those caused by some central nervous system disturbance. Changes in neural reflexes secondary to cerebral vascular accidents and other conditions related to aging of the central nervous system must be ruled out in each circumstance. In the elderly, neurologic conditions arise that may affect this complex series of events that is necessary for the control of normal swallowing. These neurologic conditions should be ruled out before swallowing difficulties are attributed to a primary upper esophageal disorder.

The response of the lower esophageal segment to the normal progression of relaxation and contractions necessary for normal swallowing may be completely absent or markedly altered in the elderly. There is a universal decrease in amplitude of contraction in the lower esophageal segment of the elderly person, and peristaltic waves are weaker and progress more slowly in the elderly. These changes suggest a degree of neuromuscular inadequacy and simulate those findings seen in well-known pathologic conditions of achalasia, hiatal hernia, and reflux esophagitis. Spontaneous gastroesophageal reflux can occur as a result of an inadequate resting pressure of the lower esophageal segment, and this may then lead to an associated true pathologic condition.

Stomach

The major effects of aging upon the stomach predominantly relate to changes in gastric emptying, neuromuscular degenerative changes, and diminished acid secretion, pepsin secretion, mucosal atrophy, and muscular strength.

The stomach is another organ in which the changes that may be due to aging are difficult to separate from those changes that are the effects of various degrees of disease states. Because many of these conditions increase in frequency with age, it is not uncommon to attribute symptoms from some true pathologic condition to an "old stomach" (40, 41).

There is some evidence that gastric emptying is prolonged or delayed with advancing age. The ill effects of this delay are difficult to demonstrate and evaluate. Sophisticated studies designed to compare gastric emptying in the young with the elderly have failed to show any associated significant digestive aberrations (42–44). It is tempting to attribute many of the "dyspepsias" of aging to poor gastric emptying, but no hard scientific evidence supports this notion.

The gastric mucosa gradually becomes atrophic as age progresses, but histologic studies have been inconsistent in relating advancing age to specific changes, such as chronic atrophic gastritis, gastric atrophy, and mucosal aberrations (45–47). Gastric acid output (GAO) declines gradually with age (45) in both basal and peak acid output. This is apt to be more marked among women than men, but in neither is frank achlorhydria or serious hypochlorhydria a common problem. When these conditions exist, a true pathologic explanation must always be sought.

Pepsin secretion tends to be decreased in those cases in which mucosal atrophy is significant and pepsin secretory levels tend to mirror the histologic picture (48). As previously stated, it is difficult to attribute much significance to this relationship between mucosal atrophy and aging.

Chronic gastritis, atrophic gastritis, and acute gastritis, which may be more common in the elderly than in the young, should all be considered true disease processes and not the natural consequences of aging.

Small Bowel

There is a reduction in the height of the villi of the small intestinal mucosa that begins to develop around age 60 in most individuals. (49). These changes lead to a reduction in the mucosal surface area, the result of which is a decrease in absorption of d-xylose, carbohydrates, and calcium. The amount of decrease in absorption of these substances varies markedly, does not usually become significant until past age 70 or older, and may not be clinically important even at those advanced ages (50, 51). Histologic evidence of aging has also been noticed as early as age 40. In these instances, the parenchyma of the mucosa and some of the healthy smooth muscles of the intestinal wall are all replaced in part by fibrous connective tissue (52). See Chapter 23 for a more complete discussion of this subject.

Colon

The aging colon shows a consistent abnormality of the muscularis propria. The thickness of the colon wall and the amount of elastin it contains normally increase with age (53). These changes, along with a weakness of the muscularis propria at the site of arterial and venous passageways through the muscle layers, allow the expression of diverticular disease. Diverticulosis is the most common disorder of the colon attributable to the aging process (54). Drummond first described the mechanism whereby intestinal and colonic diverticuli develop (55). In his description of the situation, colonic or intestinal mucosa and submucosa herniate alongside the neurovascular bundle, penetrating the bowel's muscular wall in a manner not unlike the hernia sac when it passes alongside the spermatic cord in an indirect hernia. (See Figure 25.1) Increased intraluminal pressure, motility disorders, and thickening of the tinea coli have all been implicated as etiologic contributors to the development of diverticular disease in the aging colon (56).

The mucosa of the aging colon may show a variety of changes, none of which appears to affect the absorptive ability of the large bowel. Microscopic evidence of the increasing thickness of the muscle layers occurs throughout life. The greatest increase occurs in the last trimester of fetal development and the first 3 months after birth (53).

A slow increase in muscular thickness continues to occur until approximately the sixth decade of life. Then the process becomes more rapid again, involves both circular and longitudinal muscles, is associated with an increase in fibrosis, and a slight increase in elastin is noticed. The elastin increase appears to occur more in the longitudinal layer (tinea coli) than in the circular (54). Many of the bowel complaints associated with aging (i.e., constipation, hard stool, fecal impaction, megacolon, sigmoid volvulus, and abuse of laxatives) can in part be related to these muscular changes (57).

The familiar allegation that the aging colon becomes atrophic and the musculature becomes thin and atonic is a myth. Manometric studies of the aging colon and anorectal pressures in the elderly fail to show such an age-related abnormality (58).

Liver

At or near age 50, the liver accounts for about 2.5% of total body weight (59, 60). From that point on, it gradually decreases both in relative and absolute size until at age 90 it represents only 1.6% of total body weight. Blood flow to and from the liver may show a corresponding decrease as the relative liver size changes (61). Microscopic and morphologic changes relate to an increased mean volume in liver cells and decreased number of hepatocytes associated with the atrophy of aging. Liver cell nuclei increase in size from age 30 onward, and mitochondria decrease in number but increase in volume, as do lysosomes. This suggests that fewer cells are doing the work in old age that many cells did some years before. This may be due to the decreased ability to grow new hepatocytes by cell division (62). A mild ductal proliferation associated with minimal inflammatory response

may be seen in biopsies from aging livers (63). The results of most conventional liver function tests are not altered by increased age. Some sophisticated liver clearance tests (BSP, antipyrine) may be altered by the aging liver's decreased capacity for storage. There is a marked decrease in BSP stored in cells that have increased nuclear DNA, i.e., the old large liver cells. Ethanol elimination is not affected by age (64).

Detoxification, demethalization, conjugation, and hepatic extraction of most compounds do not appear to be affected by increased age. Synthesis of body proteins and of clotting factors may be decreased because of reduced protein-binding capacity in the aged liver. This is usually not a problem under normal conditions, and homeostasis is not generally affected. However, in times of stress, enzymes in the aging liver cannot increase their activities much beyond that necessary to maintain normal function (65). Poor nutrition also seems to exert an undue influence upon the aged liver's ability to respond to stress, disease, and increased metabolic demands (41).

Gallbladder and Bile Ducts

The incidence of gallstones increases with age in most Western Societies. In Britain and the United States, over 30% of women and 20% of men over age 80 will have gallstones (66). Valdivieso et al. in 1978 concluded that aging modifies the proportion of biliary lipids and cholesterol (67). This leads to the situation in which lipids super-saturate the bile to a lithogenic level at some point during the aging process. There is no evidence that the gallbladder contractibility, absorptive abilities, or any mucosal function is altered by aging to a degree that gallstone formation would be more likely. The mechanism by which more cholesterol-saturated bile is produced with increased age is quite unclear.

Pancreas

There appears to be little change in the size of the pancreas as age progresses, although some reports of dilatation, ectasia, and the overall increased size of the main pancreatic duct and its major branches are seen in normal elderly individuals (68). Concomitant with this ductal change, the gland generally declines in weight beginning around age 70. A small percentage of elderly individuals will have an incomplete stenosis of the pancreatic duct that causes no symptoms and reflects no underlying pathology. Therefore, pancreatograms in elderly patients should be interpreted with caution (41). No microscopic picture that could be called typical evidence of senile changes has been described, although perilobular fibrosis may occur and lead to some atrophy of the entire gland (69, 70). There may be a slight decrease in lipase, amylase, and trypsin measured in the pancreatic juice of the elderly individual following infusion of pancreozymin (71). The absorption of fat sometimes seen in elderly individuals may be slightly impaired due to a slight decrease in pancreatic lipase (72). The addition of lipase to the fat meal in elderly subjects seems to abolish this defect (73). Others have failed to show a difference between fat absorption in healthy older and healthy younger individuals (74).

HEMATOPOIETIC SYSTEM

Spleen

The weight of the human spleen decreases with old age due to involution, fibrosis, and possibly to multiple small infarcted areas. A slight hypofunction of the spleen in the elderly can be measured by the increased percentage of pitted erythrocytes seen in the peripheral blood and the decreased ability of the spleen to remove heat-damaged erythrocytes from circulation. This evidence of hypofunction is felt to be caused by a reduction of splenic tissue volume (75). It may also have some effect upon the elderly patient's decreased ability to deal with pneumococcal and similar infections.

Hematology

The major effects of aging in the hematopoietic system are related to the degranulation and reduced chemotaxis of the peripheral blood granulocytes. There is some evidence to suggest that these changes are due to a reduced ability to produce cyclic AMP by the marrow cells of elderly patients (76). This may affect the ability of the granulocytes and the monocytes to

phagocytize bacteria, fungi, and other foreign material (77). It has been previously recognized that the numbers of monocytes and other phagocytes decrease in numbers after age 70. Additional evidence for a decreased ability of these leukocytes to perform in a normal manner is now being gathered. Also after age 70, the bone marrow demonstrates a decline in the actual production of myelocytes, platelets, and perhaps granulocytes. Red blood cells continue to be produced with normal functional ability but also in slightly fewer numbers. Anemia is not thought to be a normal feature of aging. The fact that non-anemic elderly patients will show some reduction in hematopoiesis suggests that age will likely contribute to the defect of anemia when some other underlying pathologic condition exists (78). When anemia occurs in the elderly, another pathologic condition should always be sought. Iron deficiency and the anemia of chronic disease are the two most frequent underlying causes of anemia in the elderly (79).

Lymphocytes appear to remain in normal numbers in the peripheral circulation of elderly patients, and the results of their laboratory reports are not significantly different from the counts reported from young controls or from lymphocyte counts from elderly anemic individuals. Neutrophil counts in the anemic elderly were markedly decreased when compared to young controls and were slightly decreased in non-anemic elderly (78).

IMMUNOLOGY

Many changes occur in the immune system as age progresses. The most dramatic of these is the involution of the thymus gland. Another reported change is that of a concomitant decrease in the number of suppressor T-cell lymphocytes and an increase in the number of helper T-cell lymphocytes. This results in a functional impairment of T-cell mediated immunity and an increased susceptibility to infections, such as pneumococcus, influenza, tetanus, etc. (80).

Lymphocytes arise from the thymus gland, which undergoes a gradual secondary involution beginning at about age 40. This adult involutional change may be a major cause of immunosenescence. By age 60, mature T-lymphocyte populations actually begin to decline (81).

As a result of decreased numbers of thymocytes, which are known to differentiate into mature T-lymphocytes, the gradual involution of the thymus gland materially affects humorally mediated immune response. Pneumococcal pneumonia and tetanus infections are materially affected by this aspect of immunosenescence (81).

An associated increase in autoimmune activity is often noticed with increased age. This autoimmune response has been suggested as an explanation for pernicious anemia, susceptibility to neoplasms, and an acceleration of the aging process itself (80). T-cells have also been noticed to have an impaired proliferative response to Interleukin-2. Interleukin-2 is a T-lymphocyte growth factor that possesses an immuno-enhancing property. Its actual production is decreased in the elderly, which causes a decrease in cellular immunity in these individuals (80, 81).

The total number of B-cell lymphocytes produced by the bone marrow and the total amount of immuoglobulin produced by the elderly hematopoietic system remain unchanged, but there seems to be a defect in immunoglobulin production. An apparent paradox in antibody production in the elderly exists. Studies show a decreased production of antibodies to foreign antigens and increased production of autoantibody. Weksler suggests that this may be due to increased activity of most suppressor T-cells that regulate antibody production to foreign antigens and a concomitant decrease in activity of a subpopulation of suppressor T-cells that regulate autoantibody production (82).

Several agents have been demonstrated to improve the immune responses in the elderly. They include vitamin C, isoprinosine, immucytal, tuftsin, and Interleukin-2, as mentioned before. All of these have been tested in studies that are encouraging, although clear evidence of consistent clinical benefits remains to be shown.

GENITOURINARY TRACT

There is a gradual loss in mass, weight, and size of the kidney after age 50. From birth to maturation, the combined weight of the two kidneys increases from about 45–50 g to 250–270 g by the age of 40 –50 (83). From that point,

the combined weight of both kidneys gradually declines until at age 90 +, the usual weight will be 180–185 g. Dunnill and Halley have shown that this loss after age 50 is due to an absolute volume loss that is caused primarily by cortical tissue loss with relative sparing of the renal medulla (84). The cortical loss is due to two main changes of the arteriolar-glomerular apparatus. One of these senescent changes is a "collapse" of the glomerular tuft and the obliteration of the preglomerular arteriole. The other is the development of a shunt around the sclerotic glomerulus between the afferent and efferent arterioles (85). This maintains good perfusion of the medulla and the collecting system parenchyma (86).

Renal function changes related to aging are mostly due to decreased renal blood flow, decreased glomerular filtration rate (GFR), decreased ability to consume sodium, and a decreased ability to concentrate urine (86, 87). These altered abilities of the elderly patient's kidney to concentrate urine and to conserve water are due primarily to decreased GFR and an age-related impairment in solute conservation. These deficiencies are likely due to a defect in the transport of $Na+$, $Cl-$, urea, and water from tubular lumina to the medullary interstitial space (88). It remains unclear what role the aging adrenal cortex and a declining aldosterone level in the elderly may play in this process (89).

As will be noted in subsequent chapters, fluid balance, electrolyte balance, drug dosage, and the use of diuretics all become an issue of great importance when the intrepid surgeon treads upon the thin ice of surgical management of the elderly. Preoperative preparation, intraoperative speed and gentleness, and vigilant postoperative care are all necessary components of avoiding renal failure in the ill elderly patient who requires a major surgical procedure.

INTEGUMENT

The organization of the collagen fibers in the dermis changes gradually with aging. In the young dermis, discrete bundles of coiled interlaced and contorted collagen fibers are seen in the relaxed skin. These coils straighten as the skin is stretched and "recoil" as the skin is relaxed. In the dermis of older subjects, the collagen is in sheets and no longer in individual bundles, and the collagen fibrils are mostly straight even in the relaxed state. A baby's skin will stretch to 40%–60% more than its resting length, but by age 65, it can be stretched only 15%–20% more than its resting length. It has lost its elastic properties as it has aged (90).

Skin regrowth is measured by the ability of the epidermis to regrow dermal-epidermal skin ridges of the fingers and finger pads. When the ridges are abraided of "fingerprints" and the regrowth measured, it has been found that the elderly regrowth potential is the same as in all healthy subjects from every age group after childhood.

The thinning of the skin in the elderly is a common observation and is due to a similar process as is seen in younger individuals who are on corticosteroid therapy (91–93). This thinning has been shown to be due to actual loss of primary collagen and also possibly to a loss of ability of fibroblasts to produce new collagen.

Collagen and elastin in the dermis are both affected by age. Soluble collagen decreases and insoluble collagen increases. Elastin increases, but the elastic quality of the elastin fibers decreases with age. As the body ages, collagenous structures undergo "maturation" and polymerization with markedly increased numbers and types of co-valent cross-links. This cross-link theory of aging is one that appears on many lists of hypotheses designed to explain the limitations imposed upon the human organism by the changing molecular structures within the aging body (6). This concept is described earlier in this chapter.

The adnexal structures also begin to show evidence of aging after age 65 with thinning of scalp, axillary and pubic hair and by exhibiting a decreased ability to secrete oil and sweat from the appropriate glands.

CENTRAL NERVOUS SYSTEM

The most striking and widely known change that occurs within the central nervous system as a result of aging is a loss of brain weight (94). There is a concomitant decrease in volume, with widening of sulci, deepening of sulci, narrowing of gyri, and a steady increase in the size of the ventricles with age. It is not surprising that the microscopic and morphologic correlates to

those findings are that of cortical cell loss (95). Cortical thickness decreases, neuronal cells in the cortex are lost at random, and glial cells increase in number along with the size of their processes. The cerebellum, basal ganglia, brain stem, thalamus, spinal cord, and cranial nerves have all been studied, and the consensus remains that there is a general, overall central nervous system-wide loss of neurons with advancing age (96). It is generally agreed that the constant cell loss begins at an early age and continues throughout life (94).

The normal process of aging in the central nervous system is clinically productive of subtle changes and functional losses that make findings associated with aging more difficult to separate from true pathologic processes than in other systems. (See Chapter 34)

The actual counting of cell loss is difficult. There is a noticeable lack of dependable methods and a recognized difficulty in interpretation of the findings due to our inability to study the same individual over a long time. A loss of extracellular substance is often seen with aging, along with a concomitant spurious increase in cell counts. Poor correlation has been shown between the actual or even the calculated cell loss and the measurable functional aspects of aging.

Atrophy of the cortical gyri is common in old age and is seen especially in the senile demented. Correlated functional losses, which can be shown in these individuals, are in short term memory, emotional expression, and intellectual capacity. Histochemically and cytologically there is found to be cytoplasmic shrinkage of nerve cells with a deposition of brown lipofuscin pigment. Most of the studies have been done with the cerebral cortex (especially in the two granular layers); the basal ganglia; the brain stem nuclei, such as locus ceruleus; cerebellar nuclei, such as dentate; all three cortical layers; and in the inferior olive of the medulla. Functional deficits are as would be expected from the anatomic sites: higher function in cortex, emotionalism etc. in hypothalamus, abnormal motor activity in basal ganglia, sleepiness in locu ceruleus, ataxia in cerebellar system and olive. Fe^{++} changes are noted to occur with aging in the spinal cord and in the white tracts and spinal ganglia. Proprioception is not markedly diminished nor is tactile sense (97).

Blood flow is altered in aging in proportion to changes in the vessels. When reduced it may be correlated with psychological functional deficits. Senile dementia and Alzheimer's disease are pathologic and are always associated with severe cell loss.

In one excellent review of the subject by Samorajski, many of the morphologic changes seen in the old adult human brain are correlated to such disease entities as Alzheimer's disease, atherosclerosis, and senile dementias (98). The control of aging by the hypothalamus as proposed by Dilman (99) and as refined by Everitt (100) is covered by Samorajski's fine review.

As will be noted in subsequent chapters, many of the uncorrectable effects of aging, some of the age-related dementias, and the tendency of the general public and many physicians to expect all old people to have central nervous system changes may lull us into failing to recognize, diagnose, and treat correctable lesions, such as tumors, aneurysms, and extracranial vascular problems, in otherwise healthy elderly patients.

AUTONOMIC NERVOUS SYSTEM

Not much is known about age changes of the parasympathetic and sympathetic nervous system. A cell loss occurs that is progressive as is seen in the central nervous system. Pfeifer and his co-workers reviewed 103 normal males and found an age-related increase of cardiovascular sympathetic nervous system activity and a decrease of activity of the cardiac parasympathetic nervous system (101). These changes in response to adrenergic stimulation and to blocking drugs suggest that the increase in cardiovascular sympathetic activity may occur as compensation for an age-related decrease in barorecepter sensitivity. Neuroendocrine changes also occur. Metabolic changes in the liver may account for many of these findings because of alterations in drug responsiveness and to toxic synergy.

PERIPHERAL NERVOUS SYSTEM

Age-related changes in proprioception have been the subject of relatively little study. Changes are reported in tactile and proprioceptive sensation in elderly individuals (102, 103). In a study of 29 subjects of all ages with normal knee joints, Skinner and his colleagues found that aging is associated with a decline in joint-position sense, but they could not determine if these deficiencies were actually the result of the aging process (103). Kokmen and co-workers found a decrease in joint motion sensation in normal elderly subjects. No significant changes in nerve fiber numbers have been reported, but reflex time is diminished with age (97).

ENDOCRINOLOGY

Many age-related changes in various types of hormone levels have been reported, but the physiologic consequences of these changes are not well-defined in many cases. The subjects used for many of the well-known endocrinologic studies on aging are hospitalized patients, or they are those who are categorized as "apparently" or "fairly" healthy. In many cases there is no way to identify those elderly patients who may have mild or unrecognized, significant, pathologic endocrine conditions. Therefore, some of the reported endocrine changes that have been attributed to senility may not be due to the truly normal process of aging but to prevalent pathologic conditions.

Endocrine Pancreas

The non-diabetic elderly person will show signs of impaired glucose tolerance much more often than the young; in fact, one study reported 9 out of 20 elderly patients (mean age, 80 years) had abnormal oral glucose tolerance tests as opposed to no abnormal tests in 20 patients in their twenties (104). This relative glucose intolerance that appears with aging is independent of obesity (105) and gender (104) and is not related to a deficiency of endogenous insulin. This can be shown by the fact that elderly patients do not have deficient insulin secretion (104, 106), but actually have increased arterial insulin levels (107). The elderly individuals can be shown to have a degree of insulin resistance, which is not due to altered insulin binding to cell membrane receptors, but is in part due to a reduction in the capacity of the glucose uptake system (104). This may involve and be the result of a reduction in the number of glucose transporters or metabolic systems (106). One study suggests that a diet that eliminates sugar and is moderately calorie-restricting may delay the onset or reduce the degree of age-related glucose intolerance (108).

The endocrine response to mild hypoglycemia appears to be preserved in the elderly. Both glucagon and adrenal hormones respond normally to moderate insulin-induced hypoglycemia (109). Likewise, basal arterial levels of glucagon do not change with age, but the elderly respond to glucagon with greater glucose production than do the young (110).

Thyroid

The aged thyroid shows some degree of atrophy, fibrosis, increased nodularity, decreased follicle size, increased amount of interfollicular connective tissue, and reduction in total gland weight (111). By the eighth decade of life, 20% of apparently healthy subjects in one study showed increased levels of antithyroglobulin and antimicrosomal antibody, which are both associated with autoimmune hypothyroidism (111). The elderly have a lower serum level of the thyroid hormone T_4 and free T_4 index than the young, but T_3 and free T_3 are not decreased significantly until after age 60 in men and after age 80 in women (112). The decrease in T_3, when it finally occurs, is believed to be due to declining peripheral conversion of T_4 to T_3 (113). A significant number of healthy elderly patients show elevated TSH levels (112, 113). It is not clear from current data whether these changes in hormone levels have physiologic consequences in the elderly (114) or represent a forerunner or predisposition to true hypothyroidism (112).

The parathyroid glands and calcitonin-producing cells are of particular interest in the elderly because osteoporosis is such a widespread problem in this segment of the population. Berlyne hypothesized that a decreasing glomerular filtration rate, which is found in the healthy elderly, could lead to a decrease in the serum calcium level (115). This may be due to phosphorus retention or to a decreased renal production of active vitamin D. A low concentration of vitamin D would in turn increase the secretion of parathyroid hormone and thereby lead to

osteoporosis (115). Other work has shown that total serum calcium does decrease with age, but it is not clear whether the parathyroid hormone levels actually rise with age when the variable glomerular filtration rates of the elderly are controlled (116, 117). Berlyne's hypothesis has not been confirmed. Serum calcitonin, the co-regulator of calcium homeostasis, seems to increase with age (118).

Male Reproductive Endocrine System

The major age-related change in the male reproductive hormone system is a decrease in testosterone levels both in serum and in the tissue of the testis. This gradual fall of testosterone production begins at age 40 despite increasing LH and FSH levels and a fall in metabolic clearance of testosterone (119). Takahishi and Baker suggest that the etiology is a primary decline in function of the testis (119, 120). They believe that there is evidence to show that the problem is caused by a reduced supply of mitochondrial steroid precursors in the Leydig cell (119, 120). Estrodial levels fall in aging men despite an increase in conversion of testosterone to estrodial. The sex hormone binding globulin also rises (119). Kinsey and his colleagues reported that 75% of 80-year-old men were impotent, but this figure likely includes a large proportion of men impotent due to causes other than normal aging (121). (See Chapter 26)

Female Reproductive Endocrine System

With the onset of menopause, women experience a marked decline in serum estrogen levels as both the ovary and the adrenal gland diminish and then stop secreting estrogens. Only the conversion of androstenedione to estrogen, which occurs primarily in fat tissue, provides estrogen to the elderly postmenopausal woman. Circulating levels of luteinizing hormone and follicle-stimulating hormone from the pituitary are elevated in the postmenopausal woman. This is thought to be due to the greatly reduced estrogen level and the loss of the usual feedback inhibition upon the pituitary for the secretion of luteinizing and follicle-stimulating hormone (122).

Pituitary System

There are interesting similarities between pituitary responses in the aged and the depressed patient. Both the diurnal cortisol nadir and the maximum peak occur earlier in the day in the aged. This correlates with the frequently reported earlier bedtime and early awakening time in the elderly. These "sleep disturbances" are also frequently reported in patients with endogenous depression (123). The sensitivity of the hypothalamic-pituitary complex to inhibition by dexamathasone rises in the elderly. This is also seen in patients with endogenous depression, stress, atherosclerosis, and endometrial and prostate carcinoma (124).

There appears to be no difference in prolactin secretion (125) or number of prolactin-secreting cells (126) in the pituitary gland of the elderly. Likewise, the elderly show no difference in basal β-endorphin levels or the response of this hormone to a cold pressor test (immersion of a hand in 4° C water) (127). There is, however, a decreased response of growth hormone to synthetic growth hormone releasing factor in the elderly (128). As is the case with many of the endocrine alterations and non-alterations seen in aging, the physiologic significance of these pituitary changes is not entirely clear.

Renin-Aldosterone System

Aldosterone levels are lower in the aged both before and after sodium depletion (128, 130), but the difference is much greater when the patient is upright than when recumbent (130). This report agrees with the cardiovascular literature findings discussed earlier in this chapter. Renin falls with aging, possibly due to decreased conversion of inactive to active renin (129).

Plasma noradrenalin levels in the elderly are higher than in the young, and the elderly show a greater increase in noradrenalin in response to stress (131). This may be due to diminished adrenergic receptor sensitivity, because the elderly have been found to have a diminished response to beta blockade (132). This increased noradrenalin in the aged can confuse the attempt to diagnose the etiology of hypertension, and the possible diminution of adrenergic receptor sensitivity would affect the reaction of the elderly

to the many adrenergic agonist and antagonist drugs (131).

EYE AND VISUAL SYSTEM

In the eye itself there are changes in all parts: increased opacity of the cornea, increased rigidity of the lens, delayed pupillary reflex time, reduced removal time of aqueous humor, and an increase in glaucoma. Changes in vitreous humor (floaters, etc) become troublesome. The most important retinal changes are those of vascular origin, and macular degeneration often occurs, which may be idiopathic or may be related to hypertension. Optic nerve fibers are reduced in number significantly with age. Several subjective changes that are universally reported include hypermetropia, decreased acuity, and reduction of visual fields, especially the upper half and peripherally (133).

The changes in the cornea that are most characteristic of aging are arcus senilis and corneal opacity. The former is an annular lipid deposit near the limbus, and the latter is a centralized loss of corneal clarity. The cornea becomes more fragile and less sensitive with age and leaves the eye more susceptible to injury without the patient's becoming aware of its occurrence (134).

The anterior chamber becomes shallow as the aging lens gradually enlarges. It has been shown that an 80-year-old lens is three times the size of a newborn lens (135). As the anterior chamber becomes more shallow, the chamber angle becomes narrow and closes, causing acute closed-angle glaucoma, a condition rare in patients under age 60.

Senile cataracts are present when the crystalline lens loses its normal transparency with age, and there is alteration of passage of light through the lens. Other causes of cataracts are genetic, congenital, metabolic, traumatic, toxic, and unknown (136). The diagnosis of senile cataract is made in persons over 45–50 years of age when other causes are ruled out. Cataracts account for about 9% of all blindness and are the third leading cause of blindness in the United States. According to the Framington Eye Study, the incidence of senile lens changes increases from approximately 10% of persons aged 55–59 years to a level of 37% for people in the 75–79 year age group. Senile cataracts, on the other hand, progress from about 1% for those persons 55–59 years of age to an incidence of 15% in the 75–79 year age group (137). Factors that increase the risk and incidence are demographic, geographic, and disease related. Nutritional deficiency, diabetes, hypertension, increased serum phospholipids, and decreased hand grip strength were all found in the Framingham Eye Study to bear a positive relationship to cataracts (138). Ionizing and infrared radiation and possibly ultraviolet and microwave radiation are thought to be significant risk factors (139).

Senile macular degeneration of the retina accounts for most forms of blindness in the United States and has a peak age incidence of 50–70 years (140). Subretinal deposits of pigment excreted from the retina and picked up in choriocapillaries are associated with neovascular changes that occur beneath the retina. An opaque membrane is then found beneath the retinal pigment epithelium. These neovascular membranes may be cauterized with the argon laser. If treated before the fovea is involved, blindness may be avoided.

The optic nerve fibers are reduced significantly in number by age 70 (estimated loss of approximately 400,000 fibers during 70 years) (141). Optic radiation, however, is not affected. There are cosmetic defects of the lids with increased laxity, loss of elasticity, demachalosis, entropion, extropion, dry eye, pterygium, xanthelosis, and skin neoplasms, all of which increase with age (135).

EAR

External Ear

Changes in the external ear are largely the results of aging skin and cartilage. Atrophy and itching may occur in the external auditory canal, and these changes are exacerbated by the effects of aging on the sebaceous glands and ceruminal glands (142). Biopsies have shown a decrease in the number of ceruminal glands in the ear canals of older persons (143). Tragi, the large hairs found in the external auditory canals of most males, become coarser and longer as early as the fourth decade of life.

Middle Ear

Middle ear changes are mostly in the incudomalleal and incudostapedial joints of the ossicles. Etholm and Belal studied the joint changes that occur during the human life span and found that the earliest changes were fraying, fibrillation, and vacuolation in the articular cartilages (144). These were followed by hyalinization of the joint capsule, cartilaginous thinning and calcification, and, occasionally, narrowing of the joint space. All subjects over 70 years of age showed moderate to severe arthritic changes in these joints. Surprisingly, these changes were not found to affect sound transmission. The earlier reports of *conductive* hearing losses associated with aging (145, 146) are now in question and are believed to have been inaccurate because of the faulty testing equipment and techniques of the past (142).

Inner Ear

Inner ear changes associated with aging are largely responsible for the gradual hearing loss experienced by more than 25 million people in the United States over the age of 65 years (142). Many of these individuals have one of the four major types of presbycusis. This aging disorder involves loss of speech processing and discrimination, as well as loss of perception of pure tones. *Sensory* presbycusis involves atrophy of the organ of Corti, especially in the basal coil where high tones are recorded and in the auditory nerve where there is loss of fibers. *Neural* presbycusis results from a loss of the cochlear neurons and may begin at any age. *Strial* presbycusis usually begins in middle to older age. With strial presbycusis, spotty atrophy of the stria vascularis occurs. In those situations of documented hearing loss for which adequate explanatory degenerative changes cannot be found, a category called *cochlear conductive* presbycusis has been established (142).

Vestibular changes are also common in the aged and result in dizziness, loss of balance, and vertigo. Less is known about the effects of aging upon the vestibular portion of the inner ear than is known about the cochlea. It is known, however, that in individuals older than 74 years a 40% decrease in the number of myelinated vestibular nerve fibers should be expected (147).

Similarly, Rosenhall found a 20%–40% decrease in the number of hair cells in the cristae and maculae in older individuals (148). (For a more detailed discussion, see Chapter 13.)

MUSCLE

A loss of muscle strength is associated with aging. This is, in part, due to altered nutrition and physical activities in older individuals, rather than a direct effect of aging. In a report by Moller, the muscles of apparently healthy, elderly individuals were studied and compared to subjects 30–40 years younger (149). The elderly muscles were found to have elevated levels of sodium, chloride, and extracellular water. Total concentrations of essential amino acids were lower in elderly women and higher in elderly men than in their younger counterparts. A 5% decrease in total adenine nucleotides and phosphocreatine was observed in the elderly group while the concentrations of creatinine and myoglobin were increased. After a 6-week period of physical training, a percentage of the elderly subjects were studied again and found to show a decrease in creatinine, an increase in ATP/ADP and phosphocreatine/total creatinine ratios, and unchanged concentrations of myoglobin. They concluded that the changes in skeletal muscle associated with aging could in part be due to physical inactivity. They found more advanced muscle deterioriation in elderly subjects with lung disease and liver cirrhosis.

There is also evidence that the number of muscle fibers decreases with age (150). This decrease appears to be more prominent in women than in men (151). Inokuchi and his colleagues found that the proportion and the cross-sectional area of type II fibers were significantly diminished in elderly males compared to younger subjects (152). Only minor enzymatic changes were identified in these subjects, and these were felt to be reflective of the change in type II fibers. Isometric and dynamic strength in the knee-extensor muscles declined with increasing age and correlated with the loss of type II fibers. An increase in total reflex time was also apparent.

BONE

All parameters of bone strength are altered with aging and disuse. Torsion, tension, and fracture resistance are all reduced. Fractures are more common in the elderly because a decrease in tensile energy absorption accompanies aging (153). The bone changes related to aging are no different between elderly men and women except in the postmenopausal woman with advanced osteoporosis.

With aging, the metabolism of osteoblasts and osteoclasts is diminished (154). Compact bone tends to become spongy, the cortex is thinned, and the marrow cavity is enlarged. There is less red marrow and more yellow marrow. Red marrow persists until very old age in the skull, ribs, vertebrae, pelvic bones, and proximal long bones. This accounts for the prevalence of and preference of certain tumors for these areas as sites of metastasis. Loss of bone mass from the fourth to the fifth decade is estimated to be 20% (155) and is associated with an age-related increase in parathyroid activity (156). The increase in parathyroid activity may occur in response to an age-related decrease in calcium absorption. Loss of teeth and absorption of alveolar bone are very common in the elderly.

Osteoporosis is a very common degenerative condition associated with aging. This disorder involves a general loss of vertebral bone substance and a greater loss of horizontal trabecular components, resulting in reduced capability of the vertebral bodies to bear weight (157). The severity of this disorder and the rate at which it progresses are both greater in elderly women than in elderly men. Tsai and his co-workers have hypothosized that elderly women have abnormal vitamin D metabolism that results in decreased calcium absorption, which in turn stimulates increased parathyroid hormone secretion (156). The parathyroid hormone stimulates increased bone turnover that, because of diminished bone formation in the elderly, results in a loss of bone mass. Their study was directed toward senile osteoporosis and excluded consideration of postmenopausal osteoporosis.

SUMMARY

Each organ system that is affected by particular changes as a result of aging will be discussed in subsequent chapters. We have attempted here to introduce the concept of aging, and we have also made an effort to mention those areas in each organ system that are most vulnerable to the passage of time. It will be the intent of the contributors of those chapters that follow to relate the changes of aging to the practice of the art and science of surgery.

REFERENCES

1. Hayflick L, Moorehead PS: The serial cultivation of human diploid cell strains. *Exp Cell Res* 25:585–621, 1961.
2. Harmon D: Aging: a theory based on free radical and radiatio chemistry. *J Gerontol* 11:298–300, 1956.
3. Orgel L: The maintenance of accuracy of protein synthesis and its relevance to aging. *Proc Natl Acad Sci* 49:517–521, 1963.
4. Burnet FM: An immunologic approach to aging. *Lancet* 2:358–360, 1970.
5. Landfield PW, Baskin RK, Pitler TA: Brain aging correlates: retardation by hormonal-pharmological treatments. *Science* 214:581–584, 1981.
6. Bjorksten J: The crosslinkage theory of aging. *J Am Geriatr Soc* 16:408–427, 1968.
7. Hayflick L: Aging under glass. *Exp Gerontol* 5:291–303, 1970.
8. Hayflick L: The biology of human aging. *Am Med Sci* 265:432–445, 1973.
9. McCay CM, Crowell MF, Maynard LA: The effect of retarded growth upon length of lifespan and upon ultimate body size. *J Nutr* 10:63–79, 1935.
10. Goodrick C: The effects of exercise on longevity and behavior of hybrid mice which differ in coat color. *J Gerontol* 29:129–133, 1974.
11. Hayflick L: The biology of human aging. *Plast Recons Surg* 64:536–550, 1981.
12. Mazess RB: Health and longevity in Vilcabomba, Ecuador. *JAMA* 240:1781, 1978.
13. Medvedev ZA: Caucasus and Altay longevity: a biologic or social problem. *Gerontologist* 14:381–387, 1974.
14. Schneider EL, Reed JD: Life extension. *N Engl J Med* 312:1159–1167, 1985.
15. Lidman D: Histopathology of human extremital arteries throughout life including measurements of systolic pressures in ankle and arm. *Acta Chir Scand* 148:575–580, 1982.
16. Mackay EH, Banks J, Sykes B, Lee G deJ: Structural basis for the changing physical properties of human pulmonary vessels with age. *Thorax* 33:335–344, 1978.
17. Warnock ML, Kunzmann A: Changes with age in muscular pulmonary arteries. *Arch Pathol Lab Med* 101:175–179, 1977.
18. Banks J, Booth FVML, MacKay EH, Rajogopalen B, Lee G deJ: The physical behavior of human pulmonary arteries and veins. *Clin Sci* 55:477–484, 1978.
19. Roach MR, Burton AC: The effect of age on the elasticity of human iliac arteries. *Can J Biochem Physiol* 37:557–570, 1959.
20. Newman DL, Lallewood RC: The effect of age on the distensibility of the abdominal aorta of man. *Surg Gynecol Obstet* 147:211–214, 1978.
21. Landowne M, Brondfoneuener M, Shock N: The relation of age to certain measures of performance of the heart and the circulation. *Circulation* 12:567–576, 1955.
22. Vargas E, Lye M, Faragher EB, Goddard C, Moser B, Davies J: Cardiovascular haemodynamics and the response of vasopressin, aldosterone, plasma renin activity and plasma catecholamines to head-up tilt in young and old healthy subjects. *Age Aging* 15:17–28, 1986.
23. Pomerance A: Cardiac pathology in the elderly. In Nobley RJ, Rothbaun DH (eds): *Geriatric Cardiology vol 12. Cardiovascular Clinics.* Philadelphia, FA Davis Co, 1981, pp 9–54.
24. Reiner L, Mazzoleni A, Rodriguez FL, Freudenthal RR: The weight of the human heart. I. Normal cases. *Arch Pathol* 68:58–73, 1959.
25. McMillan JB, Len M: The aging heart. I. Endocardium. *J Gerontol* 14:268–283, 1959.
26. Gerstenblith G, Frederiksen J, Yin FCP, Fortuin NJ, Lakatto EG, Weisfeldt ML: Echocardiographic assessment of a normal adult aging population. *Circulation* 56:273–278, 1977.
27. Harrison TR, Dixon K, Russell RO, Bidwai PS, Coleman HN: The relation of age to the duration of contraction, ejection, and relaxation of the normal human heart. *Am Heart J* 67:190–199, 1964.
28. Petrofsky JS, Lind AR: Aging, isometric strength and endurance, and cardiovascular responses to static effort. *J Appl Physiol* 38:91–95, 1975.
29. Gribbin B, Pickering T, Sleight P, Peto R: Effect of age and high blood pressure on baroreflex sensitivity in man. *Circ Res* 29:424–431, 1971.
30. Camm AJ, Evans KE, Ward DE, Martin A: The rhythm of the heart in active elderly subjects. *Am Heart J* 99:598–603, 1980.
31. Kantelip JP, Sage E, Duchene-Marulloz P: Findings on ambulatory electrocardiographic monitoring in subjects older than 80 years. *Am J Cardiol* 57:398–401, 1986.
32. Wahba WM: Influence of aging on lung function —

clinical significance of changes from age twenty. *Anesth Analg* 62:764–776, 1983.

33. Dhar S, Shastri SR, Lenora RAK: Aging and the respiratory system. *Med Clin N Am* 60:1121–1139, 1976.

34. Pelzer AM, Thomson ML: Effect of age, sex, stature and smoking habits on human airway conductance. *J Appl Physiol* 21:496–476, 1966.

35. Fowler RW: Ageing and lung function. *Age Aging* 14:209–215, 1985.

36. Thurlbeck WM, Angus GE: Growth and aging of the normal human lung. *Chest* 67:3S–7S, 1975.

37. Smith P, Heath D: The ultrastructure of age-associated intimal fibrosis in pulmonary blood vessels. *J Pathol* 130:247–253, 1980.

38. Khan TA, Shragge BW, Crispin JS, Lind JF: Esophageal motility in the elderly. *Digest Dis* 22:1049–1054, 1977.

39. Pelemans W, Vantrappen G: Oesophageal disease in the elderly. *Clin Gastroenterol* 14:635–656, 1985.

40. James OFW: Gastrointestinal and liver function in old age. *Clin Gastroenterol* 12:671–691, 1983.

41. Steinheber FU: Ageing and the stomach. *Clin Gastroenterol* 14:657–688, 1985.

42. Webster SGP, Leeming JT: Assessment of small bowel function in the elderly using a modified xylose tolerance test. *Gut* 16:109–113, 1975.

43. Evans MA, Triggs EJ, Cheung M: Gastric emptying rate in the elderly. Implications for drug therapy. *J Am Geriatr Soc* 29:201–205, 1981.

44. Kramer PA, Chapron DJ, Benson J, Mercik SA: Tetracycline absorption in elderly patients with achlorhydria. *Clin Pharm Thera* 23:467–472, 1978.

45. Andrews GR, Haneman B, Arnold BJ, Booth JC, Taylor K: Atrophic gastritis in the aged. *Aust Ann Med* 16:230–235, 1967.

46. Bird T, Hall MRP, Schade ROK: Gastric histology and its relation to anaemia in the elderly. *Gerontology* 23:309–321, 1977.

47. Giacosa A, Cheli R: Correlations anatomo-secretories gastriques en fonction de l'age chez des sujets ayant une muqueuse fundique normale. *Gastroenterologie Clinique et Biologique* 3:647–650, 1979.

48. Bock OAA, Arapakis G, Witts LJ, Richards CD: The serum pepsinogen level with special reference to the histology of the gastric mucosa. *Gut* 4:106–111, 1963.

49. Montgomery RD, Hainey MR, Ross IN, et al: The ageing gut: a study of intestinal absorption in relation to nutrition in the elderly. *Q J Med* 47:197–211, 1978.

50. Feibusch J, Holt PR: Impaired absorptive capacity for carbohydrates in the elderly. *Am J Clin Nutr* 32:942, 1979.

51. Holt PR: The small intestine. *Clin Gastroenterol* 14:689–723, 1985.

52. Schuster MM: Disorders of the aging GI system. *Hosp Pract* 11:95–103, 1976.

53. Pace JL: A detailed study of musculature of the human large intestine. PhD thesis, University of London, 1966.

54. Whiteway J, Morson BC: Pathology of the ageing—diverticular disease. *Clin Gastroenterol* 14:829–846, 1985.

55. Drummond H: Sacculi of the large intestine with special reference to their relations to the blood vessels of the bowel wall. *Br J Surg* 4:407–413, 1916.

56. Hodgson J: Transverse taeniamyotomy for diverticular disease. *Dis Colon Rect* 16:283–289, 1973.

57. Brocklehurst JC: Colonic disease in the elderly. *Clin Gastroenterol* 14:725–747, 1985.

58. Loening-Baucke V, Anuras S: Effects of age and sex on anorectal manometry. *Am J Gastroenterol* 80:50–53, 1985.

59. Calloway NO, Foley CF, Lagerbloom P: Uncertainties in geriatric data II: Organ size. *J Am Geriat Soc* 13:20–28, 1965.

60. Thompson EN, Williams R: Effect of age on liver function with particular reference to bromsulphthalein excretion. *Gut* 6:266–269, 1965.

61. Skaunic V, Hulek P, Martinkova J: Changes in kinetics of exogenous dyes in the aging process. In Kitani K (ed): *Liver and Ageing*. Amsterdam, Elsevier North Holland, 1978, pp 115–130.

62. Tauchi H, Sato T: Hepatic cells of the aged. In Kitani K (ed): *Liver and Ageing*. Amsterdam, Elsevier North Holland, 1978, pp. 3–19.

63. Schaffner F, Popper H: Non-specific reactive hepatitis in aged and infirm people. *Am J Dig Dis* 4:389–399, 1959.

64. Vestal RE, McGuire FA, Tobin JD, Andres R, Norris AH, Mezey E: Ageing and ethanol metabolism. *Clin Pharm Thera* 21:343–354, 1977.

65. Salem SAM, Rajjayabun P, Shepherd AM, Stevenson IH: Reduced induction of drug metabolism in the elderly. *Age Aging* 7:68–73, 1978.

66. Bateson MC, Bouchier IAD: Prevalence of gallstones in Dundee: a necropsy study. *Br Med J* 4:427–430, 1975.

67. Valdivieso V, Palma R, Wunkaus R, Antezana C, Severin C, Contreras A: Effect of ageing on biliary lipid composition and bile acid metabolism in normal Chilean women. *Gastroenterology* 74:871–874, 1978.

68. Weill-Bousson M, Bushcer P, Geisler F: Pancreas du sujet age. Aspects anatomopathologiques. *Annals de Gastroenterologie et d'Hepatologie* 15:568–573, 1979.

69. Walters MNI: Studies on the pancreas. I. Non-specific pancreatic ductular ectasia. *Am J Pathol* 19:973–981, 1964.

70. Schmitz-Moormann P, Himmelmann GW, Brandes HJ, Folsch UR, Lorenz-Meyer H, Malchow H, Soehendra M, Wienbeck M: Quantitative assessment of pancreatitis-like lesions in humans without pancreatic disease. In Gyr KE, Singer MV, Sarles H (eds): *Pancreatitis Concepts and Classification*. Amsterdam/New York, Elsevier, 1984, pp 67–70.

71. Moessner J, Pusch HJ, Koch W: Die Exkretorische pankreas funktion altersveranderungen Ja oder Nein? *Aktuelle Gerontologie* 12:40–43, 1982.

72. Laugier R, Sarles H: The pancreas. *Clin Gastroenterol* 14:749–756, 1985.

73. Citi S, Salvini L: The intestinal absorption of [131]labelled olein and triolein, of [58]Co vitamin B and ^{59}Fe, in aged subjects. *J Gerontol* 12:123–126, 1961.

74. McEvoy A: Investigation of intestinal malabsorption in the elderly. In Evans JG, Caird FE (eds): *Advanced Geriatric Medicine 2*. London, Pitman, 1982, pp 100–110.

75. Zago MA, Figueiredo MA, Covas DT, Bottura C: Aspects of splenic hypofunction in old age. *Klin Wochenschr* 63:590–592, 1985.

76. McLaughlin B, O'Malley K, Cotter TG: Age-related differences in granulocyte chemotaxis and degranulation. *Clin Sci* 70:59–62, 1986.

77. Nielsen H, Blom J, Larsen SO: Human blood monocyte function in relation to age. *Acta Path Microbiol Immunol Scand* 92:5–10, 1984.

78. Lipschitz DA, Udupa KB, Milton KY, Thompson CO: Effect of age on hematopoiesis in man. *Blood* 63:502–509, 1984.

79. Lewis R: Anemia—a common but never a normal concomitant of aging. *Geriatrics* 31:53–60, 1976.

80. Busby J, Caranasos GJ: Immune function, autoimmunity, and selective immunoprophylaxis in the aged. *Med Clin N Am* 69:465–474, 1985.

81. Delafuente JC: Immunosenescence. Clinical and pharmacologic considerations. *Med Clin N Am* 69:475–486, 1985.

82. Weksler MD: Senescence of the immune system. *Med Clin N Am* 67:263–272, 1983.

83. Roessle R, Roulet F: Nieren. In *Mass und Zahl in der Pathologie*. Berlin, J. Springer, 1932, pp 63–66.

84. Dunnill MS, Halley W: Some observations on the quantitative anatomy of the kidney. *J Pathol* 110:113–121, 1973.

85. Takazakura E, Sawabu K, Hande A, Takada A, Shinoda A, Takeucha J: Intrarenal vascular changes with age and disease. *Kidney Int* 2:224–230, 1972.

86. Epstein M: Effects of aging on the kidney. *Fed Proc* 38:168–172, 1979.

87. Shock NW: Current trends in research on the physiological aspects of aging. *J Am Geriatr Soc* 15:995–1000, 1967.

88. Rowe JW, Shock NW, DeFronzo RA: The influence of age on the renal response to water deprivation in man. *Nephron* 17:270–278, 1976.

89. Weidmann P, De-Myttenaere-Bursztein S, Maxwell MH, DeLima J: Effect of aging on plasma renin and aldosterone in normal man. *Kidney Int* 8:325–333, 1975.

90. Millington PF, Wilkinson R: Changes in skin with age. *Scand J Clin Lab Invest* 34(Suppl 141):52–53, 1973.

91. McConkey B, Fraser GM, Bligh AS, Whiteley H: Transparent skin and osteoporosis. *Lancet* 1:693–695, 1963.

92. Shuster S, Bottoms E: Senile degeneration of skin collagen. *Clin Sci* 25:487–491, 1963.

93. Ryckwaert A, Parot S, Tamisier S: Variations, selon l'age el le sexe, de l'epaisseur du pli cutane mesure du dos de la main. *Rev Frac Etud Clin Biol* 12:803–806, 1967.

94. Long DM: Aging in the nervous system. *Neurosurgery* 17:348–354, 1985.

95. Brizzee KR: Gross morphometric analyses and quantitative histology of the aging brain. *Adv Behav Biol* 16:401–423, 1975.

96. Kaack B, Ordy JM, Trapp B: Changes in limbic, neuroendocrine and autonomic systems, adaptation, homeostasis during aging. *Adv Behav Biol* 16:209–231, 1975.

97. Kokmen E, Bossemeyer RW, Barney J, Williams WJ: Neurological manifestations of aging. *J Gerontol* 32:411–419, 1977.

98. Samorajski T: How the human brain responds to aging. *J Am Geriatr Soc* 24:4–11, 1976.

99. Dilman VM: Age-associated elevation of hypothalamic threshold to feedback control and its role in development, ageing, and disease. *Lancet* 1:1211–1219, 1971.

100. Everitt AV: The hypothalamic-pituitary control of ageing and age related pathology. *Exp Gerontol* 8:265–277, 1973.

101. Pfeifer MA, Weinberg CR, Cook D, Best JD, Reenan A, Halter JB: Differential changes of autonomic nervous system function with age in man. *Am J Med* 75:249–258, 1983.

102. Kaplan FS, Nixon JE, Reitz M, Rindfleish L, Tucker J: Age-related changes in proprioception and sensation of joint position. *Acta Orthop Scand* 56:72–74, 1985.

103. Skinner HB, Barrack RL, Cook SD: Age-related decline in proprioception. *Clin Ortho Rel Res* 184:208–211, 1984.

104. McConnell JG, Buchanon KD, Ardill J, Stout RW: Glucose tolerance in the elderly: the role of insulin and its receptor. *Euro J Clin Invest* 12:55–61, 1982.

105. Chen M, Bergman RN, Pacini G, Porte D: Pathogenesis of age-related glucose intolerance in man: insulin resistance and decreased B-cell function. *J Clin Endocrinol Metab* 60:13–20, 1985.

106. Fink RI, Wallace P, Olefsky JM: Effects of aging on glucose-mediated glucose disposal and glucose transport. *J Clin Invest* 77:2034–2041, 1986.

107. Fink RI, Revers RR, Kolterman OG, Olefsky JM: The metabolic clearance of insulin and the feedback inhibition of insulin secretion are altered with aging. *Diabetes* 34:275–280, 1985.

108. Grobin W: Progressive deterioration of glucose transport in the aged. *J Am Geriatr Soc* 23:31–37, 1975.

109. Meneilly GS, Miraker KL, Young JB, Landsberg L, Rowe JW: Counter-regulatory responses to insulin-induced glucose reduction in the elderly. *J Clin Endocrinol Metab* 61:178–182, 1985.

110. Simonson DC, DeFronzo RA: Glucagon physiology and aging: evidence for enhanced hepatic sensitivity. *Diabetologia* 25:1–7, 1983.

111. Sirota DK: Thyroid function and dysfunction in the elderly: a brief review. *Mt Sinai J Med* 47:126–131, 1980.

112. Sawin CT, Chopra D, Azizi F, Mannix JE, Bacharach P: The aging thyroid; increased prevalence of elevated serum thyropropin levels in the elderly. *JAMA* 242:247–250, 1979.

113. Harmon SM, Wehmann RE, Blackman MR: Pituitary-thyroid hormone economy in healthy aging men: basal indices of thyroid function and thyrotropin responses to constant infusions of thyrotropin releasing hormone. *J Clin Endocrinol Metab* 58:320–326, 1984.

114. Ingbar SH: Effect of aging on thyroid economy in man. *J Am Geriatr Soc* 24:49–53, 1976.

115. Berlyne GM, BenAri J, Kucheleusky A, Idelman A, Galinsky D, Hirsch M, Shainkir B, Yagil R, Zlotnik M: The aetiology of senile osteoporosis: secondary hyperparathyroidism due to renal failure. *Q J Med* 44:501–521, 1975.

116. Marcus R, Madriug P, Young G: Age-related changes in parathyroid hormone and parathyroid hormone action in normal humans. *J Clin Endocrinol Metab* 58:223–230, 1984.

117. Gallagher JC, Riggs BL, Jerpbok CM, Arnaud CD: The effect of age on serum immunoreactive parathyroid hormone in normal and osteoporotic women. *J Lab Clin Med* 95:373–385, 1980.

118. Ross BA, Bergeron G, Guggenheim K: Maturational increases in plasma calcitonin related to gastrointestinal function. *Clin Res* 398A, 1977.

119. Baker HWG, Bwger HG, de Hretser DM, Hudson B, O'Conner S, Wong C, Mirouics A, Court J, Dunlop M, Rennie GC: Changes in the pituitary-testicular system with age. *Clin Endocrinol* 5:349–372, 1976.

120. Takahashi J, Higashi Y, LaNasa JA, Yoshida KI, Winters SJ, Oshima H, Troen P: Studies of the human testis. XVIII. Simultaneous measurement of nine intratesticular steroids: evidence for reduced mitochondrial function in testis of elderly men. *J Clin Endocrinol Metab* 56:1178–1187, 1983.

121. Kinsey AC, Pomeroy WB, Martin CE: *Sexual Behavior in the Human Male.* Philadelphia, WB Saunders, 1948.

122. Monroe SE, Menon KMJ: Changes in reproductive hormone secretion during the climacteric and post-menopausal periods. *Clin Obstet Gynecol* 20:113–122, 1977.

123. Sherman B, Wysham C, Pfohl B: Age-related changes in the circadian rhythm of plasma cortisol in man. *J Clin Endocrinol Metab* 61:439–443, 1985.

124. Dilman VM, Ostroumova MN, Tsyrlina EV: Hypothalamic mechanisms of ageing and of specific age pathology. II. On the sensitivity threshold of hypothalamo-pituitary complex to homeostatic stimuli in adaptive homeostasis. *Exp Gerontol* 14:175–181, 1978.

125. Mongioi A, Vicari E, D'agata R: The prolactin-secreting system in relation to aging. *J Endocrinol Invest* 8:33–39, 1985.

126. Kovacs K, Ryan N, Horrath E, Penz G, Ezrin C: Prolactin cells of the human pituitary gland in old age. *J Gerontol* 32:534–540, 1977.

127. Casale G, Pecorini M, Cuzzoni G, deNicola P: Beta-endorphin and cold pressor test in the aged. *Gerontology* 31:101–105, 1985.

128. Shibasaki T, Shizume K, Nakahara M, Masuda A, Jibiki K, Demura H, Wakabayashi I, Ling N: Age-related changes in plasma growth hormone response to growth hormone-releasing factor in man. *J Clin Endocrinol Metab* 58:212-214, 1984.

129. Tsunoda K, Abe K, Goto T, Yasujima M, Sato M, Omata K, Seino M, Yoshinaga K: Effect of age on the renin-angiotensin-aldosterone system in normal subjects: simultaneous measurement of active and inactive renin, renin-substrate and aldosterone in plasma. *J Clin Endocrinol Metab* 62:384–389, 1986.

130. Hegstad R, Brown, R, Jiang NS, Kao P, Weinshilboum R, Strong C, Wisgerhof M: Aging and aldosterone. *Am J Med* 74:442–448, 1983.

131. Ziegler MG, Lake CR, Kopin IJ: Plasma noradrenaline increases with age. *Nature* 261:333–335, 1976.

132. Conway J, Wheeler R, Sunnerstedt R: Sympathetic nervous activity during exercise in relation to age. *Cardiovasc Res* 5:577–581, 1971.

133. Haas A, Flammer J, Schneider U: Influence of age on the visual fields of normal subjects. *Am J Ophthalmol* 101:199–203, 1986.

134. Millodot M, Owens H: The influence of age on the fragility of the cornea. *Acta Ophthalmol* 62:819–824, 1984.

135. Wuest FC, Sayther KD, Carlson CA, Wicklund PE: The aging eye. *Minn Med* 59:540–546, 1976.

136. Leske MC, Sperduto RD: The epidemiology of senile cataracts: a review. *Am J Epidemiol* 118:152–165, 1983.

137. Podgor MJ, Leske MC, Ederer F: Incidence estimates for lens changes, macular changes, open-angle glaucoma and diabetic retinopathy. *Am J Epidemiol* 118:206–212, 1983.

138. Kahn HA, Leibowitz HM, Ganley JP, Kini MM, Colton T, Nickerson RS, Dawber TR: The Framingham Eye Study. II. Association of ophthalmic pathology with variables previously measured in the Framingham Heart Study. *Am J Epidemiol* 106:33–41, 1977.

139. Taylor HR: The environment and the lens. *Br J Ophthalmol* 64:303- 310, 1980.

140. Weingeist TA: Macular degeneration associated with aging. *J Iowa Med Soc* 73:502–505, 1983.

141. Balazsi AG, Rootman J, Drance SM, Schulzer M, Douglas GR: The effect of age on the nerve fiber population of the human optic nerve. *Am J Ophthalmol* 97:760–766, 1984.

142. Anderson RG, Meyerhoff WL: Otologic manifestations of aging. *Otolaryngol Clin North Am* 15:353–369, 1982.

143. Perry ET: *The Human Ear Canal.* Springfield, Illinois, Charles C Thomas Publishers, 1957, pp 57–70.

144. Etholm B, Belal A: Senile changes in the middle ear joints. *Ann Otol* 83:49–54, 1974.

145. Glorig A, Davis H: Age, noise, and hearing loss. *Ann Otol* 70:556- 571, 1961.

146. Rosen S: Presbycusis study of a relatively noise-free

population in Sudan. *Ann Otol* 71:727–743, 1962.

147. Bergstrom B: Morphology of the vestibular nerve. *Acta Otolaryngol* 76:173–179, 1973.

148. Rosenhall U: Degenerative patterns in the aging human vestibular neuro-epithelia. *Acta Otolaryngol* 76:208–220, 1973.

149. Moller P: Skeletal muscle adaptation to aging and to respiratory and liver failure. *Acta Med Scand* 654:1–40, 1981.

150. Grimby G, Saltin B: Mini-review. The ageing muscle. *Clin Physiol* 3:209–218, 1983.

151. Essen-Gustavsson B, Borges O: Histochemical and metabolic characteristics of human skeletal muscle in relation to age. *Acta Physiol Scand* 126:107–114, 1986.

152. Inokuchi S, Ishikawa H, Iwamoto S, Kimura T: Age-related changes in the histological composition of the rectus abdominis muscle of the adult human. *Hum Biol* 47:231–249, 1975.

153. Burnstein AH, Reilly DT, Martens M: Aging of bone tissue: mechanical properties. *J Bone Joint Surg* 58A:82–86, 1976.

154. Schmidt UJ, Kalbe I, Sielaff F: Bone aging. *Adv Exp Med Biol* 53:371–374,1975.

155. Sharpe WD: Age changes in human bone: an overview. *Bull NY Acad Med* 55:757–773, 1979.

156. Tsai KS, Heath H, Kumar R, Riggs BL: Impaired vitamin D metabolism with aging in women. *J Clin Invest* 73:1668–1672, 1984.

157. Twomey L, Taylor J, Furniss B: Age changes in the bone density and structure of the lumbar vertebral column. *J Anat* 136:15–25, 1983.

Chapter 3

The Management of Perioperative Medical Problems in the Aged

Michael J. Lichtenstein, M.D., M.Sc., F. Tremaine Billings, M.D., M.A.C.P.

The care of the geriatric patient is characterized by its multidisciplinary focus, more so than any other area of medical practice. The surgeon, internist/geriatrician, nurse, and social worker all bring the skills of their respective professions to bear on the total care of the hospitalized elderly. Full geriatric assessment focuses on the five domains of functional capabilities (activities of daily living), mental functioning, physical health, social supports, and economic resources (1). Recognition of the importance of each of these domains can aid the surgeon in planning operations and the smooth care of the aged patient when hospitalization is necessary. This chapter focuses primarily on the domain of physical health—how to recognize the aged person who is at increased risk of perioperative medical complications and what may be done about them preoperatively. The aging process, with its concomitant physiologic changes, makes major surgical procedures more risky in the elderly than comparable procedures are in younger people. Age, by itself, is never an absolute contraindication for the surgical correction of a problem. The ability to identify those aged individuals who are at higher risk preoperatively will result in more viligant and effective care, allowing proper decisions to be made in a timely manner.

It is impossible to discuss all of the potential medical problems that may occur in the perioperative period of the elderly patient. In this chapter, we will review those conditions and complications that occur most frequently and those that are of a magnitude so serious as to increase substantially the morbidity and mortality in the surgical care of the elderly.

MEDICAL CONSULTATION

There is excellent evidence that aged patients assessed and treated by geriatric teams are more frequently discharged home, functionally more independent, than those who do not receive these services (2–4). In the first report of the effectiveness of a special inpatient geriatric evaluation unit, 80% of those treated in the unit were discharged home compared to 62% of controls (2). In addition 48% of those in the evaluation unit had improvement in ambulation compared to 24% of controls (2). Among aged persons hospitalized for more than a week in a Veteran's Administration Hospital, 47% did not have problems interfering with their discharge, 17% had a terminal illness, 12% had advanced dementia, and 15% had persistent unstable medical problems (3). The remaining 9% were deemed eligible for admission to a geriatric evaluation unit: These persons were entered into a randomized trial in which both the study unit group and the control group were comparable at the outset of the study. A higher proportion of those admitted to the special unit were discharged home (73%) compared to controls (53%). After the initial hospital discharge the evaluation unit patients had fewer rehospitalizations (35% vs 50%), fewer mean nursing home days (26 days vs 56 days), and a lower 1-year mortality rate (24% vs 48%) when compared to the controls (3). The geriatric evaluation unit also resulted in a 19% reduction in institutional costs per year of survival per person (3).

Goldman et al. at the Massachusetts General Hospital (7, 8) were the first ones to make findings related to the cardiovascular system that may be elicited and observed during a preoperative evaluation. The critical question to be answered is, "Which ones of these findings are useful in identifying the person at increased risk of a cardiac complication?"

Geriatric consultation services may also be effective in improving the outcome of the hospitalized elderly. During a trial of a geriatric consultation team, the average monthly census of elderly patients fell 21% due to decreases in the length of stay (4). The census reduction was brought about by a variety of medical, social, and rehabilitative interventions aimed at solving "system issues" and overcoming barriers to the discharge of patients (4). Geriatric consultation services contribute substantial input to the care of older patients. A randomized trial of such a consultation service found that physicians in the control group identified only 27% of the actions that would have been recommended by the consult team (5). The areas most frequently neglected were those of polypharmacy, sensory impairment, confusion, and depression. Overall, 72% of the geriatric team's recommendations were followed, with compliance on recommendations for preventing instability and falls (95%) and discharge planning (94%) being highest (5).

The message to surgeons with the frail aged patient who needs an operation is to avail themselves of the services of a geriatric evaluation team. The input of such a team early in the hospitalization of the elderly patient is likely to add substantially to the quality of total hospital care, improve functioning and survival, and as a bonus, reduce the cost of institutional care for these aged persons.

EVALUATION OF MEDICAL PROBLEMS

Cardiovascular System

Nearly 50% of all postoperative deaths that occur in aged patients are attributable to cardiovascular disease (6). Because of its clinical importance, considerable effort has been placed on developing prediction rules to help us identify preoperatively those persons who are at increased risk for cardiovascular complications

(7–11). Prediction rules are derived from systematic clinical observations. These rules are designed to reduce the uncertainty inherent in medical practice by defining how to use commonly seen clinical findings to make predictions (12). There are numerous signs, symptoms, and preoperative determinations of the presence of a wide range of specific factors and findings that may have a bearing on the cardiovascular status postoperatively. After following a consecutive series of 1,001 adults over the age of 40 years, they determined (using multivariate techniques) that there were nine clinical features that were independent correlates of life-threatening and fatal cardiac complications. These features included (a) preoperative third heart sound or jugular venous distension; (b) a documented myocardial infarction within the preceding 6 months; (c) more than five premature ventricular contractions per minute recorded at any time before operation; (d) a cardiac rhythm other than sinus or the presence of premature atrial contractions found on the preoperative electrocardiogram; (e) age over 70 years; (f) intraperitoneal, intrathoracic, or aortic operation; (g) emergency operation; (h) significant aortic valvular stenosis; (i) and a "poor" general medical condition (defined in Table 3.1). Importantly, and somewhat surprisingly, factors that did not carry any predictive value for postoperative cardiac complications included smoking, glucose intolerance, hyperlipidemia, peripheral vascular disease, and angina pectoris (8).

Detsky et al. at Toronto General Hospital (11, 12) validated and modified the predictions rule developed by the MGH group in a consecutive sample of 455 patients. The clinically important preoperative features and their corresponding scoring weights are presented in Table 3.1. The findings of the Canadians are similar to those of the MGH study, but differ in several important ways. The TGH study excludes S3 gallops or jugular venous distension and type of operation as predictive of postoperative cardiac complications; it includes angina pectoris and pulmonary edema as predictive factors.

These prediction rules are useful in that they enable physicians to estimate, during the preoperative period, the probability of postsurgical cardiovascular complications. To use them effectively, two pieces of information are

Table 3.1 Multifactorial Index for Clinical Prediction Rule for Determining Cardiac Risk Preoperatively[a]

Factor	Points
Coronary Artery Disease	
Myocardial infarction within 6 months	10
Myocardial infarction more than 6 months	5
Canadian Cardiovascular Society angina	
Class III — angina after walking 1 to 2 blocks on level ground	10
Class IV — inability to carry on any physical activity without discomfort	20
Unstable angina within 6 months	10
Alveolar Pulmonary Edema	
Within 1 week	10
Ever	5
Valvular Disease	
Suspected critical aortic stenosis	20
Arrhythmias	
Rhythm other than sinus or sinus plus atrial premature beats on last preop ECG	5
More than five premature ventricular contractions per minute at any time prior to surgery	5
Poor General Medical Status[b]	5
Age over 70 Years	5
Emergency Operation	10

[a]From Detsky AS, et al.: Predicting cardiac complications in patients undergoing non-cardiac surgery. *J Gen Intern Med* 1:211-219, 1986.
[b]Poor medical status defined as pO2 less than 60 mmHg, pCO2 greater than 50 mmHg, K+ less than 3 mEq/l, BUN greater than 50 mg/dl, Creatinine greater than 3 mg/dl, abnormal SGOT, signs of chronic liver disease, or bedridden from noncardiac causes.

Table 3.2 Clinical Scores and Likelihood Ratios Derived From the Multifactorial Index for Determining Cardiac Risk Preoperatively[a]

| | Likelihood Ratios | | |
| | Major | Minor | All |
Class (Points)	Surgery	Surgery	Surgery
I (0–15)	0.42	0.39	0.43
II (16–30)	3.58	2.75	3.38
III (31–)	14.93	12.20	10.60

[a]From Detsky AS, et al.: Predicting cardiac complications in patients undergoing non-cardiac surgery. *J Gen Intern Med* 1:211-219, 1986.

needed: *first,* a knowledge of local prevailing cardiovascular complication rates by type of operation (e.g., the myocardial infarction rate may be 8% for intraperitoneal procedures and only 2% for cataract operations). These complication rates are the a priori probabilities that an individual undergoing a specific procedure will have cardiovascular problems. These probabilities will vary from institution to institution. For example, a hospital in which a large volume of coronary artery bypass grafting procedures are done may have lower complication rates for that type of operation than a hospital in which only a few such cases are done each month. The *second* bit of needed information is a knowledge of how well the prediction rule works in the local

setting, i.e., given a certain type of operation and the score from the prediction rule, what is the probability that the patient will suffer cardiovascular complications (13)?

To answer this last question, one needs to contrast the proportion of patients with and without postoperative cardiovascular complications who display a given score on the prediction rule. This contrast produces a likelihood ratio, which is the odds that a given level of a diagnostic test result (in this case the score from a prediction rule) would be expected in a patient with (as opposed to without) the target disorder (14). The a priori odds for cardiovascular complications multiplied by the likelihood ratio yields a revised odds that can then be converted to an estimate of the individual's probability of having a cardiovascular complication.

To use the prediction rule, the features itemized in Table 3.1 are assessed in the patient and a score is derived. The scores can be divided into three classes: low, intermediate, and high risk. These are given with the associated likelihood ratios derived from the Toronto study (11) in Table 3.2. As an alternative to multiplying the preoperative odds of a cardiovascular complication by the likelihood ratio to obtain the revised risk estimate, a nomogram can be used (Figure 3.1). To use the nomogram, anchor a straight edge at the value on the pretest side of the nomogram (the a priori probability of a complication). Direct the straight edge through the center of the nomogram indicating the patient's prediction rule score and the associated likelihood ratio. The value where the straight edge intercepts the right-hand column denotes the post-test probability of perioperative cardiac complications for that patient.

Although these prediction rules add a signifi-

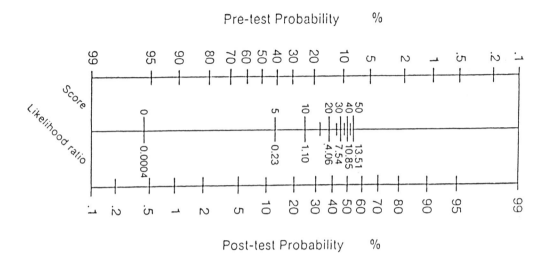

Pre-test Probability   %

Post-test Probability   %

"AVERAGE RISK FOR PATIENTS WITH INDEX SCORE"

Figure 3.1 Likelihood ratio nomogram. Anchor a straight edge at the value on the pre-test side of the nomogram determined by the surgical procedure. Direct the straight edge through the point in the center column reflecting the patient's prediction rule score and associated likelihood ratio. The point where the straight edge meets the right hand column denotes the post-test probability for the patient, i.e., the risk of a perioperative cardiac complication. (From Detsky AS, et al: Predicting cardiac complications in patients undergoing non-cardiac surgery. *J Gen Intern Med* 1:211–219, 1986 and Detsky AS, et al: Cardiac assessment for patients undergoing non-cardiac surgery: a multifactorial clinical risk index. *Arch Intern Med* 146:2131–2134, 1986.)

cant amount of predictive information about the likelihood of complications, they should be used cautiously as an initial estimate of the patient's risk. This caution arises for two reasons. First, complication rates vary from institution to institution. Second, observer variability in assessing the clinical features needed to derive the score and in assessing complications may limit the precision of the prediction rule. Results obtained at one location may not be generally applicable in another. Nevertheless, the prediction rule is useful and can be combined with other non-invasive test information.

Non-invasive exercise testing and dipyridamole-thallium scanning have been assessed as aids in determining the risk of perioperative cardiovascular complications. A study of dipyridamole-thallium scanning was performed in 48 patients (mean age, 63 years) admitted for elective vascular operations (15). In this series of patients 8 of 16 (50%) with thallium redistribution suffered cardiac complications compared to 0 of 32 (0%) without thallium redistribution. The

authors point out that in their series the cardiac complications were unrelated to age, prior history of chest pain, prior myocardial infarction, or whether the surgical procedure was intra-abdominal. Thus, in older individuals undergoing peripheral vascular procedures and in whom a prediction rule does not indicate problems, a dipyridamole-thallium scan may uncover a "silent" clinical problem that may require further evaluation preoperatively (15).

Bicycle exercise has been assessed as an adjunct to preoperative screening for cardiac risk in aged patients (10). A series of 155 persons who were greater than 65 years old and who were scheduled for elective abdominal or noncardiac procedures was screened using the prediction rule developed at MGH (7). Of the 59 patients with one or more of the prediction rule indicators, 16 (27%) had a perioperative cardiac problem. The remaining 96 patients without any prediction rule indicators underwent bicycle exercise testing. In the 31 persons unable to exercise 2 minutes, 6 (19%) had cardiac complications compared to only 1 of 65 (2%) of persons who were able to exercise for the full time. Thus, in the absence of any of the indicators from the MGH decision rule, an inability to do 2 minutes of bicycle exercise in the supine position to stimulate a heart rate of 99 beats/minute identified five of the six aged patients missed by the ''rule'' who subsequently had cardiac complications (10).

What steps can and should the surgeon take to reduce the risk of perioperative cardiac complications? The following suggestions are offered as a working guide to reduce the risk of perioperative cardiac complications:

1. Have an accurate, updated knowledge of the cardiac complication rates for various procedures done in the institution in which you are working.
2. Apply the prediction rules to each aged patient to estimate that individual's perioperative cardiac risk. Reassess the need for and timing of the elective operation:
   a. If an ''emergency'' can be stabilized and performed as an elective procedure, do so,
   b. If critical aortic valvular stenosis is present, this should be corrected first,
   c. If the patient has had a myocardial infarction within the 6 months prior to the planned operation, a delay of the procedure for as long as possible until six months after the myocardial infarction may be beneficial,
   d. Anti-anginal therapy and treatment for congestive heart failure should be optimized preoperatively,
   e. An electrocardiogram should be obtained on all aged patients preoperatively. The yield of recognizing abnormalities is great enough to be clinically worthwhile (16, 17). If the heart is not in sinus rhythm, preoperative evaluation and reasonable attempts to regain sinus rhythm should be undertaken,
   f. When possible, steps to reverse ''poor medical status'' (see Table 3.1) should be taken, as described below.
3. Elderly persons who do not have an increased risk as assessed by the prediction rules should be further tested if doubt still exists regarding the precise cardiac status:

   a. Among persons scheduled to have peripheral vascular procedures, dipyridamole-thallium scanning may detect those persons who are at increased risk.
   b. As a functional assessment, bicycle exercise testing can help detect aged persons who are at increased risk for perioperative cardiovascular complications.

Postoperatively, the surgical team must be especially alert to the possible development of a myocardial infarction. Greater reliance must be placed on clinical examination and ECG changes. Alterations in enzyme patterns (with the exception of subfractionation of creatinine-phosphokinase (CPK)) will be masked by the post-surgical changes. The signs and symptoms seen on presentation of myocardial infarction change with increasing age (18). When persons aged 70–74 years old are compared with those over 85 years old, the incidence of chest pain in myocardial infarction decreases (79% vs 66%), breathlessness remains the same (43% in both age groups), acute confusion increases (3% vs 19%), sweating decreases (33% vs 14%), stroke increases (2% vs 7%), and syncope increases (8% vs 18%). There always must be a high index of suspicion to determine the presence of myocardial infarction in older persons when symptoms and signs considered less typical of the usual presentation of myocardial infarction occur.

Pulmonary System

It is essential for the surgeon who is planning to do an operation upon an older individual to understand the pathophysiologic respiratory changes that may accompany aging. The stress of the surgical procedure on postoperative pulmonary function may exceed the ventilatory reserve of the elderly individual, and it may send him or her into respiratory failure. Three main areas of anatomic and structural changes occur that are associated with age and that lead to a number of important physiologic functional changes. These structural changes are (1) the loss of pulmonary alveolar elastic recoil, (2) alterations in the chest wall compliance and an associated decrease in respiratory muscle strength, and (3) loss of pulmonary alveolar surface area (19–22).

Loss of elastic recoil of bronchioles and alveoli

results in decreased support for the small airways, increased airway resistance, and premature airway closure during expiration. This results in "gas trapping" and an increased closing volume (relative to total lung capacity), with an accompanying decrease in vital capacity (the volume of gas expired in a maximal expiration following a maximal inspiration) in elderly persons. A second consequence of early airway closure on expiration is a redistribution of ventilation. If a concomitant shift in perfusion does not occur, ventilation-perfusion mismatch results, which accounts in part for the widened arteriolar-alveolar gradient seen in many aged individuals (20, 21).

During the process of aging, the chest wall becomes less compliant. Calcification of the costal cartilages results in decreased flexibility and mobility of the rib cage. These changes, coupled with kyphosis and loss of vertebral interspace height, lead to diminished outward expansion of the chest, which normally aids in the expansion of the lung. Consequently, inspiratory capacity of the lung is decreased. The altered shape of the chest wall is associated with weakened respiratory muscles. This contributes to the loss of expiratory reserve volume and the usual concomitant increase in residual volume found in most elderly persons (20-22).

The loss of alveolar surface area results in increased alveolar dead space, ventilation-perfusion mismatch, an increase in the arteriolar-alveolar oxygen gradient, and consequently a reduced arterial oxygen tension. The decline in oxygen tension with increasing age is constant and may be estimated by the equation:

$$PaO2 = 109 \ mmHg - 0.43 \ (age \ in \ years)$$

When this equation is used, the measured PaO2 should be within 8.2 mmHg of the calculated PaO2 95% of the time (19). If the actual gap is wider than the predicted level, another process may be superimposed on the effects attributable to aging alone.

The accumulation of these physiologic changes accounts for the increased risk of postoperative pulmonary complications in the aged. The decreased vital capacity that regularly occurs with aging is reduced further by the effect of abdominal or thoracic surgical procedures. Upper abdominal incisions and operative procedures

decrease the vital capacity to a greater extent than will lower abdominal procedures because the incision and pain of the former interfere in a more direct way with the diaphragmatic function (23). This may lead to atelectasis and hypoxemia. The increased closing volume in older persons may result in an increased difficulty in weaning them from ventilator support postoperatively. On the first postoperative day, there is usually a 20% decline in tidal volume and a 26% increase in respiratory rate so that minute ventilation usually remains constant (24). With increased closing volumes, the tendency to take rapid shallow breaths leads to further airway collapse and subsequently to hypoxemia (19).

A fourth area of structural change that occurs with aging has few functional consequences, but it does increase the risk for postoperative pulmonary problems. The elderly patients have more mucous-producing cells and fewer ciliated cells lining their upper respiratory tracts than younger people. The aged also have decreased cough reflex responses to stimulation of the upper airways. Compared to younger persons, they will cough with less volume, with weaker force, and with diminished flow rates. The observed decrease in effective mucociliatory transport and cough mechanisms results in a combination of factors that will cause difficulty in clearing secretions, can produce atelectasis, and may lead to a significantly increased risk of pulmonary infections (20).

In addition to the age-related physiologic changes there are a number of other risk factors that generally increase the risk of postoperative pulmonary complications. These include cigarette smoking, obesity, and the type and length of the proposed surgical procedure (24-26). Smokers have higher rates of pulmonary complications than non-smokers. In the elderly, smoking compounds the physiologic effects of the aging process. The mucociliatory transport is further damaged, the alveolar septae are damaged, the elasticity of the airways is reduced, and the closing volumes are increased (19). As persons age there is, on the average, an increase in weight and percentage of body fat content (22). Obese persons are at an increased risk for developing pulmonary complications because of their decreased functional residual capacity and because their expiratory reserve volumes are diminished. The added weight of the fat on the chest wall and the resistance to movement of the diaphragm by the increased abdominal mass lower the compliance of the entire respiratory system (19). These restrictive forces to thoracic expansion are increased in the recumbent position. Obesity may also result in resting hypoxemia due to ventilation-perfusion mismatching. The type and duration of the surgical procedure play an important role in the development of postoperative pneumonia (26). Persons with operations lasting more than 4 hours are known to have a five-fold increase in risk for pneumonia compared with those whose procedures last less than 2 hours (40% vs 8%). Compared to lower abdominal operations, thoracic procedures may carry an eight-fold increase in risk (40% vs 5%) and upper abdominal operations a three-fold increase in risk (17% vs 5%) for the likelihood of developing postoperative pneumonia. Other factors that may predispose patients to an increased risk for postoperative pneumonia include poor nutrition (relative risk of 2.8 for persons with serum albumin less than 3.0 mg/dl) and length of preoperative stay (relative risk of 3.9 for persons hospitalized more than a week prior to a surgical procedure). As in the assessment of cardiovascular risk, these latter items are indicators of a poor medical status and are confounded with the patient's underlying illnesses.

Having identified the reasons for the high rate of pulmonary complications expected to occur postoperatively in the elderly, what can be done to minimize the pulmonary risks of operative surgical care? The following suggestions are made to reduce the risk of postoperative pulmonary complications:

1. Admission history should focus carefully on respiratory symptoms. Respiratory symptoms will frequently confound the symptoms of chronic heart disease; indeed, individuals may be breathless because of increased left ventricular pressure and subsequent increased pulmonary venous pressure with decreased pulmonary compliance. The careful preoperative pulmonary history should focus upon:
   a. Functional activity—what is the most vigorous activity that the individual usually undertakes (e.g.,making beds, gardening), how long does it take to accomplish this task, and does the task ever affect breathing (try to avoid asking leading questions about becoming "short of breath"). Between 10% to 25% of persons over age 65 will have breathlessness with less than "normal" exercise (27).
   b. Nocturnal breathlessness may occur in 3%–6% of persons over 65 years old (27). This symptom may indicate some degree of left ventricular dysfunction and may be assessed in an unbiased way by asking the following questions in sequence:
      1. What time do you usually go to bed at night?
      2. How long does it usually take you to fall asleep?
      3. What time do you usually get up in the morning?
      4. Between the time you fall asleep and the time you get up in the morning, is your sleep disturbed for any reason? If the answer to this question is no, then ask:
         a. Do you ever have to get up to go to the bathroom during the nighttime?
         b. Does your breathing ever change during the night or when you get up to use the bathroom?
      5. What position do you actually sleep in at nighttime?
   c. Tobacco use—type of tobacco used, amount of tobacco used, duration of tobacco use, current user vs ex-user
   d. Symptoms of cough, wheezes, sputum production, and hemoptysis

2. Cardiovascular and pulmonary function can be further assessed using a 6-minute walk test. In this test, the distance that the individual can walk on level ground in 6 minutes is measured. This simple test helps discriminate between persons who have no evident disease (mean distance walked = 683 meters) and those with grade II (mean distance walked = 558 meters) and grade III heart failure (mean distance walked = 402 meters) (28). The 6-minute walk test is reproducible and has been validated against other measures of breathlessness in persons with chronic obstructive pulmonary disease

(29). Some caution should be used in performing and interpreting this test because age-adjusted reference ranges have not yet been established.

3. A routine chest radiograph is not indicated preoperatively solely on the basis of age alone. However, because the prevalence of pulmonary and chest symptoms is so high in the elderly, many older patients will require preoperative roentgenograms (30). A preoperative radiograph is indicated routinely in anyone scheduled to undergo intrathoracic procedures (30).

4. Aged persons with any abnormality discovered through history, physical exam, functional exercise testing, or on chest radiograph should undergo further pulmonary assessment.

   a. Pulmonary function testing—spirometry. This is indicated if the patient is obese, has a history of cigarette smoking/tobacco use and a cough, is scheduled for upper abdominal or thoracic operation, or has a history of pulmonary disease. Spirometric values that indicate a high risk of morbidity and mortality include a forced expiratory volume at 1 second (FEV 1) of less than 2 liters and a maximal breathing capacity less than 50% of predicted (24).

   b. Arterial blood gases—An arterial pCO_2 greater than 45 mmHg indicates decreased ventilatory capacity and increases the risk of postoperative pulmonary complications (24). In the prediction rules for postoperative cardiovascular complications, an arterial pO_2 less than 60 mmHg or a pCO_2 greater than 50 mmHg were markers for poor general medical status and added to the cardiac risk of the procedure (7, 11).

   c. Regional lung function and perfusion studies are indicated in persons with pulmonary insufficiency who are to undergo partial lung resection (24). The use of these radionuclide ventilation-perfusion scans allows for prediction of postoperative pulmonary function and therefore an estimate of how well the patient is likely to tolerate the proposed pulmonary resection.

5. Preoperative interventions to reduce the risk of postoperative pulmonary complications should include:

   a. Smoking cessation in those who use tobacco products
   b. Weight loss in the overweight
   c. Optimization of pulmonary function:
      1. Management of any underlying cardiac disease, especially full compensation of heart failure
      2. Antibiotics, humidification, and postural drainage for patients with chronic cough and bronchitis, (There is a critical need to decrease sputum production in these persons preoperatively.)
      3. Asthmatic symptoms—that is, any reversible component of airway obstruction due to bronchospasm—should be treated.

   d. Education regarding the importance of deep breathing postoperatively can aid in preventing pulmonary complications. Randomized controlled trials comparing deep breathing exercises, incentive spirometry, intermittent positive pressure breathing (IPPB), and control groups have demonstrated that using deep breathing exercises alone may reduce the pulmonary complication rate from 48% to 22% following abdominal operations (31). Incentive spirometry, when the patient is trained and has practiced preoperatively, produces a similar reduction in postoperative pulmonary complications. It was also associated with a significant shorter length of hospital stay following upper abdominal operations when compared to controls (8.6 vs 13.0 days). The length of stay following upper abdominal surgical procedures was also reduced in persons receiving IPPB, but this group was the only group to suffer pulmonary complications that were attributable to respiratory therapy (31).

6. Postoperative prevention of pulmonary complications have also been studied using randomized trials. Although it is clear that incentive spirometry and deep breathing exercises are beneficial when they are begun preoperatively, continuous positive airway

pressure (CPAP) or positive expiratory pressure (PEP) administered intermittently by mask further reduce pulmonary complications postoperatively (32). CPAP- and PEP-treated patients had a lower incidence of atelectasis, better gas exchange, and better preservation of lung volumes following upper abdominal procedures when compared to patients who were treated only by incentive spirometry (32). The PEP mask was as effective as the CPAP device in preventing atelectasis. The simplicity of the PEP mask (exhalation against a one-way valve with a set amount of resistance) makes it safer than other forms of respiratory therapy, and it is suitable for self-administration by the patient (32).

Deep Venous Thrombosis

Deep venous thrombosis is a frequent postoperative complication in the elderly. Its likelihood of occurrence depends in part on the type of operation performed, complicating about 5% of vaginal hysterectomies and 10% of transurethral prostatectomies on one end of the spectrum, and complicating more than 50% of hip arthroplasties at the other end (33). The probability of a patient's developing venous thrombosis increases with age. In community surveys comparing those patients over 46 years old with those less than 46 years old, the rates for developing deep venous thrombosis are 22 vs 4 per 10,000 men per year and 27 vs 15 per 10,000 women per year (34). In the postoperative setting, deep venous thrombosis developed in 24% of persons 40 to 60 years old and in 47% of persons 61 to 80 years old (35). The risk of developing deep venous thrombosis is also increased by a prior history of thromboembolic disease, regardless of the clinical setting (34, 35). Other factors that increase the risk of deep venous thrombosis occurring in the postoperative period are obesity and the presence of varicose veins (35).

The clinical diagnosis of deep venous thrombosis is unreliable. Only about 50% of postoperative patients with radiographically proven venous thrombosis will have clinical signs and symptoms that may alert the physicians to the presence of the problem (33). The key to managing this problem and its sequelae therefore lies

in the prevention of venous thrombosis. Prevention of this complication may be aided by early mobilization following the operation, by the use of elastic support stockings, or by the use of intermittent external pneumatic compression of the legs (33). Deep venous thrombosis may be prevented pharmacologically in one of two ways, either by the use of low dose heparin or by the use of a two-step low dose coumadin protocol.

Heparin administered in doses of 5,000 units subcutaneously every 8 hours has been shown to reduce overall mortality in a hospitalized general medicine setting (36). Heparin prevents deep venous thrombosis and reduces mortality in aged stroke victims (37). Numerous studies have demonstrated a reduced incidence of deep venous thrombosis when subcutaneous heparin is used postoperatively (38). Thus in a variety of settings, with a variety of clinical problems, low dose heparin has proved very effective in lowering the risk of venous thromboembolism and has saved lives. The largest, randomized, controlled trial of low dose heparin in the perioperative period was designed to test whether pulmonary emboli could be prevented (38). In this study 4,121 adult patients were randomized either to receive 5,000 units of heparin 2 hours preoperatively and then every 8 hours for 6 days or to serve as controls. The results were impressive. Isotopically proven venous thrombosis (using 125-I fibrinogen scans) occurred in 8% of the heparin-treated group compared to 25% of the controls. There were 180 postoperative deaths (100 in the control group, 80 in the heparin group), and autopsy rates were similar in both groups. At post-mortem examination, 24 deep venous thromboses were found in 72 (33%) control cases compared to 6 thromboses in 53 (11%) heparin-treated cases. The intraoperative and postoperative transfusion requirements for the two groups were similar. The heparin-treated group had more wound hematomas than the control group (8% vs 6%), but of the 9 deaths that were attributed to bleeding, 5 occurred in the control group and 4 in the heparin treated group (38). Therefore, low-dose subcutaneous heparin has been shown to be an effective, safe form of therapy for the prevention of deep venous thrombosis and subsequent pulmonary embolism in the operative setting.

A two-step low dose coumadin regimen may also be effective in preventing postoperative deep venous thrombosis (39). The use of coumadin should be tempered with caution because the risk of serious bleeding increases with age and is as high as 10% in persons over 70 years old (40). The two-step coumadin protocol is designed to prevent the development of deep venous thrombosis without causing excessive bleeding. This protocol has been tested in a randomized trial of 100 persons (mean age 66 years) scheduled to undergo elective hip or knee replacement (39). Patients were randomized to receive coumadin or dextran. The coumadin was begun 10 to 14 days preoperatively and adjusted so that the patient's prothrombin time was 1–3 seconds longer than the control time. Postoperatively, the coumadin dosage was increased so that the prothrombin time was 1.5 times greater than the control. Venograms (performed during the fifth to seventh postoperative day) indicated the presence of deep venous thrombosis in 11 of 53 (21%) studied patients receiving coumadin compared to 19 of 37 (51%) studied patients receiving dextran. Only 2% of the studied coumadin patients had proximal venous thrombosis compared to 16% studied dextran patients. In addition, there were no differences between the two groups with regard to intraoperative or postoperative bleeding complications, transfusion requirements, and lowest postoperative hematocrit (39). Thus, for elective orthopedic procedures, in persons without prior hemorrhagic risk factors and in those refraining from taking other drugs that would affect platelet function, a two-step low dose coumadin protocol is effective in halving the risk of developing deep venous thrombosis.

In the event that deep venous thrombosis has not been prevented, the first challenge is to make a timely and correct diagnosis. As stated above, clinical findings are notoriously unreliable; not only are they insensitive (i.e., fail to identify correctly persons with thrombosis), they are also non-specific (i.e., fail to rule out correctly persons without thrombosis) (41). Contrast venography has been the standard by which to diagnose deep venous thrombosis, but the venogram study itself may cause a phlebitis in 3%–10% of studied subjects (33). Impedance plethysmography and 125-I fibrinogen scanning are two non-invasive tests that can aid the accurate diagnosis of deep venous thrombosis. Plethysmography measures flow through the femoral-popliteal venous system as a function of blood-volume-induced changes in electrical resistance. 125-I fibrinogen detects the development of new clot formation and is most sensitive and specific for detecting calf thrombosis; it requires measurement at 24 and 72 hours following injection of the marker. To establish the usefulness of plethysmography and 125-I fibrinogen scanning, 274 patients with suspected deep venous thrombosis were studied: 114 were confirmed to have thrombosis and 160 were "ruled out" using contrast venography (42). A combination of either a positive plethysmogram or a positive fibrinogen scan correctly identified 103 of the 114 persons with thrombosis (sensitivity of 90%). Of the 78 persons with proximal thrombosis, 74 had positive plethysmograms (95%), and the remaining 4 were detected by fibrinogen scan. Of the 36 persons with thrombosis limited to the calf veins, 11 were missed by both tests, 5 were detected by both tests, 5 were detected by plethysmogram, and 15 were detected by fibrinogen scan alone. Thus, the combined testing correctly identified all persons with proximal thrombosis and 69% of those with calf vein thrombosis. Patients who were missed by both tests had symptoms lasting 7 days or more before presenting for evaluation. Among the 160 persons with negative venograms, a combination of a negative plethysmogram and a negative fibrinogen scan correctly identified 152 persons (specifically of 95%). Therefore, plethysmography and 125-I fibrinogen scanning are safe, reliable studies for the diagnosis of an initial episode of deep venous thrombosis (42).

In persons with normal plethysmograms, serial use of this study is also an effective means of evaluating persons with deep venous thrombosis; that is, a second different study may not be necessary (43, 44). Of 289 patients presenting with clinical evidence for deep venous thrombosis but in whom serial plethysemography was negative, none died of venous thromboembolism or presented with suspected pulmonary emboli during a 6-month follow-up (43). A randomized trial compared serial plethysmography (test repeated 1, 3, 5, 10, and 14 days after presentation) with a combined testing approach (plethysmography and 125-I fibrinogen scanning). At inital screening, six deep venous thromboses were detected in 311 (2%) patients receiving serial plethysmograms compared to 30 of 323 (9%) receiving the combined approach (44). This increased percentage in the combined group was due primarily to calf vein thrombosis. During long-term follow-up, only 2% of patients in each group developed deep venous thrombosis, and no patient died of pulmonary emboli. Serial impedance plethysmography, because of its non-invasive nature, ease of accomplishment at the bedside, and quick reporting of results, should be the test of choice in evaluating persons for initial episodes of proximal venous thromboembolism (44).

The non-invasive tests have also been utilized in the evaluation of recurrent deep venous thrombosis, a situation in which the diagnostic tests may not perform as well. In a cohort study of 270 persons with suspected acute recurrent venous thromboembolism, impedance plethysmography was evaluated (45). Of the 181 persons with negative plethysmography and negative 125-I fibrinogen leg scans, 3 (2%) died during follow-up (none with a pulmonary embolus). The 89 persons with initial abnormalities were treated for deep venous thrombosis, and on follow-up, 18 (20%) died (4 from a pulmonary embolus). Because a prior history of deep venous thrombosis is a risk factor for recurrence in the perioperative period, plethysmography and 125-I fibrinogen scanning are reliable tests for the detection of an acute recurrence in this setting— full anticoagulation may be safely withheld from persons with negative tests (45).

Once the diagnosis of deep venous thrombosis has been made, a decision to treat is based partly on the location of the thrombosis. Distal thrombi may be less likely to embolize than thrombi in the femoral-popliteal system (46). However, the likelihood of propagation of a calf thrombosis into the proximal system is about 20% in hospitalized patients (47). In persons who cannot be followed serially by plethysmography in order to detect the development of proximal thrombosis, it may not be safe to withhold therapy (44). Once a decision has been made to treat, the patient initially should be anticoagulated fully with a bolus of 5,000 units of heparin followed by a continuous intravenous infusion of heparin (1,250 units per hour) for 10 days. The efficacy of this regimen has been tested against a protocol of intermittent subcutaneous heparin in a randomized controlled trial (48). In this study 19% of patients on the intermittent heparin regimen developed recurrent venous thrombosis on follow-up compared to only 5% who received the continuous heparin infusion. On the seventh day of heparin treatment, patients should be started on coumadin. The coumadin should be continued for 3 months. It may be used in a less intensive regimen where prothrombin times are maintained at 1.5 times greater than control, rather than 2.0–2.5 times the control. A randomized trial of this less intense long-term program for the treatment of deep venous thrombosis with coumadin had fewer bleeding complications (4% vs 22% in the more intensively treated group) and was equally effective in preventing recurrent thrombosis (2% in each group) (49). Because the elderly are at increased risk for bleeding complications while taking coumadin, the ability to use this drug effectively in lower doses for the prevention and treatment of deep venous thrombosis is a boon to the management of this life-threatening problem.

Pulmonary Embolism

The true incidence of pulmonary emboli is difficult to ascertain. In the mid-1970s, estimates of 630,000 pulmonary emboli occurring per year in the United States were published (50). Of the 90% who survived the first hour of their embolism, it was estimated that a correct diagnosis was made in only 30% (or in about 160,000 persons). The overall case-fatality ratio for pulmonary embolism was placed at 32%, with the majority of deaths thought to occur in persons who never had the diagnosis made (50). If a firm diagnosis was made then the case-fatality ratio was placed at 8% (50). Two recent autopsy series have suggested that the incidence of fatal pulmonary embolism has been decreasing (51, 52). Although it cannot be stated with absolute certainty, both investigative teams suggested that the general adoption in the 1970s of the use of subcutaneous heparin as a prophylactic measure in the perioperative setting may have accounted in part for the observed decline in pulmonary emboli as a cause of death (51, 52). The use of anticoagulants increased from 4% of hospitalized patients to 12% of such patients between 1973 and 1976 in one report (52).

As with deep venous thrombosis, the key to managing pulmonary embolism is to prevent its occurrence. In a British multicenter trial, 5,000 units of heparin subcutaneously administered 2 hours preoperatively and then every 8 hours for 7 days postoperatively was effective in preventing pulmonary embolism (38). More than 4,000 patients scheduled to undergo elective operations were randomized to receive the heparin treatment or to be in a control group. Sixteen of 72 (22%) patients who underwent necropsy from the control group had pulmonary emboli compared to 2 of 53 (4%) from the heparin-treated group. The average age of the control group of patients with necropsy-proven pulmonary embolism was 69 years. In addition, 24 patients in the control group and 8 patients in the heparin treated group were treated for clinically suspected pulmonary emboli. Again, the two groups were comparable with respect to blood loss, transfusion requirements, and postoperative fall in hemoglobin. Thus, subcutaneous low dose heparin is a safe, effective means of preventing pulmonary embolism in older persons scheduled to undergo elective surgical procedures.

Should pulmonary embolism be suspected postoperatively, the diagnosis should be made as firmly as possible because the risks of full anticoagulation increase with advancing age. Undue reliance was placed on the clinical findings and ventilation-perfusion scanning in the past (53). We contend that a patient who is a candidate for full anticoagulation requires pulmonary angiography to establish or refute the diagnosis with any certainty. Clinically, pulmonary embolism may present with circulatory collapse (10%) or syncope (9%), pulmonary infarction with hemoptysis (25%), pleuritic pain and no hemoptysis (41%), uncomplicated embolism characterized by dyspnea (12%), or non-pleuritic pain with tachypnea (3%) (54). The most frequently occurring symptoms are dyspnea (84%), pleuritic pain (84%), apprehension (63%), and cough (50%). Although these may be fairly sensitive symptoms, their specificity is undetermined; that is, there are numerous other conditions that may present with these same symptoms. Hemoptysis occurred in only 28% of patients with embolism (54). Either dyspnea or tachypnea (greater than 20 breaths/minute) was present in 96% of persons, and dyspnea, tachypnea, or deep venous thrombosis were present in 99% of persons with pulmonary emboli. Although not firmly established, the total absence of dyspnea, tachypnea, or deep venous thrombosis makes the diagnosis of pulmonary emboli unlikely (54). Also, the true value of each of these symptoms in an older population, where the clinical manifestations of any disease may be altered, has not been established fully.

Other preliminary tests that may add information about pulmonary embolism include the routine chest roentgenogram and arterial blood gases (55). A clear chest film in the setting of sudden breathlessness and a lowered pO_2 may favor the diagnosis of pulmonary embolism. Atelectasis is a common postoperative roentgenogram finding; the chances of having a totally clear chest film (especially after upper abdominal or thoracic procedures) in this setting is remote. Arterial oxygen levels tend to decline with age and are also lowered postoperatively, so minor changes in oxygenation should be cautiously interpreted in this setting. These tests are likely to lack specificity in aiding the diagnosis of pulmonary embolism in the elderly in the immediate postoperative time period.

Ventilation-perfusion scans may be helpful in determining those patients who should then have pulmonary arteriography (56). About 7% of patients with proven pulmonary emboli will have subsegmental defects on scan compared to 48% of persons without pulmonary emboli. Given a perfusion scan that shows only subsegmental defects, the probability of the patient having emboli is about 9% (low probability). Thirty-three percent of persons with pulmonary emboli will have segmental perfusion deficits compared with 22% of persons without emboli; given a perfusion scan that shows only segmental defects, the probability of the patient having pulmonary emboli is 50% (intermediate probability). Lobar perfusion defects occur in about 52% of persons with emboli compared to 8% without; nearly 80% of persons with this perfusion pattern will have pulmonary emboli (high probability). Coupling the perfusion deficits with mismatched ventilation will increase the predictive value of the nuclear medicine study (56). The greatest value of the perfusion study is in helping to rule out pulmonary emboli: Patients with no abnormalities or subsegmental defects without ventilation mismatch are unlikely to have emboli. Angiography to confirm the diagnosis is recommended when the nuclear medicine study shows (a) a single defect involving a lobe or lung; (b) multiple segmental or segmental and subsegmental defects and no ventilation study; (c) multiple subsegmental defects associated with normal ventilation; (d) perfusion defects matching radiographic abnormalities; and (e) multiple perfusion defects, some of which have mismatched ventilation (56). To repeat, pulmonary angiography is mandatory to confirm or refute the diagnosis of pulmonary embolism in the elderly because the risk of serious bleeding while on full anticoagulation is about 10% (40).

Elderly patients who suffer pulmonary embolism in the immediate postoperative period are not often candidates for thrombolytic therapy. Those with a firm diagnosis should be fully anticoagulated with a continuous intravenous infusion of heparin for 10 to 14 days followed by 3 months of oral anticoagulant therapy.

High Blood Pressure

Essential hypertension is pathophysiologically characterized by increased peripheral vascular resistance with normal cardiac output. This is the most prevalent form of high blood pressure in middle age and is clinically recognized by an elevated diastolic and systolic pressure. The Hypertension Detection and Follow-up Program (HDFP) noted that 42% of persons aged 60–69 years will have diastolic pressures greater than 90 mmHg and 51% will have systolics greater than 140 mmHg when initially screened (57).

As persons age, a second pathophysiologic process contributes to the elevation of systolic pressure. Loss of arterial complicance results in raised systolic pressure (greater than 160 mmHg) with diastolic pressures less than 90–95 mmHg. The prevalence of isolated systolic hypertension is 7%–12% in the 60–69 year old age group, but is present in 25%–40% of those 75 years or older (58). Although isolated systolic hypertension carries a two- to five-fold increase in risk of death, to date there has been no published evidence from controlled trials to suggest that treating this form of high blood pressure in the aged results

in fewer strokes, myocardial infarctions, or deaths.

A third problem encountered when defining high blood pressure in the aged is the phenomenon of "pseudohypertension." This condition occurs when an inappropriately high cuff pressure is needed to compress a sclerotic calcified artery (59). The true prevalence of this entity is not known, but it may result in average falsely elevated blood pressure readings of 16 mmHg for both systolic and diastolic endpoints. Persons with "pseudohypertension" may be clinically recognized by palpation of the radial or brachial artery after occlusion by a sphygmomanometer cuff. Palpation of the pulseless artery ("Osler's maneuver") implies that the person may have "pseudohypertension" (59). An aged person may have essential hypertension, isolated systolic hypertension, "pseudohypertension," or combinations of these entities with varying severity. The surgeon must decide which form of high blood pressure predominates and how severe it is before electing to begin antihypertensive therapy or proceding with an elective surgical procedure.

There is still a case for conservative management of elevated blood pressure in persons over 65 years old. The Society of Actuaries' 1979 Build and Blood Pressure Study (60) demonstrates that the age-adjusted relative risk associated with a given level of blood pressure tends to decrease with age (the attributable risk increases, however). Men aged 60–69 years with diastolic pressures of 93–97 mmHg have a 20% excess mortality; this contrasts sharply with the 132% increase in mortality in 30–39 year old men with similar diastolic pressures. Men aged 60–69 years with diastolic pressures of 98–102 mmHg have age adjusted relative risks similar to 30–49 year olds with diastolics of 83–92 mmHg—levels that few would consider treating in light of present evidence for drug treatment of mild hypertension (61). The findings of the Build and Blood Pressure Study are reinforced by observations in general practice in which 704 hypertensive patients were followed without treatment over a 20-year period (1949–1969) (62). Utilizing a criterion of a sitting diastolic pressure of 100 mmHg to diagnose hypertension, the relative risks associated with this level of pressure in men were 7.5 in those aged 30–49 years, 4.9 in those aged 40–49, 2.2 in those 50–59, 1.2 in those 60–69, and 0.9 in those over 70 years old (62). The relative risks were generally lower in women. There is reasonable observational evidence that high blood pressure in the aged does not carry the same risk as it does in younger individuals.

Once raised blood pressure is recognized in an aged person, can it safely be lowered? The EWPHE study has shown that persons over 60 years old with average systolic pressures of 180 mmHg and average diastolics of 100 mmHg can have their blood pressure lowered about 20/10 mmHg using hydrochlorthiazide, with or without aldomet (63). This reduction in blood pressure was accompanied by significant increases in serum creatinine (0.2 mg/dl), uric acid (2.2 mg/dl), and glucose (17 mg/dl). Although no adverse outcomes were attributed to these chemical changes, the possibility exists that they might offset some of the benefits achieved by lowering blood pressure with thiazide diuretics.

The risk of adverse drug reactions must also be balanced against the benefits of treatment. The true incidence of adverse reactions from antihypertensive agents in the elderly is not known, but some evidence is available. Adverse drug reactions were noted in 248 (15%) of 2,000 consecutive admissions to British geriatric units (64). Of these, 209 (84%) of the reactions were felt to have contributed to the need for admission. Diuretics accounted for 60 of these adverse reactions. The risk of an adverse reaction to diuretics (percent of all those receiving this class of drug) was 8%. Although other hypotensive agents accounted for only 18 adverse reactions in this series, the risk associated with this group was 13%. Full recovery occurred in only 73% of those with adverse reactions to hypotensive or diuretic agents. More information is needed on the risks of antihypertensive therapy to assess adequately the net benefit of treatment in the elderly.

Does lowering blood pressure in aged patients confer any long term benefit to these individuals? Three studies all have shown a reduction in fatal or non-fatal cardiovascular events in persons over 60 years old who were receiving antihypertensive therapy. Each study by itself fails to provide conclusive proof of benefit. The direction of change is the same in all three studies,

and taken in aggregate, there is some evidence of modest improvement in outcome in those older persons receiving active treatment. The HDFP study (initial diastolic pressures of 90–104 mmHg) showed a 17% reduction in all-cause mortality in the 60–69 year old subgroup (57). The Australian trial of treating mild hypertension (initial diastolics of 95–104 mmHg) showed a 39% reduction in trial endpoints in the actively treated 60–69 year old subgroup. To date, the EWPHE trial is the only published randomized controlled trial specifically designed to look at the effect of antihypertensive therapy in the aged (66). In this study, 36% of subjects who entered into the study dropped out of treatment, and 15% were lost to follow-up. Overall, the benefit of treatment was modest; there was no evidence for improvement in all-cause mortality (cardiac deaths were diminished, but the rate of strokes remained unchanged). With these qualifications in mind, the group that stayed in the study and on the protocol did experience a decrease in all-cause mortality compared to controls (52 vs 70 deaths/1,000 person years) (66). The EWPHE study has also demonstrated a decrease in efficacy of drug therapy with advancing age (67), reinforcing the observational studies that suggest that there are lower levels of relative risk associated with a given blood pressure level in the elderly. There was no evidence of treatment benefit in persons over 80 years old; this subgroup of patients in the EWPHE study was 90% female. None of the three studies (57, 65, 66) provides sufficient data to allow evaluation of any differences between the sexes. Women have lower rates of cardiovascular disease than men and outnumber men after age 60.

At the present time, there is insufficient evidence to allow us to recommend drug therapy of raised blood pressure in asymptomatic persons over 70 years old. Exceptions to this position might include persons with symptoms of cerebrovascular insufficiency, heart failure, or diastolic (phase 5) blood pressures greater than 105 mmHg. If the decision is made to lower blood pressure pharmacologically in an aged person in the perioperative setting, supine and upright (standing) blood pressures should be monitored to avoid orthostatic hypotension and to minimize the risk of syncope. Initial antihypertensive therapy should be done with a low dose of a thiazide diuretic (68). Patients should be monitored closely for compliance with and understanding of their drug regimen, for possible adverse drug reactions, and for changes in serum electrolytes. Drug therapy should not necessarily be pushed vigorously in this group in order to lower the blood pressure to an arbitrary level; rather, the surgeon and internist should balance the amelioration of the symptoms for which the drugs were prescribed against side effect, cost, and inconvenience. For the aged person with high blood pressure, the principle of "first do no harm" is paramount.

Diabetes Mellitus

Glucose tolerance worsens with age primarily because of increased peripheral resistance to the effect of insulin (69). If standard criteria for a 2-hour post-prandial blood glucose level were used, then nearly half of all persons over age 70 would be considered to have chemical diabetes (69). Although the prevalence of diabetes increases with age, it is unlikely that it ever reaches a level of 50% in any age group. Diabetes is the most common endocrinologic disorder of the elderly, with estimates of its incidence in Western countries placed at 8% (70). Most aged diabetics are non-insulin-dependent; their symptoms and/or blood glucose levels are adequately controlled with diet and/or oral hypoglycemic agents. When a patient with diabetes is in need of an operation, whatever the type, with or without infection, the stress of the procedure and the events leading up to it usually increase the severity of the patient's glucose intolerance.

In managing the diabetic in the perioperative period, the surgeon wants to avoid three complications. These are hyperosmolar nonketotic coma, diabetic ketoacidosis, and hypoglycemia.

Hyperosmolar nonketotic coma is characterized by markedly elevated blood glucose levels (700 mg% or greater), elevated serum osmolarity (300 mOsm/kg or greater), extracellular volume depletion (hypotension, lack of sweating, prerenal azotemia), and neurologic signs (lethargy, confusion, stupor, or coma). Preoperatively the elderly patient may present with this problem (e.g., an elderly woman with a fractured hip who had been unable to move and feed herself for 2 days in her apartment before being found by relatives). Postoperatively hyperosmolar nonketotic coma may occur if the patient has not been adequately hydrated intravenously before fluids and food are being taken by mouth. The key to the proper management of this problem is the prompt institution of intravenous hydration with normal saline. Persons with hyperosmolar coma are very sensitive to insulin and should be managed with no more than 10 units of regular insulin initially. Once the patient is rendered hemodynamically stable, the intravenous fluid formula may be changed to half normal saline. The goal of therapy should be to replace one-half of the fluid deficit in the first 24 hours and to maintain a serum glucose level in the 200–250 mg/dl range. In the elderly patient, replacement of fluid too rapidly can result in pulmonary edema and the worsening of neurologic signs (69).

Diabetic ketoacidosis is characterized by a metabolic acidosis, hyperglycemia, dehydration, and tachypnea. This complication, like hyperosmolar nonketotic coma, may be present in the preoperative setting, or it may develop postoperatively if the elderly diabetic patient is not adequately hydrated or if insulin is withheld too long from an insulin dependent elderly patient. The mainstays of management again consist of prompt rehydration (again, initially with normal saline) and insulin. Insulin should be administered in an initial bolus of 0.10–0.15 units/kg intravenously followed by a continuous intravenous infusion of 0.10–0.15 units/kg/hr. Arterial blood gases, electrolytes, and serum glucose levels should be monitored every 1–2 hours until the ketoacidosis has resolved. While initially hyperkalemic, persons in diabetic ketoacidosis may develop hypokalemia because they are total body potassium depleted. As the acidosis is corrected, the patient may require potassium replacement.

Significant hypoglycemia is far worse in the elderly diabetic than hyperglycemia, and it should be avoided at all costs. In the aged, hypoglycemia may be difficult to suspect because of the absence or blunting of the usual peripheral symptoms (sweating, hunger, tachycardia). Also, persons who are mildly demented or who have other forms of cognitive impairment may not recognize and report these symptoms (69). Often, hypoglycemia may present solely as a worsening of confusion. Hypoglycemia generally results from a relative overuse of insulin or oral hypoglycemics. Postoperatively this may occur when the patient receives regular maintenance insulin dosages before he or she is able to take adequate calories in food by mouth. Decreases in memory, vision, and motor coordination may have impaired the elderly patient's ability to remember or see how much insulin to take and to administer an accurate dose of insulin. Postoperative insulin injections ideally should be given by the nursing staff, or the patients should be monitored very closely to be certain that they can properly self-administer a proper dose of insulin.

The key points to avoiding most of these complications in the elderly diabetic are those of ensuring adequate hydration and the judicious administration of insulin. The ideal management of diabetes during planned surgical treatment consists of keeping the patient slightly hyperglycemic with mild glycosuria. In the insulin-dependent person, an intravenous infusion of 5% dextrose and half normal saline should be started on the day of the proposed operation. Half of the patient's usual daily dose of insulin should be administered subcutaneously, with the other half placed in the intravenous fluids. The non-insulin-dependent diabetic should have an intravenous infusion of normal saline, and such patients may not require insulin. If insulin is administered to these patients, then they too should receive additional intravenous glucose to avoid episodes of hypoglycemia. The blood glucose level and the presence of glycosuria should be monitored throughout the intraoperative period. Should glucose control become necessary, continuous intravenous administration of regular insulin (0.10 unit/kg/hr) during the operation and in the immediate postoperative period will achieve better results than will intramuscular or subcutaneous injections (71).

Postoperatively, "finger stick" blood glucose levels should be determined every 4–6 hours. A sliding scale of regular insulin administered subcutaneously may be used to maintain glucose control until the patient is eating and drinking normally and can be returned to the preoperative regimen of insulin or oral hypoglycemic agents.

Renal Problems

Renal insufficiency associated with surgical procedures in the elderly can usually be foreseen and prevented by preoperative evaluation of renal function and by the examination of the genitourinary organs. Determination of blood urea nitrogen and serum creatinine levels and the results of a urinalysis should give the necessary information to assess renal function. Important preventable causes of perioperative renal insufficiency and steps to correct them include cessation of administration of nephrotoxic drugs, correction of prerenal azotemia, and relief of obstructive uropathy.

Glomerular filtration declines with age. Because muscle mass, the source of creatinine, also declines with age, the true deficit in glomerular filtration ability may not be accurately reflected in the serum creatinine level (72). This becomes important clinically when the administration of nephrotoxic drugs that depend on the kidneys for excretion (e.g., aminoglycosides) are needed. The dosage schedules for these drugs will require adjustments based on measured or calculated estimates of creatinine clearance. Creatinine clearance (ml/min) may be calculated by using the following formula:

$$\frac{(140 - age\ (yrs))\ (weight\ (kgs))}{(72)\ (serum\ creatinine(mg/dl))}$$

Nomograms are available that may be used to adjust the dosage of antibiotics according to the creatinine clearance (73). At the first sign or indication of renal insufficiency occurring postoperatively, the surgical team should carefully review the medication list and eliminate or appropriately reduce any nephrotoxic agents from the drug regimen.

Prerenal azotemia is usually the result of hypovolemia or hypoxia of the kidney. Recognition of this situation is aided by the measurement of urine electrolytes and osmolarity (74). Urinary sodium concentrations of less than 20 mEq/liter and osmolarity of greater than 500 mOsm/liter indicate that the tubular-concentrating mechanisms of the kidneys are still intact and that the azotemia is likely to be due to a prerenal mechanism. Therapy of this problem involves correction of the causes of hypoxemia and the judicious rehydration of the patient.

Obstructive uropathy is of particular importance in aged men because the frequency of prostatic hypertrophy is high in this group. A careful urologic history and physical exam will usually be adequate to evaluate this problem preoperatively. Preoperative placement of Foley catheters is usually recommended for most major operations so that obstruction should not be a problem during the procedure or in the immediate postoperative recovery period and so that accurate urinary output data are available.

Hepatic Problems

The liver does not change appreciably in size and weight with advancing age; however, hepatic blood flow diminishes (1.5% per year) and age-related decreases in albumin levels are seen. These two factors have implications for the clearance and bioavailability of drugs (75), implying that certain drugs will be more available in an active unbound state and less readily cleared from the body in most elderly individuals.

There is little direct evidence for the unfavorable influence of the aging liver upon morbidity and mortality associated with surgical procedures in the aged, but there is ample information that true hepatic insufficiency is a dangerous companion to operations (76). Among persons with liver disease, the presence of ascites, infection, and an albumin level less than 3 mg/dl, a bilirubin level greater than 3 mg/dl, or prolonged coagulation studies all carry a 50%–60% mortality rate when superimposed on the stress of surgical trauma (compared to a 7%–22% mortality when these factors are absent) (77). If active primary liver disease is identified in an aged person scheduled for a surgical procedure, consideration should be given to delaying the operation until the problem can be corrected if possible (through adequate nutrition and removal of hepatotoxins).

A word about alcohol use and alcoholic liver disease in the elderly is important. Older individuals may be more sensitive to alcohol because of higher peak serum levels post-ingestion due to an decreased amount of lean body mass and a decreased volume of distribution (78). Although the presentation of alcoholic liver disease in the elderly patient is similar to that in the young, preliminary evidence suggests a higher mortality in the aged (48% at 1 year) (79). The prevalence of alcohol dependency among older persons scheduled for a surgical procedure and the impact this has on surgical outcome are as yet unknown. Care must be taken to elicit a careful history, not only concerning alcohol ingestion but also behavioral problems (such as falls, confusion, memory lapses) that may indicate problems with alcohol dependency. If there is any suspicion that alcohol use is a problem, the patient should be watched carefully for signs of alcohol withdrawal and treated appropriately if they emerge (80).

Medications

Elderly patients frequently suffer from multiple chronic diseases that involve several organ systems. As increasing numbers of chronic diseases are present, more and more drugs are prescribed (81). People aged 25–44 years fill an average of slightly more than 5 prescriptions per person per year, whereas those over 65 years old fill an average of 12 prescriptions per person per year. The number of adverse reactions to drugs rises in direct proportion to the number of drugs taken: 4% when 1 to 5 drugs are prescribed, 7% for 6 to 11 drugs, and 24% when 11 to 15 medications are taken concurrently (82).

The activity of a drug in the body, whether therapeutic or toxic, depends upon the plasma concentration of that drug. The plasma concentration in turn depends upon the size of the dose and its frequency of administration, the absorption rate, the volume in which the drug is distributed, and the rate of clearance from the body. These factors that govern the pharmacodynamics of drugs are altered by the aging process. The proportion of body fat increases, and lean body mass and total body water tend to decrease as persons age. These changes will alter the distribution of certain drugs. For example, fat-soluble drugs (such as benzodiazepines and phenothiazines) have a delayed onset of action in the elderly, but their effect may be prolonged because they are accumulated and then released in relatively increased amounts of body fat (83–85).

Blood perfusion to most organs declines with increasing age. Because drugs are eliminated from the body primarily through renal excretion or by hepatic metabolic action, decreased perfusion through these organs can lead to increased plasma drug levels. Decreased perfusion and changes in acid-base concentrations in the stomach and intestine can also lead to unpredictable absorption rates of orally administered drugs (86).

All of these potential problems are exaggerated and become unpredictable before, during, and after surgical procedures as intravenous fluids (with possible changes in electrolyte levels) and blood products are administered. Changes in blood pressure occur intraoperatively, thus altering organ perfusion. Deprivation of food occurs (often compounded by nasogastric suctioning), which has the potential for producing malnutrition over varying periods of time. Under these circumstances it is important to monitor carefully drug usage in the perioperative period by clinical observations for toxic effects, by plasma levels when possible, and by the electrocardiographic changes when appropriate (87).

Because of the vulnerability of the aged patient to adverse drug reactions and the increased frequency with which they occur, the following suggestions are made to reduce the risk of these problems: (85,88)

1. Periodic (daily) review should be made of the medication regimen that the patient is receiving while in the hospital.
2. After careful clinical assessment consider whether any unnecessary drug is being prescribed or whether any additional medication is indicated. At this point take into account any factors that might alter the patient's responsiveness to the drug.
3. Simplify the dose and drug regimen as much as possible. Start with the lowest effective dose possible; it is easier to build up to a therapeutic dose than to remove a drug and deal with an adverse reaction due to overtreatment.
4. Consider non-pharmacologic forms of therapy whenever possible; for example, sodium restriction as the first intervention, rather than a drug, when it is deemed necessary to lower the patient's blood pressure.
5. Avoid inappropriate or over-energetic therapy when the patient's physical and mental disabilities indicate the possibility of a less active therapeutic role.

Adherence to these simple guidelines will help avoid the iatrogenic problem of adverse drug reactions and their attendant morbidity.

CONCLUSIONS

When carefully evaluated and adequately prepared for the treatment of surgically correctable conditions, elderly patients will be able to tolerate most reasonably planned surgical procedures. Diligent attention to the details of maintaining a stable physiologic environment during and following the operation is critical to the success of surgical treatment of the aged patient. When these principles are followed and when good surgical judgement is used, the elderly patient will be found to be surprisingly tolerant of most major surgical procedures. Age alone should not eliminate the elderly patient from surgical consideration.

REFERENCES

1. Williams ME: Geriatric assessment. *Ann Intern Med* 104:720-721, 1986.
2. Lefton E, Bonstelle S, Frengley JD: Success with an inpatient geriatric unit: a controlled study of outcome and followup. *J Am Geriatr Soc* 31:149-155, 1983.
3. Rubenstein LZ, Josephson KR, Wieland GD, English PA, Sayre JA, Kane RL: Effectiveness of a geriatric evaluation unit: a randomized clinical trial. *N Engl J Med* 311:1664-1670, 1984.
4. Barker WH, Williams TF, Zimmer JG, Van Buren C, Vincent SJ, Pickrel SG: Geriatric consultation teams in acute hospitals: impact on back-up of elderly patients. *J Am Geriatr Soc* 33:422-428, 1985.
5. Allen CM, Becker PM, McVey LJ, Saltz C, Feussner JR, Cohen HJ: A randomized, controlled trial of geriatric consultation teams: compliance with recommendations. *JAMA* 255:2617-2621, 1986.
6. Cole W: Medical differences between the young and the aged. *J Am* Geriatr Soc 18:589-614, 1970.
7. Goldman L, Caldera DL, Nussbaum SR, Southwick FS, Krogstad D, Murray B, Burke DS, O'Malley TA, Goroll AH, Caplan CH, Nolan J, Carabello B, Slater EE: Multifactorial index of cardiac risk in noncardiac surgical procedures. *N Engl J Med* 297:845-850, 1977.
8. Goldman L, Caldera DL, Southwick FS, Nussbaum SR, Murray B, O'Malley TA, Goroll AH, Caplan CH, Nolan J, Burke DS, Krogstad D, Carabello G, Slater EE: Cardiac risk factors and complications in non-cardiac surgery. *Medicine* 57:357-370, 1978.
9. Goldman L: Cardiac risk and complications of non-cardiac surgery. *Ann Intern Med* 95:504-513, 1983.
10. Gerson MC, Hurst JM, Hertzberg VS, Doogan PA,

Cochran MB, Lim SP, McCall N, Adolph RJ: Cardiac prognosis in non-cardiac geriatric surgery. *Ann Intern Med* 103:832–837, 1985.

11. Detsky AS, Abrams HB, McLaughlin JR, Drucker DJ, Sasson Z, Johnston N, Scott JG, Forbath N, Hilliard JR: Predicting cardiac complications in patients undergoing non-cardiac surgery. *J Gen Intern Med* 1:211–219, 1986.

12. Detsky AS, Abrams HB, Forbath N, Scott JG, Hilliard JR: Cardiac assessment for patients undergoing non-cardiac surgery: a multifactorial clinical risk index. *Arch Intern Med* 146:2131–2134, 1986.

13. Wasson JH, Sox HC, Neff RK, Goldman L: Clinical prediction rules: applications and methodological standards. *N Engl J Med* 313:793–799, 1985.

14. Sackett DJ, Haynes RB, Tugwell P: *Clinical Epidemiology: A Basic Science for Clinical Medicine.* Boston, Little, Brown & Co, 1985.

15. Boucher CA, Brewster DC, Darling RC, Okada D, Strauss HW, Pohost GM: Determiniation of cardiac risk by dipyridamole imaging before peripheral vascular surgery. *N Engl J Med* 312:389–394, 1985.

16. Moorman JR, Hlatky MA, Eddy DM, Wagner GS: The yield of the routine admission electrocardiogram: a study in a general medical service. *Ann Intern Med* 103:590–595, 1985.

17. Goldberger AL, O'Konski M: Utility of the routine electrocardiogram before surgery and on general hospital admission: critical review and new guidelines. *Ann Intern Med* 105:552–557, 1986.

18. Bayer AJ, Chadha JS, Faraq RR, Pathy MSJ: Changing presentation of myocardial infarction with increasing old age. *J Am Geriatr Soc* 34:263–266, 1986.

19. Hedley-Whyte J, Burgess GE, Feeley TW, Miller MG (eds): *Applied Physiology of Respiratory Care.* Boston, Little, Brown & Co, 1976.

20. Levitzky MG: Effects of aging on the respiratory system. *The Physiologist* 27:102–107, 1984.

21. Wahba WM: Influence of aging on lung function—clinical significance of changes from age twenty. *Anesth Analg* 62:764–776, 1983.

22. Fowler RW: Ageing and lung function. *Age Ageing* 14:209–215, 1985. 23. Bendixen HH, Egbert LD, Hedley-Whyte J, Laver MB, Pontoppidan H (eds): *Respiratory Care.* St. Louis, CV Mosby, 1965.

23. Bendixen HH, Egbert LD, Hedley-Whyte J, Laver MB, Pontoppidan H (eds): *Respiratory Care,* St. Louis, CV Mosby, 1965.

24. Tisi GM: Preoperative evaluation of pulmonary function: validity, indications, and benefits. *Am Rev Respir Dis* 119:293–310, 1979.

25. Garibaldi RA, Britt MR, Coleman MD, Reading JC, Pace NL: Risk factors for postoperative pneumonia. *Am J Med* 70:677–680, 1981.

26. Hale WE, Perkins LL, May FE, Marks RG, Stewart RB: Symptom prevalence in the elderly: an evaluation of age, sex, disease, and medication use. *J Am Geriatr Soc* 34:333–340, 1986.

27. Wiren JE, Janzon L: Risk factors for postoperative respiratory complications and their predictive value. *Acta Chir Scand* 148:479–484, 1982.

28. Lipkin DP, Scriven AJ, Crake T, Poole-Wilson PA: Six minute walking test for assessing exercise capacity in chronic heart failure. *Br Med J* 292:653–655, 1986.

29. Guyatt GH, Thompson PJ, Berman LB, Sullivan MJ, Townsend M, Jones NL, Pugsley SO: How should we measure function in patients with chronic heart and lung disease? *J Chron Dis* 1985; 38:517–524.

30. Tape TG, Mushlin AI: The utility of routine chest radiographs. *Ann Intern Med* 104:663–670, 1986.

31. Celli BR, Rodriguez KS, Snider GL: A controlled trial of intermittent positive pressure breathing, incentive spirometry, and deep breathing exercises in preventing pulmonary complications after abdominal surgery. *Am Rev Respir Dis* 130:12–13, 1984.

32. Rickstein SE, Bengtsson A, Soderberg C, Thorden M, Kvist H: Effects of periodic positive airway pressure by mask on postoperative pulmonary function. *Chest* 89:774–781, 1986.

33. Becker DM: Venous thromboembolism: epidemiology, diagnosis, and prevention. *J Gen Intern Med* 1:402–411, 1986.

34. Coon WW, Willis PW, Keller JB: Venous thromboembolism and other venous disease in the Tecumseh Community Health Study. *Circulation* 48:839–846, 1973.

35. Kakkar VV, Howe CT, Nicolaides AN, Renney JTG, Clarke MB: Deep vein thrombosis of the leg: is there a "high risk" group? *Am J Surg* 120:527–530, 1970.

36. Halkin H, Goldberg J, Modan M, Modan B: Reduction of mortality in general medical in-patients by low-dose heparin prophylaxis. *Ann Intern Med* 96:561–565, 1982.

37. McCarthy ST, Turner J: Low-dose subcutaneous heparin in the prevention of deep-vein thrombosis and pulmonary emboli following acute stroke. *Age Ageing* 15:84–88, 1986.

38. Kakker VV, Corrigan TP, Fossard DP, Sutherland I, Shelton MG, Thirlwall J: Prevention of fatal postoperative pulmonary embolism by low doses of heparin: an international multicenter trial. *Lancet* 2:45–51, 1975.

39. Francis CW, Marder VJ, Evarts CM, Yaukoolbodi S: Two-step warfarin therapy: prevention of postoperative venous thrombosis without excessive bleeding. *JAMA* 249:374–378, 1983.

40. Coon WW, Willis PW: Hemorrhagic complications of anticoagulant therapy. *Arch Intern Med* 133:386–392, 1974.

41. Sandler DA, Duncan JS, Ward P, Lamont AC, Sherriff S, Martin JF, Blake GM, Ramsey LE, Ross B, Walton L: Diagnosis of deep-vein thrombosis: comparison of clinical evaluation, ultrasound, plethysmography, and venoscan with x-ray evaluation. *Lancet* 2:716–719, 1984.

42. Hull R, Hirsh J, Sackett DK, Taylor DW, Carter C, Turpie AGG, Zielinsky A, Powers P, Gent M: Replacement of venography in suspected venous thrombosis by impedance plethysmography and 125-I fibrinogen leg scanning. *Ann Intern Med* 94:12–15, 1981.

43. Huisman MV, Buller HR, TenCate JW, Vreeken J: Seri-

al impedance plethysmography for suspected deep venous thrombosis in outpatients: The Amsterdam general practitioner study. *N Engl J Med* 314:823–828, 1986.

44. Hull RD, Hirsh J, Carter CH, Jay RM, Ockelford PA, Buller HR, Turpie AG, Powers P, Kinch D, Dodd PE, Gill GJ, LeClerc JR, Gent M: Diagnostic efficacy of impedance plethysmography for clinically suspected deep-vein thrombosis. *Ann Intern Med* 102:21–28, 1985.

45. Hull RD, Carter CJ, Jay RN, Ockelford PA, Hirsh J, Turpie AG, Zielinsky A, Gent M, Powers PJ: The diagnosis of acute recurrent, deep-vein thrombosis: a diagnostic challenge. *Circulation* 67:901–906, 1983.

46. Moser KM, LeMoine JR: Is embolic risk conditioned by location of deep venous thrombosis? *Ann Intern Med* 94:439–444, 1981.

47. Hirsh J: Venous thromboembolism: diagnosis, treatment, prevention. *Hosp Pract* 10:53–62, 1975.

48. Hull RD, Raskob GE, Hirsh J, Jay RM, LeClerc JR, Geerts WH, Rosenbloom D, Sackett DL, Anderson C, Harrison L, Gent M: Continuous intravenous heparin compared with intermittent subcutaneous heparin in the initial treatment of proximal vein thrombosis. *N Engl J Med* 315:1109–1114, 1986.

49. Hull R, Hirsh J, Jay R, Carter C, England C, Gent M, Turpie AGG, McLaughlin D, Dodd P, Thomas M, Raskob G, Ockelford P: Different intensities of oral anticoagulant therapy in the treatment of proximal vein thrombosis. *N Engl J Med* 307:1676–1681, 1982.

50. Dalen JE, Alpert JS: Natural history of pulmonary embolism. *Prog Cardiovasc Dis* 17:259–270, 1975.

51. Ruckley CV, Thurston C: Pulmonary embolism in surgical patients: 1959–1979. *Br Med J* 284:1100–1102, 1982.

52. Dismukes SE, Wagner EH: Pulmonary embolism as a cause of death: the changing mortality in hospitalized patients. *JAMA* 255:2039-2042, 1986.

53. Robin ED: Overdiagnosis and overtreatment of pulmonary embolism: the emperor may have no clothes. *Ann Intern Med* 87:775–781, 1977.

54. Stein PD, Willis PW, DeMets DL: History and physical examination in acute pulmonary embolism in patients without preexisting cardiac or pulmonary disease. *Am J Cardiol* 47:218–223, 1981.

55. Stein PD, Willis PW, Dalen JE: Importance of clinical assessment in selecting patients for pulmonary arteriography. *Am J Cardiol* 43:669–671, 1979.

56. McNeil BJ: A diagnostic strategy using ventilation-perfusion studies in patients suspect for pulmonary embolism. *J Nucl Med* 17:613–616, 1976.

57. Curb JD, Borhani NO, Schnaper H, Kass E, Entwisle G, Williams W, Berman R: Detection and treatment of hypertension in older individuals. *Am J Epidemiol* 121:371–376, 1985.

58. Lichtenstein MJ: Isolated systolic hypertension: how common? how risky? *South Med J* 78:972–978, 1985.

59. Messerli FH, Ventura HO, Amodeo C: Osler's maneuver and pseudohypertension. *N Engl J Med* 312:1548–1551, 1985.

60. Society of Actuaries and Life Insurance Medical Directors of America: *Build and Blood Pressure Study 1979.* Recording and Statistical Corporation, 1980.

61. Medical Research Council Working Party. MRC trial of treatment of mild hypertension: principal results. *Br Med J* 291:97–104, 1985.

62. Fry J: Natural history of hypertension: a case for selective non-treatment. *Lancet* 2:431–433, 1974.

63. Amery A, Beard K, Birkenhager W, Bulpitt C, Clement D, Derayttere M, DeSchaepdryver A, Dollery C, Fagard R, Forette F, Forte J, Hamdy R, Henry JF, Joosens JV, Leonetti G, Lund-Johnson P, O'Malley K, Petrie JC, Strasser T, Tuomilehto J, Williams B: Antihypertensive therapy in patients above 60 years. Eighth interim report of the European Working Party on High Blood Pressure in the Elderly (EWPHE). *Curr Med Res Opin* 8(Suppl 1):5–18, 1982.

64. Williamson J, Chopin JM: Adverse reactions to prescribed drugs in the elderly: a multicenter investigation. *Age Ageing* 9:73–80, 1980.

65. Management Committee. Treatment of mild hypertension in the elderly. *Med J Aust* 2:398–402, 1981.

66. Amery A, Birkenhager W, Brixho P, Bulpitt C, Clement D, Derayttere M, DeSchaepdryver A, Dollery C, Fagard R, Forette F, Forte J, Hamdy R, Henry JF, Joosens JV, Leonetti G, Lund-Johnson P, O'Malley K, Petrie JC, Strasser T, Tuomilehto J, Williams B: Mortality and morbidity results from the European Working Party on High Blood Pressure in the Elderly trial. *Lancet* 1:1349–1354, 1985.

67. Amery A, Birkenhager W, Brixho P, Bulpitt C, Clement D, Derayttere M, DeSchaepdryver A, Dollery C, Fagard R, Forette F, Forte J, Hamdy R, Henry JF, Joosens JV, Leonetti G, Lund-Johnson P, O'Malley K, Petrie JC, Strasser T, Tuomilehto J, Williams B: Efficacy of antihypertensive drug treatment according to age, sex, blood pressure, and previous cardiovascular disease in patients over the age of 60. *Lancet* 2:589–592, 1986.

68. The Working Group on Hypertension in the Elderly: Statement on Hypertension in the Elderly. *JAMA* 256:70–74, 1986.

69. Rowe JW, Besdine RW: Endocrine and metabolic systems. In Rowe JW, Besdine RW (eds): *Health and Disease in Old Age.* Boston, Little, Brown & Co, 1982, pp 137–156.

70. Morley JE: The aging endocrine system: evaluation and treatment of age related disorders. *Postgrad Med* 73:107–120, 1983.

71. Meyer EJ, Lorenzi M, Bohannon NV, Amend W, Federiska NJ, Salvotierra O, Forsham PH: Diabetic management by insulin infusion during major surgery. *Am J Surg* 137:323–330, 1979.

72. Rowe JW: Renal system. In Rowe JW, Besdine RW (eds): *Health and Disease in Old Age.* Boston, Little, Brown & Co, 1982, pp 165–183.

73. Bryan CS, Stone WJ: Antimicrobial dosage in renal failure: a unifying nomogram. *Clin Neph* 7:81–84, 1977.

74. Miller TR, Anderson RJ, Stuart LL, Henrich WL, Berns

AS, Gabow PA, Schrier RW: Urinary diagnostic indices in acute renal failure: a prospective study. *Ann Intern Med* 89:47–50, 1978.

75. James OFW: Drugs and the aging liver. *J Hepatology* 1:431–435, 1985.

76. Doberneck RC, Sterling WA, Allison DC: Morbidity and mortality after operation in non-bleeding cirrhotic patients. *Am J Surg* 146:306–309, 1983.

77. Garrison RN, Cryer HM, Howard DA, Polk HC: Classification of risk factors for abdominal operations in patients with hepatic cirrhosis. *Ann Surg* 199:648–655, 1984.

78. Vestal RE, McGuire EA, Tobin JD: Aging and ethanol metabolism. *Clin Pharmacol Ther* 21:343–354, 1977.

79. Woodhouse KW, James OFW: Alcoholic liver disease in the elderly: presentation and outcome. *Age Ageing* 14:113–118, 1985.

80. Sellers EM, Kalant H: Alcohol intoxication and with-

81. Covington TR, Walker JI (eds): *Current Geriatric Therapy.* Philadelphia, WB Saunders, 1984.

82. Cluff LE, Thornton EF, Seidl LG: Studies on the epidemiology of adverse drug reactions. *JAMA* 188:976–983, 1964.

83. Greenblatt DJ, Sellers EM, Shader RI: Drug disposition in old age. *N Engl J Med* 37:51–55, 1982.

84. Sloan RW: How to minimize side effects of psychoactive drugs. *Geriatrics* 306:1081–1088, 1982.

85. Everitt DE, Avorn J: Drug prescribing for the elderly. *Arch Intern Med* 95:711–722, 1986.

86. Ouslander JF: Drug therapy in the elderly. *Ann Intern Med* 95:711–722, 1981.

87. Berardi L: Geriatric medicine. *Med Clin N Am* 67:315–332, 1983.

88. Working Party on Medication in the Elderly: Medication for the elderly. *J Roy Coll Phys* (London) 18:7–17, 1984.

Chapter 4

Health Information Management Services for the Elderly

Wanda G. McKnight, A.R.T., Mary G. Wallace, R.R.A.

As discussed throughout this book, elderly patients have medical and surgical needs that are unique to them because of their age and the aging process. This chapter will address the ways in which the management of medical information can best assist the caregivers in their efforts to respond to the needs of the elderly, particularly those with surgical problems.

Most of the popular, sophisticated medical information systems are designed for acute care needs or for large ambulatory care settings. Medical information management in the long-term care setting is much more cumbersome and much harder to standardize. It is easier to manage when automated systems are used for the information about the extended periods of care, but many long-term care facilities cannot afford the cost of a computer system for medical or clinical information management. The peculiar problem of information management in long-term care settings is outside the scope of this chapter and will only be discussed as it relates to acute care situations.

IMPORTANT ASPECTS OF MEDICAL INFORMATION DOCUMENTATION FOR THE ELDERLY

The importance of accurate medical record documentation is well established (1, 2). The basic medical record documentation practices adhered to routinely should be expanded slightly to provide a comprehensive view of the elderly patient's health status. The Canadian Task Force on the Periodic Health Examination has suggested inclusion of the following items in the medical assessment of an elderly individual (3).

Although the following documentation guide appears to be a bit elementary, a review of the records of many elderly patients will prove that even these simple guidelines are not always followed.

History and Physical Documentation

A comprehensive assessment of an elderly person should include:

Updated Socioeconomic History:
1. Changes in occupation/financial resources;
2. Health of the spouse;
3. How groceries are obtained;
4. Type of housing and location of bedroom and bathroom.

Health Habits:
1. Use of seat belts;
2. Diet;
3. Exercise;
4. Use of alcohol and tobacco;
5. Careful history of prescription and nonprescription drug use; note particularly if the patient is taking any long- acting benzodiazepines commonly prescribed for sleep or anxiety;
6. Immunization record: tetanus (every 10 years) (4), influenza (yearly) (5);
7. Papanicolaou smear for cervical cancer detection (every 5 years after age 35) (6).

Review of Body Systems: Changes in
1. Vision;
2. Hearing;
3. Urinary frequency;
4. Ability to perform activities of daily living;
5. Occurrence of incontinence, constipation, falls, and accidents.

50

Physical Examination
1. Weight should be noted.
2. Blood pressure should be checked with patient lying and standing; careful observation of the patient's transfers from the chair and to the examining table should be part of every examination.
3. Skin should be checked for neoplasm, the incidence of which increases with aging.
4. Gross tests of visual acuity, visual fields, and auditory acuity are adequate in the absence of symptoms.
5. Oral cavity—Note presence or absence of oral cancer, dental caries, periodontal disease.
6. Cardiovascular—Note signs of early congestive heart failure, as well as the harsh systolic murmur of calcific aortic stenosis.
7. Extremities—Careful examination of feet may reveal reversible causes of disability; check for peripheral neuropathy.
8. Assessment of depressive symptomatology and cognitive ability is necessary.

Preoperative Assessment

Accurate history and physical examination must not be just limited to the patient, but should include consideration of the family and the patient's support team as well. Combining the information and details from all of these sources can sometimes supply data that will be life saving. The preoperative physical examination must be perceptive. It must be done in such a way as to allow the physician to predict and envision potential operative and postoperative complications. The clinician must take into consideration any findings of the physiologic changes of aging, the known tendency for different illnesses to present with the same or similar symptoms, and the inability of many elderly patients to give a reliable history. The clinical aspects of preoperative assessment are discussed in detail in Chapter 3.

It is imperative that the medical records from all of the elderly patient's previous hospitalizations be reviewed to obtain as accurate information about past conditions and operative procedures as possible. If the patient has been treated at another facility, photocopies of those medical records should be obtained; with information to include any of the following that may be available: discharge summaries, operative records, pathology reports, and daily/weekly weight and vital signs, eating habits, activities, and medications if patient is transferred from a long-term care facility.

In addition to the usual preoperative assessment that includes a complete medical history, present and future surgical care may be enhanced by including the following special items in the elderly patient's medical record.

Dietary History and Current Nutritional Status (7):
1. Special dietary restrictions;
2. History of weight loss;
3. Record of daily weights;
4. Comparative arm muscle circumference and triceps skin fold measurements (8).

Pharmacological Assessment:
The use of over-the-counter drugs should be evaluated, especially the use of tricyclic antidepressants that can interact with certain anesthetics, such as halothane and pancuronium bromide.

Assessment of Organ Systems
A. *Cardiovascular:* Presence/Absence of:
   1. Congestive heart failure;
   2. Arrhythmias;
   3. Significant valvular disease;
   4. Hyper- and hypotension.
B. *Respiratory System:*
   1. Chronic bronchitis;
   2. Potential for pulmonary embolism (examination of deep leg veins).
C. *Gastrointestinal Disorders:*
   1. Esophageal motility;
   2. Gastrointestinal blood loss;
   3. Jaundice.
D. *Genitourinary Assessment:*
   1. Infection of genitourinary tract;
   2. Presence/absence of obstructive uropathy;
   3. Dysuria, incontinence.
E. *Neurologic Assessment*
F. *Dental Evaluation:*
   1. Limitations of the temporomandibular joint;
   2. Presence of mouth pathology for anesthesia purposes.

PREVENTION-ORIENTED MEDICAL RECORD

Many family practitioners have endorsed the concept of preventive medicine, and its value is theoretically enhanced many times in the care of the elderly. Prevention-oriented medical records consist of three main components: immunizations, periodic health maintenance, and patient education (9). These records may be of interest to the surgeon who is caring for an elderly patient.

A problem list form can be used to maintain allergy, medication, and immunization histories. It is a good idea for the patient to have a copy of at least his or her immunization record. Accurate maintenance of this form is extremely important in the elderly because of their less-than-optimal response to infections and disease.

A record of family history and a personal history are also important aspects of a preventive medical record. Together with laboratory and x-ray findings, they complete the periodic health maintenance component of the record. These items are often documented in the form of flow charts, rather than in narrative summaries in the family practice office.

Finally the chart should contain a checklist reminder to the physician of patient education items. In some settings, the use of a separate patient teaching record may be a useful tool. Such a record can be divided into special sections for diet, medication, follow-up instructions, and special instructions. This type of form is generally used by nursing departments, but it just as easily could be used as a multidisciplinary form. Especially in the older patient, repeated, careful instructions are necessary if the patient's rehabilitation and recovery are to be smooth and if complications are to be prevented.

LEGAL ASPECTS OF MEDICAL RECORDS

Informed Consent

As with so many other issues mentioned in this book, the importance of obtaining a meaningful informed consent is amplified in the care of the elderly patient. Because there are laws that give the individual the right to determine what should be and what should not be done to his or her body, it is reasonable to expect that having an operation will be an intelligent decision made with the knowledge and understanding of what will need to be done and under what circumstances. This understanding must include comprehension of the risks, the possible good and bad outcomes, and the alternative treatment and its risks (10). Providing this information should be the responsibility of the physician. The hospital may also be accountable in situations where procedures are being done that are flagrant extensions beyond the informed consent.

The courts, in fact, require and have ruled that both physicians and hospitals have a duty to the patient for complete description of the therapy including risks (disclosure). Failure to inform the patient of the risks of proposed treatment and of any reasonable alternatives and options would be considered malpractice. For their legal protection, physicians should always document somewhere in the medical record, preferably in the progress notes, that they have discussed the procedure and the risks with the patient prior to the operation or prior to any significant procedure (11). There are two guiding factors that are useful to remember when all parties are deciding how far to proceed with disclosure and to what extent there is a duty to inform when the need for medical treatment is obvious. As a rule, the fullest disclosure of the facts and the risks involved that is possible and within reason should always be given. Only in an emergency, in urgent situations in which the time for such disclosure would jeopardize the patient's health or life, or when the patient waives the right to disclosure is complete disclosure not required (10).

If a patient shows any unwillingness to undergo a procedure and a hospital employee knowingly proceeds to carry out the procedure, the hospital and its employee would be held liable. If, on the other hand, a patient *willingly* undergoes a surgical procedure, the hospital would have no obligation to determine whether or not an informed consent was given by the patient to the physician. It is strongly recommended, however, that the hospital do whatever is necessary to be assured that proper consents have been obtained (10).

It is unlikely that a hospital would be held liable for failing to obtain an informed consent under an emergency situation. This would also be true for an unanticipated treatment while a patient is anesthetized and being cared for under the direction of a physician or several physicians.

If a patient does not understand the language of the hospital personnel and the physician, an interpreter must inform the patient in his or her own language and document the consent form in the same language as is best understood by the patient and also in English (11).

Oral Consent

There is no legal requirement that a consent for surgical procedures must be in writing and signed by the patient. Consent may be established by proof of a conversation between physician and patient. Or, it may be shown by the obvious fact that the patient submitted without objection to the treatment that he or she was told would be performed. There are inherent difficulties, however, in relying totally upon a verbal understanding (10). Two examples of these difficulties are the lack of documentation of the consent and the reliance upon the memory and integrity of the parties involved.

Consent by Telephone

The use of the telephone to obtain consent for a surgical procedure will always have certain disadvantages if it becomes necessary to prove the identity of the person with whom the conversation took place. The conversation should be recorded, if possible. Having another person listen to a telephone conversation is of doubtful value if neither the hospital employee nor the so-called witness can identify the voice (10).

In case of an emergency when delay in treatment may be hazardous to the life of the patient, telephone consent would be only a slight risk because the circumstances may then be such as to make consent superfluous. Whenever possible, a written confirmation of consent by telephone should be obtained and the circumstances of the telephone consent recorded in the patient's chart. Some hospitals use a recording device that is attached to the telephone for documenting such conversations. The voice identity problem is usually resolved by the recording.

Consent by Telegram

Telegrams granting permission for treatment are more reliable than telephone calls, because there is some written record to support the authority to proceed with the proposed therapy. However, if it becomes necessary to prove the identity of the telegram sender, some problems may arise. Although there is some calculated risk in depending on the telegram's validity, this method of obtaining authorization for treatment may be a necessary expediency when patients come from long distances and are unaccompanied by relatives or friends. The use of this standard medium of communication may be regarded as the application of such "reasonable care" and "good faith" as to constitute a legal defense against the possibility of a future lawsuit (10, 11).

The telegram should become part of the patient's record, as should any other consent from the patient or his or her representatives. Whenever possible, an effort should be made to confirm the consent subsequently in writing and on the usual form.

Who Must Consent

There are laws that allow us to assume that a patient is competent if there is no evidence to the contrary. If a patient is transferred from a long-term care facility to an acute care hospital for surgical treatment, he or she should have been evaluated for competency by the referring physician utilizing an appropriate questionnaire. The physician and acute care hospital should have proper identification of the patient's guardian in the event the patient is not competent. If there is a guardian, he or she is responsible for signing the consent form (10).

If a guardian has not been appointed by the court, the "next-of-kin" would be the most appropriate individual to consent to a surgical procedure. In some instances, it may be difficult to locate the next-of-kin, and telephone and/or telegram consents would again be necessary.

If the guardian and/or next-of-kin cannot be located and the procedure to be performed is elective in nature, the physician should postpone the procedure if a delay in treatment would not increase the risk for the patient. It may be necessary for the patient's condition to be "life threatening'' before the procedure can be performed if appropriate consent for an elective procedure cannot be obtained. Court approval to proceed may be obtained in some cases when all else fails.

Right to Refuse Treatment

The refusal of a patient to submit to treatment may become a problem for the hospital, the physician, and the nurse. The fact that it is medical treatment that is forced upon a patient, rather than physical violence, does not alter the elements of law related to assault and battery. A surgical procedure is a technical battery regardless of its result, unless there is expressed or implied consent or desire by the patient.

The ''right'' to refuse to consent to medical care is a troubling concept. It is an established principle of law, nevertheless, that every human being of adult years and of sound mind has the right to determine what shall be done and what shall not be done with and to his or her own body. The patient may choose whether to be treated or not to be treated and to what extent, no matter how necessary the medical care nor how imminent the danger to life or health if he or she fails to submit to treatment. If the physician relies upon the patient's refusal of treatment and the patient is later ruled to be incompetent at the time of refusal, the physician would be liable for malpractice for failing to advise the family or the appropriate guardian of the necessity of treatment. If the patient is proved to have been competent at the time of refusal and the physician has relied upon the consent of the spouse or other members of the family for authority to treat the patient against his or her will, the physician may still be found to have committed an assault and battery. Most courts have maintained that no one else has the authority to consent for an adult who is in full possession of his or her mental faculties (10).

If the patient, legal guardian, and the next-of-kin refuse treatment, a consent form refusing care should be completed and signed. The physician and the hospital must make every effort to inform the patient why they recommend treatment; however, if patients continue to refuse treatment, they should sign a form stating that they were informed but refused. If patients have refused the treatment and refused to sign the form, a report should be prepared and attached to their medical record outlining the circumstances. This should be written by the physician and witnessed by two other people.

Orders Not to Resuscitate

Do Not Resuscitate (DNR) orders are used in many facilities and have become a common topic of discussion among medicolegal authorities. These orders are written only in situations of unremitting disease when death is imminent. Competent and incompetent (through a guardian) patients have the legal right to decline resuscitative measures in these situations.

Some authors have recommended the establishment of an ad hoc committee within a hospital to consult and advise on cases in which DNR orders are being contemplated (12). This approach requires the involvement of many persons outside the doctor-patient-nurse relationship and the careful and complete documentation of the entire situation in the medical record.

The authors and editors would submit, however, that it is possible to allow a terminally ill patient to die with dignity without the furor and commotion of an ad hoc committee. If the surgeon has established good rapport and clear communication with the patient and family, the decision not to resuscitate the patient can be gradually and intelligently made between the doctor, the patient, and the family. The decision of the parties involved should indeed be recorded in the patient's medical record in the form of a progress note. When the patient then experiences a sudden cessation of heart or lung function and the doctor is called, the doctor and the family know what is to happen and they are prepared for it. This has been evident in many situations of which we have both personal and professional knowledge. The absolute *key* ingredient is the physician's rapport with the patient and family. We do not recommend the routine use of DNR orders for the simple reason that they tend to remove the physician prematurely from any participation in the last moments of his or her patient's life.

Withdrawing Treatment

Another situation of great interest to medicolegal professionals is the case of withdrawing life-

LIVING WILL

I,_____, willfully and voluntarily make known my desire that my dying shall not be artificially prolonged under the circumstance set forth below, and do hereby declare:

If at any time I should have a terminal condition and my attending physician has determined that there can be no recovery from such condition and my death is imminent, where the application of life-prolonging procedures would serve only to artificially prolong the dying process, I direct that such procedures be withheld or withdrawn, and that I be permitted to die naturally with only the administration of medications or the performance of any medical procedure deemed necessary to provide me with comfortable care or to alleviate pain.

In the absence of my ability to give directions regarding the use of such life-prolonging procedures, it is my intention that this declaration shall be honored by my family and physician as the final expression of my legal right to refuse medical or surgical treatment and accept the consequences of such refusal.

I understand the full import of this declaration, and I am emotionally and mentally competent to make this declaration. In acknowledgement whereof, I do hereinafter affix my signature on this _____ day of _____, 19____.

_____
Declarant

We, the subscribing witnesses hereto, are personally acquainted with and subscribe our names hereto at the request of the declarant, an adult, whom we believe to be of sound mind, fully aware of the action taken herein and its possible consequence.

We the undersigned witnesses further declare that we are not related to the declarant by blood or marriage; that we are not entitled to any portion of the estate of the declarant upon his decease under any will or codicil thereto presently existing or by operation of law then existing; that we are not the attending physician, an employee of the attending physician or a health facility in which the declarant is a patient; and that we are not a person who, at the present time, has a claim against any portion of the estate of the declarant upon his death.

_____
Witness

_____
Witness

Subscribed, sworn to and acknowledged before me by _____, the declarant, and subscribed and sworn to before me by _____ and _____, witnesses, this _____ day of _____, 19____.

_____
Notary Public

Figure 4.1. A sample living will.

support systems as a form of treatment. When this is the wish of a patient or family, informed consent is necessary, and proper documentation of such consent is critical. The record should also reflect that the patients, their families, or their legal representatives have reached their decisions voluntarily and with a full understanding of the consequences (13).

Living Wills

At this time, at least 11 states have some form of legislation recognizing ''living wills'' or patient directives. These states now include Alabama, Arkansas, California, Idaho, Kansas, Nevada, New Mexico, North Carolina, Oregon, Texas, and Washington.

The living will is a legal document that allows persons, while they are competent, to inform their family and physician of their preferred kind of terminal care. The legal premise for this document is the recognition that adults have a fundamental right to control decisions relating to their personal medical care, including withholding or withdrawing life-support systems. A sample living will is shown in Figure 4.1.

The statutes pertaining to living wills vary, of course, from state to state. Generally speaking, however, the will/directive when properly drawn must be signed by the patient in the presence of two witnesses who are neither relatives nor entitled to any portion of the patient's estate. It may not be witnessed by the attending physician or any personnel of the health care facility in which the person is a patient. In several states, there is a required 2-week waiting period before the will can be executed. Should the patient become incompetent within those 2 weeks, the will is not considered valid (10).

The scope of this issue cannot be covered within this chapter, but physicians should become familiar with the laws pertaining to living wills, especially those within the state of their practice. The wills or directives should always, however, become a permanent part of the patient's medical record. Failure to follow the direction of a properly written living will has been ruled to constitute unprofessional conduct.

INFORMATION NEEDS FOR POSTDISCHARGE CARE

A large percentage of elderly surgical patients will require some degree of medical care after they are discharged from the hospital, even if it is needed only for a short time. In 1985, the American Medical Record Association (AMRA) began a Home Care Project that was funded by the W.K. Kellogg Foundation. The end result of this study was a model for home care record forms and guidelines. The package is compatible with Health Care Financing Administration guidelines. It is hoped that the project will ultimately result in the standardization of health care records for home health care agencies. Until such time, the surgeon, in the interest of the patient, must be cognizant of the fact that basic accepted medical record practices pertaining to release of information, use of a problem list, care plans, and documentation standards are not necessarily the norm among home care agencies. The Medicare-approved agencies, however, tend to be further developed in their record keeping and quality assurance practices. The surgeon, then, should take care to ensure that the home care nurses and other caregivers understand the needs of each individual patient and the goals of treatment. In the interest of the patient, the surgeon should remain aware of the patient's home care status.

The extra effort to attend to these details on the surgeon's part may seem unnecessary and a potential waste of time, but it may be very important for the patient's recovery. According to the Home Care Project Survey conducted by AMRA, only one-fourth of the home care agencies studied performed quality assurance studies based on objective criteria (14). Annual home health care program evaluations and clinical

record reviews are required by Medicare, and they are performed by most facilities. In order to know of his or her patient's progress, the surgeon may need to see the patient more often postoperatively when home care is being used because, even in institutionally based agencies, 42% of the agencies provide no home care information to the in-patient record.

Transfer information for patients needing institutionalized skilled care ideally should include the transfer of a current history and physical examination, a discharge summary detailing the diagnosis, summary of the course of treatment, medications and dosages, diet and activity restrictions, significant lab and x-ray findings, the current treatment plan, and the expectations for the patient's progress (15). A referral or transfer form is sometimes required, but the space available on the form may not be sufficient for all of the information if detailed care will be needed.

NEW HEALTH RECORD TECHNOLOGIES

The American Medical Record Association has designed a Health Record Core Data Set that outlines the necessary components of an institution's database (16). The items have been carefully defined and, pertinent to our purpose in this chapter, can enhance sharing of information among health care facilities by providing what is known as the longitudinal record. The elderly patient is more likely than the younger patient to need various levels of care and to be transferred from one facility to the other. Moreover, careful documentation of follow-up care is extremely important in the elderly patient in whom a postoperative complication might be poorly tolerated.

New technologies affecting the medical record field could have a very positive impact on the medical and surgical care of the elderly. Personal Health Cards (also called Memory or Smart Cards) have been developed that can be carried in a purse or wallet. Through an embossing process, a magnetic strip or a microprocessor chip is embedded that details a medical history, diagnosis, procedures, lab test results, medications, and other important medical information. The card is easily updated, is relatively reliable, and, by its nature, is secure confidentially. The Personal Health Card now is being evaluated in several settings. If it proves successful, it could greatly enhance the elderly patient's health care. Ideally elderly persons who carry a personal health card have on their person all of the medical information of their past, including ambulatory care events, acute and long-term care events, and other information necessary to enable a new caregiver to care safely and effectively for them even if they are unconscious, in an unfamiliar setting, or unaware of their medical history. An additional benefit of this system is the avoidance of serious medical errors that can result from the transfer of information among facilities (17, 18).

Although these cards are the result of new technology, the concept of a portable, personal health record has been a subject of interest for some time. Sherman and Libow have evaluated a portable medical record system in elderly patients (19). Chronically ill, ambulatory, mentally clear patients in the study wore a bracelet and carried a wallet card during their routine physician office visits. On the bracelet, one major diagnosis that could be important in an emergency situation was imprinted, as was the phrase, "See wallet card for vital facts." On the wallet card was the following information: patient's name and address, recent discharge date, all surgical and medical problems, all current medications, all allergies, and the name and telephone number of the next of kin. The patients were asked to show these items to their physician at the time of the initial visit and to continue to wear and carry them throughout the study period. The patients were very accepting of the system; twenty of 23 participated until the end of the study. The physicians were later contacted to ascertain their opinions of the system. Ninety-one percent of the physicians thought the system was useful for the elderly population and that it would be especially so for the mentally debilitated patient. However, in only 50% of the patients' visits was the bracelet noticed and in only 30% was the wallet card seen. Further study of these innovative medical information systems and their usefulness will be important for the future health care of the elderly.

PROSPECTIVE PAYMENT SYSTEM

The evolution of the prospective payment system for Medicare providers has had a great impact on the management of medical information for the elderly patient. The current practice involves the assignment of diagnosis-related groups (DRGs) for patient billing. The DRG is assigned based upon the principal diagnosis and procedure, and the reimbursement for hospital services is determined by it. The stated diagnoses and procedures that appear in a patient's record have therefore assumed a new importance for the financial aspect of the patient's care. Although the DRG system of determining reimbursement will certainly be modified in coming years as new systems develop, most health industry leaders believe that prospective payment is here to stay.

Assigning a Principal Diagnosis

The regulation for Public Law 98–21 specifies that "all hospitals subject to the prospective payment system will be paid, for inpatient services provided, a specific amount for each discharge based on the case's classification into one of the 468 diagnosis-related groups (DRGs). Every hospital discharge case will fit into a DRG category and no case will apply to more than one category," (20).

This assignment is based on:
1. Principal diagnosis;
2. Secondary diagnoses (if any);
3. Procedures performed;
4. Age, sex, and discharge status.

As mentioned earlier, the assignment of a case to a particular DRG determines the amount that will be paid to the hospital for the treatment and care of a patient. It is important that this assignment be done honestly, systematically, and uniformly. The Health Systems (HSI) Grouper is the automated classification system endorsed by HCFA that assigns discharge diagnoses to their proper DRGs using the essential information specified above.

Medicare Transmittal Number 387, effective May 15, 1984, states: "The principal diagnosis is the condition, established after study, to be chiefly responsible for admission of the patient." The words *after study* in this definition are very significant and cannot be ignored when selecting the principal diagnosis. Patients are frequently admitted to hospitals with a group of symptoms that require further study before a definitive diagnosis can be identified. For example, a patient may have the following admitting diagnosis and diagnosis after study.

Admitting Diagnosis
Severe abdominal pain;
Unexplained convulsions;
Ascites;
Jaundice.
Diagnosis after Study
Diverticulitis with perforation;
Metastatic carcinoma of brain;
Cirrhosis of liver;
Obstruction of common duct.

Other diagnoses that relate to the current hospitalization should be documented on the medical record. "Other diagnoses" cover two types of conditions:

1. Those co-existing at admission—diabetes, epilepsy, renal failure;
2. Those that develop subsequently—wound disruption, urinary tract infection, myocardial infarction.

These diagnoses, which are referred to as co-morbid conditions and complications, are significant in determining the DRG. A substantial complication or comorbidity is defined as: "a condition that because of its presence with a specific principal diagnosis could cause an increase in length of stay by at least 75 percent of the patients," (20).

Medical record documentation should indicate that the patient received medication, other therapy, or diagnostic evaluation for each co-morbidity or complication listed (20).

The Effect of Prospective Payment on Surgical Care

The above-mentioned guidelines have had a major impact on the financial aspects of surgical care, and they should be of concern to all surgeons. These guidelines also have the potential to affect seriously and negatively surgical care for all Medicare recipients. The medical profession should and must not allow this negative effect to become a reality. Our older citizens, and indeed all Americans, have grown to expect that medical care would not be denied to anyone in this country because of financial status. Granted, there is growing concern about the rising cost of health care, but few among us would be willing to allow a family member or friend to be denied needed medical care because of cost.

The situation facing the health care industry in general and the medical profession in particular is therefore quite difficult. We must work within the rules and regulations of third party payers but only to the degree that they do not negatively affect patient care. The medical profession can best respond to this dilemma by taking the time to question each determination that seems inappropriate or unfair.

The importance of the medical record documentation and its reflection of the appropriate principal diagnosis and procedure cannot be overstated. In fact, the Medicare program has gone so far as to require that physicians sign an attestation statement and a fraud and abuse statement that reads:

I certify that the identification of the principal and secondary diagnoses and the procedures performed is accurate and complete to the best of my knowlege. Notice: Intentional misrepresentation, concealment, or falsification of the information may, in the case of a Medicare beneficiary, be punishable by imprisonment, fine, or civil penalty.

It is unfortunate that the publicly supported Medicare program has been allowed to grow in power and importance to the point that its proprietors have been allowed to alienate the physicians upon whom the elderly depend.

All third party payers, including Medicare, now have medical directors who are ultimately responsible for determining the "approval" or "disapproval" of claims for health care. In the authors' experience, direct communication between the attending physician and the medical director has resulted more often than not in the reversal of a negative determination. This conversation, usually by telephone, is generally unpleasant because it has the potential of placing the attending physician in the position of defending his or her actions to an unknown and unsolicited overseer. From a larger perspective, however, this can be an opportunity for the physician to make the statement that insurance companies, federal or private, *cannot* engage in the practice of medicine. The caring physician will take the time to make this effort on behalf of the patient and will, in a broader sense, contribute to the survival of the health care industry as we have come to know it.

REFERENCES

1. Greenlaw J: Documentation of patient care: an often underestimated responsibility. *Law Med Health Care* 10:172–174, 1982.
2. Broccolo BM: The importance of proper medical record entries. *Topics Health Care Management* 2:67–75, 1981.
3. Carnes M: Preventive health care for the elderly. *Wisconsin Med J* 82:15–18, 1983.
4. Canadian Task Force on the Periodic Health Examination. *Can Med Assoc J* 121:1193–1254, 1979.
5. Recommendation of the immunization practices advisory committee, influenza vaccines, 1982–1983. *Morbidity and Mortality Weekly Report:* 31:26, 1982.
6. Lowther CP, MacLeod RMD, Williamson J: Evaluation of early diagnostic services for the elderly. *Br Med J* 3:275–277, 1970.
7. Organ CH, Finn MP: The importance of nutritional support for the geriatric surgical patient. *Geriatrics* 32:77–84, 1977.
8. Martorell R, Yarbrough C, Lechtig A: Upper arm anthropometric indicators of nutritional status. *Am J Clin Nutr* 29:46–53, 1976.
9. Sloane P: A prevention oriented medical record. *J Fam Pract* 9:89–96, 1979.
10. Rozovsky FA: *Consent to Treatment.* Boston, Little, Brown, and Co, 1984.
11. Hayt E: *Medical-Legal Aspects of Hospital Records*, ed 2. Berwyn IL, Physician's Record Company, 1977.
12. Rabkin MT, Gillerman G, Rice NR: Orders not to resuscitate. *N Engl J Med* 295:364–366, 1976.
13. Kaufer DS, Steinberg ER, Toney SD: Revising medical record forms: an empirical model and test. *JAMRA* 55:34–40, 1984.
14. Miller S: Home care project survey data. *JAMRA* 56:21–24, 1985.
15. Huffman E: *Medical Record Management*, ed 8. Berwyn, IL, Physician's Record Company, 1985.
16. Schraffenberger LA: Health record core data set. *JAMRA* 57:47–50, 1986.
17. Miller EB, Elliott D: Errors and omissions in diagnostic records on admission of patients to a nursing home. *J Am Geriatr Soc* 24:108–116, 1976.
18. Libow LS: Another type of iatrogenic problem. *Geriatrics* 33:92–99, 1978.
19. Sherman FT, Libow LS: A portable medical record system for the elderly. *JAMA* 242:57–59, 1979.
20. Finnegan R: *Coding for Prospective Payment.* Chicago, American Medical Record Association, 1984.

Chapter 5

Anesthetic Considerations in the Aged Patient

Bradley E. Smith, M.D., W. Jerry Merrell, M.D.

In 1900 only 4% of Americans were 65 years of age or older, but in 1987 about 12% of the population are over the age of 65, and less than 1% are age 85 and over. The median age of Americans in 1986 was 31.5 years, but projections indicate a median age of 36 by the year 2000 and 39 by 2010. Projections indicate that, by 2036, 22% of the population will be over the age of 65 and approximately 4% will be over the age of 85 (1). Various observers have estimated that in the range of 50% of people aged 50 years and older will require a surgical procedure at least once during the balance of their life.

It has been estimated that currently approximately 25% of all surgical procedures in the United States involve patients over the age of 65. These aging patients formerly presented a foreboding surgical prognosis. As recently as 1960, overall perioperative and postoperative surgical mortality was reported to be 19.3% in elderly patients, dropping to 13.3% in 1972 and 6.2% in 1979 (2). Yet mortality is still very high in the elderly group (3). Recent data from Great Britain showed that 50% of all intraoperative deaths occurred in elderly patients, although the elderly group represented only 5% of the surgical caseload (4).

A recent study reported that death within 7 days of receiving a general anesthetic and having a surgical procedure occurred in 1% of postsurgical patients between the ages of 21 and 50, in 4.4% between the ages of 61 and 70, 6.8% in patients 71–80, and in 8.2% of patients over the age of 80 (5).

Another report states that patients from 65 to 70 years of age have an overall perioperative surgical complication rate of 60%, and those surgical patients greater than 75 years in age have a 73% chance of some perisurgical complication. The chance of a life threatening complication developing is approximately 12% in the age group 65–74 and 33% in the surgical patient above 75 years (6).

This increased mortality rate from the anesthetic-surgical experience is due to a combination of three major factors. Of course, the type of operation required in progressing age is more frequently likely due to a potentially fatal condition. In particular, the incidence of advanced cancer, major vascular illness, and some manifestation of the end stage of chronic and acute surgical illness all take their toll. This is such an obvious factor that it will not be explored in this chapter. On the other hand, two other factors that have a direct bearing on the conduct of anesthesia are extremely important in the etiology of the high-risk and difficult management of anesthesia in the elderly. First, the physiologic changes common to progressing age in many cases lead to profound alterations in the pharmacology of the anesthetic agents. Second, there is an increasing incidence with advancing age of chronic pathology that also directly affects the response of the body to the stresses of anesthesia. In one study the average geriatric patient presented to the hospital for a surgical procedure with a total of six diseases present (7). In the same report, the incidence of mortality after the procedure appeared to be directly related to pre-existing conditions, such as cardiac and mental diseases (7). The perioperative mortality rate increases from approximately 15% in the fourth decade and 22% in the fifth decade to over 30% in the sixth and seventh decades. It is axiomatic that careful examination of the patient to discover pre-existing pathologic conditions and to evalu-

60

ate to what extent the aging process in the individual patient coincides with the patient's chronologic age will allow the anesthesiologist and the surgeon to prepare for, circumvent, and minimize many of the dreaded complications of general anesthesia and surgical therapy in the elderly patient.

PHYSIOLOGIC CHANGES OF AGING

Metabolic Rate

There is roughly a 1% decrease in basal metabolic rate each year after age 30 (8).

Central Nervous System

Brain function is commonly held to deteriorate progressively with age, but much evidence indicates this is a selective decline and that most changes commonly associated with "aging" have to do with pathologic changes, such as infarctions due to emboli, blood extravasation, or occlusions of the end branches of cerebral blood flow by arteriosclerotic vascular disease leading to chronic insufficient vascularity (9). Cerebral pressure is decreased in the elderly, as is brain oxygen perfusion consumption (10). Some studies imply a decrease in success of autoregulation of cerebral blood flow that is progressive with age (11). In the elderly patient this may be accentuated by accommodation to chronically elevated arterial pressures in chronic hypertensive patients, possibly resulting in a greater tendency toward perfusion defects during periods of hypotension that may occur with anesthesia (12).

Most inhalation and intravenous anesthetics, sedatives, and narcotics appear to share a reduced requirement (lowered threshold of initial activity) in the aged. This may result from reduction in the numbers of surviving neuronal cells, reduction in the insulating qualities of the neurons, relative decreases in some neurotransmitter substances, or a change in the quantity or sensitivity of various receptors, particularly alpha- and beta- adrenergic receptors in both brain and cardiovascular sites, both end receptors, and in the substantia gelatinosa (13–15).

There is some evidence that the blood-brain barrier is less efficient in the elderly. A classic example is the greater ease of onset of atropine and scopolamine "psychosis" in elderly patients than in younger ones, possibly due to achievement of higher active drug levels in the brain substance in the elderly.

The receptor site of activity of diazepam, GABA (gamma amino butyric acid) receptor is more sensitive in the elderly. Therefore, the older patient may be more sensitive to diazepam (16).

Protective autonomic reflexes of the trachea, pharynx, larynx, and airway are well known to be progressively less effective as age advances (17), thus leading to far more frequent aspiration of vomitus, secretions, or foreign substances and decreased vigor in clearing upper airways by coughing (18).

Cardiovascular System

Cardiac index decreases about 1% per year over age 30. However, resting stroke volume ordinarily is little changed with aging, although cardiovascular response to stress may be reduced. Unlike young patients, who typically increase the ejection and stroke volume under cardiovascular stress, the elderly patients are unable to respond in that way.

Cardiac output declines approximately 1% per year, but a relatively high proportion of the output is routed to the brain. This may lead to some of the findings of increased sensitivity of elderly patients to inhalation anesthetics.

Heart rate in the elderly is frequently reduced. In fact, the tachycardic response to atropine and similar drugs is much attenuated in the elderly. The expected responses to sudden changes in posture or intrathoracic pressure often are not seen at all in the elderly due to the marked decrease in baroreceptor and other homeostatic reflex responses.

Respiratory Function

Structural changes, such as kyphosis, frequently result in restrictive decreases in vital capacity and lung volume. There is a progressive decrease in maximum breathing capacity, total lung capacity, and vital capacity consistent with the progressive loss of elasticity of cartilaginous structures and decrease in muscularity of the diaphragm and intercostal muscles (19). In addition, respiratory rate, tidal volume, minute volume, and maximum diffusing capacity of the lung for oxygen are all decreased progressively with age (20, 21).

Anatomic dead space, residual volume, functional residual capacity, and total lung capacity increase progressively with age, often mimicking or actually involving emphysema (22). Lung "closing volume" increases progressively with age due to the functional deterioration of the terminal elements of the lung's architecture (19). Thus, progressively greater portions of tidal ventilation in the elderly routinely take place at lung volumes below the closing volume, leading to air trapping, ventilation-perfusion mismatch, and often a gradual decline of the resting arterial oxygen values.

There may be less efficient compensation for increased pulmonary shunting in the elderly due to a less efficient hypoxic pulmonary vasoconstrictor reflex mechanism (23).

The aged are less able to respond successfully to hypercarbia and hypoxia (24, 25). In one study displacement of 15 mm to the right elicited little ventilatory response (26). Central control of respiration is even further impaired than in younger patients by the use of narcotics or other respiratory-depressant agents, such as inhalation anesthetics (26).

Obviously, postoperative hypoventilation and inability to "clear" secretions are more likely in the elderly because of the above changes.

Hepatic Function

Most laboratory liver function values of the elderly remain within the same normal limits as for younger patients. Specifically, coagulation-related values, SGOT, SGPT, and alkaline phosphatase are within normal ranges (27).

Liver blood flow at age 65 is reduced to about 40% less than the liver blood flow in the same patient at age 30. (Part of this reduction is due to the relative decrease in cardiac output.) In addition, the mass of the liver is decreased by about 20% in old age. Liver microsomal enzymes, important in oxidizing drugs, are less active in older patients. The phenomena of enzyme induction and glucuronidation are also impaired in older patients. However, acetylation and alcohol dehydrogenase enzymes are preserved at near normal activity in the elderly liver.

The conversion by the liver of lipid-soluble drugs to water-soluble metabolites by conjugation is therefore hindered. This may lead to an increased duration of action for many lipid-soluble drugs, including many anesthetics and sedatives (28, 29).

Renal Function

Renal blood flow and glomerular filtration rate declines steadily past the age of 30, thus resulting in a hindrance to excretion of drugs and metabolic breakdown products. Glomerular filtration rate averages 120 ml/min/1.73m^2 at age 20, but only 60 ml at age 90. Renal plasma flow is decreased by about 50% at age 65 compared to age 30. Geriatric patients exhibit the same serum creatinine level as their younger counterparts because, even though there is reduced renal excretion of creatinine, there is also relatively less skeletal muscle mass producing creatinine, resulting in a net normal serum level (28). However, the reduced renal clearance in elderly patients affects many drugs related to anesthesia. For example, vecuronium, a non-depolarizing muscle relaxant, must be infused at a lower rate (30).

Although proximal tubular function may remain essentially unchanged, concentrating ability and other distal tubular functions are progressively impaired, particularly resulting in decreased ability to excrete acid. Therefore, a greater urinary volume is necessary when an acid solute load is expected. Urinary volume in these circumstances should be maintained at 1.0 ml/kg/hr (31).

Body Composition and Compartments

Increased Body Fat in the Elderly

Intracellular water gradually decreases with age, along with a gradual increase of approximately 10% in body fat. Thus elderly patients often store a greater proportion of inhaled or intravenous anesthetics due to the proportionate increase of the fat reservoir to which these highly lipid-soluble substances are attached. This can lead both to prolonged somnolence in some cases and to the production of an increased percentage of secondary metabolic breakdown products, which are at times toxic, from these stored agents.

Decreased Serum Protein

During aging a progressive fall in serum albumin levels (32) is seen, but with a relative increase in alpha$_1$-acid glycoprotein proportion of circulating protein.

PHARMACOLOGY OF AGING

Drug Interactions

Thirty percent of all prescriptions written in this country are said to be utilized by the elderly (33). Furthermore, perhaps 70% of the elderly population frequently use additional over-the-counter medications compared with only about 10% of the adult population under age 65 (34). Therefore, it may be estimated that elderly patients present at least a three-fold increased possibility for the presence of drugs that may be involved in drug actions, in addition to various physiologic predilections toward exacerbating these interactions (4). In Great Britain, a report showed that elderly patients demonstrated an incidence of in-hospital drug reactions of 15.4% versus only 6.3% for younger adult patients (35).

Therefore, a history of the use of corticosteroid, antihypertensive, anticoagulant, beta-blocker, monoamine oxidase inhibitor, tricyclic antidepressant, and antidiabetic drugs should be sought in every geriatric patient before the administration of anesthetic drugs.

The anesthetist must be alert for increased duration of action of non-depolarizing neuromuscular blockade, which can be caused by chronic ingestion of propranolol or the calcium channel blockers, synergism between opioids and tranquilizers, a decreased effect of digitalis in the presence of halogenated anesthetics, and other reasons.

A history of the following drugs should alert the anesthesiologist to possible drug interactions.

1. Digitalis and diuretics—hypo-k-lemia;
2. Quinidine—prolongation of the action of succinylcholine;
3. Antibiotics—prolongation of the action of non-depolarizing muscle relaxants, particularly prominent with kanamycin, gentamycin, neomycin, streptomycin, and other similar drugs;
4. Monoamine oxidase inhibitors—should be discontinued 10–14 days before anesthesia;
5. Echothiophate eyedrops—potentiation of succinylcholine and ester- type local anesthetic drugs by inhibition of circulating pseudocholinesterase;
6. Tricyclic antidepressants—interference with myocardial conduction; should be discontinued 48–72 hours before anesthesia;
7. Alcohol—potential hepatic disease, potential delerium tremens, also potential resistance to thiobarbiturates during anesthesia induction.

In the elderly, drug actions may be altered by two major categories of effects. Alteration in drug receptors, either because of decreased sensitivity or decreased population, may reduce drug sensitivity in the elderly. Such changes are referred to as pharmacodynamic effects. Alternately, changes in drug absorption, distribution, metabolism, and elimination are also frequent in elderly patients. These are called pharmacokinetic effects (36). Age-related pharmacokinetic changes appear to be more frequent in altering drug response in the elderly than are pharmacodynamic changes. Clinicians caring for these patients should therefore be aware of the therapeutic implications of age-related pharmacokinetic and pharmacodynamic changes in drug effects.

Absorption

Changes in drug absorption are most significant in the case of medications administered orally. Elderly patients usually have an increased gastric pH due to decreased gastric secretion. Gastric emptying is also delayed in these individuals. Consequently, absorption of organic acids (for example, aspirin) may be impaired. However, the extent of the effects of these changes in the gastrointestinal system on drug absorption has not been totally outlined.

Intestinal motility and splanchnic blood flow have also been found to decrease with age. These effects are probably exaggerated in most patients who are receiving anticholinergic or narcotic drugs. Because of these changes in gastrointestinal physiology, it is prudent to allow sufficient time for absorption of orally administered agents (for example, many premedicants) before their effect is needed during induction or maintenance of anesthesia.

Distribution

Many of the alterations in drug response described in elderly patients are produced by changes in drug distribution (37). Distribution changes are most frequently related either to alterations in body composition or drug-binding characteristics. Drugs can be bound in plasma, to red cells, or to various plasma proteins. In the elderly, there is a larger proportion of metabolically inactive tissue, and in addition, a smaller proportion of body mass is made up of water. Therefore, lipophilic compounds appear to distribute into a larger volume than in younger patients of the same total body weight, whereas hydrophilic (polar) compounds appear to distribute into a smaller effective volume than in younger individuals of a similar weight. This relative change in proportionate distribution between lipid and hydrophilic areas can be termed an "apparent increase of the volume of distribution (Vd)" when lipid-soluble agents are administered to the elderly. This leads to a prolongation of drug elimination half-life of lipid-soluble agents in the elderly.

Diazepam, a lipophilic drug, illustrates the practical significance of this distribution phenomenon. The rate at which the concentration of diazepam disappears from the circulating blood ("clearance") is similar in elderly patients and in younger patients. However, the apparent volume of distribution is increased in the elderly because of the usual relative increase in body fat. The increase in diazepam volume of distribution, in turn, causes a dramatic fourfold increase in elimination half-life from 20 hours at age 20 to approximately 80 hours at age 80. In contrast, oxazepam (Serax) and lorazepam (Ativan) are two commonly used benzodiazepines that are far more hydrophilic than diazepam (Valium). The pharmacologic disposition of these two agents has been shown to be very similar in elderly and younger patients. Recent clinical experience suggests that an even newer benzodiazepine, midazolam (Versed), is appropriate for incremental intravenous use in elderly patients due to its relative hydrophilic qualities and relatively normal clearance rate and half-life (38–40).

In contrast to lipophilic agents, the volume of distribution (Vd) of water-soluble compounds is generally decreased with age. If drug clearance is unchanged, a diminished Vd will lead to a decreased elimination half-life and also higher peak plasma levels. Because pharmacologic response is related to plasma drug concentration, a decrease in Vd could produce exaggerated drug effects, as well as an increased incidence of adverse drug reactions.

Ethanol is a frequently quoted example of this effect in the elderly. Because body water is usually diminished in older patients, volume of distribution of ethyl alcohol (water soluble) is diminished, and consequently blood alcohol levels are frequently higher in older men after ingestion of similar doses of alcohol than in younger men. However, the rate of metabolism and excretion of alcohol (the "clearance") is relatively normal, and alcohol dehydrogenase enzyme has normal activity.

Drug distribution is also affected by age-related changes in protein composition. Albumin concentrations usually decrease progressively with increasing age, but concentrations of alpha$_1$-acid glycoprotein (AAG) and the serum globulins are often increased in the elderly. As the amount of drug bound to protein increases, the amount of free drug in plasma ("free fraction") decreases. The free fraction of highly protein-bound acidic compounds is often increased in the elderly because these substances are often tightly bound to albumin. However, the free fraction of highly protein-bound basic compounds is often lower in the elderly because these compounds usually bind specifically to AAG and not to albumin. AAG levels also increase during chronic illness and malnutrition. Proteinuria and liver dysfunction often further lower serum albumin concentrations.

Drugs that are particularly bound to alpha$_1$-acid glycoprotein include propranolol, local anesthetics, such as lidocaine, and procainamide. Therefore, equal doses may actually result in lower circulating free active portions of these drugs in older patients.

Thiopental (Pentothal), the most commonly used anesthetic induction agent, is highly bound to albumin. Therefore, the dose of thiopental must be severely monitored and limited in elderly patients, because lower albumin levels lead to greater concentrations of the unbound, active thiopental. In addition, the volume of distribution is greatly increased in the elderly, and the elimination half-life is much longer. Loss of lid reflex is often found at 70% of the dose required for the same endpoints in younger patients. These effects are felt to be due to distribution in the elderly patient and not due to impaired metabolism or increased drug sensitivity (41, 42).

Metabolism

Drug distribution is not the only variable that determines pharmacokinetic disposition. Elimination half-life is related to the volume of drug distribution and to systemic blood clearance by the following relationship:

$$T\ 1/2\ =\ Vd\ *0.693/C$$

where T 1/2 = elimination half-life. From the equation, it is apparent that decreasing systemic clearance causes a prolongation in elimination half-life. Drug clearance in turn is determined by drug metabolism and elimination by organs, such as the liver, kidney, and lung. Some compounds are metabolized by plasma cholinesterase. Representative drugs include procaine (Novocaine), tetracaine (Pontocaine), succinylcholine (Anectine), trimetaphan (Arfonad), and the yet to be released ultra-short-acting beta-blockers, such as esmolol. Yet, most drug metabolism is largely a function of the liver.

As a rule the liver transforms drugs into more polar compounds to facilitiate elimination of these compounds by the body. In the process of transformation, drugs can be changed into active or inactive compounds. There are two major determinants of hepatic drug metabolism: liver blood flow and intrinsic enzymatic activity. Hepatic clearance of many drugs decreases with age because of age-related decreases in hepatic blood flow, hepatic mass, and enzymatic activity. Such factors as malnutrition, use of other drugs, and cigarette smoking can also alter drug metabolism by inhibition or induction of hepatic enzyme systems (43).

Alteration of drug excretion by the kidney can also impair drug clearance rates. The decrease of renal blood flow with age results in a decreased clearance of compounds eliminated by the kidney. The elimination of pancuronium bromide (Pavulon) (44) and gallamine (Flaxedil)

may be impaired in the elderly with decreased renal function because of the drugs' dependence upon glomerular filtration and excretion. Administration of the same dose by weight that would ordinarily be administered to a younger patient results in similar pharmacologic effect after the initial dose. However, subsequent dose requirements are decreased, and the duration of action is prolonged. Neuromuscular transmission should be carefully monitored during the use of these agents, and subsequent doses should be reduced according to the observed response in elderly patients.

In addition, decreased renal function in the elderly can lead to accumulation of drug metabolites that may have secondary toxic or depressing effects in the body. The accumulation of active drug metabolites is often clinically important in the case of methyldopa (Aldomet), morphine, triamterine (Diazide), spirinolactone (Aldactazide), levodopa (Larodopa), and acetylated sulfonamides.

PHARMACOLOGY OF INDIVIDUAL DRUGS

Propranolol

Propranolol exhibits decreased first-pass metabolism in the elderly because of decreased liver function. Therefore, blood levels are three to four times higher in 75-year-old patients than in younger patients, when propranolol is taken orally. However, distribution and elimination are almost identical in the elderly at the elevated level. Blood levels achieved by intravenous administration of propranolol during the maintenance of anesthesia are unaltered, although similar blood levels may be more effective due to a decreased population of beta-receptors in the aged.

Lidocaine

Lidocaine behaves similarly to diazepam, reaching lower plasma concentrations because of an apparent increased volume of distribution, but the clearance rate is unchanged. In one study, half-life was 80 minutes in young adults and 139 minutes in elderly patients (45).

Pancuronium

Pancuronium exhibits no changes in absorption, distribution, or metabolism, but its elimination is impaired in the elderly, because a great proportion of the elimination depends upon excretion by the kidney and glomerular filtration rate is progressively decreased in the elderly. Therefore, its half-life is increased by approximately 100% in patients above 75 years of age, and there is an increased duration of action. Studies have shown that neuromuscular endplate receptor sensitivity in patients between the ages of 65 and 75 is equal to that in young patients. However there is some increased sensitivity of the receptors in patients above the age of 75 (46, 47).

Other Non-Depolarizing Muscle Relaxants

Except for gallamine and pancuronium, the non-depolarizing muscle relaxants are not excreted by the kidney. Nonetheless, their activities are markedly altered. Although receptor sensitivity is not altered until after age 75, at which time the sensitivity increases, duration of action is greatly changed. One study reports that half-life of metocurine is 269 minutes in young patients versus 530 minutes in the elderly. Half-life of d-tubocurarine was reported to be 173 minutes in young patients and 268 minutes in elderly patients. The volume of distribution with both metocurine and d-tubocurarine was found to be approximately one-half that in young adults with both agents, thus resulting in much higher plasma concentrations of similar doses of the agents in elderly patients. Probably due to decreased hepatic activity, clearance with metocurine was found to be 0.36 ml/kg/min in the elderly and 1.1 ml/kg/min in young adults, and with d-tubocurarine it was 0.8 ml/kg/min in the elderly and 1.7 ml/kg/min in young adults. Therefore, in elderly patients higher blood levels are achieved by the same dose. Clearance is decreased and the half-life is vastly increased, leading both to more profound muscle relaxation and prolonged duration of activity of similar doses (48).

Etomidate

The dose of etomidate required to reach EEG stage III is decreased; however, "sensitivity" to etomidate does not appear to change with age. The volume of distribution is decreased with age, and the clearance rate is reduced with age; therefore, the active concentration achieved by a given dose is greater and acts longer in the aged (49). Etomidate appears to cause somewhat less cardiovascular depression than thiopental in the elderly, but the anesthesiologist should be careful in dosing etomidate in the elderly because reports have suggested a markedly decreased affinity for the binding of etomidate to plasma proteins, thus leading to a much higher effective plasma concentration of free drug (50).

Fluorinated Inhalational Anesthetics

MAC (minimum alveolar concentration of an inhalation anesthetic required to obviate gross motor response during a surgical skin incision) is reduced in the elderly. These changes parallel those known to take place in cerebral oxygen consumption, cerebral blood flow, and neuronal density (51–53).

Meperidine

Due to decreased number of plasma proteins in the elderly to which it ordinarily binds, administration of meperidine in the elderly results in a marked increase in free (active) plasma drug concentration (54). Although respiratory depression from the same relative dose of meperidine is greater in the aged, achieved blood levels are similar to those seen in younger patients. This is not due to a difference in narcotic receptors, but rather the active (unbound) "free fraction" is much greater in the elderly due to decreased binding even when blood levels are similar (55).

Morphine

Medullary respiratory center CO_2 responsiveness to morphine was recently measured and shown to exhibit a slope of 1.7 in unmedicated young adults and 10.0 after morphine medication (10 mg/70 kg). In elderly patients, the slope was 13.6 before medication and 9.1 after a similar dosage of morphine medication (56).

Narcotics are well tolerated by the cardiovascular system, at least in somewhat reduced dosage, but they have accentuated respiratory-depressant qualities for a prolonged period in the postoperative period.

Fentanyl

The elimination half-life of fentanyl, a powerful narcotic utilized during the maintenance of anesthesia, is three to four times longer in the elderly (57, 58). In addition, the apparent volume of distribution was found to be reduced in the elderly to approximately one-half that in young adults. Therefore, similarly administered doses achieve a much more profound narcotic level in the elderly (59, 60).

ANESTHETIC MANAGEMENT

Preoperative Evaluation of the Elderly

One study demonstrated that 86.5% of elderly patients who had been ''cleared'' for anesthesia and a surgical procedure by usual evaluations actually had demonstrated pathologic hemodynamic, respiratory, or oxygen transport mechanisms (61). For example, 44% were found to have abnormally low blood oxygen levels, and 8% of those (previously ''cleared'' for surgery) exhibited arterial pO_2 below 50 mmHg. Left ventricular function was studied in this same group of ''cleared'' patients; 22.3% had poor left ventricular function evidenced by assessing left ventricular stroke work index versus pulmonary capillary wedge pressure. Only 24% had normal myocardial contractility, whereas another 22.3% had demonstrably poor left ventricular function.

Another study of 1,000 elderly patients admitted for surgical therapy found that hypertension was noted in 47%; renal disease in 31%; atherosclerosis in 27%; pulmonary disease in 28%; cardiomegaly in 14%; and congestive heart failure, angina, cerebrovascular accidents, diabetes, and liver disease each were present in from 6% to 9% of these patients (62).

Evaluation of anesthetic risk in elderly patients with cardiac or vascular disease can be aided by utilization of the cardiac risk index proposed by Goldman (63, 64). Factors contributing to increased perioperative mortality include myocardial infarction within the past 6 months, one of a number of tests displaying myocardial dysfunction, jugular venous distention (elevated central venous pressure), presence of cardiac arrhythmia, and age greater than 70 years.

Myocardial infarction associated with general anesthesia and a surgical procedure carries a much higher mortality rate than for patients admitted through the emergency room with myocardial infarction. Certainly all authors agree that elective operations should be postponed until 6 months after the last previous myocardial infarction. Several studies agree that assiduous monitoring of the elderly patients with a history of myocardial infarction or other vascular disease and alert reaction to developing symptoms can markedly reduce the severity and incidence of reinfarction in the immediate postoperative period.

Airways

Assessment of the adequacy of the airway and anatomic access to the trachea and airway should be particularly careful in the aged. Arthritis or deterioration of nucleus pulposi in the cervical vertebrae or arthritis in the temporal mandibular joint may affect intubation. Pyorrhea is more common in the aged and may lead to easy dislodging of teeth, which may then be aspirated into the airway. These conditions should be carefully assessed in advance and preventive measures taken when necessary. During the preoperative visit the patient should be asked to demonstrate a full range of motion of the neck and mandible. A potential for nerve damage due to hyperextension of the neck leading to pressure of arthritic or deformed vertebral processes onto nerve roots should be carefully assessed in advance and avoided. A history of paresthesias with movement of the neck or chronic symptoms of osteoarthritis or rheumatoid arthritis in the neck should alert one to the possible necessity for special precautions and procedures.

Cardiovascular Diseases

Coronary artery disease may exist in as many as 65% of the elderly population (65), and the aortic valve has been found to be calcified in 26% of elderly patients by postmortem study, whereas aortic stenosis was found in only 9% (66).

Partially as a result of chronic hypertension, intravascular volume is usually decreased, thus potentially synergizing with the tendency of many anesthetic agents to cause hypotension. However, peripheral vascular resistance is usually elevated both due to the high incidence of arteriosclerosis and to the natural tendency toward loss of elasticity in arterial walls. Despite conflicting practices in former times, most anesthesiologists today continue most types of antihypertensive medication at routine doses until the day of operation and return to them as soon as possible after the operation. However, most agree that it is best to diagnose thoroughly the cause of hypertension and to bring it under satisfactory control by medication before an elective surgical procedure is attempted. In those patients receiving various diuretics, punctilious attention should be paid to replacement of any depleted total body potassium stores.

Most modern anesthesiologists also recommend continuing the patient's accustomed level of beta-block and calcium block medications up to the day of the operation. Although the beta-blockers exhibit little interference with narcotic-based general anesthesia, they synergize somewhat with the inhalational anesthetics in the depression of the myocardium (67). However, extensive recent research has demonstrated the very prominent potentiation of myocardial-depressant effects caused by the combination of most current inhalation anesthetics (but not of narcotic based general anesthesia) and a wide variety of modern calcium channel blockers. The anesthesiologist should be aware of the presence of these medications and should exercise caution in dosage of the inhalation anesthetics accordingly. Continuing intravenous infusion of nitroglycerine during the preoperative period is a practical and desirable plan to avert severe angina, but hypotension is a common complication. Therefore, careful monitoring is recommended during such use.

Elderly patients with uncompensated or unstable congestive heart failure frequently require invasive monitoring to detect signs of sudden deterioration occurring under anesthesia. The weakening effects of inhalation anesthetics on the myocardium of the congestive failure patient are pronounced and may be deadly. Even with the use of narcotic anesthesia, which spares the myocardium to a great extent, alterations in preload or afterload to the heart due to the surgical procedure or to pain or surgical stress may quickly worsen the cardiac failure. Therefore, constant monitoring of pulmonary artery pressures and

pulmonary artery occluded (wedge) pressures along with cardiac output is almost indispensable during all but the briefest of anesthetic and surgical procedures in such patients.

Supraventricular arrhythmias are common in the elderly, but should never be disregarded. Premature atrial contractions and disturbances of the electrocardiographic P-wave are often early indicators of pulmonary hypertension or incipient atrial fibrillation. Atrial fibrillation is usually accompanied by from 15% to 30% decrease in cardiac output due to loss of efficiency of ventricular filling. In many elderly patients who already have a compromised cardiac reserve, such loss of cardiac output may be life threatening.

Common practice today usually avoids "prophylactic" digitalization. Premature ventricular contractions are of course much more frequent in the elderly; however a change in the incidence of premature beats or a change in the source of the ectopic beat as judged from electrocardiographic evidence may signify a worsening condition, cardiac ischemia, or recent myocardial infarction. AV-nodal disturbances may indicate an impending deterioration.

Premedication

Due to the unpredictability of dosage schedules and sensitivity of the elderly to respiratory-depressant effects of narcotics and other respiratory depressants, all such drugs should be reduced in dosage or totally eliminated in the preoperative medication (68). Oral (but never intramuscular) diazepam in similar doses to those used for younger patients is frequently found to be a useful preoperative medication in elderly patients who are without severe pain.

Induction of Anesthesia

Previously mentioned pharmacologic sensitivities to thiobarbiturates and the inhalation anesthetics require a much slower, more careful induction of any type of anesthesia in the aged; the use of smaller doses and concentrations; and careful monitoring of the physiology during slow induction. Blood volume is frequently decreased in the elderly. Because of poor eating habits, chronic disease, and not infrequently because of the doctor's "nothing by mouth" orders after midnight the previous night, these patients are quite commonly dehydrated and additionally hypovolemic. Many anesthesiologists advocate prophylactic acute intravenous hydration with 5–10 mg of balanced salt solution per kg of body weight just before induction of anesthesia. Others use maintenance intravenous fluids overnight the evening before the operation.

Maintenance

The type of anesthesia for elderly patients depends somewhat upon the type of operation and the particular physiologic condition of the specific patient being considered. Although nitrous oxide-narcotic-tranquilizer-muscle relaxant techniques have perhaps the least degree of depressant effect on the myocardium, they do not offer the advantage of decreasing workload on the heart by reducing peripheral vascular resistance, as is the case with some of the inhalation anesthetics, such as isoflurane. In addition, isoflurane stabilizes the heart against arrhythmias, much unlike the narcotic-based anesthesia.

Induction of anesthesia with inhalation anesthetics is often dangerously accelerated because of lower cardiac output and lower myocardial reserve leading to a decreased transit rate of blood through the pulmonary circulation. This leads in turn to an enhanced diffusion of soluble-inhalation anesthetics into the blood and eventually therefore to a higher anesthetic content in the blood ejected from the left heart bound for the brain. In some elderly patients, this effect is somewhat reduced by an increased degree of intrapulmonary shunting. This increased speed of inhalation induction can, of course, be circumvented by intentionally limiting the inhalational anesthetic concentration during the induction phase in these elderly patients.

Because MAC is reduced in the elderly, inhalation anesthetic maintenance requirements are usually somewhat lower in elderly than in younger adult patients. Frequently today a combination of low dose narcotics and reduced concentration inhalation anesthetics is utilized in order to receive the benefits of both and to minimize the side effects of each type.

Regional Anesthesia

The general desirability of major regional anesthesia, such as subarachnoid (spinal) block and epidural block, in comparison to modern endotracheal general anesthesia has been debated vigorously for several decades (69–74). Indicators of success for regional block anesthesia, such as lower perioperative mortality, lesser postoperative hypoxemia, early ambulation, lesser incidence of thromboembolism, and lower incidence of resulting mental changes after the surgical procedure, have been utilized in this study (75). Obviously, many operations are not in regions easily conducive to the use of major regional anesthesia care. Even for such operations as hip fractures, subtle practical anesthetic management problems lead to a narrowing of distinctions between the two methods.

Regional anesthesia properly retains great popularity for some specific operations and might be argued to offer advantages in a wider range of surgical procedures than is commonly seen in today's practice. Transurethral resection of the prostate is a typical example of an operation in which there can be excellent application of the technique of subarachnoid anesthesia. This technique does little to disturb the patient's physiology, ability to respond to the minimal blood loss of the operation, or respiratory, cardiac, and brain function.

However, during the use of major regional anesthetic procedures in elderly patients, extensive sympathetic block may lead to some difficulty in the maintenance of normal blood pressure. A bradycardia due to high sympathetic block also may be more frequent than in young patients. Establishment of major epidural block in the aged requires reduction in the dose of local anesthetic to be injected into the epidural space (76–78).

There seems to be an analogous reduction in the requirement for local anesthetic to establish subarachnoid block in the elderly, and a reduction of doses and volumes by approximately one-third is the common clinical practice. In addition, many anesthesiologists preclude the use of epinephrine in subarachnoid block for elderly patients, because of the fear of induction of ischemia in spinal arteries nourishing the spinal cord, which might very well lead to neuropathy or paraplegia.

The ability to converse with the patient during the operation can be an excellent indicator of continuing good cerebral function and a monitor of the lack of symptoms attributable to angina or any other stress responses. However, when elderly patients become pained or frightened during the course of regional anesthesia and a surgical procedure, they may require sedation, which may then bring on the attendant complications of the medication being used, particularly respiratory and cardiovascular depressions.

Perioperative Hypothermia in the Elderly

Along with the progressive decline in the metabolic rate associated with increasing age, a progressive impairment of the central thermal regulatory system of the body also develops (79). This can be accentuated further by various drug actions. For example, neuromuscular blocking agents may reduce heat production by reducing the ability to shiver, whereas beta-adrenergic agonists and inhalation anesthetics may actively cause skin vasodilitation leading to extra heat radiation. Hypothermia in the elderly may be due to a variety of causes, including decreased heat production, increased heat loss, and derangement of the central heat regulatory mechanism. Neurologic disease, including diabetic retinopathy, peripheral neuropathy, or central damage due to cerebral vascular accident, may impair transmission from skin thermal receptors.

Several physical factors in the operating suite lead to hypothermia in elderly patients who already may be deprived of intrinsic heat preservation mechanisms. These include the habitually cold air conditioning and rapid air turnover of operating rooms. The additional depression of the brain thermostatic center by general anesthetics, the blocking of peripheral autonomic vasoconstriction that usually functions to conserve heat, and the actively dilating of skin vasculature caused by several anesthetic agents further contribute to hypothermia. Shivering to produce heat is reduced by muscle relaxants and by the usual administration of various amounts of cold blood and fluids; these factors also contribute to heat loss and the blocked ability to respond. However, perhaps a major factor is the almost universal use of unheated, cold dry gases for ventilation and respiration.

Several studies indicate that elderly patients routinely drop their body temperatures. In our operating suite, temperatures as low as 90 °F in elderly patients undergoing intraperitoneal procedures were not at all uncommon before the technique of heating and humidifying all respiratory gases was added to the other standard methods already in use. During the recovery period, attempts to increase body heat frequently lead to the excessive utilization of oxygen, hypertension, tachycardia, increased cardiac output, and severe evidences of stress (80). Furthermore, some evidence indicates there is a higher incidence of thromboembolism when operations are performed under cold ambient conditions. It is strongly advocated that heated anesthetic gases be used for all elderly patients undergoing general anesthesia for more than short periods and that this provision should be instituted in all operating rooms.

RECOVERY ROOM CARE

A large percentage of elderly patients, due to such factors as increased intrapulmonary shunting and increased respiratory-depressant effect of drugs, require enrichment of the inhaled oxygen atmosphere during transport to and while resident in the recovery room in order to avoid oxygen desaturation. A semi-sitting position improves the ease and effectiveness of ventilation, and early encouragement to movement, speech, and coughing helps to avoid pulmonary atelectasis and vascular thromboembolism. Particular attention should be paid in the recovery room to lingering hypoventilation. Pertinent measurements of respiratory volumes and blood gas values should be offered on very lenient indications. In elderly patients in particular, narcotics can be demonstrated to have lingering effects at surprisingly long intervals after the last lingering effects would have been expected to have passed in younger patients.

ANESTHETIC MANAGEMENT OF SOME REPRESENTATIVE CONDITIONS

Carotid Endarterectomy

Perioperative mortality and morbidity in the

course of carotid endarterectomy vary from 1% in patients with no major medical problems to 10% in patients with major medical problems or unstable neurologic deficits secondary to vascular disturbances (81). Elderly patients presenting for this procedure generally have the same wide spectrum of diseases as other elderly patients, but in addition can have a greater incidence of myocardial ischemia and myocardial infarction, cardiac arrhythmias, and compensated heart failure. Those conditions must be stabilized preoperatively in order to minimize perioperative risk.

The choice of anesthesia for this procedure varies among institutions, with some relying on major regional block anesthesia of the cervical epidural area or the cervical plexus, or on local anesthesia. However, general anesthesia appears to achieve better patient acceptance and is used extensively in many areas of the country. It also allows concurrent use of intentional depression of cerebral metabolic rate by the heavy use of barbiturate or inhalation anesthetics in an attempt to minimize ischemic damage during intentional carotid cross clamping.

Under regional anesthesia, however, patients can offer verbal response, helping to define the extent of ischemia as it develops during the endarterectomy procedure, and emergence agitation and hypertension are often minimized (82). Yet, when, as occasionally occurs, such patients become frightened or disoriented during the operation, institution of general anesthesia and the attainment of an adequate airway may not only be difficult but also frankly dangerous after the patient has been positioned and the procedure has begun.

When general anesthesia is chosen, drugs that generally support or increase cerebral blood flow yet decrease cerebral metabolic rate are desirable. Some medical centers prefer barbiturate drugs in large doses because of their beneficial effect on decreasing cerebral metabolic rate. However, hypotension and even cerebral hypoperfusion may result from the overall cardiovascular side effects of these drugs. Although some have therefore recommended ketamine for this use, due to its assistance with the maintenance of cerebral blood flow, most anesthesiologists reject it because of the dangers of enhancement of hypertension, postoperative anesthetic excite-

ment, and the occasional excitement reaction episodes during anesthesia that can occur in elderly patients.

Because halothane and to a lesser extent other inhalation anesthetics increase intracerebral pressure, these agents have not been popular for this operation. However, "light anesthesia" with these agents can be used successfully, particularly with careful clinical monitoring. Potent inhalation anesthetics have the advantage of increasing cerebral blood flow while decreasing cerebral metabolic rate. Isoflurane is frequently avoided in these patients even though it has a very favorable effect on cerebral metabolism and evidence of protecting cerebral cortical activity. Because of its tendency to cause peripheral vasodilitation, sometimes along with relative hypotension, in patients that have a history of accommodation to their chronic hypertension, it is to be used very selectively (83).

Intravenous narcotic-based anesthetics generally exhibit less peripheral dilitation and myocardial depression and therefore aid in maintenance of blood pressure (84). On the other hand, blood pressure sometimes is inordinately high even with large doses of these agents. The use of nitrous oxide has become somewhat controversial due to its various vascular and toxic side effects. Yet, it is still a standard basal anesthetic agent in many institutions and is utilized along with low concentrations of fluorinated anesthetics or with non-depolarizing muscle relaxants to reduce the requirement for general anesthetic agents. Metocurine, atracurium, or vecuronium are current favorites because of their relatively more favorable cardiovascular effect in the elderly, chronic hypertensive patients.

Anesthetic Management of the Elderly Diabetic

In diabetics, a variety of perioperative problems are of interest to the anesthesiologist (85). These include diabetic ketoacidosis, the hyperosmolar syndrome, lactic acidosis, and hypoglycemia. These patients should be carefully examined preoperatively for evidence of diabetic retinopathy, diabetic nephropathy, peripheral neuropathies, cardiac and particularly peripheral vascular disease, and chronic hypertension. Risk of cardiac and cerebral infarction appears greater in patients with diabetic vascular disease, and it now appears that they tolerate hypotension less successfully than non-diabetic patients. Survival from infarction is decreased in diabetics. An interesting and fortunately rare syndrome includes sudden cardiac arrest due to diabetic neuropathy of the autonomic nervous system. Because of these conditions, the patient should be carefully evaluated for the status of the heart and peripheral circulation before anesthesia (86).

The most common concern in diabetics is management of the blood sugar. Hyperglycemia can be regulated to relatively low normal levels by the frequent intraoperative use of blood glucose estimations. The availability of easy to use semi-quantitative devices makes it practical for the anesthesiologist to evaluate resulting blood glucose levels fairly frequently during anesthesia.

Hyperglycemia should also be assiduously avoided because of the likelihood of a hyperosmolar syndrome leading to dehydration of the brain and severe neurologic symptoms and hypovolemia. The mortality rate for nonketotic hyperosmolar syndrome may be as great as 50% (87). Initial treatment with 2 L of rapidly administered half-normal saline is often recommended. This is usually followed by hypotonic saline at the rate of 1 L every 2 hours while carefully monitoring central venous pressure. This syndrome may be further accelerated by the concurrent administration of steroids and diuretics, the presence of infections, during cerebral vascular accidents, or during total parenteral alimentation. Serum bicarbonate levels may be decreased in this situation, but blood urea nitrogen is usually elevated due to the hypovolemia and pre-renal azotemia. Serum osmolarity is usually above 320 mosmol/kg. Blood glucose levels exceed 600 mg/dl (88).

Patients already presenting with diabetic ketoacidosis should, whenever possible, be slowly resuscitated with insulin and adequate systemic fluids, and when necessary, antacid therapy such as bicarbonate should be used. Treatment of diabetic ketoacidosis consists of intravenous infusion of 20–50 units of insulin, with extremely careful monitoring of blood glucose levels, followed by infusion of titrated increments of 1–10 intravenous units of insulin per hour. Meanwhile, careful attention should be given to the maintenance and restoration of normal serum potassium levels. When emergency surgical procedures are necessary in patients exhibiting diabetic ketoacidosis, frequent arterial blood gases and aggressive use of carefully monitored, incremental doses of intravenous insulin and fluid therapy are highly recommended.

Extreme hypoglycemia can be a consequence of residual insulin activity from previously administered long-acting preparations. Patients often become symptomatic when blood glucose levels decrease below 50 mg/dl. When this occurs during anesthesia, there are frequently few warning signs. Increased blood pressure, sweating, and tachycardia sometimes give warning, but in elderly patients, these are quite unreliable during general anesthesia. Therefore, constant infusion of small amounts of dextrose throughout the operation is important in elderly diabetic patients, and frequent monitoring of blood glucose levels is important even in elderly patients thought to present with only mild diabetes.

In order to prevent this important complication, many anesthesiologists advocate removal of at least more severe diabetic patients from all long-acting insulin preparations at least 2 days before major surgical procedures are to be done. Replacement of long-acting preparations with multiple dose usage of crystalline insulin and the use of a sliding urinary scale for dose regulation of insulin are recommended. However, at a intelligent minimum, most anesthesiologists recommend reduction in the preoperative dose of long-acting insulin preparations followed by frequent blood glucose analysis during the operation and in the immediate postoperative period, with appropriate reaction for high or low readings.

Some anesthesiologists prefer using major regional anesthesia where applicable in diabetic patients because they feel that the re-establishment of a preoperative maintenance plan is easier and that the hyperglycemic stress response after intraperitoneal procedures may be reduced by spinal or epidural anesthesia (89). However, many are concerned with both pre-existing neuropathy, which may later be confused as an anesthetic complication, and the patency of diabetic spinal blood vessels, which might be more susceptible to occlusion by the irritation of the subarachnoid medication. Further impairment of these vessels theoretically might lead to enhancement of the present level of neuropathy, or it might even lead to disastrous spinal cord ischemia.

When general anesthesia is required, rapid sequence tracheal intubation has been advocated by some who feel that aspiration of gastric contents may be more frequent in this patient group because of manifestations of autonomic neuropathy in some diabetic patients (89).

In former times, the use of diethyl ether frequently led to hyperglycemia in diabetics, but there is no current evidence for a particular preference among modern inhalation anesthetics. However, whether narcotic-based intravenous anesthesia or inhalation anesthesia is chosen, sufficient doses, concentrations, and anesthetic depths are advisable for reducing the stress reaction, cortisol and catecholamine release, and therefore the secondary disturbances in the glucose and insulin levels (89).

Major Vascular Procedures

In addition to the usual range of diseases found in other elderly patients, nearly half of patients who are presenting for abdominal aortic aneurysm resection will give a history of previous myocardial infarction. One-half also exhibit chronic obstructive pulmonary disease, and nearly 70% are chronic smokers. Five to 10% of these patients may exhibit symptoms of congestive heart failure, and such patients have been said to account for a four-fold increase in cardiac complications (90). Thus, both anesthetic and postoperative management of these patients must include consideration of methods to minimize the effects of these conditions (91).

Routine coronary angiography in a group of patients about to undergo vascular surgical procedures showed that up to 30% had significant coronary artery disease despite a normal resting electrocardiogram. Patients with myocardial infarction account for approximately 50% of early postoperative deaths from vascular operations, and the mortality rate of reinfarction during this postoperative period is as high as 70% (92, 93). Evaluation of cardiac function in patients with other suspect symptoms is advocated, and it has been noted that an ejection fraction of less than 35% is associated with a four-fold increase in the incidence of postoperative myocardial infarction. Renal function is frequently depressed in patients who have abdominal aneurysms due to renal vascular embarrassment. In the elderly patient, there may also be evidence of concurrent diabetes, hypertension, or other manifestations of vascular diseases. Renal dysfunction may have been accentuated by the various diagnostic tests, bowel preparation, and fluid restriction leading to further decrease in urine flow. Intraoperative renal vascular compromise may be superimposed upon this condition. Careful peripheral neurologic evaluation should be carried out in order to gauge the potential effects of peripheral nervous system and spinal cord ischemia during cross clamping of the aorta.

The choice of anesthesia for vascular procedures remains controversial, although there appears to be no clear-cut advantages either of major regional or general anesthesia. Many anesthesiologists do not use major regional anesthesia in the presence of preoperative heparinization because of the fear of epidural or subarachnoid bleeding from the needle necessary to institute the block. Such bleeding may result in serious neurologic complications. Although the incidence of this complication is quite low, its physical, social, and legal implications are formidable. Unless a distinct advantage can be demonstrated for the regional anesthetic over general anesthesia, the latter is preferred.

In the absence of heparinization, continuous epidural anesthesia minimizes the pulmonary effects of anesthesia in cases of chronic obstructive pulmonary disease. In these patients it provides a pathway for continued postoperative analgesia via the epidural catheter by the use of either a low concentration of local anesthetic or small doses of narcotics. Such treatment minimizes the respiratory complications of all abdominal operations and provides excellent pain relief. However, central nervous system narcotics on rare occasions will lead to profound delayed central nervous system respiratory depression, and patients so treated should be carefully monitored for respiratory adequacy. During aortic cross clamping, considerable myocardial ischemia can develop due to increased work and afterload (94). Therefore, the infusion of vasodilators, including nitroglycerin or sodium nitroprusside, during the cross clamping to reduce these effects is becoming very popular. Some vascular teams advocate the routine prophylactic use of bicarbonate to counteract lactic acid return from the periphery just after clamping, and some also recommend prophylactic fluid or blood boluses to be given just before unclamping the aorta. At any rate, this portion of the operation must be monitored very alertly, and the surgeon must be ready to return the cross clamp to the aorta for complete or partial clamping if the systemic pressure nourishing the coronary and brain vessels falls uncontrollably. Minimally incremental doses of potent alpha-vasoconstrictor drugs are sometimes used here to promote vascular tone in the legs immediately after cross clamping, but under no circumstances should these drugs be continued chronically.

Orthopedic Procedures

The use of various types of brachial plexus blocks, including interscalene blocks, supraclavicular brachial block, and axillary blocks, is particularly appropriate in arm operations and procedures. Older patients appear to tolerate these procedures perhaps even better than younger ones. However, particular caution must be taken to guard against the inadvertent induction of a pneumothorax during the block procedure because a high percentage of elderly patients may already have compromised pulmonary and cardiovascular function and can tolerate a pneumothorax less easily. As previously mentioned, many of the local anesthetic agents exhibit longer duration of systemic activity in the elderly, and this extends to some extent to their local actions.

Most patients in the lateral position during certain hip operations require sedation because of the discomfort of the prolonged pressure on the unanesthetized portions of the upper body and from the psychologic strain of being in this necessary position. In addition, in this position, ventilation is often impaired even in the awake state. When sedation is added to the major regional anesthesia, hypoventilation is almost certain, if not the rule, often leading to oxygen desaturation. The addition of narcotic drugs accentuates this tendency. The same problem may be solved under general anesthesia by the use of inhalation anesthetics that are quickly breathed out and dissipated following the end of the operations, thereby removing their respiratory-depressant effects. In addition, the endotracheal intubation allows, by positive pressure breathing, avoidance of oxygen desaturation and hypercapnia.

Major hip operations can frequently be managed with continuous spinal anesthesia administered through a tiny plastic catheter placed into the subarachnoid space. Although this technique has nearly disappeared in use with younger patients, it has done so largely out of the fear of infection (which admittedly could be disastrous, but whose incidence is almost nil in modern times) and the fear of postdural puncture headaches. Postdural puncture headaches are quite rare in elderly patients in direct proportion to advancing age, and therefore this consideration may be less important than feared by some.

The use of general anesthesia in orthopedic patients is a matter of individual choice, but it is subject to the same considerations as general anesthesia for other elderly patients.

SUMMARY

Anesthesia in elderly patients presents the surgical care team with a range of difficult problems. These include unusual responses to anesthesia when compared to younger adults that are caused by alterations in the physiology of elderly patients. The prevalence of pathologic conditions other than the surgical condition, when combined with the anesthetic, gives rise to the need for special precautions and aftercare. Both "normal" aging processes and pathologic conditions call forth very altered pharmacologic responses to many of the anesthetic drugs. In many cases, different kinds of responses are predicted by altered neurologic tissue composition and depression of receptor sensitivity. More commonly, the duration of action and the dose-response magnitude may simply be altered by body compartment variations from young adults or from depressed organ blood flow or excretion functions. In addition, elderly patients have a distinctly different psychology, and many anesthetic procedures and techniques that might be used in younger patients are not acceptable to some elderly patients.

Therefore, anesthesia for the elderly patient must be attempted only after careful evaluation of the health of the individual patient, the physical and psychological needs of the patient, and the special requirements imposed by the surgical procedure. Anesthesia and surgically related perioperative mortality and morbidity are declining at an encouragingly rapid rate due to acquisition of new knowledge bearing on these questions and the continuing development of new and more appropriate drugs. It can be anticipated that in the near future necessary surgical procedures can be offered to patients of unlimited age with an even greater degree of confidence.

Acknowledgement. The authors are grateful to Ms. Ann Holbrook and Mrs. Joy Lyerly for editorial assistance.

REFERENCES

1. Rothstein M: Biochemical studies of aging. *Chem Engi News* 64:26–39, 1986.
2. Djokovic JL, Hedley-Whyte J: Prediction of outcome of surgery and anesthesia in patients over 80. *JAMA* 242:2301–2306, 1979.
3. Ziffren SE: Comparison of mortality rates for various surgical operations according to age groups, 1951–1977. *J Am Geriatr Soc* 27:433–438, 1979.
4. Davenport HT: Anaesthesia for the geriatric patient. *Can Anaesth Soc J* 30:S51-S55, 1983.
5. Marx GF, Mateo CV, Orkin L: Computer analysis of post anesthetic deaths. *Anesthesiology* 59:54–58, 1983.
6. Seymour DG, Pringle R: Post-operative complications in the elderly surgical patient. *Gerontology* 29:262–270, 1983.
7. Wilson LA, Lawson IR, Proass W: Multiple disorders in the elderly: a clinical and statistical study. *Lancet* 2:841–843, 1962,
8. Evans TI: The physiologic basis of geriatric general anesthesia. *Anaesth Intensive Care* 1:319–322, 1973.
9. Earnst MP, Heaton RK, Wilkinson WE, Manke WR: Cortical atrophy, ventricular enlargement and intellectual impairment in the aged. *Neurology* 24:1138–1143, 1979.
10. Kety SS: Human cerebral blood flow and oxygen consumption as related to aging. *J Chronic Dis* 3:478–486, 1956.
11. Fujishima M, Sadoshima A, Ogatha J, Yoshida F, Shiokawa O, Ibayashi S, Omae T: Autoregulation of cerebral blood flow in young and spontaneously hypertensive rats (SHR). *Gerontology* 30:30–36, 1984.
12. Naritomi H, Meyer JS, Sakai F, Yamaguchi F, Shaw T: Effects of advancing age on regional cerebral blood flow. Studies in normal subjects and subjects with risk factors for atherothrombic stroke. *Arch Neurol* 36:410–416, 1979.
13. Dax EM: Receptors and associated membrane events in aging. *Rev Biol Res Aging* 2:315–336, 1985.
14. Feldman RD, Limbird LE, Nadeau J, Robertson D, Wood AJJ: Alterations in leukocyte beta-receptor affinity with aging. A potential explanation for altered beta-adrenergic sentivity in the elderly. *N Engl J Med* 310:815–819, 1984.
15. Vestal RE, Wood AJJ, Shand DG: Reduced beta-adrenoceptor sensitivity in the elderly. *Clin Pharmacol Ther* 26:181–186, 1979.
16. Ochs HR, Greenblatt DJ, Divoll M, Abernathy DR, Feyerabend H, Dengler HJ: Diazepam kinetics in relation to age and sex. *Pharmacology* 23:24–30, 1981.
17. Pontoppidan H, Beecher HK: Progressive loss of protective reflexes in the airway with the advance of age. *JAMA* 174:2209–2213, 1960.
18. Pfeifer MA, Weinberg CR, Cook D, Best JD, Reenan A, Halter JB: Differential changes of autonomic nervous system function with age in man. *Am J Med* 75:249–257, 1983.
19. Pontoppidan H, Geffins B, Lowenstein A: Acute respiratory failure in the adult. *N Engl J Med* 287:690–698, 1972.
20. Fowler RW: Ageing and lung function. *Age Ageing* 14:209–215, 1985.
21. Schmidt CD, Dickman ML, Gardner RM, Brough FK: Spirometric standards for healthy elderly men and women. *Am Rev Respir Dis* 108:933–939, 1973.
22. Tenney SM, Miller RM: Dead space ventilation in old age. *J Appl Physiol* 9:321, 1956.
23. Wahba WM: Influence of aging on lung function-clinical significance of changes from age twenty. *Anesth Analg* 62:764–776, 1983.
24. Brischetto MJ, Millman RP, Peterson DD, Silage DA, Pack AI: Effect of aging on ventilatory response to exercise and CO2. *J Appl Physiol: Respirat Environ Exercise Physiol* 56:1143–1150, 1984.
25. Yamamoto M, Meyer JJ, Sakai F, Yamaguchi F: Aging and cerebral vasodilator response to hypercarbia. *Arch Neurol* 37:489–496, 1980.
26. Kronenberg RS, Drage CW: Attenuation of the ventilatory and heart rate responses to hypoxia and hypercapnia with aging in normal men. *J Clin Invest* 52:1812–1819, 1973.
27. Lubin JR, Millward BA, Coles JA, Croker JR: Value of profiling liver function in the elderly. *Postgrad Med J* 59:763–766, 1983.
28. Rowe JW, Andres R, Tobin JD, Norris AH, Shock NW: The effect of age on creatinine clearance in man—a cross-sectional and longitudinal study. *J Gerontol* 31:155–163, 1976.
29. Thompson EN, William R: Effect of age on liver function with particular reference to bromsulphalein excretion. *Gut* 6:266–269, 1965.
30. D-Hollander A, Massaux F, Nevelsteen M, Agonston S: Age dependent dose response relationship of ORGNC-45 in anesthetized patients. *Br J Anaesth* 54:653–659, 1982.

31. Janis KM: Anesthesia for the geriatric patient. *ASA Refresher Courses in Anesthesiology* 7:143–154, 1979.

32. Greenblatt DJ: Reduced serum albumin concentration in the elderly. *J Am Geriatr Soc* 27:20–22, 1979.

33. Thompson TL, Moran MG, Nies AS: Psychotropic drug use in the elderly. *N Engl J Med* 308:134–138, 1983.

34. Guttman D: Patterns of legal drug use by older Americans. *Addict Dis* 3:337–356, 1977.

35. Hurwitz N: Predisposing factors in adverse reactions to drugs. *Br Med J* 1:536–539,1969.

36. Richey DP, Bender AD: Pharmacokinetic consequences of aging. *Ann Rev Pharmacol Toxicol* 17:49–65, 1977.

37. Greenblatt DJ, Sellers EM, Shader PI: Drug disposition in old age. *N Engl J Med* 306:1081–1088, 1982.

38. Kanto J, Aaltonen L, Himberg J-J, Hovi-Viander M: Midazolam as an intravenous induction agent in the elderly: a clinical and pharmacokinetic study. *Anesth Analg* 65:15–20, 1986.

39. Dundee JW, Halliday NJ, Loughran PG, Harper KW: The influence of age on the onset of anaesthesia with midazolam. *Anaesthesia* 40:441-443, 1985.

40. Greenblatt DJ, Abernathy DR, Locniskar A, Harmatz JS, Limjuco RA, Shader RI: Effect of age, gender, and obesity on midazolam kinetics. *Anesthesiology* 61:27–35, 1984.

41. Homer TD, Stanski DR: The effect of increasing age on thiopental disposition and anesthetic requirement. *Anesthesiology* 62:714–724, 1985.

42. Jung D, Mayersohn M, Perrier D, Calkins J, Saunders R: Thiopental disposition as a function of age in female patients undergoing surgery. *Anesthesiology* 56:263–268, 1982.

43. Klotz U, Avant GR, Hoyumpa A, Schenker S, Wilkinson GR: The effects of age and liver disease on the disposition and elimination of diazepam in adult man. *J Clin Invest* 55:347–350, 1975.

44. Somogyi A: PanCuronium plasma clearance and age. *Br J Anaesth* 52:360, 1980.

45. Nation RL, Trigg EJ: Lignocaine kinetics in cardiac patients and aged subjects. *Br J Clinic Pharmac* 4:439–448, 1977.

46. Duvaldestin P, Saada J, Berger JL, D'Hollander A, Desmonts JM: Pharmacokinetics, pharmacodynamics, and dose-response relationships of pancuronium in control and elderly subjects. *Anesthesiology* 56:36–40, 1982.

47. McLeod K, Hull CJ, Watson MJ: Effects of ageing on the pharmacokinetics of pancuronium. *Br J Anaesth* 51:435–438, 1979.

48. Mateo RS, Backus WW, McDaniel DD, Brotherton WP, Abraham R, Diaz J: Pharmacokinetics and pharmacodynamics of d-tubocurarine and metocurine in the elderly. *Anesth Analg* 64:23–29, 1985.

49. Arden JR, Holley FO, Stanski DR: Increased sensitivity to etomidate in the elderly: initial distribution versus altered brain response. *Anesthesiology* 65:19–27, 1986.

50. Dagnino J, Prys-Roberts C: Anesthesia in the aged hypertensive patient. In Stephen CR, Assaf RAE (eds): *Geriatric Anesthesia.* Boston, Butterworth Publishing Co, 1986, pg 264.

51. Munson ES, Hoffman JC, Eger EIII: Use of cyclopropane to test generality of anesthetic requirement in the elderly. *Anesth Analg* 63:998–1000, 1984.

52. Stevens WC, Dolan WM, Gibbons RT, White A, Eger EIII, Miller RD, De Jong RH, Elashoff RM: Minimum alveolar concentrations (MAC) of isoflurane with and without nitrous oxide in patients of various ages. *Anesthesiology* 42:197–200, 1975.

53. Gregory GA, Eger EIII, Munson ES: Relationship between age and halothane requirement in man. *Anesthesiology* 30:488–491, 1969.

54. Mather LE, Tucker GT, Pflug AE, Lindop MJ, Wilkerson C: Meperidine kinetics in man, intravenous injection in surgical patients and volunteers. *Clin Pharmacol Ther* 17:21–30, 1975.

55. Herman RJ, McAllister CB, Branch RA, Wilkerson GR: Effects of age on meperidine disposition. *Clin Pharmacol Ther* 37:19–24, 1985.

56. Daykin AP, Bowen DJ, Saunders DA, Norman J: Respiratory depression after morphine in the elderly. A comparison with younger subjects. *Anaesthesia* 41:910–914, 1986.

57. Schmucher DL: Alterations in drug disposition. In Stephen CR, Assaf RAE (eds): *Geriatric Anesthesia.* Boston, Butterworth Publishing Co, 1986, pp. 155–188.

58. Bently JB, Borel JD, Nenad RE Jr., Gillespie TJ: Age and fentanyl pharmacokinetics. *Anesth Analg* 61:968–971, 1982.

59. Helmers H, Van Peer A, Woestenborghs R, Noorduin H, Heykants J: Alfentanil kinetics in the elderly. *Clin Pharmacol Ther* 36:239–243, 1984.

60. Singleton MA, Rosen JI, Fisher DM: Pharmacokinetics of fentanyl in the elderly. *Anesthesiology* 63:A372, 1985.

61. Del Guercio LRM, Cohn JD: Monitoring operative risk in the elderly. *JAMA* 243:1350–1355, 1980.

62. Stephen CR: Risk factors and outcome in elderly patients and epidemiologic study. In Stephen CR, Assaf RAE (eds): *Geriatric Anesthesia.* Boston, Butterworth Publishing Co, 1986, pp. 345–362.

63. Goldman L, Caldera DL: Risk of general anesthesia and elective surgery in the hypertensive patient. *Anesthesiology* 50:285–292, 1979.

64. Goldman L, Caldera DL, Nussbaum SR, Southwick FS, Krogstad D, Murray B, Burke DS, O'Malley TA, Goroll AH, Caplan CH, Nolan J, Carabello B, Slater EE: Multifactorial index of cardiac risk in noncardiac surgical procedures. *N Engl J Med* 297:845–850, 1977.

65. Fisch C: Electrocardiogram in the aged: an independent marker of heart disease. *Am J Med* 70:4–6, 1981.

66. Pomerance A: Cardiac pathology in the elderly. *Cardiovasc Clin* 12:5–9, 1981.

67. Slogoff S, Keats AS, Hibbs CW, Edmonds CH, Bragg DA: Failure of general anesthesia to potentiate propranolol activity. *Anesthesiology* 47:504–508, 1977.

68. Muravchick S: Effect of age and premedication on thiopental sleep dose. *Anesthesiology* 61:333–336, 1984.

69. Riis J, Lomholt B, Haxholdt O, Kehlet H, Valentin N, Danielsen U, Dyrberg V: Immediate and long-term men-

tal recovery from general versus epidural anesthesia in elderly patients. *Acta Anaesthesiol Scand* 27:44–49, 1983.

70. Modig J, Borg T, Karlstrom G: Thromboembolism after total hip replacement: Role of epidural and general anesthesia. *Anesth Analg* 62:174–180, 1983.

71. Mann RAM, Bisset WIK: Anaesthesia for lower limb amputation. A comparison of spinal analgesia and general anaesthesia in the elderly. *Anaesthesia* 38:1185–1191, 1983.

72. Hole A, Terjesen T, Brevik H: Epidural versus general anaesthesia for total hip arthroplasty in elderly patients. *Acta Anaesthesiol Scand* 24:279–287, 1980.

73. Davis FM, Laurenson VG: Spinal anaesthesia or general anaesthesia for emergency hip surgery in elderly patients. *Anaesth Intensive Care* 9:352–356, 1981.

74. Bigler D, Adelhoj B, Petring OU, Pederson NO, Busch P, Kalhke P: Mental function and morbidity after acute hip surgery during spinal and general anaesthesia. *Anaesthesia* 40:672–676, 1985.

75. McKenzie PF, Wishart HY, Smith O: Long term outcome after repair of fractured neck of femur. *Br J Anaesth* 56:581–584, 1984.

76. Bromage PR: Ageing and epidural dose requirements. *Br J Anaesth* 41:1016–1022, 1969.

77. Park WY, Hagins FM, Rivat EL, Magnamara TE: Age and epidural dose response in adult men. *Anesthesiology* 56:318–320, 1982.

78. Anderson S, Cold GE: Dose response studies in elderly patients subjected to epidural analgesia. *Acta Anaesthesiol Scand* 25:279–281, 1981.

79. Collins KJ, Easton JC, Exton-Smith AN: The ageing nervous system: impairment of thermoregulation. *Adv Med* 18:250–257, 1982.

80. Heymann AD: The effect of incidental hypothermia on elderly surgical patients. *J Gerontol* 32:46–48, 1977.

81. Bove EL, Fry WJ, Gross WS, Stanley JC: Hypotension and hypertension as consequences of baroreceptor dysfunction following carotid endarterectomy. *Surgery* 85:633–637, 1979.

82. Balestrieri FJ, Brough DS, Stullken EH, Davis CH, McWhorter JM, Howard G: Hemodynamic events associated with regional anesthesia for carotid endarterectomy. (Abstract) *Anesth Analg* 64:195, 1985.

83. Campkin TV, Honigsberger L, Smith IS: Isoflurane: effect on the encephalogram during carotid endarterectomy. *Anaesthesia* 40:188–191, 1985.

84. Lee JK, Hanowell S, Kim YD, Macnamara TE: Morphine-induced respiratory depression following bilateral carotid endarterectomy. *Anesth Analg* 60:64–65, 1981.

85. Gallina DL, Mordes JP, Rossini AA: Surgery in the diabetic patient. *Compr Ther* 9:8–16, 1983.

86. Lipson LG: Introduction: Diabetes in the elderly: a multifaceted problem. *Am J Med* 80 (Suppl 5A):1–2, 1986.

87. Podolsky S: Hyperosmolar nonketotic coma in the elderly diabetic. *Med Clin N Am* 62:815–828, 1978.

88. Lipson LG: Diabetes in the elderly: diagnosis, pathogenesis, and therapy. *Am J Med* 80(Suppl 5A):10–21, 1986.

89. Brown EM, Brown M: Management of the elderly diabetic patient during anesthesia. *Clin Anesthesiol* 4:881–898, 1986.

90. Goldman L: Cardiac risks and complications of noncardiac surgery. *Ann Surg* 198:780–791, 1983.

91. Young AE, Sandberg GW, Couch NP: The reduction of mortality of abdominal aortic aneurysm resection. *Am J Surg* 134:585–590, 1977.

92. Davison JK: Anesthesia for major vascular procedures in the elderly. *Clin Anesthesiol* 4:931–957, 1986.

93. Rao TKL, Jacobs KH, El-Etr AA: Reinfarction following anesthesia in patients with myocardial infarction. *Anesthesiology* 59:499–505, 1983.

94. Attia RR, Murphy JD, Snider M, Lappas DG, Darling RC, Lowenstein E: Myocardial ischemia due to infrarenal aortic crossclamping during surgery in patients with severe coronary artery disease. *Circulation* 53:961–965, 1976.

Chapter 6

Medical Oncology in the Elderly

John D. Hainsworth, M.D.

The treatment of some types of advanced inoperable cancer has improved greatly during the last 20 years, due to the development of effective systemic chemotherapy. Some cancers (e.g., Hodgkin's disease, non-Hodgkin's lymphomas, testicular cancer, ovarian cancer) are potentially curable with chemotherapeutic measures, whereas appropriate treatment of many other advanced neoplasms results in relief of symptoms and prolongation of survival. In spite of these improvements, systemic chemotherapy has, until recently, been considered to be a therapeutic option primarily for young and middle-aged adults. Elderly patients have been considered poor candidates for systemic chemotherapy, primarily for two reasons. First, most types of cancer that responded well in early trials of chemotherapy occur primarily in children or in young adults. Conversely, several cancer types that increase in incidence with age (e.g., colon, pancreas, prostate, lung) have been relatively insensitive to chemotherapy. Second, the use of cytotoxic drugs is associated with side effects, particularly when these drugs are used in combinations. It has been assumed that the toxicity of these drugs would be increased in elderly patients and that any benefit caused by tumoricidal activity would be negated by unmanageable side effects.

Recently, increased attention has begun to be focused on the treatment of advanced cancer in the elderly. The side effects of chemotherapy in the elderly have not been as formidable as once feared, and some elderly patients with Hodgkin's disease, high-grade non-Hodgkin's lymphoma, ovarian cancer, and small cell lung cancer have been cured with systemic combination chemotherapy originally proven to be effective in younger patients (1–4). Nevertheless, coexistent medical problems and particular susceptibility to specific chemotherapy-related side effects often necessitate modifications in therapy of aged cancer patients. In addition, some cancers (e.g., breast cancer) have different natural histories in elderly versus younger adults; specific therapy has evolved in the elderly that is based on the differences in tumor biology and the responsiveness to systemic therapy.

This chapter contains a brief documentation of the increased cancer incidence in the elderly, along with some current speculations regarding the molecular and biologic basis for this increased incidence. The use of systemic treatment for advanced cancer in elderly patients and how it differs from treatment of the same cancers in younger adults are discussed in detail. Specific problems involving the use of cytotoxic drugs and radiation therapy in the elderly will be considered, followed by a discussion of several tumor types in which the tumor biology and/or therapy is distinctive in the elderly.

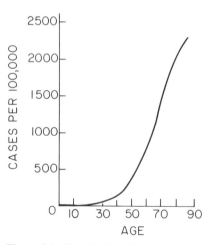

Figure 6.1   Relationship of age and cancer incidence. (Data from The Surveillance, Epidemiology, and End Results Program of the Biometry Branch, NCI.)

78

Table 6.1 Average Annual Age-Adjusted Cancer Incidence Rates per 100,000: Surveillance, Epidemiology, and End Results 1979–1981

Primary Site	Males Age in Years 45–64	Males Age in Years 65	Males Ratio Over 65/45–64	Females Age in Years 45–64	Females Age in Years 65	Females Ratio Over 65/45–65
Lung	151	482.5	3.2	70.3	128.6	1.8
Colon	50.9	278.8	5.5	45.2	216.3	4.8
Female breast	—	—	—	200.6	332.3	1.7
Prostate	61.0	635.2	10.4	—	—	—
Pancreas	16.8	69.1	4.1	11.1	48.8	4.4
Urinary bladder	38.8	185.6	4.8	11.1	44.7	4.0
All sites	586.7	2468.2	4.2	609.7	1401.1	2.3

CANCER INCIDENCE AND MORTALITY RATES IN THE ELDERLY

Cancer is one of the most serious and pervasive illnesses affecting persons 65 years of age and over. Approximately 50% of all cancers occur in patients who are older than 65 years, even though this age group currently comprises only 12% of the population (5). In addition, 60% of all cancer deaths occur after 65 years of age; the median age for all cancer deaths is 67.9 years (5). Figure 6.1 reveals the striking increase in cancer incidence with advancing age. The increase is particularly rapid after age 40 and continues to rise steadily thereafter. Further increases in cancer incidence are predicted in the future, paralleling the steadily increasing percentage of elderly people in this country.

Although certain types of cancers occur only in children and young adults, these neoplasms are rare and account for only a small fraction of the total cancer incidence. In contradistinction, most of the common types of cancer occur rarely in children and young adults and increase in incidence in the elderly (Table 6.1).

Conflicting data exist concerning the prognosis of specific cancer types in elderly when compared to younger adults. Holmes reviewed the stages of 30,991 cancer patients diagnosed between 1944 and 1977 in the regional cancer registry of Kansas and western Missouri (6). He found a significant correlation between advanced stage at diagnosis and advanced age for cancers originating at many sites, including breast, cervix, ovary, uterus, urinary bladder, stomach, and kidney. Various explanations for the later stage at diagnosis in the elderly include patient delay in seeking medical attention, increased difficulty in recognizing symptoms of cancer in the eld-

erly, reluctance of the physician to refer the elderly for treatment, and poor access by the elderly to the health care system.

The majority of current evidence, however, indicates that, for most cancer types, 5-year survival is not significantly different in the elderly age group than it is in the younger adult population. Table 6.2 shows the 5-year survival rates for several types of cancer in patients age 65 and over when compared to those age 45 to 64 as compiled by the National Cancer Institute from 1973 to 1979 (5). Elderly patients with carcinoma of the cervix, carcinoma of the endometrium, or non-Hodgkin's lymphoma have significantly worse survival than do younger adults with these diseases. The performance of regular Papanicolaou smears has been shown to decrease after the age of 40, and this delay in diagnosis presumably explains the shorter survival of elderly patients with cervical or endometrial cancers (7, 8). Successful systemic treatment of non-Hodgkin's lymphomas in young adults is responsible for the difference in survival with this disease (see below). Other cancer types show no marked differences in 5-year survival rates of elderly versus younger adults, implying that delayed diagnosis is not a major factor in the elderly.

PATHOGENESIS OF CARCINOMA IN THE ELDERLY

The precise events occurring at a molecular biologic level that give rise to a cancer are still unknown. A variety of chromosomal alterations have been suggested, including conventional mutations, movement of transposable genetic ele-

Table 6.2 Five Year Relative Survival Rates for Selected Primary Cancer Sites in Elderly>65 versus Younger Adults: Surveillance, Epidemiology, and End Results, 1973-1979

Primary Site	Males		Females	
	45–64	Over 65	45–64	Over 65
Lung	11	8	16	11
Colon	49	47	51	49
Female breast	—	—	72	72
Prostate	69	64	—	—
Pancreas	2	2	3	2
Urinary bladder	79	66	77	63
Non-Hodgkin's lymphoma	58	35	58	35
Uterine cervix	—	—	62	50
Uterine corpus	—	—	91	75
All sites	37	38	57	45

ments, and the changing expression of various regulatory genes. With the tremendous recent advances in biologic technology, it seems likely that many of the basic mechanisms responsible for cancer development will be elucidated within the decade.

The explanation for the increased incidence of cancer in the elderly is also unknown, although several hypotheses exist. The best known of these hypotheses is the concept of "immune surveillance," first proposed in 1970 by Sir MacFarlane Burnet (9). According to this theory, one function of the normal immune system is to eliminate abnormal cells that are capable of giving rise to malignant tumors. With advancing age, the immune system becomes less efficient in this function, allowing cancers to develop with greater frequency. Changes in immune function with advancing age are now well documented. Involution of the thymus, which begins during adolescence, results in decreased numbers of regulatory T cells (10) and a decreased proliferative T-cell response to various mitogens (11). Clinically, these changes result in impaired delayed cutaneous hypersensitivity in the majority of elderly patients (12). In addition, humoral immune responses also decline with age; impaired interaction between T and B lymphocytes, rather than any intrinsic defect in B cell function, is responsible (13). The increased incidence of certain types of cancer in association with immunosuppression (drug-induced, congenital, or acquired) also supports the likelihood of a connection between the development of cancer and the immune system (14).

The "immune surveillance" concept, however, is not sufficient in itself to explain the age-related increase in cancer incidence. Although persons who are immunosuppressed are at increased risk for certain types of cancer (in particular, lymphoproliferative neoplasms), their incidence of other cancers is not increased (15). Furthermore, the risk of cancer does not rise after thymectomy. Most current research on tumorogenesis is centered on fundamental chromosomal alterations, rather than changes in the host immune system.

The process of aging is also associated with genomic rearrangements; these chromosomal changes may be responsible for increased malignant transformation. Several inherited disorders that involve abnormalities in DNA repair or recombination have a high incidence of cancer development (16); these same diseases also have early onset and accelerated progression of biologic aging in one or more organ systems (17). Although aging cells maintain a grossly stable diploid karyotype on cytogenetic analysis, subtle changes in DNA content of older cells have been identified (18, 19). These age-related DNA abnormalities may prove to be intimately involved in the process of carcinogenesis.

Finally, there are some investigators who doubt that advanced age per se is associated with an increased susceptibility to the process of carcinogenesis (20, 21). Rather, they postulate that the development of cancer is the final step in a multi-step process of carcinogenesis that results from cumulative, life-long exposure to carcinogens. Some epidemiologic data support this concept; the development of lung cancer in smokers and of mesothelioma following asbestos exposure both depend upon the dose and duration of exposure to the carcinogen, rather than upon patient age (22, 23).

It is likely that increased mutagenicity of aged cells, alterations in immune function, and cumulative exposure to various carcinogens all play a role in the increased incidence of cancer in the elderly. Identification of the relative importance of each of these factors awaits further advances in the understanding of carcinogenesis.

THE USE OF CYTOTOXIC DRUGS IN THE ELDERLY

All drugs in current use for the systemic treatment of cancer, with the exception of a few hormonal agents, are cytotoxic agents. These drugs interfere with cell replication in a variety of ways, including direct damage to DNA (alkylating agents), inhibition of synthesis of DNA/RNA precursors (antimetabolites), and interference with the mitotic mechanism (vinca alkaloids). Because cell replication is very similar in normal and neoplastic cells, the therapeutic/toxic ratio of most antineoplastic agents is low, and side effects occur frequently with the use of these agents. Cancer patients with poor physical performance status at the time of treatment have been repeatedly shown to experience more severe side effects when these agents are used.

Based on this observation, it has been assumed that the use of antineoplastic agents in elderly patients would cause prohibitive side effects. In fact, many cooperative cancer study groups have excluded patients over the age of 70 from chemotherapy trials and have routinely reduced doses of cytotoxic drugs in patients between 60–70 years of age (24). However, as chemotherapeutic treatments have become the standard of care in the optimal therapy of many types of neoplasms, the feasibility of treating elderly patients has become a subject of renewed interest. It is now clear that some types of combination chemotherapy are well tolerated by elderly patients, although certain drugs must be used with caution. The very intensive treatment regimens used in potentially curable neoplasms (e.g., non-Hodgkin's lymphomas, acute leukemia) remain difficult to administer safely in the aged patient.

Single Agents

Specific chemotherapy-related side effects that are seen more commonly in elderly patients are listed in Table 6.3. These side effects are not peculiar to the elderly, but are seen with greater frequency and are more severe than in younger patients.

Although many of the antineoplastic drugs cause myelosuppression, only methotrexate and the nitrosoureas have been particularly myelo-

Table 6.3 Antineoplastic Drugs Associated with Increased Toxicity in the Elderly

Drug	Toxicity Increased in Elderly	Comment	References
Methotrexate	Myelosuppression	Decreased glomerular filtration rate causes delayed excretion.	24, 25
Doxorubicin (Adriamycin)	Congestive heart failure	Pre-existing heart disease increases risk.	26, 27
Bleomycin	Pulmonary fibrosis	Pre-existing lung disease increases risk.	28
Vinca alkaloids (vincristine, vinblastine)	Neurotoxicity	Pre-existing neurologic dysfunction increases risk.	29
Nitrosoureas	Myelosuppression		24
Glucocorticoids	Hyperglycemia		

toxic in the elderly (24). Myelosuppression due to methotrexate is related to the dose administered and the duration of exposure; the decreased glomerular filtration rate in most elderly patients delays excretion of methotrexate, increases duration of exposure, and therefore results in increased myelosuppression (30). Methotrexate can be used safely in elderly patients when the dose is modified based on the creatinine clearance (31). The nitrosoureas can be associated with prolonged myelosuppression even in young patients, and this side effect is worse in the elderly. This class of agents should be avoided in the elderly or used at significantly reduced doses.

Cardiotoxicity associated with the use of doxorubicin (Adriamycin) is a serious complication and is seen with increased frequency in the elderly (26, 27). Cumulative doxorubicin dose remains the most significant predictor of cardiotoxicity, and elderly patients have a low incidence of problems with a total dose less than 450 mg/m². The increased incidence of congestive heart failure in elderly patients is probably related to pre-existing cardiac problems. Patients with significant congestive heart failure (i.e., ejection fraction less than 40%) are poor candidates for doxorubicin administered by the standard dosing schedule (i.e., large doses at 3-week intervals). These patients may tolerate administration of low-dose doxorubicin on a weekly basis, which has been associated with a reduced incidence of cardiotoxicity (32).

Bleomycin is associated with pulmonary fibrosis, which increases in incidence and severity when the cumulative bleomycin dose exceeds 300 units. This side effect occurs with increased incidence in elderly patients and is probably related to pre-existent chronic pulmonary disease. Although bleomycin-induced pulmonary fibrosis is irreversible, its development can be monitored with serial pulmonary function tests; particularly important is the measurement of diffusing capacity (DLCO). Patients of any age who have severe restrictive lung disease should not receive bleomycin therapy.

The vinca alkaloids (vincristine, vinblastine) can be associated with neurotoxicity, which is also related to the cumulative dose. Peripheral neuropathy is the most common manifestation of neurotoxicity and is seen with greater frequency

and severity in the elderly, particularly in those with pre-existing neurologic deficits. Although vinca-alkaloid-induced neurotoxicity is slowly reversible, it can be very disabling; the vinca alkaloids should therefore be used with great caution in the elderly and should be discontinued if significant peripheral neuropathy develops.

Combination Chemotherapy

The treatment of elderly patients with combination chemotherapy regimens has been approached with some trepidation in the past, and as a result, data regarding side effects are limited. However, a recent retrospective review by the Eastern Cooperative Oncology Group (ECOG) revealed surprisingly few problems in elderly versus younger patients and has provided impetus for inclusion of the elderly in current drug trials (24). Nineteen combination chemotherapy regimens used in studies involving eight different types of cancer were retrospectively reviewed, and elderly patients (over 70 years) were found to have identical rates of severe toxicity as their younger counterparts, with the exception of increased myelosuppression associated with methotrexate and methyl-CCNU (discussed above) (24). In addition, elderly patients had similar tumor response rates and survival rates when compared to the younger patients. It was recommended that physiologic functional parameters, such as measures of renal, liver, and bone marrow function, or physical performance status be the basis of patient selection for chemotherapy, rather than age.

Although the ECOG study provides important data, several factors may limit the strength of its conclusions. Most of the types of cancer studied were relatively unresponsive to chemotherapy, and the regimens used were of moderate intensity. In addition, only a minority of the patients in each study group were older than 70 years (e.g., 10% of lung cancer patients), indicating a probable selection bias with inclusion of only unusually healthy elderly patients. Nevertheless, the data from this study have led to the increased willingness of investigators to consider the inclusion of elderly patients in many cooperative group studies, and further data will be available from those trials in the near future.

The treatment of elderly patients with the intensive combination chemotherapy regimens used in the treatment of potentially curable neoplasms has been especially difficult. In these demanding regimens, drugs are administered in maximally tolerated doses, and the interval between doses is minimized. The duration of treatment in these rigorous protocols is only 4–6 months, and the significant acute toxicity encountered during treatment is considered to be acceptable because long-term survival is the goal of treatment. Decreases in drug dosage and delays between doses have consistently resulted in lower cure rates. Specific problems with these intensive regimens when used in elderly patients include increased severity and duration of myelosuppression, declining physical performance status, severe muscular weakness, anorexia, and weight loss. These problems necessitate dose reductions and delays between doses and invariably result in lower cure rates. Difficulties encountered in the course of administering intensive regimens of combination chemotherapy are discussed more specifically in the sections on Hodgkin's disease, non-Hodgkin's lymphoma, and acute leukemia.

In summary, the use of combination chemotherapy is feasible and beneficial in many elderly patients. Regimens of moderate intensity that are used to produce tumor remissions and prolongation of survival (e.g., those used in metastatic breast cancer) can be used with similar results and toxicity in patients of all ages. Certain chemotherapeutic agents must be used with caution in the elderly, particularly if specific organ dysfunction exists prior to treatment. (Table 6.3) Although some elderly patients with Hodgkin's disease, non-Hodgkin's lymphoma, and acute leukemia can be cured with chemotherapy regimens, the very intensive treatments required to cure these neoplasms are difficult to administer in the aged patient, and the results are still inferior in the elderly. However, because other curative modalities do not exist for these diseases, all elderly patients with reasonably good general health sould be considered for an attempt at curative chemotherapy.

Radiation Therapy

Radiation therapy currently plays an integral role in the treatment of many cancers. Although most frequently used to provide relief of local symptoms in patients with advanced cancer, radiation therapy may be used as the primary curative modality in several malignancies, including testicular seminoma, early stage Hodgkin's disease, and some types of carcinomas of the head and neck, uterus, cervix, and endometrium. Radiation therapy can produce distinctive acute and chronic tissue toxicity. Although radiation tolerance in elderly patients has not been specifically studied, it is generally accepted that the tolerance of normal tissues to irradiation is about 10%–15% less in elderly patients. Acute radiation effects are found largely on tissues with rapid rates of cell renewal, such as bone marrow, skin, oropharyngeal mucosa, gastrointestinal tract, vaginal mucosa, and bladder mucosa. Acute radiation damage to these tissues depends not only on the radiation dose but also on the rate of administration. Short breaks between doses of radiation or decreases in radiation fraction size can allow sufficient time for tissue repair and can minimize acute toxicity. With modern radiotherapy equipment, acute toxicities can usually be minimized, particularly in patients in whom a relatively low, palliative dose of radiation is being administered. In addition to direct tissue effects, elderly patients are also more prone to experience constitutional symptoms, such as fatigue, weakness, anorexia, and weight loss, during courses of radiotherapy.

The chronic side effects of radiotherapy are potentially more serious and are much more dependent on total dose of radiation administered. Late effects include tissue necrosis, fibrosis, fistula formation, non-healing ulceration, and damage to specific organs. Unfortunately, the effective tumoricidal radiation doses for some tumor types (e.g., head and neck cancers, cervical cancer, non-small cell lung cancer) are very close to those doses that will produce major chronic tissue damage. In elderly patients whose tissues are less tolerant of large doses of radiation, side effects are more frequent. In addition, pre-existing impairment of specific organs can enhance their susceptibility to chronic radiation damage. An example of this problem, which is frequently encountered, is the difficulty in administering palliative doses of radiation therapy to elderly patients with non-small cell lung cancer in the face of significant pre-existing underlying pulmonary emphysema.

In spite of the mildly increased risk for chronic side effects, most elderly patients are able to receive radiation therapy without major problems. Tumor response to radiotherapy in the elderly seems to be identical to that in younger patients. The decision to use radiotherapy in either a palliative or a potentially curative role in the treatment of cancer should not be made on the basis of age.

CANCERS WITH DISTINCTIVE CLINICAL FEATURES AND/OR THERAPEUTIC CONSIDERATIONS IN THE ELDERLY

Breast Cancer

In recent years, recognition of a number of clinical and pathologic prognostic factors has helped to explain the long-observed heterogeneity of patients with breast cancer. Age at the time of diagnosis is an important determinant of both tumor biology and prognosis; it is therefore not surprising that treatment recommendations for elderly women with breast cancer differ from those in younger women. The primary surgical therapy of breast cancer in elderly women is discussed elsewhere in this text. (See Chapter 14) This section will highlight some of the differences in tumor biology and discuss recommended systemic therapy in elderly women with advanced breast cancer.

Tumor Biology

The clinical profiles of young and old women with breast cancer are contrasted in Table 6.4. Considerable overlap exists; however, the differ-

Table 6.4 Clinical Profile of Young versus Elderly Patients with Breast Cancer

Clinical Feature	Young	Old
Estrogen receptor	Negative	Positive
Histopathology	Poorly differentiated	Well differentiated
Growth rate	Fast	Slow
Metastatic sites	Viscera	Bone, soft tissue
Prognosis	Poor	Good

ences in the parameters listed are substantial and help in part to explain the differences in response to therapy.

The measurement of cytosolic estrogen receptor levels in breast cancer cells is of great value both prognostically and therapeutically. Estrogen receptors are present (greater than 10 fm/g) in approximately 50% of patients with breast cancer; however, the incidence of estrogen receptor positivity increases steadily with age. Sixty percent of postmenopausal women have cancers that are estrogen receptor positive; this figure rises to 70%–80% in women over the age of 75 (33). The estrogen receptor status of the tumor is the most powerful predictor of hormonal responsiveness; 60% of patients with estrogen receptor positive tumors respond to hormonal therapy, whereas fewer than 10% of those with estrogen receptor negative tumors respond (34). Therefore, hormonal therapy is much more frequently an effective therapeutic option in elderly patients with metastatic breast cancer than it is in the younger patient.

The presence of estrogen receptors in malignant breast tumors is also a favorable prognostic factor, independent of therapy. Although the status of the axillary lymph nodes at the time of primary therapy remains the most important prognostic factor, patients whose tumors have estrogen receptors present have a lower recurrence rate than do those tumors of similar stage that lack estrogen receptors. In patients with stage II breast cancer and whose tumors have positive estrogen receptors, the prognostic importance of estrogen receptor status outweighs the importance of axillary lymph node status. These patients have comparable or slightly better survival than do patients with stage I estrogen receptor negative tumors (35, 36). In addition, patients with estrogen receptor positive tumors that do recur have a longer disease-free interval (mastectomy to recurrence) and a longer survival with metastatic disease than do patients whose tumors are estrogen receptor negative (34, 37).

The other clinical and pathologic features, listed in Table 6.4, are related to estrogen receptor status of the tumor, as well as to patient age. Histologically, well-differentiated tumors are much more likely to be estrogen receptor positive (38); these tumors also have a lower rate of

Table 6.5 Adjuvant Chemotherapy for Breast Cancer: Comparison of Results in Premenopausal and Postmenopausal Women

Trial	Follow-Up Yr	Premenopausal Total	Premenopausal 1–3 Nodes	Premenopausal More than 3 Nodes	Postmenopausal Total	Postmenopausal 1–3 Nodes	Postmenopausal More than 3 Nodes
NSABP[a] (44)	5						
L-PAM[b]		60	75	40	48	60	35
Placebo		40	52	30	52	68	35
Milan (45)	8						
CMF[c] × 12 mos		56	71	26	37	40	30
No treatment		33	43	6	34	38	25
Southwest Oncology Group (46)	4						
L-PAM		51	64	41	54	72	40
CMFVP[d]		75	90	67	73	89	60

[a]NASBP=National Surgical Adjuvant Breast Program
[b]L-PAM=Alkeran
[c]CMF=Cyclophosphamide, methotrexate, 5-fluorouracil
[d]CMFVP=CMF + vincristine, prednisone

proliferative activity (39). Sites of recurrence are also related to estrogen receptor status. Recurrences in bone and soft tissue are more frequent in women with estrogen receptor positive tumors, whereas visceral, particularly hepatic, involvement is seen more frequently in patients with estrogen receptor negative tumors (40, 41).

Two important prognostic factors are not age dependent. First, the stage at diagnosis is similar in young and elderly women. Second, the progesterone receptor status of the tumor, which is an independent prognostic variable, is unrelated to age (42, 43). Many elderly patients therefore have adverse prognostic features at the time of diagnosis, and the cancer will recur despite optimal primary therapy.

Adjuvant Therapy

The administration of systemic therapy to breast cancer patients at risk for recurrence after primary surgical therapy (i.e., patients with involved axillary lymph nodes) has altered the natural history of breast cancer. Several large randomized studies have demonstrated 15%–20% improvement in disease-free survival and overall survival rates at 5–10 years in patients who received adjuvant chemotherapy when compared with those who received no treatment following primary therapy (44–46). However, premenopausal women have derived the major benefits from these treatments, whereas identical chemotherapy in postmenopausal patients has been less effective. Table 6.5 compares the results of adjuvant chemotherapy in premenopausal and postmenopausal women. Two large trials demonstrated no benefit in postmenopausal women, whereas a consistent benefit was demonstrated in premenopausal patients.

The relative lack of efficacy of adjuvant chemotherapy in the postmenopausal age group is incompletely explained, but is probably related to a number of factors. The dose and scheduling of adjuvant chemotherapy have been important, with regimens of increased intensity producing better results (47). In one large study, postmenopausal women receiving adjuvant cyclophosphamide, methotrexate, and 5-fluorouracil (CMF) were found to have received lower doses because of poor tolerance; postmenopausal women receiving greater than 75% of the planned dose were found to have survival benefits equivalent to those observed in premenopausal patients (48). However, this dose-response relationship has not been sufficient

Table 6.6 Adjuvant Tamoxifen Therapy in Postmenopausal Women with Stage II Breast Cancer[a]

Group	Tamoxifen Dose mg/day	Duration of Tamoxifen mos	Other Treatment	Median Follow-Up mos	Increase in Relapse-Free Survival	Increase in Overall Survival
Nolvadex trial (51)	20	24	Rad Rx	35	Yes	No
Pritchard et al. (52)	30	24	Rad Rx	37	Yes	No
Wallgren (53)	40	24	None	30	Yes	No
Ribeiro and Palmer (54)	20	12	Rad Rx	—	Yes	No
Cummings et al. (55)	20	24	None	41	Yes	No

[a]All trials contain more than 150 women.

to explain the inferior results in postmenopausal women in other studies. It is likely that the distinctive biology of breast cancer occurring in elderly women also plays a role. The NSABP adjuvant studies have shown a lack of benefit from adjuvant chemotherapy in women with well-differentiated tumors (most common in elderly women), whereas women with poorly differentiated tumors derive benefit from adjuvant chemotherapy regardless of age (49). In a randomized prospective trial, the Ludwig Breast Cancer Study Group (Switzerland) found no benefit when chemotherapy was added to hormonal adjuvant therapy in postmenopausal women with estrogen receptor positive tumors, but documented a marked benefit from chemotherapy in postmenopausal women whose tumors were estrogen receptor negative (50). These data indicate that some subsets of postmenopausal breast cancer patients are likely to benefit from adjuvant chemotherapy. However, definitive recommendations await the results of randomized trials that are currently in progress.

Adjuvant hormonal therapy is an attractive option in postmenopausal women, because of the high frequency of tumors with estrogen receptor positivity and the early discouraging results with adjuvant chemotherapy in this group. Several large randomized trials comparing adjuvant tamoxifen to no treatment in postmenopausal women have been reported and are summarized in Table 6.6. Although these trials have differed slightly in design (dose and duration of tamoxifen administration, use of postoperative chest wall irradiation), all have demonstrated an increase in disease-free survival in the tamoxifen-treated groups. Predictably, patients who had tumors with high levels of estrogen receptors derived the greatest benefit. In most studies, patients with three or more axillary lymph nodes involved with metastases derived greater benefit than did those with fewer than three involved nodes when compared to similar patients who received no treatment. Although increase in overall survival has not been reported, this may be due to short follow-up time, because many elderly women who relapse with breast cancer live several years with metastatic disease. If the differences in disease-free survival persist, overall survival benefits should emerge with further follow-up.

In summary, adjuvant therapy in postmenopausal women with stage II breast cancer differs from that proven effective in premenopausal women, probably due to the different tumor biology in these two groups. Adjuvant hormonal therapy with tamoxifen is effective in prolonging relapse-free survival in postmenopausal women with stage II estrogen receptor positive breast cancer and is the treatment of choice. There is no evidence that higher doses than the standard 20 mg/day improve results; the optimal duration of tamoxifen therapy is not yet clear, but it should be at least 24 months. The role of adjuvant chemotherapy in postmenopausal women is also unclear. However, it is probable that postmenopausal women with estrogen receptor negative tumors benefit from adjuvant chemotherapy if the treatment can be given according to prescribed dose and schedule. At the present time, there is no evidence to suggest that combined chemo-hormonal therapy is of any greater benefit than either modality used singly for any subset of postmenopausal women. There is also no evidence that postmenopausal women with stage I breast cancer should receive or will benefit from adjuvant therapy.

Metastatic Disease

The guidelines for therapy of metastatic breast cancer in elderly women do not differ appreciably from those currently used in younger women. At present, metastatic breast cancer is considered to be an incurable disease, although appropriate treatment can palliate symptoms, provide meaningful remissions, and prolong survival in many patients. The general goal of therapy for metastatic breast cancer is to provide patients with the best and longest remissions possible while minimizing the side effects of the palliative treatment. In patients with hormonally responsive tumors, hormonal therapy usually provides longer remissions with less toxicity than does chemotherapy, and it should always be the first type of systemic therapy considered for estrogen receptor positive tumors in postmenopausal women. Even postmenopausal women whose tumors are estrogen receptor negative but who have clinical features suggestive of estrogen positive tumors (e.g., well-differentiated histology, long disease-free interval, soft tissue or bone metastases) should be considered for a trial of hormonal therapy because estrogen receptor determinations in breast tumors sometimes give false negative results for a variety of reasons (56). Patients should receive a trial of hor-

monal therapy for 4–6 weeks; patients whose tumors respond favorably should then continue therapy as long as the response persists. Tamoxifen is usually the first drug used for hormonal therapy of breast cancer in postmenopausal women because of its ease of administration. Patients who have a relapse after an initial response to hormonal therapy often can achieve a second hormonal response with a different agent (e.g., progesterone, aminoglutethimide). The average duration of the first hormonal response is approximately 18 months; however, some patients will have remissions that last several years.

Chemotherapy should be considered in patients whose tumors have become refractory to hormonal therapy or in those patients who have estrogen receptor negative tumors with visceral metastases. As in younger patients, chemotherapy with a combination of agents yields higher response rates and remissions of longer duration (57). The problems with chemotherapy tolerance in elderly patients have been discussed earlier. In general, regimens that are used for palliative treatment of breast cancer are of mild to moderate toxicity and can usually be tolerated by elderly patients. If doxorubicin (Adriamycin) is to be used, a low-dose, weekly schedule is usually tolerated better than a higher dose given every 3 weeks. Approximately 60% of patients achieve a remission with initial chemotherapy; average remission duration is 12 months.

The patient with metastatic breast cancer, therefore, usually receives a series of treatments with various hormonal and/or chemotherapeutic agents and can have a series of remissions to sequential treatments. The use of combined chemotherapy and hormonal therapy or the use of more than one hormonal agent simultaneously has not been shown to increase remission duration or overall survival and should be avoided (58).

Hodgkin's Disease

The natural history and prognosis of Hodgkin's disease have been radically changed by the development of effective radiotherapy techniques and active combination chemotherapy. Optimal therapy now produces long-term disease-free survival in 75% of patients, whereas this disease was formerly uniformly fatal. Although the malignant cell of origin of Hodgkin's disease is still unknown, most current evidence suggests that the Reed-Sternberg cell is a monocyte-derived cell that is involved in antigen processing in the T-lymphocyte system. Important differences between young and elderly patients with respect to the clinical features and treatment results have been appreciated only recently.

Hodgkin's disease is one of the few diseases that demonstrates a bimodal age incidence pattern, with the largest incidence peak occurring in young adults and a second small peak in the fifth and sixth decades of life. Several differences have been observed in the clinical and pathologic features of Hodgkin's disease in these two age groups. *First,* the histology differs, with young adults having a higher incidence of nodular sclerosing and lymphocyte-predominant subtypes, whereas elderly adults more often have tumors with mixed cellularity or lymphocyte-depleted histologic features (59). *Second,* a higher percentage of elderly patients with Hodgkin's disease have advanced stages (III or IV) at the time of diagnosis. This may be partially related to delay by older patients in seeking medical aid, but is more probably related to the higher incidence of histologically unfavorable tumors in elderly patients (60). *Third,* several epidemiologic features distinguish young from elderly persons who develop Hodgkin's disease. Factors in the childhood environment associated with a higher incidence of Hodgkin's disease in the young age group include later age of exposure to common viruses, small sibship size, higher level of parental education, and living in single-family houses (61). None of these factors seems important in the elderly age group; in fact, the socioeconomic background of elderly people with Hodgkin's disease was somewhat below average (61, 62). These differences have led to continued speculation that the etiology of Hodgkin's disease differs in the young and elderly age groups. Although the true etiology remains unknown, many feel that Hodgkin's disease in young adults develops as the result of an abnormal response to certain viral exposures, whereas Hodgkin's disease in the elderly develops by a mechanism more similar to the development of other lymphomas in this age group (61, 62).

Prior to the development of curative therapy for Hodgkin's disease, median survival in elderly patients was significantly worse than in younger patients (60). This finding was not surprising because the higher stage and more unfavorable histologic tumor types are seen in the elderly age group. However, even with the highly effective treatments currently available, age continues to be an independent prognostic factor (1, 63–66). In a large Swedish study, the 5-year survival estimate was 28% in patients older than 50 years compared to 74% in younger patients (65). In this study, marked differences persisted even in patients with clinical stages I and II (95% versus 55% actuarial 5-year survival) (67). Other groups reported more optimistic data for their elderly patients with early stage Hodgkin's disease. The group at Stanford University has reported an 86% 5-year survival in a small group of elderly patients with Hodgkin's disease who had pathologic stages I to IIIA disease and who were treated with definitive radiotherapy (1). They stressed the importance of strict pathologic staging with laparotomy to determine optimal treatment in these patients. They found that their patients with "early" stage Hodgkin's disease diagnosed on the basis of clinical staging alone had a much lower survival with radiotherapy (35%).

Results of treatment in elderly patients with advanced stage Hodgkin's disease (i.e., stages IIIB, IV) are inferior to treatment results in younger patients in all series. Difficulty in administering combination chemotherapy at optimal dose and on the correct schedule has been commonly reported. In one report, only 8 of 18 elderly patients were able to receive 70% or more of the ideal calculated doses (1). Because the dose of the chemotherapy has proven to be a critical factor in the outcome of treatment of advanced Hodgkin's disease, this problem in elderly patients is almost certainly a contributing factor to the lower cure rates. In addition, the possibility that Hodgkin's disease in the elderly is a biologically distinct and different entity must be considered and may also partially explain the different treatment results.

In spite of the inferior results of treatment in elderly patients, Hodgkin's disease nevertheless is a curable disease in some aged patients. Elderly patients with Hodgkin's disease should be carefully staged, including a staging laparotomy in patients with clinical stage I or II disease. Following staging, all patients should be considered for appropriate curative therapy, which usually includes radiotherapy for stages I and II and either chemotherapy or combined modality therapy (radiotherapy plus chemotherapy) for stages III and IV. Radiotherapy and chemotherapy techniques should be identical to those used in younger patients; some elderly patients will tolerate a full course of therapy and may achieve long-term survival.

Non-Hodgkin's Lymphoma

During the past 15 years, substantial progress has been made in both the understanding and the management of the non-Hodgkin's lymphomas. Improved pathologic techniques have enabled recognition of several types of non-Hodgkin's lymphoma, each with a definable cell of origin and distinctive clinical behavior. Treatment for the high-grade, or aggressive, lymphomas has improved greatly; formerly, this group of lymphomas was uniformly fatal with a median survival of 5–6 months. Fifty to 70% of patients can now be cured with appropriate systemic chemotherapy (68–70).

The spectrum of non-Hodgkin's lymphoma in elderly patients is different from that of younger adults, because indolent (low-grade) lymphomas occur much more frequently in the elderly. Recognition and appropriate management of these lymphomas are important. Prolonged survival without treatment occurs in many patients. In addition, the treatment of high-grade lymphomas poses special problems in the elderly because curative regimens for these lymphomas are very intensive.

Indolent Lymphomas

Approximately 70% of lymphomas developing in patients over 60 years of age can be categorized as "indolent" or low grade. Histologically most of these lymphomas retain nodular characteristics, reminiscent of the nodules seen in normal lymph nodes. Immunologic typing has revealed that most of these lymphomas are derived from B cells. Individual malignant cells are usually small and can either be cleaved cells derived from the follicular centers of the lymph nodes or have small round nuclei similar to the "normal appearing" lymphocytes seen in chronic lymphocytic leukemia. Clinical presentation is variable, but most patients initially develop asymptomatic enlarging lymph nodes in multiple lymph node groups. Fluctuation in size of the lymph nodes is common, and spontaneous decrease in lymph node size is observed in 20%–25% of patients. The majority of patients have asymptomatic bone marrow involvement with lymphoma at the time of diagnosis. Extranodal sites of involvement are uncommon early in the disease course, but can become problematic in the later stages.

Although these lymphomas are sensitive to available chemotherapeutic agents and to radiation therapy, these treatments are not curative in patients with indolent lymphomas. Even patients who achieve complete responses to therapy invariably relapse. In one recent series of patients with low-grade non-Hodgkin's lymphomas who were initially followed without treatment until symptoms occurred, actuarial survival was 82% at 5 years and 73% at 10 years (71). Because of the remarkable longevity of many patients with indolent lymphomas, vigorous systemic therapy is no longer employed.

Indications for treatment in this group of patients include local symptoms due to bulky adenopathy, cytopenias due to bone marrow involvement, symptomatic extranodal involvement (e.g., gastrointestinal, lung), or constitutional symptoms (e.g., fever, sweats, weight loss). Optimal treatment varies according to the clinical situation; local symptoms can often be effectively managed with a course of local radiation therapy, whereas systemic problems are usually managed with short courses of chemotherapy. Due to the indolent nature of many of these lymphomas, chemotherapy-induced partial remissions can provide prolonged palliation. Because achievement of complete remission is not an important goal, fewer drugs can be used at lower dosages. Therefore, effective management of these low-grade lymphomas is possible in elderly patients in whom local radiotherapy and moderate doses of chemotherapy are well tolerated. Because prolonged survival is the rule in these patients, careful follow-up and appropriate treatment of intercurrent problems are essential.

High-Grade Lymphomas

Most lymphomas in this group are included in the diffuse histiocytic and undifferentiated lymphoma categories in the Rappaport classification system. Almost all non-Hodgkin's lymphomas developing in young patients (less than 40 years of age) are high grade, compared to only 30% of all lymphomas in elderly patients. Although potentially curative treatments are available even for patients with advanced stages, the effective treatment of high-grade lymphomas in the elderly has been very difficult. Curative regimens for these lymphomas are among the most intensive chemotherapy regimens used in medical oncology and involve multiple cytotoxic agents given at frequent intervals (2, 68, 69). Attempts to use these regimens in elderly patients have resulted in marked toxicity and increased treatment-related mortality when compared to younger age groups (2, 71). Dose reductions and prolongation of the intervals between doses are often necessary due to poor tolerance. However, achievement of complete remission and long-term survival is possible in some elderly patients, and due to the dismal prognosis without effective treatment, elderly patients without other severe problems should be considered for an attempt at curative therapy. Currently, attempts are being made to design effective regimens that exclude drugs particularly problematic in the elderly (e.g., vincristine, doxorubicin).

In summary, the treatment of high-grade lymphoma in the elderly is fraught with difficulties, but curative treatment can be administered to some patients. Unlike breast cancer and Hodgkin's disease in the elderly, there is no suggestion that different tumor biology is responsible for the the lower complete response rates; rather, inferior results are due to our inability to administer effective treatment to many elderly patients.

Acute Leukemia

The treatment of adult acute leukemia has improved steadily in recent years, so that 70%–80% of patients currently achieve complete remission (72). A variety of very intensive regimens have resulted in 20%–40% 5-year relapse-free survival (73–75). In patients receiving optimal chemotherapy, age is the most important determinant of complete response rate and overall survival. Complete responses are currently achieved in greater than 80% of young adults (16–40 years of age), in 65% of patients aged 40–60 years, and in only 30%–55% of patients over the age of 60 (76). Although some groups have reported a similar survival for all adults who achieve complete remission, others have noted shorter median duration of complete remission in elderly patients (77).

Inferior results in the treatment of acute leukemia in elderly patients are primarily due to difficulty in administering the necessary treatment. Successful remission induction in acute leukemia requires 4 to 6 weeks of chemotherapy-induced bone marrow aplasia. Serious infection and/or bleeding during this period occurs with great frequency in elderly patients; early mortality from these complications is the major explanation for the lower complete response rate and shorter median survival in elderly patients. Even after obtaining a complete remission, further intensive treatment is necessary to maximize remission duration. Again, elderly patients are unable to tolerate this type of therapy well. Allogeneic bone marrow transplantation following the achievement of a complete remission is considered by most to be the treatment of choice in young adults with acute leukemia (75). Prohibitive problems with graft versus host disease occur in patients over 40 years of age, and therefore this treatment is not available to elderly patients (78, 79).

Currently, the achievement of complete remission remains the only treatment outcome that offers patients a chance for prolonged survival with this disease. Although less intensive chemotherapy produces bone marrow aplasia of shorter duration, this type of therapy is also much less effective in producing complete remissions. Therefore, if acute leukemia is to be treated in an elderly patient, the initial treatment should be similar to that which has proven most useful in younger patients. Meticulous attention must be paid to early identification and treatment of infection, and intensive platelet support during marrow aplasia must be provided. In spite of the best available supportive care, a higher incidence of complications will occur in elderly patients. Once complete remission is achieved, elderly patients should be given further treatments to prolong remission if these can be tolerated; the optimal regimen for this purpose in elderly patients is unclear.

Ovarian Carcinoma

Adenocarcinoma of the ovary is usually advanced when diagnosed and remains the leading cause of death among cancers of the female genitourinary tract. Treatment with cisplatin-based combination chemotherapy regimens can produce surgically documented complete remissions in 19%–35% of women with intra-abdominal spread of tumor (i.e., stage III or IV) (3, 80). Many women achieving complete remissions have been followed for more than 5 years without evidence of relapse; approximately 10%–15% of all women with advanced ovarian cancer can therefore be cured with combination chemotherapy.

The incidence of ovarian cancer increases with age, and at the present time, there is no evidence for any distinctive tumor biology that is age related. Elderly women can be treated with the drug combinations necessary to achieve optimal results, and complete remissions have been documented in women over the age of 70. Therefore, treatment of advanced ovarian cancer should not be modified because of age; all elderly patients who have advanced ovarian cancer and who are not completely bedridden should be considered candidates for this therapy.

Small Cell Lung Cancer

Combination chemotherapy is effective in prolonging survival in patients with small cell carcinoma of the lung. With optimal therapy, median survival is approximately 12 months compared to a median survival of 2–3 months in untreated patients. Ten to 20% of patients with limited stage small cell lung cancer (confined to the chest at diagnosis) survive more than 2 years following chemotherapy, and many of these 2-year survivors are cured (4). As with ovarian cancer, the incidence of small cell lung cancer increases with age, and therefore, most of the information concerning chemotherapeutic results in this disease has been obtained in patients older than 50 years. Elderly patients seem to have a similar natural history and response to treatment to younger patients and should therefore be con-

sidered for the same combination chemotherapy treatments. Because the regimens used to treat small cell lung cancer are intensive, elderly patients will have a higher incidence of certain side effects, including severe myelosuppression, peripheral neuropathy from vincristine, and generalized constitutional symptoms (fatigue, anorexia, weight loss). The use of reduced drug doses results in shorter remission duration and essentially eliminates the possibility of long-term survival. Therefore, all patients should receive standard doses initially; reduced doses should be used only after poor tolerance is demonstrated.

SUMMARY AND OVERVIEW

The field of medical oncology is relatively new and continues to undergo rapid change as new systemic treatments are developed. It is therefore not surprising that problems peculiar to elderly patients with advanced malignancy are only beginning to be studied. Although this chapter has focused on differences that exist between young and elderly patients with cancer, it must be emphasized that *most* decisions in the treatment of the cancer patient should not be made on the basis of age. Surgical excision remains the only curative therapy for most types of cancer. All elderly patients with neoplasms amenable to surgical therapy should be considered for the same types of cancer operations that are offered to younger patients. Too often, elderly patients are felt to be poor candidates for radical cancer operations due to "severe" coexistent chronic medical problems. These patients receive less radical operations or nonsurgical palliative treatments and often die subsequently of metastatic cancer while their "severe" medical problems remain stable. Surgical therapy for most of the various types of cancer is discussed elsewhere in this text.

The adult malignancies for which potentially curative chemotherapy exists have been discussed separately in this chapter. Results of treatment of these neoplasms have been inferior in elderly patients. Although differences in tumor biology may play a role, the difficulties in administering intensive combination chemotherapy regimens to elderly patients are probably the major cause of treatment failure. Because cure is achievable in some elderly patients (albeit a lower percentage), all elderly patients with a reasonable performance status should receive a trial of therapy with an intensive, potentially curative regimen. Dose and scheduling of drugs are crucial when administering these regimens, and the potential for cure is lost when doses are routinely diminished. Therefore, treatment regimens should not be altered on the basis of age in patients undergoing therapy with curative intent.

The majority of patients receiving chemotherapy have incurable neoplasms and are being treated to prolong survival and/or to palliate symptoms. Chemotherapy regimens used in these situations are much less intensive than are those used in the treatment of potentially curable tumors. Recent data indicate that elderly patients tolerate most palliative chemotherapy regimens as well as do younger patients. Therefore, elderly patients who have cancers for which palliative treatments exist should be considered for a trial of chemotherapy.

Further advances in the field of medical oncology await the development of more effective and less toxic drugs. Elderly patients are now routinely included in trials of new therapeutic regimens; therefore, further improvements in our understanding of age-related differences in cancer biology and treatment are likely in the near future.

REFERENCES

1. Austin-Seymour MM, Hoppe RT, Cox RS, Rosenberg SA, Kaplan HS: Hodgkin's disease in patients over sixty years old. *Ann Intern Med* 100:13–18, 1984.
2. Klimo P, Connors JM: MACOP-B chemotherapy for the treatment of diffuse large-cell lymphoma. *Ann Intern Med* 102:596–602, 1985.
3. Greco FA, Julian CG, Richardson RL, Burnett L, Hande KR, Oldham RK: Advanced ovarian cancer—brief intensive combination chemotherapy and second-look operation. *Ob Gyn* 58:199–205, 1981.
4. Johnson BE, Ihde DC, Bunn PA, Becker B, Walsh T, Weinstein ZR, Matthews MJ, Whang-Peng J, Makuch RW, Johnston-Early A, Lichter AS, Carney DN, Cohen MH, Glatstern E, Minna JD: Patients with small-cell lung cancer treated with combination chemotherapy with or without irradiation. Data on potential cures, chronic toxicities, and late relapses after a five to eleven year followup. *Ann Intern Med* 103:430–438, 1985.
5. Young JL, Percy CL, Asire AJ (eds): Surveillance, Epidemiology, and End Results: Incidence and Mortality Data, 1973–1977. *Natl Cancer Inst Monogr* 57:1–1082, 1981.
6. Holmes FF, Hearne E: Cancer stage-to-age relationship: implications for cancer screening in the elderly. *J Am Geriatr Soc* 29:55–57, 1981.
7. Warnecke R, Graham S: Characteristics of blacks obtaining Papanicolaou smears. *Cancer* 37:2015–2025, 1976.
8. Warnecke RB, Havlicek PL, Manfredi C: Awareness and use of screening by older-aged persons. In Yancik R, Carbone PP, Patterson WB, Steel K, Terry WD (eds): *Perspectives on Prevention and Treatment of Cancer in the Elderly*. New York, Raven Press, 1983, pp 275–287.
9. Burnet FM: *Immunological Surveillance*. Oxford, Pergamon Press, 1970.
10. Schwab R, Staiano-Coico L, Weksler ME: Immunological studies in aging: IX. Quantitative differences in T lymphocyte subsets in young and old individuals. *Diag Immunol* 1:195–198, 1983.
11. Hefton JM, Darlington GJ, Casazza BA, Weksler ME: Immunologic studies of aging: V. Impaired proliferation of PHA responsive human lymphocytes in culture. *J Immunol* 125:1007–1010, 1980.
12. Makinodan T, Adler WH: Effect of aging on the differentiation and proliferation potential of cells of the immune system. *Fed Proc* 34:153, 1975.
13. Price GB, Makinodan T: Immunnologic deficiencies in senescence: I. Characterization of intrinsic deficiencies. *J Immunol* 108:403–412, 1972.
14. Gatti RA, Good RA: Aging, immunity, and malignancy. *Geriatrics* 25:158–168, 1970.
15. Magee PN: Carcinogenesis and aging. *Adv Exp Med Biol* 97:133–146, 1978.
16. Setlow RB: Repair deficient human disorders and cancer. *Nature* 271:713–717, 1978.
17. Goldstein S: Human genetic disorders which feature accelerated aging. In Schneider EL (ed): *The Genetics of Aging*, New York, Plenum Press, 1978, pp 171–224.
18. Shmookler Reis RJ, Goldstein S: Loss of reiterated DNA sequences during serial passage of human diploid fibroblasts. *Cell* 21:739–749, 1980.
19. Lipschitz DA, Goldstein S, Reis R, Weksler ME, Bressler R, Neilan BA: Cancer in the elderly: basic science and clinical aspects. *Ann Intern Med* 102:218–228, 1985.
20. Fraumeni JF, Hoover R: Immuno-surveillance and cancer: epidemiologic observations. *Natl Cancer Inst Monogr* 47:121–126, 1977.
21. Cairns J: Aging and the natural history of cancer. In Yancik R, Carbone PP, Patterson WB, Steel K, Terry WD (eds): *Perspectives on Prevention and Treatment of Cancer in the Elderly*. New York, Raven Press, 1983, pp 19–23.
22. Doll R: The age distribution of cancer: implications for

models of carcinogenesis. *J R Statist Soc* (Ser A) 134:133–166, 1971.

23. Peto J, Seidman H, Selikoff IJ: Mesothelioma mortality in asbestos workers: implications for models of carcinogenesis and risk assessment. *Br J Cancer* 45:124–135, 1982.

24. Begg CB, Carbone PP: Clinical trials and drug toxicity in the elderly. The experience of the Eastern Cooperative Oncology Group. *Cancer* 52:1986–1992, 1983.

25. Kristensen L, Wesimann K, Hutlers L: Renal function and the rate of disappearance of methotrexate from the serum. *Eur J Clin Pharmacol* 8:439–444, 1975.

26. Praga C, Beretta G, Vigo PL, Lenaz GR, Pollini C, Bonnadonna G, Canetta R, Castellani R, Villa E, Gallegher CG, vonMelchner H, Hayat M, Ribaud P, DeWasch G, Mattson W, Heinz R, Waldner R, Kolaric K, Buehner R, TenBokkel-Huyninck W, Perevodchikova NI, Manziuk LA, Senn HJ, Mayr AC: Adriamycin cardiotoxicity: a survey of 1273 patients. *Cancer Treat Rep* 63:827–837, 1979.

27. Von Hoff DD, Layard MW, Basa P, Davis HL, VonHoff AL, Rozencweig M, Muggia FM: Risk factors for doxorubicin-induced congestive heart failure. *Ann Intern Med* 91:710–717, 1979.

28. Haas CD, Coltman CA, Gottleib AJ, Haut A, Luce JK, Talley RW, Samal B, Wilson HE, Hoogstraten B: Phase II evaluation of bleomycin: a Southwest Oncology Group Study. *Cancer* 38:8–12, 1976.

29. Weiss HD, Walker MD, Wiernik PH: Neurotoxicity of commonly used antineoplastic agents. *N Engl J Med* 291:15–81, 127–133, 1974.

30. Hansen HH, Selawry OS, Holland JF, McCall CB: The variability of individual tolerance to methotrexate in cancer patients. *Br J Cancer* 25:298–305, 1971.

31. Gelman RS, Taylor SG: Cyclophosphamide, methotrexate, and 5-fluorouracil chemotherapy in women more than 65 years old with advanced breast cancer: the elimination of age trends in toxicity by using doses based on creatinine clearance. *J Clin Oncol* 2:1404–1413, 1984.

32. Torti FM, Bristow MR, Howes AE, Aston D, Stockdale FE, Carter SK, Kohler M, Brown BW, Billingham ME: Reduced cardiotoxicity of doxorubicin delivered on a weekly schedule: assessment by endomyocardial biopsy. *Ann Intern Med* 99:745–749, 1983.

33. Kiang DT, Kennedy BJ: Factors affecting estrogen receptors in breast cancer. *Cancer* 40:1571–1576, 1977.

34. Samaan NA, Buzdar AU, Aldinger KA, Schultz PN, Yang K, Romsdahl MM, Martin R: Estrogen receptor: a prognostic factor in breast cancer. *Cancer* 47:554–560, 1981.

35. Hahnel R, Woodings T, Vivian AB: Prognostic value of estrogen receptors in primary breast cancer. *Cancer* 44:671–675, 1979.

36. Cooke T, George D, Shields R: Estrogen receptors and prognosis in early breast cancer. *Lancet* 1:995–997, 1979.

37. Falkson G, Gelman RS, Pretorius FJ: Age as a prognostic factor in recurrent breast cancer. *J Clin Oncol* 4:663–671, 1986.

38. Fisher ER, Redmond CK, Liu H, Rockette H, Fisher B, Collaborating NSABP Investigators: Correlation of estrogen receptor and pathologic characteristics of invasive breast cancer. *Cancer* 45:349–353, 1980.

39. Silvestrini R, Daidone MG, DiFronzo G: Relationship between proliferative activity and estrogen receptors in breast cancer. *Cancer* 44:665–670, 1979.

40. Sherry MM, Greco FA, Johnson DH, Hainsworth JD: Metastatic breast cancer confined to the skeletal system: an indolent disease. *Am J Med* 81:381–387, 1986.

41. Rosen PP, Menendez-Botet CJ, Urban JA, Fracchia A, Schwartz MK: Estrogen receptor protein (ERP) in multiple tumor specimens from individual patients with breast cancer. *Cancer* 39:2194–2200, 1977.

42. Clark GM, McGuire WL, Hubay CA, Pearson OH, Marshall JS: Progesterone receptors as a prognostic factor in stage II breast cancer. *N Engl J Med* 309:1343–1347, 1983.

43. Fisher B, Wickerham DL, Brown A, Redmond CK: Breast cancer estrogen and progesterone receptor values: their distribution, degree of concordance, and relation to number of positive axillary nodes. *J Clin Oncol* 1:349–358, 1983.

44. Fisher B, Redmond C, Fisher ER: The contribution of recent NSABP clinical trials of primary breast cancer therapy to an understanding of tumor biology. *Cancer* 46:1009–1025, 1980.

45. Bonadonna G, Rossi A, Tancini G, Valugussa P: Adjuvant chemotherapy in breast cancer. *Lancet* 1:1157, 1983.

46. Glucksberg H, Rivkin SE, Rasmussen S, Tranum B, Gad-el-Mawla N, Costunzi J, Hoogstraten B, Athens J, Maloney T, McCracken J, Vaughn C: Combination chemotherapy (CMFVP) versus L-phenylalanine mustard (L-PAM) for operable breast cancer with positive axillary nodes. *Cancer* 50:423–434, 1982.

47. Hryniuk WM, Levine MN, Levin L: Analysis of dose intensity for chemotherapy in early (stage II) and advanced breast cancer. *NCI Monographs: Proceedings of the NIH Concsensus Development Conference of Adjuvant Chemotherapy and Endocrine Therapy for Breast Cancer.* Number 1, 1986, pp 87–95.

48. Bonadonna G, Valagussa P: Dose-response of adjuvant chemotherapy in breast cancer. *N Engl J Med* 304:10–15, 1981.

49. Fisher ER: Prognostic and therapeutic significance of pathological features of breast cancer. *NCI Monographs: Proceedings of the NIH Consensus Development Conference of Adjuvant Chemotherapy and Endocrine Therapy for Breast Cancer.* Number 1, 1986, pp 29–34.

50. Ludwig Breast Cancer Study Group: Randomized trial of chemo-endocrine therapy, endocrine therapy, and mastectomy alone in postmenopausal patients with operable breast cancer and axillary node metastasis. *Lancet* 1:1256–1260, 1984.

51. Nolvadex Adjuvant Trial Organization: Controlled trial of tamoxifen as adjuvant agent in management of early breast cancer: interim analysis at four years. *Lancet* 1:257–261, 1983.

52. Pritchard KI, Meakin JW, Boyd NF: A prospective randomized controlled trial of adjuvant tamoxifen in postmenopausal women with axillary node positive breast cancer. In Jones SE, Salmon SE (eds): *Adjuvant Therapy of Cancer IV.* Orlando, Grune & Stratton, 1984, pp 339–347.

53. Wallgren A, Breast Cancer Group of Stockholm: Treatment with Nolvadex alone and in combination with chemotherapy in postmenopausal women. In Blamey RS, Stoll BA (eds): *Adjuvant Therapy in Breast Cancer.* Macclesfield, England, Imperial Chemical Industries, 1983, pp 15–20.

54. Ribeiro G, Palmer MK: Adjuvant tamoxifen for operable carcinoma of the breast: report of clinical trial by the Christie Hospital of Holt Radium Institute. *Br Med J* 286:827–830, 1983.

55. Cummings FJ, Gray R, Davis TE, Torney DC, Harris JE, Falkson G, Arseneau J: Adjuvant tamoxifen treatment of elderly women with stage II breast cancer: a double-blind comparison with placebo. *Ann Intern Med* 103:324–329, 1985.

56. Hawkins RA, Hill A, Freedman B, Gore SM, Roberts MM, Forrest APM: Reproducibility of measurements of oestrogen receptor concentration in breast cancer. *Br J Cancer* 36:355–361, 1977.

57. Canellos GP, Pocock SJ, Taylor SG, Sears ME, Klaasen DJ, Band PR: Combination chemotherapy for metastatic breast carcinoma: prospective comparison of multiple drug therapy with L-phenylalanine mustard. *Cancer* 38:1882–1886, 1976.

58. Australian and New Zealand Breast Cancer Trials Group: A randomized trial in postmenopausal patients with advanced breast cancer comparing endocrine and cytotoxic therapy given sequentially or in combination. *J Clin Oncol* 4:186–193, 1986.

59. Hanson TAS: Histological classification and survival in Hodgkin's disease. *Cancer* 17:1595–1603, 1964.

60. Tubiana M, Attie E, Flamant R: Prognostic factors in 454 cases of Hodgkin's disease. *Cancer Res* 31:1801–1810, 1971.

61. MacMahon B: Epidemiology of Hodgkin's disease. *Cancer Res* 26:1189–1200, 1966.

62. Gutensohn NM: Social class and age at diagnosis of Hodgkin's disease: new epidemiologic evidence for the ''two-disease hypothesis.'' *Cancer Treat Rep* 66:689–695, 1982.

63. Kaplan HS: Survival and relapse rates in Hodgkin's disease: Stanford experience, 1961–71. *Natl Cancer Inst Monogr* 36:487–496, 1973.

64. Bjorkholm M, Holm G, Mellstedt H, Johansson B, Askergren J, Soderberg G: Prognostic factors in Hodgkin's disease. I. Analysis of histopathology, stage distribution, and results of therapy. *Scand J Haematol* 19:487–495, 1977.

65. Wedelin C, Bjorkholm M, Biberfeld P, Holm G, Johansson B, Mellstedt H: Prognostic factors in Hodgkin's disease with special reference to age. *Cancer* 53:1202–1208, 1984.

66. Eghbali H, Hoerni-Simon G, Mascarel I: Hodgkin's disease in the elderly: a series of 30 patients aged older than 70 years. *Cancer* 53:2191–2193, 1984.

67. Collaborative Study: Survival and complications of radiotherapy following involved and extended field therapy of Hodgkin's disease, stages I and II. *Cancer* 38:288–305, 1976.

68. Fisher RI, DeVita VT, Hubbard SM, Longo DL, Wesley R, Chabner BA, Young RC: Diffuse aggressive lymphomas: increased survival after alternating flexible sequences of ProMACE and MOPP chemotherapy. *Ann Intern Med* 98:304–309, 1983.

69. Skarin AT, Canellos GP, Rosenthal DS, Case DC, MacIntyre JM, Pinkus GS, Moloney WC, Frei Emil: Improved prognosis of diffuse histiocytic and undifferentiated lymphoma by use of high dose methotrexate alternating with standard agents (M-BACOD). *J Clin Oncol* 1:91–98, 1983.

70. Horning SJ, Rosenberg SA: The natural history of initially untreated low-grade non-Hodgkin's lymphomas. *N Engl J Med* 311:1471–1481, 1984.

71. Armitage JD, Potter JF: Aggressive chemotherapy for diffuse histiocytic lymphoma in the elderly: increased complications with advanced age. *J Am Geriatr Soc* 32:269–273, 1984.

72. Gale RP, Foon KA, Cline MJ, Zighelboim J, UCLA Acute Leukemia Study Group: Intensive chemotherapy for acute myelogenous leukemia. *Ann Intern Med* 94:753–757, 1981.

73. Peterson BA, Bloomfield CD: Long term disease-free survival in acute nonlymphocytic leukemia. *Blood* 57:1144–1147, 1981.

74. Wolff SN, Marion J, Stein RS, Flexner JM, Lazarus HM, Spitzer TR, Phillips GL, Herzig RH, Herzig GP: High-dose cytosine arabinoside and daunorubicin as consolidation therapy for acute nonlymphocytic leukemia in first remission. A pilot study. *Blood* 65:1407–1411, 1985.

75. Thomas ED, Buckner CD, Clift RA, Fefer A, Johnson FL, Neiman PE, Sale GE, Sanders JE, Singer JW, Shulman H, Storb R, Weiden PL: Marrow transplantation for acute nonlymphoblastic leukemia in first remission. *N Engl J Med* 301:597–599, 1979.

76. Wiernik PH, Glidewell OJ, Hogaland HC, Brunner KW, Spurr CL, Cuttner J, Silver RT, Carey RW, DelDuca V, Kung FH, Holland JF: A comparative trial of daunorubicin, cytosine arabinoside, and thioguanine, and a combination of the three agents for the treatment of acute myelocytic leukemia. *Med Pediatr Oncol* 6:261–277, 1979.

77. Preisler HD, Davis R, Anderson K, Dupre E: The role of maintenance therapy in the treatment of acute nonlymphocytic leukemia (ANLL). (Abstr) *Proc Am Soc Clin Oncol* 4:167, 1985.

78. Klingemann HG, Storb R, Fefer A, Deeg J, Appelbaum FR, Buckner CD, Cheever MA, Greenberg PD, Stewart PS, Sullivan KM, Witherspoon RP, Thomas ED: Bone marrow transplantation in patients aged 45 years and older. *Blood* 67:770–776, 1986.

79. Peterson BA, Bloomfield CD: Treatment of acute non-

lymphocytic leukemia in elderly patients: a prospective study of intensive chemotherapy. *Cancer* 40:647–652, 1977.

80. Louie KG, Ozols RF, Myers CE, Ostchega Y, Jankins J, Howser D, Young RC: Long-term results of a cisplatin-containing combination chemotherapy regimen for the treatment of advanced ovarian carcinoma. *J Clin Oncol* 4:1579–1585, 1986.

Chapter 7

Surgical Nursing in the Elderly

Anne Keane, Ed. D., R.N., Perry Aievoli, M.S.N., R.N.C.

Each year, ever-increasing numbers of elderly patients are undergoing major surgical procedures. This steady increase in operative experience in the elderly is due in part to an increase in their numbers in the general population, in part to the improvement in surgical techniques, and to a major degree to the success of modern postoperative monitoring and support systems. There is also a change in societal attitudes regarding the ethical acceptability of major surgical intervention in the elderly. It has been shown that even those of us at the extreme upper limits of age can survive major surgical procedures and achieve a reasonable and perhaps improved quality of life.

A SPECIAL POPULATION GROUP

The ill elderly are a population group with special physical and psychological needs. These special requirements must be taken into account if a comprehensive approach to nursing care is to be established. In addition to disease-related symptoms, the nurse must also consider symptoms of the normal physiologic changes of aging along with the concomitant psychosocial and developmental changes of the elderly. Table 7.1 summarizes the degenerative changes of old age and associated problems that the elderly must endure because of these physical changes. Aging has long been recognized as a period of losses, both physical and psychosocial. Although the healthy older adult may accommodate to many of these losses or physical restrictions, the ill, hospitalized older adult facing enormous stresses may not respond with as much resiliency as expected. As Hamner and Lalor (1) note, the response of the aged to stresses may be slower

than that of the younger counterpart, and the response may continue for a longer period of time. The elderly patient may be seen to respond to the stresses of illness, hospitalization, and surgical procedures with varying degrees of mental confusion.

Because of physical changes associated with aging, such as loss of teeth and decreased taste perception, limited financial resources, and decreased mobility, the elderly may face the prospects of an operation with a poor nutritional status. They can also be expected to exhibit a degree of impairment in pulmonary, renal, and cardiovascular function. Over 85% of those over 65 years of age will have at least one significant chronic health problem (2). Social contacts may be limited but not absent in most cases. Most older adults are able to maintain regular family contacts, and only 5% require institutional living arrangements (2).

The decision to undergo any type of surgical procedure ultimately rests with the mentally competent older patient or with the legal guardian in some instances. The nurse can act as a patient advocate by ensuring that the elderly patient and family understand the situation, the nature of the proposed procedure, and the expected risks and benefits of surgical treatment. Good communication among the nurse, the surgeon, the patient, and family members is critical. Potential communication problems may result in some instances from decreased hearing ability on the part of the elderly patient. The use of overly technical terms; the lack of patient, careful, two-way communication sessions; the failure to repeat concise information as frequently as required; and the reluctance to include the elderly client or family in the decision-making process are all common mistakes made by health care team

Table 7.1 Degenerative Changes of Old Age[a]

Physical Changes	Results	Problems
Decrease in lean body mass due to gradual decrease of bone, muscle, cartilage, and connective tissue mass	Relative increase in body fat content	Possible unacceptable change in physical appearance
Loss of bone density	Compression of bones especially in vertebral area, slight decrease in height, change in physical appearance of chin	Possible decrease in level of physical strength
Loss of cartilage	Painful joints, decreased range of motion and mobility, curved posture	
Vision changes: cataracts, glaucoma, retinal changes, presbyopia, decrease in rapidity of accommodation from light to dark, less accurate color and depth perception		Problems of safety and night driving
Hearing loss; higher tones more difficult to hear		Problems of communication and socialization
Loss of vestibular function of inner ear	Loss of balance	Problems of safety
Fewer taste buds, decrease in saliva and digestive juices, decreased reabsorption from intestine, sluggish peristalsis		Decreased appetite, increased indigestion, nutritional imbalances
Loss of teeth	Chewing problems	Difficulty with eating, unattractive facial appearance
Loss of hair pigmentation	Gray or white hair	Elderly appearance
Skin changes, pigmentation deposits, loss of elasticity	Brown spots on skin, wrinkles, sagging	Possible unacceptable changes in physical appearance

[a]From Keane A: *Developmental Issues in Cardiac Disease in People with Cardiac Problems: Nursing Concepts.* Philadelphia, McGurn Lippincott, 1981.

members. When discussing the proposed operation with the older patient and family, it is important to understand that they may have unduly fatalistic attitudes about its outcome. Frequently, older people view hospitalization and especially a surgical procedure as "a time to die." Careful, patient explanation and encouragement may help relieve some apprehension in many instances, but will not entirely remove this attitude.

Preparation of the elderly patient for an operation is more difficult if the client is confused or if the procedure is an emergency, rather than of an elective nature. In these highly stressful situations, the nurse should always offer brief explanations regarding needed cooperation with care. Attempts should be made to recognize and correct physiologic factors (dehydration, electrolyte imbalance, presence of pain) and psychological factors (noise, darkness, lack of a familiar person) that may contribute to the patient's confusion or stress. If the older person is mentally unable to consent to the proposed procedure, the nurse must ensure that appropriate legal and patient advocacy policies are followed when permission for the operation is being sought.

NURSING APPROACHES TO THE SPECIAL PROBLEMS OF THE ELDERLY

Assessment and History

Nursing care begins with a care plan that is based upon information provided through the nursing assessment and history. The American Nursing Association Standards for Gerontological Nursing Practice provide guidelines for a comprehensive history and assessment and emphasize that aging is an individual process. Normal responses due to aging alone must be understood before truly abnormal responses due to disease, and especially those conditions necessitating nursing intervention, can be identified. The plan of care must reflect not only the age of the patient and associated changes but also the problems and needs that are related to the expected surgical procedure. The plan must be individualized and related to the older adult's responses, lifestyle, and goals (3).

The nursing history should note both past and present health status. Modes of communication, patterns of coping, and patterns of daily living should be included. A comprehensive history should also include occupational background, educational level, eating habits, and support systems, such as family, friends, or social clubs.

Several special factors need to be considered when one obtains a health history from an older patient. The elderly individual is likely to have a long, detailed personal and medical history. Reminiscing, which is common in the elderly, may occur as questions tend to recall past events. Response time may be slow. Older, familiar phrases and terms may be more easily understood than contemporary slang. The health history may be more easily completed by using short, concise words or phrases. Clarifying,

summarizing, or rephrasing may be helpful in obtaining accurate information. Rushing the elderly client or rapid questioning will not facilitate obtaining the nursing history. In addition, the nurse should always allow time for the patient to ask questions of his or her own.

The environment in which the history and assessment are obtained is important to consider as well. A quiet, well-lit room can decrease many of the visual problems of the elderly and may enable the patient to hear and see clearly and thus respond more appropriately. If possible, the health history should take place in the morning to avoid the period of the day when the older patient is apt to experience fatigue (4, 5).

Several aspects of the history and assessment are particularly important for the elderly surgical patient. Careful consideration should always be given to any existing medical problems that may be expected to complicate the surgical procedure and slow the recovery progress postoperatively. Particularly important are the presence of any significant symptoms of arteriosclerotic vascular disease, history of myocardial infarction, hypertension, diabetes, or chronic obstructive pulmonary disease and any indication of renal, liver, or neurologic dysfunction. The history and assessment should be directed toward the recognition of subtle signs of the presence of congestive heart failure, the possible signs of a recent myocardial infarction, and the findings of arrhythmias, unstable angina, dyspnea, productive cough, or infections.

The neurologic evaluation of the elderly patient always includes identifying the presence of altered mental status, irritability, restlessness, or disorientation, as these may indicate the presence of significant underlying medical problems. Orientation to time, place, and person should always be recorded. A standardized assessment form may be used to obtain much of the above information. Neurologic deficits, levels of consciousness, and orientation should be accurately described and documented. This information will aid in the postoperative patient assessment and plan of care (6, 7).

When collecting this information, the use of standardized history and physical forms decreases the time required to obtain lengthy amounts of information and can increase the accuracy and completeness of the data collected.

Many such helpful forms are found in basic nursing texts, or they may be found in modified form in many hospital-based nursing units. Standardized forms can readily be adapted for use with the elderly, keeping in mind the need to use clearly worded questions. Sample questions can be written under general headings and referred to by the nurse when needed. For example, when obtaining a visual history, rather than asking about the patient's visual status (a general question), the nurse can readily see if the patient wears glasses, can obtain the date of the most recent eye examination, can ask if the patient regularly reads the newspaper, can notice if the patient readily identifies known personnel entering the room, and can check to see if he or she has difficulty reading in the evening, or sewing or engaging in other routine activites.

Needed information can also be obtained directly from the patient and family. Some unchanging data may already be available from the patient's previous medical record. However, relying solely on the patient's previous and current medical record for information is inadvisable. The initial history relating to the current episode may have been obtained during the admission period, a time of great stress for most patients. Also, the initial questioning session may have jarred the patient's memory and helped clarify information related to previous activity and present symptoms or the sequence of events leading to the present admission. Answers that are inconsistent from the initial history do not necessarily indicate that the patient is an unreliable historian. Inconsistent answers from an elderly sick person may indicate that the initial history was conducted during a highly stressful period when the patient was very tired, in pain, or frightened or possibly that the questions were asked too rapidly or that the interview was conducted in a noisy room.

Members of the older patient's existing social support network should be identified early, and they should be seen as an integral part of the health team in planning the approach to the patient's care. These supportive people may be family members or friends. If well informed, they can aid the older patient in the immediate adjustment to and preparation for the proposed operation and also help in the follow-up care and during the posthospitalization period. Finally, because they are familiar with the older patient's preoperative status, they can be helpful in identifying and recognizing subtle changes in behavior that may herald unfavorable physiologic changes.

Use of the older patient's support network is most readily accomplished if family members or friends are encouraged to remain with the patient. Many special care units have restrictive visiting policies that actively discourage extended visiting periods. Although the goals of such policies are understandable, they should be and must be modified when older patients are admitted. The presence of a familiar person can act as a stabilizing factor and serve to reorient the older patient who is probably frightened and whose sensorum may be distorted as a result of needed pain medication.

Subtle behavioral changes, such as confusion or even hallucinations, are not readily detectable unless the nurse carefully questions the patient in an effort to detect signs of their presence. Patients may fear they are "losing their minds" and actively attempt to conceal their loss of mental clarity. When the nurse is aware of these changes, he or she can act to reorient and reassure the patient. The nurse should also recognize the changed mental status as an indicator of the need to re-evaluate the patient's physiologic status (blood gases, urinary output), to determine that the patient has received adequate and appropriate pain relief, and to evaluate the surgical wound for signs of infection (increased tenderness, redness, fever, swelling, increased drainage).

Respiratory Care: Problems and Management

Changes in lung structure and function that are associated with advancing age must always be considered when planning postoperative care. Maximum breathing capacity usually decreases with increasing age, and this usually results in decreased inspiratory and expiratory ability. These changes are in part the result of atrophy and weakening of the respiratory muscles and of a stiffening and calcification of the costal cartilages. Diminished resiliency of the elastic tissue surrounding pulmonary alvcoli and some degree of associated pulmonary arterial hypertension may combine to cause alterations in pulmonary circulation. This will result in decreased oxygen-diffusing capacity across the alveolar and capillary membrane.

Changes in the proper ventilation of the alveoli occur with advancing age. These result in the under-ventilation of the alveoli, especially in the lower portion of the lungs. There is usually an uneven pattern of ventilation in the elderly, with better ventilation occurring in the upper portion of the lung. The ability to cough also diminishes with age, due to diminished muscle tone, lack of lung compliance, and decreased sensitivity to reflex stimuli (8–10). For a more detailed discussion of the anatomic and physiologic pulmonary changes see Chapters 2 and 16.

Anticipation of the respiratory care needs of the elderly surgical patient is crucial. If the surgical procedure is of an elective nature, the nurse has adequate time to teach proper coughing and deep breathing exercises and to have return demonstrations from the patient. The patient should be taught to deep breathe and cough twice before trying to expectorate mucous. He or she should be told that coughing and deep breathing sessions will occur at least hourly in the immediate postoperative period. The patient should also be shown how to decrease incisional pain associated with coughing through use of a rolled towel or pillow to splint the incisional area.

Other physical measures associated with respiratory care include frequent turning, chest clapping, and vibrating. These measures can be demonstrated to the patient, who can be told that they will assist him or her in the effort to cough. Early ambulation, including sitting on the side of the bed, sitting in the bedside chair, and gradual increases in walking distances, can be discussed with the patient. The connection can be made between these activities, the optimum respiratory care, an early recovery, and the return home.

The fact that it may be necessary to use nasotracheal suction for the patient in the immediate postoperative setting may be discussed briefly, but probably should not be stressed as it is an unpleasant procedure. Many patients connect the need for suctioning with failure to cooperate with necessary nursing care. They may even view it as punishment for not coughing! Patients can and should be told that suctioning is necessary only when they are too fatigued to cough deeply but that this is a short term intervention.

The elderly patient is more likely to learn from and cooperate with these measures if he or she can see the connection between them and a good postoperative outcome. Preoperative teaching must therefore be both content related and highly motivational. The patient should always be assured that postoperative pain and the level of fatigue will be constantly evaluated. This will increase his or her cooperation with postoperative measures. The nurse must realize that if postoperative pain is not adequately managed, if the patient is kept out of bed for overly long time periods, if respiratory toileting is done too soon after meals so as to provoke vomiting, and if the patient is not constantly reminded of the necessity of respiratory care measures, the patient's cooperation with respiratory care measures is not likely to continue.

Factors related to the actual surgical procedure, such as the length and complexity of the operation, the location of the surgical incision, and the type of anesthetic agent to be used, also affect postoperative respiratory function. Incisions within the chest wall or in the upper abdomen may contribute to respiratory difficulty. Intercostal muscles, weak and sore from the incision, are unable to function normally. Upper abdominal incisions compromise lung expansion and coughing. Changes in pulmonary function occur after anesthesia. The effects of anesthesia contribute to reduction in lung volumes and diminished gas exchange and may produce a slow monotonous breathing pattern without spontaneous deep breaths. Preoperative and postoperative medications also affect respiratory function. Narcotics, administered preoperatively, intraoperatively, or postoperatively, can result in slow, shallow respirations potentiating the breathing pattern of anesthesia (11, 12).

The nurse has important responsibilities in the immediate postoperative period. With the high incidence of postoperative pulmonary infections that occur in the elderly, nursing activities must focus on the prevention and early detection of respiratory complications. Measures to ensure adequate ventilation and aeration include the control of secretions through frequent suctioning, mechanical ventilation if needed, and adequate hydration. Seymour notes that systemic hydration and/or humidification of inspired gases may improve respiratory function in volume-depleted patients (13). Fluid overload, on the other hand, can produce pulmonary edema, and the nurse must carefully monitor the fluid volume intake and the urinary output in this situation.

Other measures to ensure adequate ventilation and aeration include frequent turning, chest physical therapy, and the use of incentive spirometry when the patient is alert enough and able to cooperate. Frequent auscultation of the lungs for the presence of rales or ronchi is necessary at regular intervals and after any of the above interventions to evaluate their effectiveness.

The ability to clear secretions and thus maintain effective ventilation is diminished by long operations and anesthesia. There are several contributing factors: depressed mucociliary transport associated with anesthesia, the drying effect of preoperatively administered atropine, and edematous mucosal tissues that are irritated by an endotracheal tube and vigorous suctioning. An additional factor is postoperative pain. Persistent pain causes a restriction of respiratory excursion and reduced chest expansion, and as a result, effective cough diminishes and secretions pool in the bronchi, alveoli, and lung tissues (11, 14). The cough reflex is depressed by too many narcotics and too much analgesia.

Postoperative pulmonary care in the elderly should be directed toward the maintenance of effective respirations, the assurance of adequate ventilation, the promotion of secretion clearance, and the judicious control of pain. Nursing interventions include frequent deep breathing and coughing exercises. Deep breathing and coughing are particularly important as they increase the capacity of the lung to take in air and distribute oxygen to tissues, and they promote clearance of airways and encourage expectoration of secretions (12). Deep breathing is most effective when inspiration is maintained for 3 seconds. These ''aerobic'' maneuvers maintain alveolar inflation and increase arterial oxygen concentration. Coughing should be completed at least twice so that the first cough loosens the mucous and the second and subsequent episodes of coughing move it out of the lung. Narcotics should be administered for pain. The quality of pain relief should be evaluated so that dosage and

Table 7.2 Measures Aimed at the Prevention of Postoperative Pulmonary Complications[a]

Preoperative Measures	Postoperative Measures
Psychological preparation and education (including return demonstration)	Physical therapy, including percussion, postural drainage, vibration and coughing
Physical training and weight reduction (may be helpful)	Use of mechanical aids—incentive spirometry, positive end expiratory pressure (PEEP), and Continuous Positive Airway Pressure (CPAP) may be necessary
Cessation of smoking for 8 weeks or more (may be helpful)	Control of secretions, including physical therapy, endotracheal suctioning, hydration, and possibly mucolytics
	Drugs to control pain, bronchospasm, infection, or emboli if present

[a]Adapted from Seymour G: *Medical Assessment of the Elderly Surgical Patient.* Rockville, MD, Aspen Publishers, 1986.

frequency of administration can be adjusted according to the patient's needs. Activities, such as deep breathing exercises and coughing, should be planned for the time of maximum analgesia and should not take place immediately after eating as this may provoke vomiting and possible aspiration of gastric contents (11, 14, 15). Other nursing interventions include frequent turning, chest physical therapy, and early ambulation—measures that are important in promoting effective ventilation and in preventing pulmonary complications.

Prevention of postoperative pulmonary complications in the elderly surgical population may also be achieved through a variety of other measures that will require careful nursing intervention and patient cooperation. Ideally, some of these measures are begun in the preoperative period, whereas others are more appropriate in the postoperative setting. Table 7.2 summarizes these interventions.

Cardiovascular Care: Problems and Management

Aging changes in heart structure and function will influence postoperative management. Fibrosis and sclerosis in the endocardium, hypertrophy of the left ventricular wall, and increased fat infiltration in and upon the right atrium and ventricle result in diminshed cardiac output. Blood flow through the coronary arteries decreases with age, as does the ability of the myocardium to utilize oxygen (16, 17). Because of these changes, the aged heart is less able to tolerate prolonged stress. Atherosclerotic processes, as well as the fragmentation and thickening of elastic tissue, contribute to a stiff, non-distensible vascular tree, and the heart is rendered unable to compensate readily for the rapid changes in circulating volume or in prolonged, elevated blood pressure and pulse rate. Changes in the structure of the sinoatrial and atrioventricular nodes include a reduction in the number of pacemaker cells and an increase in the relative amount of fibrous tissue and fat. Additionally, there is a loss of Perkinjie fibers in the bundle of His and the right and left bundle branches. These changes in the conduction system contribute to myocardial irritability, valvular and myocardial disease, and the occurrence of arrythmias (17, 18). (For a more detailed discussion of physiologic changes of the heart see Chapters 2 and 15.)

Two major effects of anesthesia and surgical procedures on the aged heart are myocardial depression and arrhythmias. Bradycardia may persist postoperatively due to the continuing depressing action of drugs used preoperatively and intraoperatively. This condition, when left uncorrected, will contribute to decreased cardiac output and result in hypotension. Tachycardia also may occur, and if it occurs in association with an increased ventricular preload accompanied by an increased myocardial contractility, it will then result in an increased myocardial oxygen demand. Increased myocardial demand may then contribute to the development of severe myocardial ischemia. Other types of dysrhythmias can occur as a result of endotracheal intubation or extubation, from the anesthetic agents used, because of the duration and type of the operative procedure, and due to the possible intraoperative occurrence of hypothermia (19).

Hypotension

Hypotension can develop postoperatively as a result of changes in the circulatory status that can be related to the anesthetic agent or from actual blood volume changes from the operation. Cardiac output, peripheral vascular resistance, and circulating blood volume are frequently altered by surgical procedures; they all will contribute to changes in blood pressure. Drugs used during anesthesia can lead to hypotension. Most general anesthetics as well as large doses of local anesthetics can depress heart function. Some anesthetic agents can also decrease peripheral vascular resistance, and some produce myocardial depression. Restrictive abdominal dressings can produce decreased venous return, with the subsequent development of hypotension. Excessive blood loss, pulmonary embolus, hypoxia, rapid position change, and arrhythmias are other causes of postoperative hypotension (19, 20).

Older patients in their eighth decade develop postoperative cardiovascular complications at a rate of 2–12 times that of patients from a younger population (13). If an emergency operation has to be done, it can be anticipated that patients 65 years and older will develop cardiovascular complications at twice the rate as would be expected from a younger population of patients who need general surgical procedures and at four times the rate of a younger population who have cardiac procedures (13).

Because of the vulnerability of the aged to postoperative cardiac complications, evaluation for these events must be thorough and must occur in the recovery room, the surgical intensive care unit, and all other nursing care areas. The status of wound dressings must be evaluated at regular intervals and their relative snugness and their likelihood of interference with adequate respirations estimated. The amount of blood loss must be carefully recorded and documented. Appropriate drainage bottles must be marked and recorded with the date and the time so that any increase in rate of drainage can be easily identified. The presence of dysrhythmias should always be noted. Ideally, a cardiac monitor is used to evaluate the presence of dysrhythmias for at least 72 hours postoperatively, the peak time for postoperative myocardial infarctions. Rapid changes of positions should be avoided, and any symptoms related to shortness of breath, changes in sensorium, or level of pain should be identified and evaluated for their significance. The level of urinary output, changes in values of blood gases, serum and urinary electrolytes, and all of the central venous and pulmonary vascular pressures are also monitored frequently in the immediate postoperative period.

Hypertension

Several factors may contribute to the development of hypertension in the postoperative period. Postoperative pain increases circulating catecholamines, resulting in elevated blood pressure. Respiratory difficulty and the development of hypercarbia (elevated arterial serum pCO_2) and hypoxia (low pO_2) also cause the release of catecholamines and a concomitant rise in blood pressure. Hypervolemia, resulting from excessive blood and fluid administration, also influences the development of hypertension. The reversal of anesthetic agents can also produce transient increases in blood pressure. Finally, postoperative shivering and restlessness cause increased oxygen utilization and catecholamine release, with a resulting increase in blood pressure (20).

Nursing Management of Cardiovascular Changes

Nursing activities related to all of these physiologic changes of the cardiovascular system include close monitoring of blood pressure, pulse rate and respiration, cardiac rhythms, and central venous pressure. Skin color and turgor can be an important gauge to internal events, especially when they are considered along with lip and nail bed color and with the temperature and the relative warmth of the skin. Skin assessment can be an important guide used to assess the efficiency of tissue perfusion.

Hypotensive states, when accurately assessed, can usually be treated with the judicious replacement of the proper colloids and fluids. The elderly patient must be closely monitored in order to avoid the cardiac and respiratory complication of cardiac failure, which can occur during the replacement of lost blood volume. Central venous pressure measurements must be constantly assessed and corrected (normal range is from 4–15 cm H_2O) (21).

Central venous pressure is not always an accurate measure of left heart function in patients with myocardial disease or in those with pulmonary hypertension. Many elderly patients have either one or both of those conditions, and in such cases, a more accurate evaluation of left-sided heart function is available through the use of a Swan-Ganz catheter to measure pulmonary artery wedge pressures. If this central venous and pulmonary arterial line is used, it is usually inserted in the femoral vein. Attention to hygiene, sterility, and to the dependent position of the leg is necessary because continued circulation is important. These patients are not permitted to have the head of their beds elevated. This is to avoid kinking of the central venous and pulmonary arterial line and to maintain a constant manometric height on the venous column.

Hypotension related to hypoxia must be corrected immediately. Proper positioning of the head and neck, suctioning to remove secretions, and the administering of oxygen are the first steps to be taken while preparations are being made for endotracheal intubation and mechanical ventillatory support if necessary. Hypotension related to arrhythmias may require administration of antiarrhythmias drugs (21, 22).

The effective treatment of hypertension includes relief of postoperative pain through the judicious administration of narcotics and a careful assessment for the possible presence of fluid overload. The correction of hypercarbia and hypoxia must be achieved by the immediate correction of the causative situation and by the promotion of effective ventilation and respiration. Frequent arterial blood gas measurements must be made to determine arterial oxygen concentration, arterial pH, and pCO_2 status. The stressed, fatigued elderly patient may require extended postoperative use of the ventilator and of an endotracheal tube. This should be converted to a tracheostomy tube, if necessary, in order to maintain adequate postoperative ventilation and respiration. Prevention of shivering postoperatively can be achieved through the use of effective rewarming techniques, including thermal blankets, heat shields, and lamps.

The prevention of shivering is extremely important as it can overwhelm the reserves of an already compromised myocardium. All wet linens should be removed immediately upon being detected, and patients should not be bathed when they are cold or if their temperatures are below normal. The use of a hyperthermia blanket, covered with a bath blanket, may help with rewarming. The temperature of the blanket should not be more than 10 degrees higher than the patient's current body temperature. This precaution will help avoid thermal burns and keep the sensation of warmth from being perceived as pain. Patients who are cold or shivering should have their heads wrapped in a towel, or they should wear a cap, for up to one-half of the body's heat production can be lost through an uncovered head (23).

Fluid and Electrolyte Balance: Problems and Management

The size of the kidneys and the number of functioning nephrons decrease with age. Changes occur in the glomeruli as the number of capillary cells and filtering surfaces are reduced. The renal vascular system may be affected both by atherosclerosis and nephrosclerosis, and the blood flow to the kidneys is consequently decreased. Associated with these changes both in the anatomic structure and in the blood flow characteristics is the resultant decreased efficiency of the functions of glomerular filtration, tubular excretion, and distal tubular reabsorption.

The regulatory mechanisms of fluid, pH, electrolyte, and nitrogen excretion all diminish with age. The kidneys have a lessened ability to excrete diluted or concentrated urine in response to changes in fluid load or in the face of increased amount of solutes. Acid-base regulatory mechanisms are usually maintained to some degree in the elderly, but are often characterized by a slower response time (8, 9). For a more detailed discussion of renal anatomic and physiologic changes see Chapters 2 and 26.

The most significant and critical function of the kidneys during a surgical experience is the maintenance and regulation of fluid balance in the postoperative period. In response to the combined stress of anesthesia and the trauma of an operative procedure, the kidneys release renin that acts as a catalyst for the production of angiotensin, a potent vasoconstrictor. Angiotensin in turn stimulates aldosterone secretion by the adrenal cortex and the antidiuretic hormone by the anterior pituitary. These mechanisms are effective in maintaining adequate intravascular volume and blood pressure. Drugs given perioperatively affect the regulatory function of the

kidney as well. Morphine, meperidine, and some barbiturates can decrease glomerular filtration rate, urine volume, and urinary solute excretion, without bringing about increased urinary concentration (24, 25).

Effective nursing intervention in the area of renal function and fluid management for the elderly surgical patient includes assessment of the patient's circulatory status, state of hydration, and urinary output. Blood pressure, central venous pressure, pulse, and level of consciousness are important and should be monitored, as well as serum osmolarity, urinary output, and urine specific gravity. Hourly and daily records of intake and output should be maintained. Daily weight, skin turgor, and integrity of mucous membranes should be noted as they are excellent gauges of hydration and are additional ways by which one may assess the general status of hydration.

Assessment of circulatory status and hydration also includes observing the patient for signs of hypo- or hypervolemia. In hypovolemia, tachycardia and/or tachypnea may be present, as well as a decreased blood pressure and a lowered central venous pressure. Skin turgor will be diminished or absent. Hypervolemia may be evidenced by a rapid, bounding pulse, and a rise in central venous pressure is the hallmark sign of this condition. Blood pressure will usually be elevated, and neck veins may be distended. Respirations may be rapid, and rales may be heard upon auscultation of breath sounds at the lung bases. Thorough nursing assessment of circulatory status also includes the monitoring of laboratory data, including blood urea ntirogen, creatinine clearance (0.6–1 mg/100 ml in women and 0.8–1.3 mg/100 in men), and serum electrolytes.

The nurse can expect to monitor the elderly patient's 24-hour intake and output for at least 3 to 7 days postoperatively, depending upon whether the surgical procedure was major, minor, elective, or emergency. Postoperative monitoring generally includes daily electrolytes and blood urea nitrogen evaluation for at least 72 hours after a major procedure and then another serum creatinine approximately 1 week postoperatively.

Accurate monitoring of intake and output will be made easier by the use of a standardized reporting form, which often will require the cooperation of the patient and family members. Family members generally want to participate in some level of their elder member's care, and they need a convenient method of recording fluid intake and output. The use of a bedside clipboard with paper and a pen attached will encourage accurate recording of fluid and food intake. A readily available card listing the capacity of cups and glasses helps increase the accuracy of such records. Family members can be taught to measure and record urine output just as easily and are usually just as willing to do this also.

Drug Therapy

Structural and functional changes of aging associated with various disease processes in the elderly can result in prolonged drug circulation time and delayed drug metabolism and/or excretion. Consequently, both the therapeutic effect and adverse responses to drugs may be altered or prolonged.

Because of the effects of aging and the associated decline in renal function and reserve, drugs excreted by the kidney require very close monitoring to prevent overdosage and toxicity. Elderly patients receiving aminoglycoside antibiotics, for example, should be monitored through assessment of hydration, documentation of intake and output, and frequent or daily review of laboratory data, such as creatinine clearance (25, 26).

Seymour suggests some guidelines to minimize the chance of postoperative nephrotoxic damage in the elderly surgical patient (13):

1. Careful attention to the dosage of all drugs (not just known nephrotoxins);
2. Adjustment of the initial dosage of aminoglycosides, considering body weight, renal function, and blood level monitoring (serum creatinine);
3. Total avoidance of some drugs, such as methacillin and tetracyclines (other than doxycycline);
4. Recognition of the wide range of potentially nephrotoxic drugs;
5. Need for close monitoring of blood urea nitrogen in the early postoperative period.

Decreased liver mass, reduction in hepatic blood flow, and somewhat suppressed enzymatic activity of hepatocytes all contribute to a diminished liver metabolism and to the continued and prolonged effect of many types of drugs and medications. Drugs, such as barbiturates, diazepam, and meperidine, that are metabolized by the detoxification process that usually depends upon the liver enzymes require close monitoring in the elderly because of the possibility of hepatic impairment in this group of patients. Assessment of patients receiving these or other drugs that are metabolized by the liver should include observation for signs of hepatic impairment, such as pruritus, jaundice, or clay-colored stools (27). These are measures that are nonspecific for the exact level of liver function, but may alert the care team that liver impairment exists or may be developing.

There are other changes associated with aging that affect drug metabolism. With increasing age, there is a gradual decrease in total body water, total muscle volume, and lean body mass and an associated relative increase in total body fat content. These changes in the relative amounts of fat and water in the body result in a preferential and uneven distribution of lipid- and water-soluble drugs. Lipid-soluble drugs, such as phenobarbital and diazepam, are stored in this extra fatty tissue. This results in an apparently lower concentration of these drugs in the body when only plasma or serum levels are obtained. As a result, there may be a longer duration of action but a less potent drug effect (27).

Certain classes of drugs, such as antihypertensives, thiazides, diuretics, anticoagulants, psychotropics, and anticholinergics, may have a special and peculiar effect on the elderly and must be used with caution. Anticholinergics—for example, atropine given preoperatively—may cause mental status changes in the elderly. Memory impairment, disorientation, delusions, hallucinations, or agitation may occur. Other anticholinergic side effects, such as urinary hesitancy and/or retention, may develop (28). Because of the decreased homeostatic ability of the elderly, such drugs as antihypertensives, diuretics, psychotropics, and others should be administered within narrowed dose levels and within guarded therapeutic ranges.

Medication programs for the elderly require close monitoring of both the drug effect and of the physiologic response of the patient to the drug. Medication types and dosage levels must be individualized and administered with caution in the elderly. Comprehensive nursing care in all age groups includes observation for medication side effects and toxicity. In the elderly, this duty is of paramount importance. Observations of altered physical and mental status and close monitoring of blood chemistries must be meticulously recorded in order not to neglect this aspect of patient assessment. Medication records should be reviewed closely and drug use monitored often in order to determine the optimum pattern and timing of drug administration (28).

Neurosensory Care: Problems and Management

With advancing age, physiologic and pathologic changes begin to occur in the central nervous system. In the fourth decade of life, muscle, peripheral nerve, and spinal cord tissue that are responsible for agility, strength, and athletic capacity begin to show gradual deterioration. Beginning as early as the third decade, brain weight declines, and there is the start of a life-long process of gradual loss of nerve cells, shrinkage of neurons, storage of lipofuscin in neurons, deposits of senile plaques about the glia, and other degenerative central nervous system changes (29). Caplan also (29) notes that, despite these documented neurologic changes of aging, differentiation of them from other common pathologic and sometimes treatable disorders that are not associated with aging alone is often difficult. As one grows older, these normal changes of aging become more pronounced and are more likely to mask an underlying true pathologic disorder. See Chapters 2 and 34 for further discussion of the anatomic and physiologic effects of aging upon the central nervous system.

Hearing and Vision

Elderly patients are likely to have decreased sensory perception related predominately to decreases in visual and auditory acuity. More than 50% of blind people are over age 65, and the majority of these are over 85 years (30). Older people have a tendency to develop presbyopia or farsightedness, and this condition causes them to have the additional visual

difficulty in adjusting from areas of brightness to darkness.

Similarly, approximately 30% of those over 65 years and 50% of people over 85 years of age have significant hearing losses (31). Both men and women experience a loss of perception for high frequency sounds, although men are affected earlier and experience a greater loss than women (31). A loss of word discrimination is common in the elderly, and this may interfere with normal conversation.

The nurse must clinically assess gross hearing status and visual acuity preoperatively in all patients. Because of the prevalence of some degree of communication deficit in both of these sensory areas in the elderly, problems related to these functions should be anticipated and prevented if possible. Although the older patient may have compensated somewhat for these deficits in his or her home environment, hospitalization and the prospect of surgical procedures may magnify the problem. As a result of these decreased levels of receptor functions, poor communication, misunderstandings, and confusion may occur. Poorly lit and unfamiliar surroundings create a hazardous environment and should be recognized and avoided to the fullest extent possible in the care of the elderly. Associated metabolic and electrolyte abnormalities in the elderly ill patient may precipitate bouts of disorientation, confusion, or even episodic hallucinations.

Efforts should be made to create a safe and comfortable environment for the ailing elderly. The older person needs about twice as much light to see things clearly as does the average young adult (32). Brock suggests that high intensity lights be focused on important objects or surfaces, rather than brightly lighting the entire room. She also recommends constant low lighting in bathrooms when bright lighting is not used (32). Older patients should always be encouraged to wear their glasses, and bright lights should not be focused on or directed toward their faces.

When talking with the hearing-impaired patient of any age, the nurse and other health care providers should remember to face the patient and speak firmly in a measured, low-pitched voice. This may be difficult for many nurses who normally have high-pitched voices. Background noises and rapid speech should be avoided. Conversation should be well organized so that multiple thoughts, directions, or instructions are not given in one session. Finally, if the elderly patient normally uses a hearing aid, he or she should be encouraged to wear it whenever possible during the hospitalization.

Confusion

It is not uncommon for the ill person to experience swings in mood, changes in behavior, problems with cognition or judgement, and apparently irrational thoughts. This may be even more apparent in the ailing elderly patient. When this occurs, elderly patients are often called "confused" and sometimes are ordered to be restrained or heavily sedated. Foreman (33) has pointed out that these interventions are usually ineffective and often worsen the "confusion." Rather than the diagnostic label of "confusion," she urges that nurses accurately describe the inappropriate behaviors, for only then can the correct therapeutic measures be directed appropriately toward alleviating or preventing these behaviors (33).

Foreman summarizes the multiple factors leading to confusion as follows (33):

1. *Systemic factors* that interfere with the optimum environment needed to support brain processes; these factors that affect brain cell metabolisms are systemic in origin and result primarily from alterations in body temperature, oxygen supply, metabolites, fluid and electrolyte imbalances, and drug toxicities.
2. *Mechanical problems,* such as vascular obstructions;
3. *Factors related to a lack of meaning in the environment* associated with life-event changes or lack of social interaction; another important factor in this category is likely to be the decreased visual or auditory acuity of the elderly, contributing to misinterpretation of minimally meaningful environmental stimuli.

When considering the multiple factors contributing to confusion in the elderly, it is clear that the nurse has the greatest potential for a major interventional role in modifying many of these systemic and environmental conditions. The nurse's role here is one of systematic assessment and evaluation of neurologic, cardiovascular, respiratory, and peripheral vascular status and the environment (33). Foreman has constructed a helpful tool, the *Algorithm for Assessment of Confusional States,* with a decision-tree approach to assessment and intervention. These are the eight steps in her algorithm (33):

1. Assess the patient;
2. Avoid fluid volume deficit;
3. Prevent respiratory insufficiency;
4. Assess alterations in temperature;
5. Prevent hyperglycemia;
6. Avoid hypoglycemia;
7. Consider drug toxicity;
8. Increase orientation.

The advantages of the standardized assessment tool developed by Foreman are that it is comprehensive, objective, and orderly. Subtle clinical signs are unlikely to be missed when this tool is followed, even by the less experienced caregiver. Early recognition of confusion in the elderly is extremely important because elderly patients have a decreased ability to compensate for even moderate physiologic changes once they have begun. Finally, the use of such an assessment tool reminds the caregiver that confusion in the ill elderly is likely to be due to some physiologic derangements that can be avoided or controlled and not necessarily the sole result of long-standing impaired and senile cerebral circulation.

Sleep

Numerous factors in the postoperative period can interfere with the elderly patient's ability to sleep. Inability to sleep can be a serious problem as sleep has both physical and mental restorative functions. Lack of sleep can therefore have an unfavorable effect on the overall physical status and progress toward recovery, including wound healing (34). It may contribute to the onset of and be the reason for confusion, irritability, and listlessness. Hayter (35) notes that stage IV sleep relaxes and rests the body physically and that after periods of strenuous exertion, there is greater need for this type of sleep. Rapid eye movement (REM) sleep restores the individual mentally and is important for learning, memory, and psychological adaptation (35). With psychological stress there is increased need for REM sleep.

Illness, operations, and the stress of hospitalization clearly increase the need for sleep, and the nurse must be a vigilant advocate for his or her patients to ensure that the elderly patient in particular has the opportunity to sleep. Contrary to popular belief, the older person does not require less sleep than the younger one (35). The sleep patterns of the elderly are different, however, from those of younger people. Older people take longer to get to sleep, awake earlier in the morning, and may nap during the day. Daytime naps do not have the same rhythms as night sleep (35). REM sleep predominates in morning naps, and stage IV sleep predominates in afternoon or evening naps (35). Because an average sleep cycle requires a minimum of 90–100 minutes, the nurse must ensure that the patient is not disturbed during periods of time established for rest. This can require a high level of organization, planning, communication, and firmness because the nurse, respiratory therapist, laboratory technician, surgeon, and others will need to coordinate their visits if the patient is to be left undisturbed for an adequate period of time. Ideally, these nap periods should not be started just before morning and evening "work rounds." However, if the sleep-deprived patient has just fallen asleep, the nurse advocate must ensure that the patient is not awakened solely for the convenience of the caregivers as it will take another 90 to 100 minutes for the patient to reestablish the sleep cycle. Finally, the nurse must realize that the use of certain drugs, such as sedatives or hypnotics, will interfere with the achievement of needed REM sleep.

Pain

Pain management in the elderly is a topic that has never been adequately studied. Many writers claim that elderly people feel less pain than younger individuals. This stereotypic notion has the potential for actually denying the elderly patient the usual benefits of care that younger patients are given. Achieving the salubrious effects of comfort, rest, and unaltered quality of life of the elderly, especially during the postoperative period should be a high priority item. Indeed, a major review of studies that compared the effects of age on pain sensitivity reveals mixed results (36). In many of the studies reviewed, the pain threshold of the elderly and their reaction to pain were found to be similar to that of other age groups. The alleviation of that similar pain deserves similar attention in all age groups.

One must always consider the special factors that affect the pain management of the elderly. It must be remembered that the renal clearance and the hepatic metabolism of narcotics and other analgesics take longer in older people than they do in younger patients. For this reason, it is common to see analgesics ordered for older patients at a lower dose (calculated according to body weight) and at longer intervals (e.g., 6 hours versus 3- to 4-hour intervals) than is customary for most patients. Even in this population group, it is important to ensure that a regular schedule of analgesic administration be achieved in the immediate postoperative period.

The attitude of nurses and other caregivers can interfere with achievement of adequate analgesia in the elderly. For example, Faherty and Grier (37) found that older postsurgical patients had less analgesic medication prescribed and administered than younger patients. Although even less than usual medication had been prescribed by the physician, nurses administered an even smaller percentage of the prescribed dosage. This finding probably reflects a lack of information by both physicians and nurses regarding proper pain management in the ill elderly.

Safety

There are numerous factors that produce problems of safety for the hospitalized elderly patient. Table 7.3 summarizes personal and environmental factors with potential for producing safety problems. The nurse's responsibility is to assess these factors and intervene accordingly.

Wound Healing: Problems and Management

Vascular insufficiency, diminished cellular response and regeneration, decreased immune response, and the possibility of a poor nutritional status are factors associated with aging that will affect wound healing. Atrophy of arterioles and capillaries in the papillary dermis and associated

Table 7.3 Factors Capable of Producing Problems of Safety in the Elderly

Personal	Environmental
Decreased auditory and visual perception	Use of restraining devices Inappropriate or or excessive use of medications
Problems of balance and coordination	Presence of complicated equipment
Decreased response time	Unfamiliar surroundings, slippery floors inadequate lighting
Altered physiologic parameters	Presence of many unfamiliar people Rushing the patient, poor communication pattern

artherosclerotic vascular changes may contribute to diminished blood flow to the skin and fascia of the surgical site. Poor nutritional status may be present and may contribute to low blood cell counts and a concomitant diminished immunologic response. As a result, leukocytes that phagocytize bacteria, engulf cellular debris, and help desolve necrotic tissue are decreased in number and in vitality. Phagocytosis may be impaired and prolonged if protein deficiency exists as well (34).

Wound repair in part depends upon the timely proliferation and differentiation of epithelial cells. With epithelialization, a protective barrier is formed over the wound, preventing bacterial invasion and continued loss of fluid and electrolytes. Fibroblasts must enter the healing wound to begin collagen formation, tissue repair, and cicatrix construction. Wound strength is increased as a collagenous matrix is produced and allowed to mature. With advanced age, there may be diminished cell replacement, cell reproduction, and collagen synthesis so that wound repair is affected. Deficiencies in serum protein and in vitamin A and C levels may also contribute to inadequate collagen synthesis so that wound strength is lessened (34).

Several other factors may also be present in patients of all age groups that can retard wound healing in postoperative periods. Vomiting can cause stretching of an abdominal wound and bleeding into the operative site. Stretching of the tissues can inhibit formation of the healthy stable fibrin framework that is necessary for cell migration and repair (38). Postoperatively, temporary contractions along the magenstrassen area of the stomach, which is the muscular "main street" pathway, may occur along the lesser curvature of the stomach wall. Air, fluid from ice chips, and gastric secretions can accumulate in the fundus and then migrate to and move along this route and on into the duodenum even when nasogastric suction is being used. This unwanted air and fluid can accumulate in a hypoactive gastrointestinal tract beyond the duodenum and cause abdominal distention (38).

Electrolyte losses also contribute to abdominal distention. Continuous gastric suctioning can result in hydrogen ion and chloride losses and can cause metabolic alkalosis. Obligatory potassium ion loss is the result of the intracellular and renal tubular response to replace the lost hydrogen ions with potassium ions. This occurs as intracellular potassium is lost to the cell and excreted through the kidneys in an attempt to correct the metabolic imbalance (38). This process may be seen as metabolic alkalosis and may have an associated, parodoxical aciduria. Decreased potassium levels then lead to hypokalemia and an associated inactivity of the smooth muscle layer of the stomach and bowel wall, paralytic ileus worsens, and abdominal distention progresses.

Normal oxygenation of the tissues, an essential component of wound healing, is affected by the surgical trauma. Actively dividing fibroblasts need an environment that has rich or at least adequate tissue oxygen tension (at least 15 mm/Hg) in order to form the collagen needed for wound repair. Excessive coughing or forced coughing can cause pulmonary alveoli to rupture, form blebs, or leak air into the pleural space and cause a pneumothorax. These situations always cause dramatic decreases in arterial and tissue oxygen tension. Forced expiration or coughing can adversely affect right atrial and pulmonary artery pressure, cause diminished venous return to the heart, and lead to reduced cardiac output. As a result of prolonged respiratory efforts, there is decreased tissue perfusion and lowered oxygen tension in the wound tissue (38). To avoid the untoward effects of prolonged postoperative hypotension with poor local wound perfusion, pain medication should not be administered until the hypotensive effects of the general anesthetic agents have been reversed. The nurse must understand, however, that the response to unrelieved pain may stimulate the stress response and cause the production of cortisol, which can lead to some delay in wound healing.

Postoperative wound care should be directed toward prevention of trauma and stretching of the wound by making efforts to avoid vomiting and abdominal distention, to promote maintenance of normal electrolyte balance, to promote effective respiration, to achieve good pain control, and to protect the wound from contamination and wetness. Withholding food or oral fluids until nausea passes and administering antiemetics before vomiting occurs may be helpful in preventing vomiting (38). Nursing care should always include assessment of abdominal distention and ascultation of the abdomen for the presence of bowel sounds. Abdominal distention can often be prevented by frequent position changes and vigorous ambulation periods. Peristalsis, deep breathing, and wound tissue oxygenation are all stimulated by these measures. Electrolyte balance can be monitored through a frequent review of laboratory data. The frequency and amounts of nasogastric irrigations should be accurately documented. Because adequate oxygenation and maintenance of normal tissue oxygen tension are such important aspects of wound healing, measures to promote effective respirations, ventilation, and oxygenation must be achieved. These measures are fully discussed in the section on respiratory care. In addition to the usual measures, many caregivers also recommend that moist, nasal oxygen be administered for the first 48 hours postoperatively in most elderly patients. This is an intervention believed to improve wound tissue perfusion. The effective use of analgesics will aid in wound healing by resting the wound. Measures to promote pain relief are discussed in the section on pain management.

Additional nursing measures may aid wound healing in aged patients. Attention should be given to maintaining wound dryness and cleanliness in an effort to minimize infection. This is particularly important in the elderly patient because of the immunologic impairment that may be associated with aging. Body temperature should be maintained at normal levels so as to prevent vasoconstriction and diminished tissue

perfusion. Fluid intake should be closely monitored for adequate volume replacement and hydration without overloading the cardiovascular system by creating temporary hypervolemia. Assistance with the physical aspects of eating meals and the pleasant conversation and companionship of a nurse at mealtime may improve the elderly patient's appetite and eating habits. The nutritional status of the elderly patient should be maintained, and providing the proper nutrients needed for wound healing should be a priority in planning the dietary program (34). Undernourished patients have difficulty mounting their cell-mediated immune defense systems (39). A diet adequate in the proper vitamins, trace elements, and minerals is essential for wound healing. Proteins, carbohydrates, and fats should be well balanced in the postoperative diet. The nurse should realize that marginal nutritional status is not uncommon in the elderly and that this is not an acceptable situation to be tolerated during the postoperative period.

REHABILITATION: PROCESS AND OUTCOMES

A comprehensive nursing approach for the elderly patient requiring a surgical procedure must include a planned program of postoperative rehabilitation. These efforts can be either preventive or restorative in nature, depending upon the patient's needs and deficits. The highly complex needs of many elderly patients will demand that a rehabilitative philosophy and approach be initiated for the patient at the time of admission to the hospital. If this is done routinely, it may be possible in many instances for the rehabilitative approach to remain largely preventive in nature.

Complete recovery from a major operation, such as an open prostatectomy or a total hip replacement, may require at least 4 to 6 months for most elderly patients (40). It is likely that the services of several members of the interdisciplinary health care team (physical therapist, social worker, nurse, and surgeon) will be required during the process of recovery, along with the active participation of the patient and family. A formal discharge plan will be necessary in most

Table 7.4 Rehabilitation Goals and Related Interventions

Goals and Interventions
1. Competence in Activities of Daily Living (ADL) Approach requires assessment of physical and psychological capacity. As physical strength increases, patient should be encouraged to assume as much independence as is realistic. Family and support network should not be excluded from care. Capability for independent living and self care management postdischarge should be identified.
2. Mobility Approach requires assessment of premorbid and current capability and an evaluation of potential for improvement. Interventions may require assistance of physical therapist during and posthospitalization. Ambulation and passive range of motion exercises are necessary.
3. Avoidance of Incontinence Approach requires obtaining history of patient's pre-disease urinary and bowel patterns and identification of postoperative patterns if different. A bowel and bladder program may be required if incontinence becomes a problem. Limitation of fluids must be evaluated in relation to hydration status. Adjustment of dietary fiber intake or inclusion of stool softeners may be indicated. Attention to the physiologic causes of confusion may be required.
4. Maintenance of Skin Integrity Approach requires regular, systematic assessment of skin integrity and pressure points, along with frequent turning and mobilization. Adequate nutrition and extra sources of protein may be required to enhance tissue repair and prevent breakdown.
5. Maintenance of Pre-Disease Level of Sexual Functioning Approach requires assessment of pre-disease functioning and an identification of patient expectations in this area. Limitations related to current operation should be identified. If necessary, patient and partner may be referred for counseling.
6. Psychological Adjustment Approach requires an assessment of patient's coping style and its adequacy. Available support during and postdischarge should be assessed. Need for referral programs to provide continued emotional support or for adult day care should be identified.

cases, and thoughtful referral for follow-up care or home care supervision may be desirable.

Several problem areas can be anticipated that will require a specific rehabilitation approach. Some of these will become evident during the hospitalization and will continue to require care after hospital discharge. Other areas will become more important to the elderly patient after discharge from the hospital has occurred. Table 7.4 summarizes major rehabilitation goals and suggested methods of interventions.

Teaching Approaches

The nursing and health care needs of many elderly patients are likely to continue following hospital discharge. Because of this, a teaching and training approach for the older patient and family may be necessary in order that some degree of self-care can be achieved. Information presented by the nurse coordinator in these teaching and training sessions should be well organized and should include only the essential aspects necessary for attaining some degree of self-care. Although this information should be verbally reviewed with the patient and the family, it should also always be presented in a simple, easy-to-read, printed format. Attention must be given to exact word usage in these instructions because many elderly patients read at approximately the sixth-grade level. In addition, the size of print used should be large, and glossy paper that reflects light should be avoided. Although it is true that many elderly people have short-term memory problems, they are usually able to learn information that they deem necessary or relevant to their situation. Reinforcement and provision for follow-through on needed information following hospital discharge can increase the success of teaching efforts. At the same time, one must not overdo the ''simplicity routine'' in those instances where very alert and intelligent elderly patients are involved. Many aged patients are alert, well educated, and have normal understanding of complex matters. They deserve the same respect and the same approach that an intelligent, younger patient would receive.

It is the less well-equipped and more dependent elderly ill who will require the most effort by the postoperative teachers and caregivers, but it is from helping these more fragile members of the ranks of our elders that the rewards of success are most gratifying.

REFERENCES

1. Hamner M, Lalor L: The aged patient in the critical care setting. *Focus Crit Care* 10:22–29, 1983.

2. Freiberg K: *Human Development: A Life-span Approach.* Monterey, CA, Wadsworth Publishing Co, 1979.
3. *Standards of Gerontological Nursing Practice.* Kansas City, MO, American Nurses' Association, 1976.
4. Mezey M, Rauckhorst L, Stokes S: The health history of the aged person. *J Gerontol Nurs* 3:47–51, 1977.
5. Rauckhorst L, Stokes S, Mezey M: Health assessment-considerations for the older individual. In Stilewell E (ed): *Readings in Gerontological Nursing.* Thorofare, NJ, Slack, Inc, 1980.
6. Carrick L: Consideration for the older surgical patient. *Geriatr Nurs* 3:43–50, 1982.
7. Johnson J: The medical evaluation and management of the elderly surgical patient. *J Am Geriatr Soc* 31:621–625, 1983.
8. Tichy A, Malansanos L: Physiological parameters of aging. *J Gerontol Nurs* 5:42–45, 1979.
9. Steinberg F: The aging of organs and organ systems. In Steinberg F (ed): *Care of the Geriatric Patient.* St. Louis, CV Mosby, 1983, p 3.
10. Roberts S: Cardiopulmonary abnormalities in aging. In Burnside I (ed): *Nursing and the Aged.* ed 2. New York, McGraw-Hill, 1981, p 232.
11. Resser N: Preoperative and postoperative care to prevent pulmonary complications. *Heart Lung* 9:57–66, 1980.
12. Podjaski J: Which post op patient faces the greatest respiratory risk? *RN* 48:44–53, 1985.
13. Seymour G: *Medical Assessment of the Elderly Surgical Patient.* Rockville, MD, Aspen Publishers, 1986.
14. Edwards V, Murphy M: Disturbances in the oxygen-carbon dioxide exchange mechanism. In Jones D, Dunbar C, Jirovec M (eds): *Medical-Surgical Nursing. A Conceptual Approach.* New York, McGraw Hill, 1982, pp 875–930.
15. Spearing C, Garrett M: Deep breathing and coughing, how to do them right. *RN* 48:52, 1985.
16. Burggraf V, Donlon B: Assessing the elderly. *Am J Nursing* 9:974– 984, 1985.
17. Shepton A: The perioperative care of the geriatric patient. *SA Med J* 63:855–860, 1983.
18. Moss A: Cardiac disease in the elderly. In Calkins E, Davis P, Ford A (eds): *The Practice of Geriatrics.* Philadelphia, WB Saunders, 1986, p 302.
19. Wlody G: Complications of anesthesia: a case study. *Crit Care Nurse* 3:50–54, 1983.
20. Webb G: Hyper and hypotension in the recovery room. *AORN J* 26:546–574, 1977.

21. Kenner C: Hemodynamic monitoring. In Kenner C, Guzzetta C, Dossey B (eds): *Critical Care Nursing Body Mind Spirit,* ed 2. Boston, Little, Brown and Co, 1985, p 73.
22. Phipps W, Daly B: Problems of the lower airway. In Phipps W, Long B, Woods N (eds): *Medical Surgical Nursing.* St. Louis, CV Mosby, 1979, p 1108.
23. Reuler J: Hypothermia: pathophysiology, clinical settings, and management. *Ann Intern Med* 89:4, 1978.
24. Marcinek M: Stress in the surgical patient. *AJN* 11:1808–1811, 1977.
25. Metheny N, Snively W: Perioperative fluids and electrolytes. *AJN* 5:840–845, 1978.
26. Giordano B, Dossey B: Acute renal failure. In Kenner C, Guzzetta C, Dossey B (eds): *Critical Care Nursing Body Mind Spirit.* ed 2. Boston, Little, Brown and Co, 1985, p 819.
27. Hayes J: Normal changes in aging and nursing implications of drug therapy. *Nurs Clin N Am* 17:253–261, 1982.
28. Bressler R, Conrad K: Clinical pharmacology. In Steinberg F (ed): *Care of the Geriatric Patient.* St. Louis, CV Mosby, 1983, p 256.
29. Caplan L: Neurology in health and disease. In Rowe J, Besdine R (eds): *Old Age.* Boston, Little, Brown and Co, 1982, pp 55–84.
30. Porth C: *Pathophysiology. Concepts of Altered Health Status.* ed 2. Philadelphia, JB Lippincott, 1986.
31. Corso J: Sensory process and age effects in normal adults. *J Gerontol* 26:90–105, 1971.
32. Brock A: Surgery. *Today's OR Nurse* 6:16–25, 1984.
33. Foreman M: Acute confusional states in the elderly: an algorithm. *Dim Crit Care Nurs* 3:207–215, 1984.
34. Bruno P, Craven R: Wound healing. *J Gerontol Nurs* 8:687–715, 1982.
35. Hayter J: The rhythm of sleep. *AJN* 3:457–461, 1980.
36. Harkins S, Kwentus J, Price D: Pain and the elderly. In Benedetti C (ed): *Advances in Pain Research and Therapy* vol 7. New York, Raven Press, 1984, pp 48–54.
37. Faherty B, Grier M: Analgesic medication for elderly people post surgery. *Nurs Res* 3:369–372, 1984.
38. Schumann D: How to help wound healing. *Nursing 80* 10:35–40, 1980.
39. Flynn M, Rovee D: Wound healing mechanisms. Influencing repair and recovery. *AJN* 10:1544–1558, 1982.
40. Pomorski M: Surgical care for the aged: the decision making process. *Nurs Clin N Am* 18:365–372, 1983.

Chapter 8

Diseases of the Adrenal Glands in the Elderly: Surgical Aspects

Jon A. van Heerden, M.B., F.R.C.S.(C), F.A.C.S., Clive S. Grant, M.D., F.A.C.S.

Is there anything different about surgical adrenal disease in the elderly, or is a discussion about diseases of the aged simply a reiteration of what is well known regarding disease entities afflicting the adrenal glands that occur in all age groups? What makes the elderly patient with adrenocortical and adrenal medullary problems *special*?

There is little doubt that the symptoms and signs of endogenous hypercortisolism (Cushing's syndrome) are quite similar in the elderly patient to these seen in younger patients. However, it is much more likely that the elderly patient will have Cushing's symptoms secondary to exogenous hypercortisolism as a result of steroid administration. This is true because of the several disease entities that may be much more common in the older population, e.g., rheumatoid arthritis, pulmonary disease, renal diseases etc. Similarly, the elderly patient might unwittingly develop exogenous hypercortisolism because of the chronic intake of self-administered "arthritis pills" that may, unbeknown to the consumer, contain steroids. A particularly difficult diagnostic conundrum is posed by the older patient with chronic renal failure —an entity that is again more common at the latter stages of life (1). Not only can hemodialysis modulate the diurnal variation in plasma cortisol (2) secretion, but renal failure per se may result in poor gastrointestinal absorption of dexamethasone (3) (which therefore should be administered intravenously in this setting), spurious overestimation of plasma cortisol, abnormal cortisol binding, and abnormal response to dexamethasone. All of these factors may make the diagnosis of endogenous hypercortisolism extremely difficult in the elderly patient.

The clinical diagnosis of hypercortisolism may also be problematic because of the changes that occur in the elderly patient's bodily habitus due to the normal aging process (Fig. 8.1), especially if chronic alcohol abuse is taking place as well.

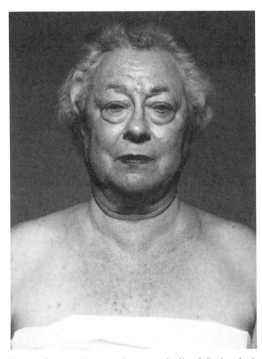

Figure 8.1. Old age or hypercortisolism? Patient had Cushing's syndrome secondary to an adrenocortical carcinoma.

113

In this latter instance, the clinical picture of a flushed face, hyperglycemia, osteoporosis, cutaneous ecchymoses, etc. can accurately mimic the picture found in patients with endogenous hypercortisolism. It should also be remembered that hypercortisolism, even to a minor degree, in the elderly may aggravate problems common to the elderly, such as hypertension, depression, senile dementia, and osteoporosis.

Are there any *distinct physiologic alterations* of the neuro-endocrine system that occur with the normal aging process?

1. Plasma noradrenalin concentrations appear to increase with advancing age. This may be as a result of reduced clearance of noradrenalin from the circulation in the aging population. When this increase is coupled to the growing evidence of a diminished responsiveness of beta-adrenoceptor-mediated function in the elderly population, it is not surprising that plasma levels will be elevated. Interestingly enough, there is little or no evidence to suggest that there is any alteration in the alpha-adrenoceptor mechanisms with increasing age. It has been postulated that the observed increase in norepinephrine levels in men, particularly over the age of 60 years, may be correlated with a marked decrease in stage IV sleep and more frequent periods of wakefulness. The decrease in receptor responsiveness may theoretically be an important mechanism for an age-related decrease in tissue sensitivity to those hormones (4–6).

2. There appears to be a steady decrease in aldosterone secretion with advancing age. This has been shown to be the result of a definite decrease in aldosterone secretion by the adrenal cortex and is not due to alterations of the metabolic clearance of aldosterone, which remains unchanged with advancing age. It is worth noting that we have encountered no patients over the age of 65 years who had primary aldosteronism.

3. Similarly, plasma renin activity declines with increasing age and is most likely the primary cause of the lowered aldosterone value usually reported in older patients. This physiologic change perhaps has the greatest importance when one is considering the diagnosis of primary hyperaldosteronism in the elderly patient. It should be appreciated that the ''normal aldosterone values'' decreases as age increases (7–8). Of interest is the fact that the adrenal circadian system appears to be totally unaffected by advancing age (9).

4. Extensive studies have taken place that were designed to evaluate the metabolic response to stress in the elderly. It has been clearly documented that plasma cortisol increase was significantly higher in the elderly than in the young controls, that the plasma renin response to stress was lower in the older age group, and that there was no change demonstrated in the renin-aldosterone and electrolyte response when older and younger patient groups were compared (10).

5. Similar studies have been performed to establish whether the immunoreactive corticotropin reserve was impaired in old age and whether a depletion of this reserve could account for the increased morbidity and mortality following operations in the elderly age group. These studies have shown that there is no decrease in the immunoreactive corticotropin reserve following various surgical procedures in the older age group (11).

Clinically, it should be remembered that the incidence of both adrenal hyper- and hypofunction is extremely low in the elderly population. Despite all of the physiologic changes enumerated above, the essential clinical features of all the surgical diseases of the adrenal glands do not basically differ from those found in younger patients. The complication rate for these surgical procedures should be anticipated to be higher in this senior population group because of the attending ravages of old age, i.e., atherosclerosis, cardiovascular heart disease, hypertension, diabetes mellitus, renal failure, etc. In an attempt to obtain objective data in our own practice, we have analyzed our experience with all of our patients over the age of 65 years of age who underwent surgical treatment for Cushing's syndrome (5 patients), adrenocortical carcinoma (5 patients), pheochromocytoma (9 patients), incidentaloma (22 patients), and primary hyperaldosteronism (0 patients) during the period 1972 through 1981.

Of cardinal importance before any surgeon recommends that an operation be performed is that he or she weigh the potential benefits of that procedure against the risks of, or alternatives to,

Table 8.1 American Society of Anesthesiologists Preoperative Evaluation Classification

Class I	A normally healthy patient
Class II	A patient with mild systemic disease
Class III	A patient with severe systemic disease that is not incapacitiating
Class IV	A patient with an incapacitating systemic disease that is a constant threat to life
Class V	A moribund patient who is not expected to survive for 24 hours with or without operation

Table 8.2 Multivariate Index of Cardiac Risk in Noncardiac Surgical Procedures[a]

Preoperative Factor	Points
1. S3 gallop, congestive heart failure	11
2. Myocardial infarction $\leq$ 6 months	10
3. Abnormal electrocardiographic rhythm other than atrial premature contractions	7
4. $\geq$ 5 premature ventricular contractions per minute	7
5. Age > 70 years	5
6. Intraperitoneal operation	3
7. Important valvular aortic stenosis	3
8. Poor general medical condition, e.g., abnormal electrolytes, renal insufficiency, chronic liver disease, chronically bedridden patient	3

	Points	Life-Threatening Complication %	Cardiac Deaths %
Class I	0–5	0.7	0.2
Class II	6–12	5	2
Class III	13–25	11	2
Class IV	$\geq$26	22	56

[a]Modified from Goldman L, et al: Multifactorial index of cardiac risk in noncardiac surgical procedures. *N Engl J Med* 297:845–850, 1977.

that operation. Multiple factors will and should influence that decision. They will include factors that will come from broad categories of circumstances, such as the expertise of the entire medical and surgical team, the medical status of the patient, and the primary and secondary diseases affecting the patient. To quantify numerically all ramifications of these categories and to produce a meaningful formula for universal application defies the current status of our sophisticated technology. Rather, this decision is the substance of individual surgical judgement. Careful, honest analysis of surgical results—one's own and those of others—is the cornerstone of this judgement.

Presuming that high quality medical care is available, one can then focus on the patient and his or her particular disease. The chronologic, and more importantly, the physiologic age of the patient is of clearly recognized importance as a determinant of operative risk (12). From an epidemiologic perspective, this issue deserves significant attention. Whereas there were 22 million people over the age of 65 in the United States just 10 years ago, the same age group is now projected to increase to over 32 million by 1995 (13). One must also be cognizant of the changing life expectancy of this elderly population. Nearly 90% of those 60 to 64 years old, 75% of people aged 70 to 74, and 50% of 80-year-olds will live another 5 years (13).

The objective assessment of operative risk accounting for age and other factors affecting physiologic status has been widely practiced by anesthesiologists in the United States for years (14). (Table 8.1) Moreover, Del Guercio and Cohn utilized preoperative invasive monitoring techniques to develop a more precise preoperative risk staging system. This has become a system that can now be used to optimize hemody-namic parameters and to lessen the operative risk (15). The American Society of Anesthesiologists (ASA) classification correlated well with these high risk patients, although the specific physiologic defect could be identified only by using the sophisticated invasive techniques. Because cardiac disease occurs frequently and is the most common cause of death in the elderly surgical patient, particular emphasis should be placed on yet another reported multifactorial assessment of cardiac risk (12). (Table 8.2) (See Chapter 3)

We included the assessment of the calculated operative risk using the ASA classification and the multifactorial cardiac risk scheme in reviewing patients who were 65 years of age or older and who underwent adrenalectomy at the Mayo Clinic between 1972 and 1981. These studies included all patients who were operated upon for

Table 8.3 Patients ≥65 Years of Age Undergoing Adrenalectomy for Cushing's Syndrome (1972–1981)

Age/ Sex	Approach[a]	Pathology	Other Intra-Abdominal Procedures	ASA Classification	Multi-fact Score	Multi-fact Class	Postoperative Complications
65/M	A	Hyperplasia	–	4	3	1	–
70/F	P	Hyperplasia	–	3	5	1	–
66/F	P	Adenoma (4 cm)	–	3	7	2	–
65/M	A	Hyperplasia	–	3	10	2	–
70/F	A	Hyperplasia	+	2	15	3	–

[a]A = abdominal; P = posterior.

Cushing's syndrome (5 patients) and nonfunctioning adrenocortical adenomas (22 patients). (Tables 8.3 and 8.4) All of these particular operations were elective. Combined ASA classifications II and III accounted for 86% of these patients, with two postoperative complications occurring in the ASA Class II and one in the ASA Class III group.

When categorized by the multifactorial scheme, Class I included 12 patients (43%); Class II, 13 patients (46%); Class III, 2 patients (8%); and there were no Class IV patients. Complications occurred in two Class I patients and one Class II patient. None of the complications

Table 8.4 Patients ≥ 65 Years of Age Undergoing Adrenalectomy for "Incidentalomas" (1972–1981)

Age/ Sex	Approach[a]	Size cm	Other Intra-Abdominal Procedures	ASA Classification	Multi-fact Score	Multi-fact Class	Postoperative Complications
66/M	A	2 and 3	+	1	3	1	–
72/F	A	8	–	3	8	2	–
78/F	A	6.5	+	2	8	2	–
66/M	A	2.0	+	3	6	2	–
66/M	A	4.0	–	3	3	1	–
73/F	A	3 and 1.5	+	3	8	2	Pulmonary embolus
65/F	A	8	–	2	3	1	Respiratory arrest induced (narcotic)
72/F	A	2.5	+	–	8	2	–
67/F	A	2.5	+	3	0	1	–
66/M	A	3.5	–	3	3	1	–
71/M	A	2.8	+	3	8	2	–
70/M	A	5	+	3	8	2	–
65/M	P	3	–	2	0	1	–
68/F	P	3	–	2	0	1	–
67/M	F	4	–	2	0	1	GI hemorrhage (colonic)
65/M	P	3	–	2	14	3	–
67/F	A	2.5	–	3	10	2	–
69/M	P	4.0	–	2	7	2	–
66/M	A	2	–	3	3	1	–
70/M	F	2	–	2	12	2	–
74/M	A	4.1	–	3	11	2	–
71/F	F	2	–	2	5	1	–

[a]A = abdominal, F = flank; P = posterior.

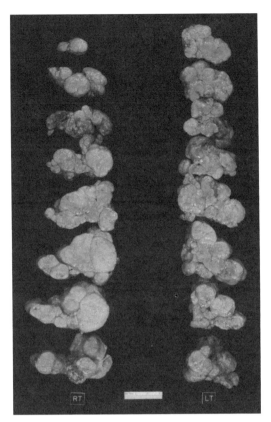

Figure 8.2. Gross appearance of bilateral micro- and macrofollicular non-ACTH-dependent adrenocortical hyperplasia.

was a life-threatening cardiac event, as might have been predicted by the low risk incurred by nearly 90% of combined Class I and II patients.

CUSHING'S SYNDROME

During the period of study (1972–1981) 83 patients underwent adrenalectomy for hypercortisolism at our institution. Of these, five (6%) were over the age of 65 years.

To establish the diagnosis of Cushing's syndrome in this elderly group was no more difficult or complex than in younger patients. All patients presented with the characteristic stigmata of Cushing's syndrome, and the standard laboratory evaluation yielded the expected results (16, 17). Despite a decreased degree of adrenocortical responsiveness in our elderly patients, the correspondingly reduced clearance rate resulted in the usual cortisol values (18). Secretion of

ACTH continues to follow the typical circadian rhythm, with normal basal levels, and brisk response to stress, and the servo feedback mechanism of the ACTH-cortisol axis is maintained (11). Abdominal computed tomography (CT) is especially valuable in imaging the adrenal glands, and by using this technique, virtually all Cushing's adrenal adenomas can be identified (19). When it is combined with chest CT scan, ectopic ACTH-producing tumors can frequently be identified (20).

Classically, endogenous hypercortisolism may be classified as follows:

1. Primary: Cushing's disease (pituitary adenoma)
2. Secondary: Cushing's syndrome
   i. Adrenocortical adenoma
   ii. Adrenocortical carcinoma
   iii. Ectopic ACTH-secreting tumor
   iv. Primary non-ACTH-dependent micro/macro-nodular adrenocortical hyperplasia (Figure 8.2)

Of these various causes, Cushing's disease accounts for approximately 70% of patients; this is exemplified in Table 8.3 where 80% (four patients) were found to have diffuse bilateral hyperplasia. In this small but representative group of patients, there was no operative mortality and no morbidity. This is quite surprising and is in contrast to our overall experience in which we encountered an operative mortality of 6% with a concomitant morbidity of 40%, principally respiratory in nature (21). In two of the four patients in whom no concomitant abdominal operative procedure was planned, the adrenal glands were explored via the posterior approach. This approach increasingly is favored by us—we continue to be impressed with the minimal postoperative morbidity that ensues following this approach and with the decrease in length of hospitalization. Although often more technically demanding, it is an approach that is "bad for the surgeon, but good for the patient!" Our current (1986) indications for the posterior approach to the adrenal glands are (a) bilateral adrenocortical hyperplasia (Cushing's disease), (b) aldosterone-producing adenomata, and (c) small (less than 4 cm) nonfunctioning adenomata. In all of these instances, naturally, no concomitant abdominal procedures should be either planned or indicated.

All patients with hypercortisolism undergoing adrenalectomy will require supplemental steroid administration. Patients who have undergone bilateral adrenalectomy are eventually tapered to a maintenance dosage of prednisone (7.5 mg in divided doses) and usually the mineralocorticoid Florinef (0.1 mg per day). Unilaterally adrenalectomized patients, we feel, should have very gradual total withdrawal of exogenous steroids. This slow withdrawal may require up to 6–12 months.

It should be stressed again that the surgical treatment of choice for Cushing's disease in any aged patient continues to be transsphenoidal hypophysectomy, which is performed with low mortality and, in our neurosurgical experience, a cure rate of 80%–85% (17). The principal indicators for adrenalectomy in the patient with Cushing's disease in our opinion are (1) pituitary surgical failures, (2) when rapid and assured control of hypercortisolism is indicated, and (3) when concomitant abdominal operations are required.

INCIDENTALOMAS (NONFUNCTIONING ADRENOCORTICAL ADENOMAS)

During the period 1972–1981, 72 patients underwent excision of nonfunctioning adrenocortical adenomata at our institution. Of these, 22 (30.0%) were over the age of 65 years.

In contrast to the well-accepted agreement about the benefits from and the value of adrenalectomy in the treatment of Cushing's syndrome, considerable controversy abounds over the proper method of management for these nonfunctioning adrenal tumors. Only slightly more than a decade ago, some investigators considered all nonfunctioning adrenal tumors to be malignant (22). However, this was prior to the advent of computed tomography and subsequent radiologic "discovery" of more small, asymptomatic adrenal tumors ("incidentalomas"). Approximately 1%–15% of normal individuals harbor these asymptomatic tumors as reported in autopsy series (23, 24). They seem to represent localized overgrowth of adrenocorti-

cal cells; they may be considered a normal part of the aging process, and they are more common in patients with hypertension, cardiovascular disease, and diabetes (25).

When such a nodule of the adrenal gland is discovered, appropriate tests should always be performed to exclude the presence of abnormal hormonal activity because unsuspected pheochromocytomas have been uncovered in this manner (26). As a minimum workup, all of these patients should have A.M./P.M. cortisol levels, urinary metanephrines, and serum potassium determinations to exclude Cushing's syndrome, pheochromocytoma, and primary hyperaldosteronism, respectively. The principal dispute then revolves about the decision of whether these tumors should be excised or simply observed with serial CT scans. A recent report seriously questions the advisability of ever using the conservative approach when four of eight incidentally discovered tumors were found to be malignant (27). With the real potential of "incubating" a cancer, caution is therefore emphasized when deciding to allow small tumors to enlarge. There is support for the aggressive approach to these lesions, but most reports advise selective surgical excision (28–30). We have taken a somewhat more aggressive approach than Copeland (28) who prefers to watch some tumors up to 6 cm. Somewhat arbitrarily, we have advised adrenalectomy for the treatment of all nonfunctioning adrenal tumors greater than 3 cm, unless other medical contraindications exist (12, 17). Additionally, we are encouraged by the discriminatory power of magnetic resonance imaging (MRI) in separating pheochromocytomas and adrenal metastases from primary cortical tumors (31, 32). Whether this modality will prove to be as valuable in distinguishing an adrenocortical carcinoma from a benign adenoma still remains to be elucidated.

As seen in Table 8.4, our "incidentalomas" varied in size from 1.5 to 8 cm and were benign adenomata in all instances. In eight patients (36%), a concomitant abdominal procedure was planned. Although there was no operative mortality, these patients did have significant postoperative morbidity, and because the pathology was both benign and nonfunctional in all of these cases, the dilemma regarding the decision for or against surgical removal is becoming readily evident. We feel (in 1986) that the indications for elective excision of incidentally discovered nonfunctional adenomas should be (a) tumors greater than 3 cm in diameter, (b) tumors that have enlarged on serial CT, (c) patient's desire (anxiety), and (d) in younger patients (less than 45 years).

ADRENAL CORTICAL CARCINOMA

Primary carcinoma of the adrenal cortex is indeed an extremely rare malignancy, accounting for only an estimated 0.2% of all cancers. This is reflected in our own experience in which, during the years 1971–1982, we saw and operated on only 25 patients with adrenocortical carcinomas, of whom only 5 (20.0%) were over the age of 65 years. Because of this rarity, by nature, few medical centers, and indeed very few individual surgeons, have had a large experience with these interesting malignant lesions. It is both intriguing and depressing to deal with these patients—intriguing because their presentation is often bizaare and depressing because the prognosis, regardless of treatment employed, is in most instances dismal.

Adrenocortical carcinoma should be suspected when one or a combination of several of the following occur:

1. A *mixed hormonal picture*—Adrenocortical carcinomas will often produce and secrete not only corticosteroids but also mineralocorticoids and sex hormones. (Figure 8.3) Usually one of these hormones produced by the cancer will cause a dominant clinical presentation, i.e., Cushing's syndrome. If carefully tested, most of these patients with adrenocortical carcinoma will be found to have a mixed hormonal picture. This is in contrast to the pure, single hormonal production of both benign adenomas and adrenocortical hyperplasia.
2. *Excessive urinary ketosteroid* production usually measuring more than 30–40 mg per 24 hours.
3. A *disproportionate ketosteroid* elevation— These latter two features suggest that there is a rapid cell turnover and an immaturity of the ongoing biochemical process.
4. *Abdominal symptoms,* and in particular, abdominal pain and the finding of an abdominal mass.

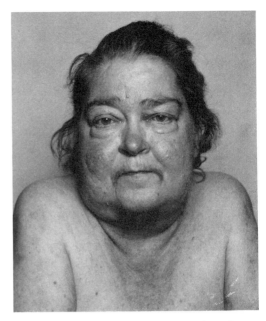

Figure 8.3. Patient with adrenocortical carcinoma; typical Cushinoid appearance with additional features of virilization.

5. *Rapid onset of disease*—This is in direct contrast to Cushing's syndrome secondary to either adrenocortical or pituitary adenoma when the onset of the disease may be so insidious that the diagnosis if often missed for a long period of time.
6. *Elevation of dehydroepiandrosterone*—This hormone precursor production is another reflection of the immaturity of the biochemical process in the rapidly growing malignancy. The malignant cells are biochemically immature and inefficient, which in turn leads to a high level of 17-ketosteroids and a high urinary level of steroid precursor metabolites.

Presentation

In a recent study, we found that 58% of adrenocortical carcinomas were functioning, whereas 42% were nonfunctioning (33). Those that presented with hormonal function were divided into Cushing's syndrome (42%), a mixed syndrome (33%), mineralocorticoid excess (11%), and miscellaneous (14%). The patients who presented with nonfunctioning tumors were diagnosed and categorized according to their presenting findings as follows: pain (33%), fa-

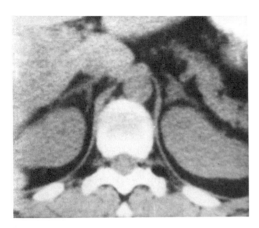

Figure 8.4. Computed tomographic scan demonstrating a normal right adrenal gland and a 9.9 cm left pheochromocytoma.

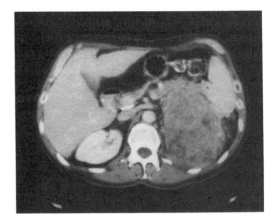

Figure 8.5. Computed tomographic scan demonstrating huge left adrenal tumor.

tigue (29%), abdominal mass (17%), unexplained weight loss (14%), and fever of unknown origin (7%).

Localization

The accurate localization of the side and exact site of adrenal tumors, in general, has been revolutionized since the advent of computed tomography in the mid-1970s. Today, computed tomography remains the modality of choice for localizing adrenal tumors and cysts of all types, although experience with magnetic resonance imaging is growing, and the early results are promising. One of the benefits of computed tomography is the ease with which the contralateral adrenal gland can be visualized. This obviates the unnecessary surgical exploration of the opposite gland in most instances, especially when a normal gland is clearly visualized by this study. (Figures 8.4-8.6)

Pathology

Most adrenocortical carcinomas are either grade 2 or grade 3 lesions (Broder's). Metastases are quite common. Usual sites of spread include local invasion (42%), followed by liver (22%), lung (23%), regional lymph nodes (5%), distal lymph nodes (3%), peritoneum (5%), bone (3%), and small bowel (2%). Most adrenocortical carcinomas are large, with most series reporting a mean diameter of 12-14 cm. (Figure 8.7) We have never encountered a malignant

adrenocortical tumor smaller than 5 cm in diameter. As it is true of most malignant endocrine tumors, the histologic diagnosis of adrenocortical carcinoma is a difficult one. This is particularly true if a needle biopsy or a small local surgical biopsy is performed. The surgeon can greatly aid the pathologist in establishing the exact diagnosis, particularly by identifying and removing suspected sites of extra-adrenal spread. All patients undergoing operation for adrenocortical carcinoma should be staged according to the criteria of McFarlane, subsequently modified by Sullivan.

T1 Tumor $\geq$ 5 cm, no invasion
T2 Tumor < 5 cm, no invasion
T3 Tumor any size, locally invading, but not involving adjacent organs

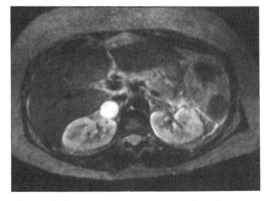

Figure 8.6. Magnetic resonance imaging scan demonstrating functioning (pheochromocytoma) right adrenal tumor.

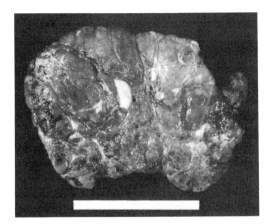

Figure 8.7. Typical gross appearance of an adrenocortical carcinoma.

T4	Tumor any size, locally invading adjacent organs
N0	No regional positive nodes
N1	Positive regional nodes
M0	No distant metastatic disease
M1	Distant metastatic disease

Stage I   T1N0M0
Stage II   T2N0M0
Stage III T1 or T2N1M0, T3N0M0
Stage IV Any T, any N, M1, T3N1, T4

Operation

The treatment of choice for all malignant adrenocortical tumors is surgical extirpation. Unfortunately, this has been possible in our experience in only 50% of patients undergoing abdominal exploration. This has also been the experience of other surgeons. At the time of resection, great care should be taken to stage the patient very accurately and not to rupture the capsule of the tumor. Rupture and spillage of the tumor virtually ensure the possibility of local recurrence in the near future.

Adjuvant Therapy

Although a great variety of protocols for adjuvant therapy have been tried, the only chemotherapeutic modality that holds promise is that of a prolonged course of Ortho'DDD, an adrenolytic agent. Approximately two-thirds of patients with nonresectable disease will respond by showing evidence of steroid suppression following the initiation of Ortho'DDD therapy. Perhaps more exciting is the prospect of using this therapy as adjuvant treatment in patients who have been "resected for cure." Some of these patients are subsequently being treated with an 18-month course of this chemotherapeutic agent. The best study supporting this concept is that by Steingart and his colleagues (34).

Survival

The overall 5-year survival of patients with malignant adrenocortical tumors in our experience has been approximately 16%. This cure rate, however, rises to 32% in the subgroup of patients resected for cure. The mean survival for patients with stages I, II, III, and IV lesions is 25, 24, 28, and 12 months, respectively. In our study of patients undergoing palliative resection, we found that this exercise afforded no increased survival when compared to exploration with biopsy alone.

Drug Dosages

1. *Adrenolytic:* Ortho'DDD (mitotane), 1–2 grams per day for 18 months
2. *Palliation:* (a) aminoglutethemide, 1–2 grams per day (principally blocks the conversion of cholesterol to pregnenalone) and (b) metyrapone, 2–6 grams per day (blocks the conversion of deoxycortisol to cortisol)

Summary of Data in Patients More than 65 Years of Age

Our experience with the five patients over the age of 65 with adrenocortical carcinoma is summarized in Table 8.5. They presented with rather classically encountered features for patients of any age with this disease. In particular, the findings were as follows:

1. The correct preoperative diagnosis was made in only two of the patients (patients 1 and 5). The modes of presentation, signs, and symptoms were vague and nonspecific in all patients. This resulted in the observed paucity of biochemical measurements recorded in the preoperative workup.
2. The mean diameter of the tumors was 13 cm.

Table 8.5 Summary of Data in Patients ≥ 65 Years of Age with Adrenocortical Carcinoma (1972–1981)

Age/Sex	Presentation	Hyper-cortisolism	Hyper-aldosteronism	Sex hormones	Size cm	Morbidity	Follow-Up
68/F	Anemia, fatigue	X[a]	0[b]	0	14	Reop for hemorrhage	Died, 2 months, metastases
65/M	Abdominal pain	0	0	0	12	None	Died, 3 months, metastases
68/F	Fever of unknown origin	0	0	0	15	None	Died, 108 months, malignant lymphoma
75/M	Fever, fatigue	0	0	0	15	Reop for hemorrhage	Alive, 144 months
65/F	Weakness	X	X	0	11	None	Died, 29 months, carcinomatosis

[a]X = not present
[b]0 = not done

3. Two patients required early reoperation for postoperative intra-abdominal hemorrhage.
4. Two of the patients died soon (60 and 90 days) after operation secondary to extensive metastases. No patients received any form of adjuvant chemo- and/or radiotherapy.
5. Somewhat atypically, two patients experienced prolonged survival (108 and 144 months, respectively).

PHEOCHROMOCYTOMA

"Although morphologically benign, it is physiologically malignant."

—Epperson

The year 1927 was a banner year for surgical endocrinology. In that year, the first insulinoma was operated upon, as was the first pheochromocytoma in North America, both by Dr. C. H. Mayo, in Rochester, Minnesota. Earlier that year, the first pheochromocytoma in the world, however, had been resected in Lausanne, Switzerland, by Professor Roux of Roux-en-Y fame. Since that time, pheochromocytoma (the great mimicker) has intrigued all investigators, due principally to its fascinating and bizarre behavior and presentation. It remains one of the six causes for surgically remedial hypertension, the others being (1) coarctation of the aorta, (2) primary hyperaldosteronism, (3) Cushing's syndrome, (4) thyrotoxicosis, and (5) renal artery stenosis.

During the period 1972–1981, 107 patients underwent surgical exploration at our institution for proven pheochromocytomas; of these 9 (8.3%) were over the age of 65 years.

Presentation

The classical presentation of a patient with a pheochromocytoma is one with bouts of paroxysmal hypertension. This unfortunately, however, only occurs in 50% of patients (35). The investigator, therefore, should be careful not to rule out the diagnosis of pheochromocytoma in a patient presenting with steadily sustained hypertension. The classical spells of paroxysmal hypertension are characterized by cardiac awareness, tachycardia, occipital headaches, anxiety, flushing, sweating, nausea, and vomiting. During these spells, a systolic blood pressure of 160–260+ mm/Hg is usually obtained. Besides having the presentation of sustained and paroxysmal hypertension, the patient with a pheochromocytoma may also present with an abdominal mass. The presence of a pheochromocytoma may be found serendipitously during the investigation of patients from families with the mutiple endocrine neoplasia type 2 syndrome.

Catecholamine Metabolism

There are three main catecholamines (dopamine, norepinephrine, and epinephrine), the metabolic pathway of which, along with their degradation products, is depicted as follows:

Tyrosine $\rightarrow$ DOPA $\rightarrow$ dopamine $\rightarrow$ norepinephrine $\rightarrow$ epinephrine

homovanillic normetanephrine metanephrine
acid (HVA)

metanephrines

vanillylmandelic acid (VMA)

Diagnosis

Although the diagnosis may be clinically suspect, the definitive diagnosis of pheochromocytoma and of a catecholamine excess depends upon the chemical demonstration of that excess. This can be performed by measuring either the degradation products (metanephrines, VMA, or HVA) or by direct measurement of the catecholamines themselves. The most reliable of all these measurements is the measurement of urinary fractionated catecholamines (dopamine, epinephrine, and norepinephrine) by high pressure liquid chromatography. The measurement of 24-hour urinary metanephrines is a good screening test and is positive in approximately 96% of patients with a pheochromocytoma. Both false positive and false negative results may, however, be obtained if the patient has received intravenous radiographic contrast material within 48 hours of metanephrine determination.

Localizing Modalities

In 1986, only two modalities for the localization of adrenal medullary tumors need to be discussed: computed tomography and 131-I metaiodobenzylguanadine (MIBG). Both of these have now supplanted all other localizing modalities. MIBG is of special interest because it is known to be concentrated only in an abnormal adrenal medulla (adrenal medullary hyperplasia or pheochromocytoma) or in a paraganglioma. When MIBG is administered, it is important to block iodine uptake by the thyroid gland by the administration of iodine 24 hours before and 7 days after the scan. We have found the MIBG scan to have a sensitivity of 79%, a specificity of 96%, and an overall accuracy of 88% (36). (Figure 8.8) The scan is of major benefit in a patient with either a suspected malignant or recurrent pheochromocytoma. Additionally, it may be of great help in a patient who is suspected of having multiple adrenal or extra-adrenal pheochromocytomas and/or paragangliomata, e.g., the MEN 2A and B syndromes, neurofibromatosis, the Carney triad (multiple paragangliomata, atrial myxomas, and gastric leiomyomas) and the von Hippel-Lindau syndrome. Perhaps most exciting, and currently under investigation, is the possiblity of utilizing MIBG as a therapeutic modality analogous to radioactive iodine treatment of metastatic follic-

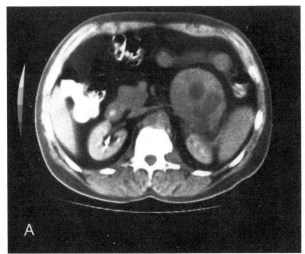

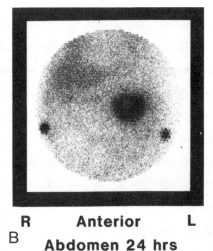

R   **Anterior**   L

Abdomen 24 hrs

Figure 8.8. **A,** Computed tomographic scan demonstrating large, partly cystic left pheochromocytoma. **B,** MIBG scan confirming A.

ular cancer in the patient with metastatic pheochromocytoma.

Magnetic resonance imaging (MRI) is the "new kid on the block" technologically. Experience is early but appears promising. Of particular importance is the ability of MRI to differentiate between functioning medullary and cortical tumors. (Figure 8.6)

Preoperative Preparation

We continue to feel that all patients with pheochromocytomas require both alpha and beta blockade preoperatively. With this pharmacologic blockade, there is no need for intravenous volume expansion. The drugs we currently recommend are phenoxybenzamine (Dibenzyline), 30–90 mg per day for 7–10 days, and propranolol (Inderal), 30 mg per day for 3 days.

This preoperative blockade requires careful monitoring in the older patient who may be less tolerant of induced changes in blood pressure. We like to aim for nasal stuffiness and postural hypotension as an end point—both being evidence of adequate alpha blockade.

Operative Strategy

The secret to the successful outcome during resection of the pheochromocytoma is to "steal the tumor away from the patient." By this is meant that there will be minimal intraoperative tumor manipulation, with early adrenal vein ligation whenever possible. Because of our support of this philosophy, we have adhered to the recommendation that all pheochromocytomas should be approached transabdominally. The posterior approach, which has been suggested by some, requires excessive intraoperative tumor manipulation for adequate exposure. This is strictly contraindicated in patients with catecholamine excess, in spite of our ability to administer adequate preoperative blockade.

A successful outcome is also predicated on the active participation of an anesthesiologist who is experienced in the management of hypertensive episodes. These intraoperative hypertensive episodes that occur commonly during tumor manipulation, despite "adequate" blockade, are best managed by the immediate infusion of sodium nitroprusside (Nipride). Both hypotension and cardiac arrhythmias (with the exception of

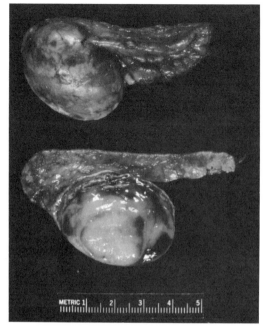

Figure 8.9. Typical gross appearance of sporadic pheochromocytoma.

sinus tachycardia) are the most uncommon problems encountered in our experience since the advent of pharmacologic blockade. Posttumor removal hypotension is mild and occurred in approximately 20%–25% of patients in our practice.

In patients with a history of cardiac disease and *particularly* in older patients (more than 55 years), we feel it is very valuable to place a Swan-Ganz catheter. The postoperative course of the majority of our patients is totally uneventful—no unusual pharmacologic or fluid manipulation is necessary—a situation that is largely due to the routine institution of preoperative alpha and beta blockade.

Pathology

Pheochromocytomas are equally distributed between the right and left adrenal glands in the sporadic situation. (Figure 8.9) Extra-adrenal tumors (paragangliomata) and bilateral tumors occur in approximately 10%–15% of patients and are more common in patients with multiple endocrine neoplasia type 2A or B syndromes (medullary thyroid carcinoma, pheochromocytoma, normal (A) and abnormal (B) phenotype

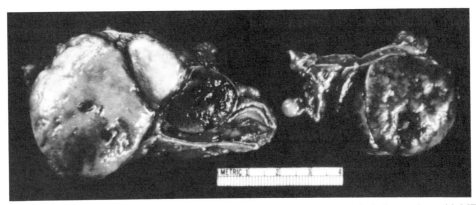

Figure 8.10. Typical bilateral tumors with associated adrenal medullary hyperplasia in a patient with MEN II.

and hyperparathyroidism) (37). (Figure 8.10) In these syndromes, the cellular pathology varies from the subtle changes of the precursor of pheochromocytoma (adrenal medullary hyperplasia) to frank bilateral tumor formation. These familial syndromes occur in approximately 10% of patients with pheochromocytoma. Approximately 10% of pheochromocytomas are malignant, with this incidence rising to close to 50% in patients with extra-adrenal tumors (paragangliomata).

Prognosis

The operative mortality is 4%–5% for patients undergoing tumor resection. In those patients with malignant pheochromocytomas, the 5-year survival rate is approximately 50%. Of importance to most patients, however, is the cure of the hypertension and the freedom from the severe paroxysmal attacks. If the preoperative hypertension were paroxysmal in nature, almost all patients can be assured of a normotensive state postoperatively. In those patients who presented with sustained hypertension, two-thirds should be rendered normotensive, with one-third requiring some form of antihypertensive medication postoperatively. Those patients with symptomatic metastatic pheochromocytoma can be well controlled with long-term phenoxybenzamine administration. In patients with benign disease, as documented by yearly urinary studies, the paroxysmal attacks cease.

Summary of Data in Patients More than 65 Years of Age with Pheochromocytoma

Our experience with the nine patients 65 years of age and older who had pheochromocytoma is summarized in Table 8.6. Several important features are worth noting:

1. In only four of the nine patients (44%) was a diagnosis of pheochromocytoma made preoperatively.
2. Catecholamine secretion, which was measured in only five patients, was elevated in all five, affirming the accuracy of catecholamine determination.
3. The operative mortality of 22% (two of nine patients) is considerably higher than the approximate 5% reported in most large series.
4. The 11% incidence of malignancy is in keeping with most other reports.
5. Of the seven surviving patients, only three remained alive at the time of follow-up. This death rate is considerably higher than that encountered in younger patients. The causes of death were cerebrovascular accident (two), myocardial infarction (one), and pulmonary emphysema (one). This has served to remind us once again about the increased risk of operation in this group of senior citizens.

In closing, a reiteration of an earlier statement in this chapter is worthwhile: "This, then, is the substance of individual surgical judgement. Careful, honest analysis of surgical results—

Table 8.6 Summary of Data in Patients ≥ 65 Years of Age with Pheochromocytoma (1972–1981)

Age/ Sex	Presentation	Catecholamines	Pathology	Operative Mortality	Follow-up
65/M	Renal stones	0	Benign, 20 cm	0	Died, 168 months, CVA
67/M	Sustained HPT	↑	Benign, 6 cm	+	Myocardial infarction
66/F	Incidental	↑	Benign, 3 cm	0	Alive, 55 months
82/M	Abdominal pain	0	Benign, 10 cm	0	Died, 36 months, emphysema
76/M	Elevated blood pressure during anesthesia	0	Benign, 6 cm	0	Died, 32 months, MI
65/M	Sustained HPT	↑	Malignant, 8 cm	+	Myocardial infarction
74/F	Pancreatic pseudocyst	0	Benign, 12 cm	0	Alive, 120 months
68/M	Elevated blood pressure during anesthesia	↑	Benign, 6 cm	0	Died, 57 months CVA
72/F	Sustained HPT	↑	Benign, 4 cm	0	Alive, 60 months

one's own and those of others—is the cornerstone of this judgement.'' This judgement is of paramount importance in the care of all surgical patients, but *particularly* in the care of the senior citizens in all of our practices.

REFERENCES

1. Sharp N, Devlin JT, Rinmer JM: Renal failure obfuscates the diagnosis of Cushing's disease. *JAMA* 256:2564–2565, 1986.
2. Wallace EZ, Rosman P, Toshav N: Pituitary-adrenocortical function in chronic renal failure: studies of episodic secretion of cortisol and dexamethasone suppressability. *J Clin Endocrinol Metab* 50:46–51, 1980.
3. Ramirez G, Gomez-Sanchez C, Meikle WA, Jubiz W: Evaluation of the hypothalamic hypophyseal adrenal axis in patients receiving long-term hemodialysis. *Arch Intern Med* 142:1448–1452, 1982.
4. Kelly J, O'Malley K: Adrenoceptor function and aging. *Clin Sci* 66:509–515, 1984.
5. Ziegler MG, Lake CR, Kopin IJ: Plasma noradrenalin increases with age. *Nature* 261:333–335, 1976.
6. Lake CR, Ziegler MG, Coleman MD, Kopin IJ: Age adjusted plasma norepinephrine levels are similar in normotensive and hypertensive subjects. *N Engl J Med* 296:208–209, 1977.
7. Hegstad R, Brown RE, Jiang NS, Kao P, Weinshilboum RM, Strong C, Wisgerhof M: Aging and aldosterone. *Am J Med* 74:442, 1983.
8. Noth RH, Lassman MN, Tan SY, Fernandez-Cruz A, Mulrow PJ: Age and the renin aldosterone system. *Arch Intern Med* 137:1414–1417, 1977.
9. Touitou Y, Sulon J, Bogden A, Touitou C, Reinberg A, Beck H, Sodoyez JC, Demey-Ponsart E, Van-Couwenberge H: Adrenal circadian system in young and elderly human subjects: a comparative study. *J Endocrinol* 93:201–210, 1982.
10. Blichert-Toft M, Christensen V, Engquist A, Fug-Moller F, Kehlet H, Madsen SN, Skovsted L, Thode J, Olgaard K: Influence of age on the endocrine-metabolic response to surgery. *Ann Surg* 190:761, 1979.
11. Blicher-Toft M, Hammer L: Immunoreactive corticotropin reserve in old age in man during and after surgical stress. *J Gerontol* 31:539–545, 1976.
12. Goldman L, Caldera DL, Nussbaum SR, Southwick FS, Krogstad D, Murray B, Burke DS, O'Malley TA, Gorroll AH, Caplan CH, Nolan J, Carabello B, Slater EE: Multifactorial index of cardiac risk in noncardiac surgical procedures. *N Engl J Med* 297:845–850, 1977.
13. Mason JH, Gau FC, Byrne MP: General Surgery. In Steinberg FU (ed) *Cowdry's The Care of the Geriatric Patient*, ed 5. St Louis, CV Mosby, 1976, pp 217–246.
14. Dodd RB: Anesthesia. In Steinberg FU (ed) *Cowdry's The Care of the Geriatric Patient*, ed 5. St Louis, CV Mosby, 1976, pp 299–325.
15. Del Guercio LRM, Cohn JD: Monitoring operative risk

in the elderly. *JAMA* 243:1350–1355, 1980.

16. Edis AJ, Grant CS, Egdahl RH: *Manual of Endocrine Surgery*, ed 2. New York, Springer-Verlag, 1984, pp 151–205.

17. Carpenter PC: Cushing's syndrome: Update of diagnosis and management. *Mayo Clin Proc* 61:49–58, 1986.

18. Ohashi M, Kato K, Nawata H, Ibayashi H: Adrenocortical responsiveness to graded ATCH infusions in normal young and elderly human subjects. *Gerontology* 32:43–51, 1986.

19. Hattery RR, Sheedy PF, Stephens DH, van Heerden JA: Computed tomography of the adrenal gland. *Semin Roentgenol* 16:290–300, 1981.

20. White FE, White MC, Drury PL, Fry IK, Besser GM: Value of computed tomography of the abdomen and chest in investigation of Cushing's syndrome. *Br Med J* 284:770–774, 1982.

21. Watson RGK, van Heerden JA, Northcutt RC, Grant CS, Ilstrup DM: Results of adrenal surgery for Cushing's syndrome: ten years' experience. *World J Surg* 1-:531–538, 1986.

22. Lewinsky BS, Grigor KM, Symington T, Neville A: The clinical and pathologic features of "non-hormonal" adrenocortical tumors. *Cancer* 33:778–790, 1974.

23. Russi S, Blumenthal HT, Gray SH: Small adenomas of the adrenal cortex in hypertension and diabetes. *Arch Intern Med* 76:284–291, 1945.

24. Dobbie JW: Adrenocortical nodular hyperplasia: the aging adrenal. *J Pathol* 99:1–18, 1969.

25. Neville AM: The nodular adrenal. *Invest Cell Pathol* 1:99–111, 1978.

26. Prinz RA, Brooks MH, Churchill R, Graner JL, Lawrence AM, Paloyan E, Sparagana M: Incidental asymptomatic adrenal masses detected by computed tomographic scanning: is operation required? *JAMA* 248:701–704, 1982.

27. Seddon JM, Baranetsky N, VanBoxel PJ: Adrenal "incidentalomas": need for surgery. *Urology* 25:1–7, 1985.

28. Copeland PM: The incidentally discovered adrenal mass. *Ann Intern Med* 98:940–945, 1983.

29. Glazer HS, Weyman PJ, Sagel SS, Levitt RG, McClennan BL: Nonfunctioning adrenal masses: incidental discovery on computed tomography. *AJR* 139:81–85, 1982.

30. Mitnick JS, Bosniak MA, Megibow AJ, Naidich DP: Nonfunctioning adrenal adenomas discovered incidentally on computed tomography. *Radiology* 148:495–499, 1983.

31. Reinig JW, Doppman JL, Dwyer AJ, Johnson AR, Knop RH: Adrenal masses differentiated by MR. *Radiology* 158:81–84, 1986.

32. Glazer GM, Woolsey EJ, Borrello J, Francis IR, Aisen AM, Bookstein F, Amendola MA, Gross MD, Bree R., Martel W: Adrenal tissue characterization using MR imaging. *Radiology* 158:73–79, 1986.

33. Henley DJ, van Heerden JA, Grant CS, Carney JA, Carpenter PC: Adrenal cortical carcinoma—a continuing challenge. *Surgery* 94:926- 931, 1983.

34. Steingart DE, Motazdy A, Noonan RA, Thompson NW: Treatment of adrenal carcinoma. *Arch Surg* 117:1142–1146, 1982.

35. Hamberger B, Russell CF, van Heerden JA, ReMine WH, Northcutt RC, Sheedy PF, Edis AJ, Ilstrup DM: Adrenal surgery trends during the seventies. *Am J Surg* 144:523–526, 1982.

36. Swenson SJ, Brown MJ, Sheps SG, Sizemore GW, Gharib H, Grant CS, van Heerden JA: Use of 131-MIBG scintigraphy in the evaluation of suspected pheochromocytoma. *Mayo Clin Proc* 60:299–304, 1985.

37. van Heerden JA, Sizemore GW, Carney JA, Grant CS, ReMine WH, Sheps SG: Surgical management of the adrenal glands in the multiple endocrine neoplasia type II syndrome. *World J Surg* 8:612–621, 1984.

Chapter 9

Surgery of Thyroid and Parathyroid Disorders in the Aged

Oliver H. Beahrs, M.D., F.A.C.S.

The diseases of the thyroid gland and the parathyroid glands are essentially the same for all age groups. However, the incidence of diseases in these two endocrine organs varies somewhat from the young to the elderly. The fact that there is an increasing number of elderly people in the United States and elsewhere in the world is somewhat responsible for the increased frequency at which some of these diseases are occurring. The absolute incidence of thyroid disorders is not increasing, just the total numbers because of the increased numbers of elderly people. In the early 1900s, about 4% of the population of the United States was over 65 years of age, whereas it is projected that by the year 2000, 17% of the population will be over 65.

Although not entirely true for each individual, it is reasonable to say that, as most persons grow older, the chance will increase that some serious pathologic change might occur. With increasing age, there is most likely a decrease of functional reserve of the endocrine organs, and this then tends to lead to some of the diseases that are seen in the elderly.

Another factor that must be considered when dealing with thyroid and parathyroid diseases in the elderly is that their symptoms often are not as clear-cut as they are with those diseases in the younger population. The possible existence of other concomitant diseases in an older person complicates the evaluation of the symptoms and delays the establishment of an appropriate diagnosis. Thyroid disorders must be considered in the differential diagnosis of almost every elderly patient's problems (1). Sirota warns that a clinician dealing with an elderly population must keep in mind that thyroid disorders of patients in that age group frequently present with manifestations more suggestive of disease entities of other organ systems than of thyroid disease (2).

In general, once thyroid or parathyroid illness is diagnosed, the management of the condition is essentially the same for all age groups. However, in the elderly, because of the risks that might be present due to coexisting disease, some of which will increase the risk of surgical treatment, the decision-making process regarding the surgical management of the problem has to be very carefully considered. Likewise, the risk of thyroid and parathyroid disease in an elderly patient has to be given some weight in the decision, as well as the anticipated longevity of the patient considering all the other medical problems that might be present.

Even though caution needs to be taken, in general, aggressive surgical management of thyroid and parathyroid conditions requiring surgical treatment should be seriously considered for the elderly patient. Definitive surgical management of a thyroid or parathyroid disorder will prevent complications from these untreated conditions that might further interfere with the well-being of the patient.

The actual chronologic age of the patient alone should never be a deciding factor in the final decision whether to operate or not operate. Instead, the physiologic age of the patient, carefully evaluated and considered, is the most important factor in making the final decision. In other words, if a patient is 80 years of age and has no evidence of any other disease process that would increase the risk of surgical treatment, age alone should not interfere with the decision to treat that patient surgically for a thyroid condition or a parathyroid condition that is or might be a potential hazard to the patient's well-being. In a

128

younger patient, it is not always necessary to be so critical when evaluating the preoperative cardiac function, pulmonary function, and other aspects of the patient's health. However, it is increasingly necessary to be very careful in the preoperative evaluation of the older patient, so that undue risks are not taken in the management of a particular problem related to the thyroid or parathyroid glands. If the outcome of any surgical treatment is in the best interest of the patient and the benefits outweigh the risks of undertaking the operation, then the procedure should be carried out.

In the elderly patient, it becomes increasingly important that the purpose and intent of the surgical treatment be carefully discussed with the patient and relatives so that some other benefits unrelated to the operation are not unduly and unrealistically anticipated. In other words, if a condition exists that, in fact, is causing no symptoms at the moment, but some symptoms of another chronic process exist, it is important for the patient to recognize that the treatment of the current asymptomatic lesion of the thyroid or parathyroid glands will not necessarily make any difference in or be any help for those other existing symptoms. The patient should be made to understand that the operation will prevent serious symptoms and drastic problems in the future that might complicate his or her well-being.

Naturally, a physician wants to provide each and every patient with the very best and the highest quality of care irrespective of socioeconomic factors. However, these factors cannot be entirely ignored and should always be given secondary importance in making a final decision as to whether the benefits of the surgical treatment in an elderly patient are justified. If longevity is predicted to be shortened because of coexisting disease, treatment of thyroid or parathyroid disease in the elderly might not be practical or required.

SPECIFIC DISEASE CONDITIONS OF THE THYROID GLAND

Conditions of the thyroid gland that are of importance and that will be discussed are those of hyper- and hypofunction resulting in either thyrotoxicosis or myxedema or hypothyroidism.

There are also inflammatory diseases, such as acute thyroiditis, lymphocytic thyroiditis, subacute or granulomatous thyroiditis (de Quervain's thyroiditis), and fibrous thyroiditis (Riedel's struma).

Neoplasms of the thyroid gland to be considered include adenomas that will be degenerative or colloid adenomas (not true neoplasms); fetal adenomas, either single or multiple; and, lastly, malignant neoplasms that include well-differentiated carcinomas, such as papillary and follicular adenocarcinoma, and the more aggressive undifferentiated cancers, such as medullary and anaplastic adenocarcinoma. Medullary adenocarcinoma can be familial or sporadic in type. Anaplastic adenocarcinoma is undifferentiated and occurs in several cellular types. In addition to the adenocarcinomas, lymphosarcoma is seen in the thyroid gland occasionally, and very rarely a metastatic cancer that is spread from some other anatomic site will be found. The most frequently occurring metastases are from a hypernephroma and a cancer of the breast.

Thyrotoxicosis

Thyrotoxicosis in the elderly is one of two types. First, exophthalmic goiter is the result of parenchymatous hypertrophy and is otherwise known as Graves' disease. Thyrotoxicosis from an adenomatous goiter has become known as Plummer's disease.

Exophthalmic goiter can occur overtly in about 1% of elderly patients and is seen more commonly in women than in men. Davis states that about 20% of hyperthyroid patients are elderly, and possibly one-third of all thyrotoxic patients are older than 60 years (3). Exophthalmus is a prominent symptom of thyrotoxicosis in younger patients, but it is not seen as often in older patients. The symptoms that do exist in the older patients are much milder. Weight loss is usually due to anorexia in the thyrotoxic elderly patient whereas it is more often associated with an increased oral intake in younger patients. Palpitations and other cardiac symptoms might predominate in the aged patient and lead to some uncertainty as to the underlying cause of the problem, in part because thyroid disease is not usually considered early on. The presence of Graves' disease can be confirmed by palpation of the thyroid gland, which is not always enlarged but which is usually firm. A bruit can be heard on auscultation. The normal thyroid gland in the elderly is somewhat larger than the thyroid gland in the young, weighing as much as 30 to 40 grams. Size alone, then, is not always important, but rather the consistency of the gland and the presence of a bruit are diagnostic.

Laboratory studies can confirm the diagnosis. Elevation of the T4 and T3 levels and radioisotope uptake determinations support the diagnosis of exophthalmic goiter. Once the diagnosis of Graves' disease is established, several forms of treatment can be considered. First, the modality most often used is ablation of the thyroid gland in part or totally with radioactive iodine. This treatment is effective in over 95% of cases. The big disadvantage is that most patients so treated will eventually become hypothyroid, requiring thyroid medication to maintain a euthyroid state. The radiation effect on the thyroid tissue is not only immediate, but is progressive. There are a few patients who have an allergy to iodine, and for that reason, an alternate method of treatment must be considered for them.

At one time, the second method, the use of antithyroid drugs, was very popular, but today they are infrequently used unless to prepare the patient for thyroidectomy. With the use of antithyroid drugs as the primary treatment, the patient can be brought to a euthyroid state, but it is necessary to continue the antithyroid drugs over a prolonged period of time. Upon discontinuance of their use, about one-half of the patients will have a recurrence of the thyrotoxicosis.

Third, surgical thyroidectomy remains a very effective method of treating Graves' disease. It is considered the treatment of choice by Simms (4). The only disadvantage of this modality is that it is an operation, and most patients, especially those in an older age group, would prefer an alternative to an operation if the results of the alternative were equally good.

Subtotal thyroidectomy, a double-lobe resection with removal of the isthmus, results in a 97% cure rate and only a 3% recurrence rate, which are essentially the same as that when radioactive iodine is used (5). One advantage of surgical therapy is that it is immediately effective, whereas with the use of radioactive iodine, the effect is somewhat delayed and is then progressive toward cure and most often beyond.

There is potential morbidity associated with a thyroidectomy. However, in the hands of surgeons who are experts in thyroid procedures, the risk of iatrogenic injury to the recurrent laryngeal nerve is almost nonexistent. However, there is about a 1% risk of hypoparathyroidism secondary to either excision of all the parathyroid tissue or interference with the blood supply to all the parathyroid glands. Katz argues for total thyroidectomy in the treatment of Graves' disease, but in general, the morbidity of this procedure is higher in the hands of most surgeons (6).

One distinct advantage of surgical resection of the thyroid is that in 3%–5% of cases, there will be found a coexisting cancer. For this reason, thyroidectomy can be argued to be the method of choice. However, it should be recognized that almost all of these incidental malignant lesions are small and papillary in cellular type. For that reason, in an elderly population, it is highly unlikely that these coexisting papillary cancers will ever become a clinical problem if the patient is treated by a nonoperative modality. Those cases that recur after surgical thyroidectomy are best treated by radioactive iodine because the risks of secondary thyroidectomy are about twice those of a primary thyroid operation.

Thyrotoxicosis secondary to a adenomatous goiter (Plummer's disease) often presents itself in the way of cardiac symptoms in an older person. Cardiac irregularity, tachycardia, and decompensation are the most common cardiac findings. If an elderly patient presents with these cardiac symptoms, it is well to evaluate thyroid function, especially if there is a palpable lesion in the thyroid gland. A radioisotope scan will usually show a hot nodule, which is an indication of hyperfunction of localized thyroid tissue. Although a hot nodule might be treated by radioactive iodine, surgical thyroidectomy is preferred unless there is a serious medical contraindication to an operation. By removing the nodular portion of the thyroid gland, the hyperfunctioning nodule is not only excised but the risk of its being a malignant neoplasm is also eliminated. Also, if the lesion is somewhat large, the risk of pressure symptoms on the airway or on the esophagus is eliminated, and the unsightly cosmetic appearance of a tumor is corrected.

Elderly patients being treated either with radioactive iodine or with thyroidectomy for thyrotoxicosis usually should be placed on a euthyroid dose of thyroid replacement therapy to prevent the development of myxedema or hypothyroidism. Patients with Graves' disease might also be placed on a small dose of iodine when they are treated surgically to reduce the chance of significant symptoms should a recurrence develop.

Thyroiditis

Riedel's Struma

Fibrous thyroiditis or *Riedel's struma* occurs infrequently, but when it does, it is almost always found in the elderly. Actually, it is seen once in about 2,000 thyroidectomies carried out for all causes. On palpation, it appears as a firm-to-hard thyroid gland that is somewhat fixed to adjacent tissues. Because of its physical characteristics, it is impossible to rule out the presence of a cancer. Even though needle or aspiration biopsy might be considered, many times the gland is so hard that in this condition, as in so many others, this diagnostic approach is unsuccessful. For this reason, and in particular to rule out the chance that a cancer is present, thyroidectomy is indicated. At the time of the operation when fibrous thyroiditis is found, it is reasonable to resect a part of the lesion and to free up the trachea. It is not essential that the total thyroid gland be removed, and no adjacent tissues that might be involved need be excised. Following the surgical procedure, in certain instances, steroids might be given with the hope that doing so will further reduce the fibrous and inflammatory process.

de Quervain's Thyroiditis

Subacute granulomatous thyroiditis or *de Quervain's thyroiditis* usually starts in one area of the thyroid gland as a painful, tender mass, and then it gradually becomes progressive to involve other parts of the thyroid gland. Most often, this thyroiditis can be identified and diagnosed by its historical and physical characteristics. Surgical treatment is not necessary. Actually, after a short period of time, varying from a few weeks to several months, the process

will "burn" itself out. Steroids will usually be of some benefit in the treatment of the worst symptoms, and they will most likely have a beneficial effect on reducing the pathologic process.

Hashimoto's Thyroiditis

Hashimoto's thyroiditis or *lymphocytic thyroiditis* is seen in older age groups much more frequently than in the young. The thyroid gland, when this process is present, can vary considerably in size. Some patients will have glands that are of about normal size and weight, and others with this disease will have a gland that weighs 100 or more grams. The gland is rubbery in consistency, and it has a nodular surface. On physical examination, this nodular surface can be felt, and the process can be suspected. Most often, the entire gland—that is, both lobes and the isthmus—is involved. When this condition is suspected, a needle biopsy, especially if it is a core biopsy, will usually but not always substantiate the diagnosis.

Unless there are symptoms related to the presence of a goiter, surgical treatment is not indicated. However, all patients with suspected Hashimoto's thyroiditis should be placed on thyroid suppression therapy using euthyroid doses of exogenous thyroxin. These patients should then be followed *very* carefully because, in a certain number of glands with lymphocytic thyroiditis, coexisting neoplasms will occur. Clark has stated that patients with Hasimoto's thyroiditis can be separated into those at low risk and those at high risk for cancer (7). Those glands having a dominant cold nodule will have a 25% chance of having cancer. In 605 cases of lymphocytic thyroiditis operated at our institution, papillary cancer coexisted in 3% of the cases, and in another 3% lymphosarcoma coexisted (8). Because of this experience, we feel that it is essential for a patient with Hashimoto's thyroiditis who is being treated medically to be followed very carefully. If the gland does not significantly diminish in size or if it becomes apparent that a discrete nodule is present or developing, then thyroidectomy should be carried out straight away and the underlying pathology treated appropriately.

If a malignant lesion is not found to be present

at the time of the surgical exploration, only a sub-total thyroidectomy is indicated. These patients should then be placed again on thyroid replacement therapy in euthyroid doses (9).

Nodular Goiter and Cancer

In the elderly, the occurrence of nodular goiter is very frequent. It has been estimated that, in women over the age of 70, 90% of thyroid glands will contain some nodules. In men over the age of 80, it is estimated that 80% of glands will be nodular.

Mortenson, in 1,000 routine necropsies, found that over 50% of the thyroid glands that he examined contained nodules and that 2.8% of these glands contained a primary cancer, whereas another 2% contained metastatic cancers (10).

Because of the frequency of the occurrence of nodular goiter, especially in the elderly, it becomes entirely impractical to consider thyroidectomy for all patients just because a nodule is present. Therefore, selection has to be based on evaluation of the nodule using historical and physical facts and biopsy information. Clark states that thyroidectomy is indicated for elderly patients in a high-risk group (11).

If a nodular goiter has been present without significant change for many years, is multinodular in type, is relatively soft, and is easily felt, it seems reasonable to follow the patient and not advise surgical removal. On the other hand, if the goiter is new, if the lesion is discrete or is thought to be a solitary or a single nodule that is increasing in size, and the nodule is firm to palpation, then it should be considered a surgical problem.

Preliminary to a final decision whether the goiter should be removed, one might occasionally consider a needle biopsy or an aspiration biopsy to determine the cellular type of lesion. If the biopsy is positive, the decision is easy! Likewise, one might consider a radioisotope scan because most cancers of the thyroid gland will show as a cold nodule; however, the presence of a hot nodule does not rule out the possibility that the lesion is a cancer. For this reason, undue emphasis should not be placed on whether the nodule is hot or cold. Considering the historical facts and physical findings, and especially if the needle biopsy shows a neoplasm, then surgical treatment is indicated. If the needle biopsy is negative

but the suspicion is still great that it is malignant, the nodule should be excised. Hamburger indicates that fewer papillary carcinomas and significantly more anaplastic and medullary carcinomas are seen in older patients (12).

At the time of the surgical procedure, if the lesion grossly in all respects appears to be benign, then either a partial lobectomy or a subtotal thyroidectomy should be carried out. On the other hand, if the lesion appears to be a malignant one, then the operation preferably should be tailored for the type of cancer that is present.

Papillary Carcinoma

If the lesion is considered to be a papillary adenocarcinoma, then it is our preference for a lobectomy to be done on the side of the lesion, with removal of the isthmus and a partial lobectomy done on the opposite side. Even though a total thyroidectomy is advocated by many, and admittedly the procedure can be carried out safely in the hands of the experts, it is not essential that a total thyroidectomy be done for papillary carcinoma. Actually, in the follow-up of 692 of our patients with papillary cancer, none died when the primary lesion was less than 1-1/2 cm in diameter over a 40-year period, and only 3% died of the cancer when the lesion was greater than 1-1/2 cm in diameter but was still contained within the thyroid gland (13). This was true even though 39% and 50% respectively had regional lymph node metastasis. Almost all of our cases were treated by less than a total thyroidectomy.

If the papillary cancer is extrathyroidal or if distant metastases are known to be present, then certainly a total thyroidectomy and postoperative radioactive iodine therapy is indicated.

If regional lymphadenopathy is present that is thought to be due to metastatic thyroid cancer, then a modified neck dissection is indicated to remove the involved lymph nodes and the adjacent tissues. Rarely is a standard radical neck dissection justified for this type of neoplasm.

Again, the reason for being conservative in the treatment of this lesion is that it has an excellent prognosis and it is best not to expose the patient to the morbidity of the more extensive surgical procedure. The average age of patients with papillary cancer is 42 years. The lesions appear to be larger in the older age group. However, it should be recognized that, if a papillary cancer is left alone long enough, 2% to 4% of all cases will undergo a more aggressive malignant transformation, change into an anaplastic cancer, and behave as such. This has been noticed to occur most often in older patients. Therefore, a papillary cancer of the thyroid in the elderly patient should be removed to reduce the chance of this occurring.

Follicular Carcinoma

Follicular cancers occur in an age group about 10 years older than those patients who have papillary cancers. The malignant characteristics of these lesions are related to the presence or absence of blood vessel and capsular invasion. They tend to spread distantly most often and only infrequently spread to the regional lymphatics. This cancer is best treated by a total thyroidectomy. By eliminating all normally functioning thyroid tissue, the patient is better prepared for radioactive iodine treatment of any residual or distant tumor, if present. This can then be done postoperatively or at any time during the follow-up period if recurrence should occur.

Medullary Carcinoma

Medullary cancer of the thyroid, of both the familial and sporadic groups, occurs in older patients. For this reason, this cancer must be considered as a possibility at the time of evaluation of any thyroid condition and should be suspected at the time of any thyroid operation. These lesions are more aggressive than either the papillary or the follicular types of thyroid cancers and are frequently multicentric. They are best treated by total thyroidectomy. This cancer spreads to the regional lymphatics, and if lymphadenopathy is present at the time of treatment, then an appropriate radical neck dissection should be carried out. In older patients, as in all patients with a medullary cancer, family members should be screened for the presence of thyroid abnormalities and, if present, treated appropriately. Medullary thyroid carcinoma can be diagnosed early using basal and poststimulation levels of calcitonin (14).

Anaplastic Carcinoma

Anaplastic adenocarcinoma occurs in older patients, is a rapidly growing cancer that invades the tissues immediately adjacent to the thyroid gland, and spreads distantly. The tumor can be suspected or diagnosed by considering some historical facts and by the physical findings. In the presence of this lesion and as it expands, there is danger of compromise of the airway. Even though the prognosis is dismally poor in the surgical management of the lesion, it is reasonable to debulk the tumor. Frequently the establishment of a tracheostomy is necessary to protect the airway. Postoperatively, radiation therapy and chemotherapy should be considered. Even though these measures are all used, most patients die of this cancer within 12 months of its diagnosis, and only about 5% will live longer than a year.

Thyroid Lymphoma

Lymphosarcoma occurs infrequently in the thyroid gland. It may be found at the time of thyroid exploration or occasionally by needle biopsy. When present, thyroidectomy is indicated, and radiation therapy is indicated postoperatively.

Tumors Metastatic to Thyroid

The possibility of a metastatic lesion must always be considered in the evaluation of an elderly patient with a thyroid problem. The most common origin of a metastatic tumor to the thyroid gland is first from a hypernephroma of the kidney and secondly from an adenocarcinoma of the breast.

Discussion

In the Mayo experience with evaluating older patients for abnormal thyroid findings, only about 10% of these patients come to surgical treatment. The others are observed because their lesions are not considered to be of surgical significance or there are medical contraindications to an operation. Even though a lesion is asymptomatic, if it is large enough to be a cosmetic problem or if it is large enough to be causing compression or deviation of the airway or compression of the esophagus, thyroidectomy should be considered to prevent these symptomatic complications.

In the best of hands, there should be no mortality to thyroidectomy if the cases are appropriately selected for surgical management. The mortality rate should be less than 1%, even though the patient is being operated upon at some risk. The morbidity of these procedures likewise should be very low. The recurrent laryngeal nerves should in all cases be identified in order to protect them from injury. They should be sacrificed only when it is absolutely necessary to do so, i.e., in order to make the operative procedure a definitive one. Also, in almost all cases, care should be taken to identify and protect parathyroid tissue and the blood supply to these glands in order to prevent postoperative tetany or chronic hypoparathyroidism. Parathyroid tissue should be sacrificed only when it is absolutely essential to the operative procedure. If normal parathyroid glands are excised by necessity in carrying out the thyroid resection, consideration should be given toward implantation of the parathyroid tissue either back into the soft tissue of the neck or into the forearm.

Finally, patients in the older age groups who have findings that are suspicious for or suggestive of thyroid pathology, whether the patient is asymptomatic or symptomatic, should be treated appropriately. The surgical management of a patient in an older age group should be no different than the management of a patient in a younger age group. With the increase in the number of older persons in our nation's population, there is the possibility that thyroid problems will be seen more frequently and that they will require both medical and surgical management.

PARATHYROID PROBLEMS IN THE ELDERLY

Several decades ago, primary hyperparathyroidism was an infrequently occurring disease, or at least it is more likely that it was clinically recognized infrequently. However, the advent of the less expensive autoanalyzer, used routinely now for determining the levels of multiple chemical components of the blood, including serum calcium and serum phosphorous levels, has resulted in the identification of hyperparathyroidism with increasing frequency. It is likely that the true occurrence of hypercalcemia secondary to hyperparathyroidism has not significantly changed over the years but that cases of elevated calcium in serum are now more often identified. The increasing identification of hypercalcemia in "asymptomatic" or borderline cases has led to a better understanding of the variety of symptoms that can occur from the elevation of calcium in the blood.

At one time, bone disease appearing as osteitis fibrosis cystica, von Recklinghausen's disease, was thought to be the primary presentation of all cases of hyperparathyroidism, along with the usual occurrence of urinary calculi. In earlier years, presentation by stone or bone disease was responsible for the diagnosis of hyperparathyroidism in well over 50% of the cases. Today, bone disease is actually seen infrequently, and even stone disease is seen less often than previously. Hypercalcemia, when discovered in the course of screening, when it is asymptomatic, or when symptoms are ill-defined, such as with neuromuscular complaints, mental disturbances, fatigue, and lethargy, creates diagnostic and management problems. Brennan has reported that studies suggest that approximately 1 to 2 patients per 1,000 in a clinic or hospital population will have primary hyperparathyroidism. In Scandinavia, there is a report that suggests that its presence might be as high as 5.2 per 1,000 (15). Block reported one-third of his cases to be over 60 years of age (16).

In a screening program at the Mayo Clinic, the instance of hypercalcemia was 0.5 per 1,000. In the course of this screening program, the age of the patient diagnosed also increased from a median of 56 years before screening was instituted to 62 years after screening had begun. This is an indication that primary hyperparathyroidism is being seen today in much older age groups.

Brennan added that perhaps the most significant recent observation has been that, among women 60 or more years of age, primary hyperparathyroidism is being diagnosed at an annual rate of 108.5 cases per 100,000, more than twice the rate for men of the same age (15).

The etiology of hyperparathyroidism is not known. The primary process might be in parathyroid tissue alone, but it has been speculated that the parathyroid pathology is secondary to some other endocrine dysfunction. The pathology of parathyroid glands is well established as either being a single or multiple adenoma involving most often a single gland but occasionally involving multiple glands or rarely the condition of hyperplasia involving all of the glands.

Paloyan and others have speculated that the adenomatous changes seen in most parathyroid tissue from hypercalcemic patients are a reflection of hyperplasia (17). Assuming this to be true, it is suggested that in surgical treatment, all four glands be either totally or partially resected, rather than for the single, obviously enlarged gland alone to be excised. Although this possibility does exist, the report by Edis and his colleagues fairly well establishes the fact that, in approximately 80% of cases, the pathology is of a single gland disease, rather than of multiple gland disease secondary to hyperplasia (18).

Recognition of the exact pathology of hyperparathyroidism becomes very important when tailoring the appropriate operation for the management of an individual case. In the elderly, because of the possibility of other aging disorders being present that will affect the serum calcium levels, careful evaluation of the patient has to be undertaken. The chance of a metastatic malignant disease being present is more likely in the elderly than in the young. The presence of osteomalacia and osteoporosis, as well as other conditions, such as prolonged immobilization, must also be considered. Because of this possibility, when hypercalcemia is found either on screening or because of symptoms being present, care has to be taken to evaluate completely the presence or absence of these other processes.

Once primary hyperparathyroidism is diagnosed, the decision has to be made whether surgical intervention is justified in each particular case. Naturally, the age of the patient becomes an important factor in the decision-making process. However, age alone should not be the only deciding factor favoring operation; the presence or absence of other diseases and the general well-being of the patient must also be considered as being most important.

Also, instead of the chronologic age of the patient alone being a deciding factor for operation, the anticipated longevity of the patient at that age must be seriously considered (19). If the symptoms are thought to be related to hypercalcemia and there is a small but very reasonable risk to parathyroidectomy, then cervical exploration should be carried out. If there are no symptoms

and the hypercalcemia has been discovered incidentally in the course of screening, it still seems reasonable to consider cervical exploration in light of the study by Purnell that indicated that, in about 3 years, symptoms became apparent in about 20% of their cases (20).

To leave hypercalcemia untreated, thereby permitting complications of bone disease and stone disease to occur in the elderly is of serious consequence. The skeletal and urinary systems might be adversely affected by other degenerative or aging diseases, and to add these complications from hypercalcemia to the others would jeopardize the patient's general condition and longevity.

In a large series of cases, the risk of mortality from surgical treatment is extremely small, and in various reports, the mortality is less than 1% and in many instances 0%. Morbidity associated with cervical exploration for parathyroid disease includes the potential risk of damage to the recurrent laryngeal nerve with its resultant vocal cord paralysis. This in turn results in changes in the voice, and it could possibly compromise the airway. In addition, depending somewhat on the extent of the parathyroid resection, hypoparathyroidism can be a postoperative complication in some patients, and this condition requires subsequent replacement therapy using a calcium supplement and/or vitamin D.

The technical aspects of parathyroid exploration are very important. There are usually four glands present, two on either side of the neck, which are typically located on the posterior aspects of the thyroid capsule on each side. The glands vary somewhat in normal size from 30 to 60 mg, but grossly they have an appearance that makes them easily identifiable. The glands are light chocolate to dark chocolate brown and well encapsulated with a vascular pedicle; the parathyroid tissue structure is very delicate in contrast to the "meaty" appearance of thyroid tissue, the pale yellow of normal fatty tissue, and the vacuolated appearance of lymphoid tissue.

If the surgeon is fully knowledgeable regarding the embryology and the anatomy of parathyroid glands and if he or she appreciates the abnormal locations where they might be present by embryologic undescent and overdescent, approximately 95% to 97% of the glands can be identified with this knowledge alone (21). With this high success rate of finding all of the glands on neck exploration, there hardly seems need to use any preoperative localizing tests to identify the position of the parathyroid tissue. The most common cause of failure to effect a cure in the course of surgical exploration is the overlooking of multiple gland disease (22). In secondary cases and certainly in tertiary cases where cervical exploration is always required, one or several localizing procedures can be used. These would include ultrasound, computed tomography, magnetic resonance, selective venous sampling, and rarely arteriography. Arteriography is best not used because of the occurrence of neurologic deficits that are seen occasionally secondarily to that procedure, especially in the elderly.

The surgical procedure for cervical exploration is not different in the elderly than the younger patient. In 80% to 90% of cases, single gland involvement will be found. In the remaining cases, primary hyperplasia is most often present. Multiple, single gland involvement occurs in only about 2% of cases, and carcinoma of parathyroid tissue occurs in less than 1% of cases. Removal of abnormal parathyroid tissue of all kinds results in normocalcemia occurring in over 95% of the cases. In the other 5% of cases, the pathology has been overlooked, a fifth gland with the adenoma is present, or an error in the preoperative diagnosis was made. If after cervical exploration, the patient remains hypercalcemic, it is well to observe the patient carefully for a period of 3 to 6 months and then to re-evaluate the basis for the hypercalcemia. If again, the diagnosis of hyperparathyroidism is established, secondary exploration is then justified in most instances.

Cohn and Silen emphasize that normal-appearing parathyroid tissue should not be resected. To do so might result in parathyroid insufficiency, and this should be prevented (23). As Donaldson has pointed out, in today's surgical environment, it is now axiomatic that, in good hands, parathyroidectomy is a safe procedure. He recommends that advanced age and multiple physical disabilities should not preclude the patient from surgical cure of a disorder that may otherwise contribute to further disabilities and loss of independence (24). Alveryd and associates consider cervical exploration to be the treatment of choice for elderly hypercalcemic patients who have nonspecific symptoms, such as neuromuscular deterioration, extreme fatigue, and lethargy (25).

In the future, if the etiology of the several pathologic changes in the parathyroid glands is better understood, then preventive measures might be taken to eliminate the need for surgical treatment. Likewise, in time, medical measures might become more effective, which also would eliminate the need for cervical exploration. In the meantime, because resection is the only effective treatment, it does seem reasonable to recommend the surgical approach to all patients in whom a diagnosis of symptomatic primary hyperparathyroidism is present. Even in those patients in whom hypercalcemia is asymptomatic but in whom it is considered to be due to parathyroid pathology and who are considered to be reasonable surgical risks, then cervical exploration should be considered.

REFERENCES

1. Gambert SR: Atypical presentation of thyroid disease in the elderly. *Geriatrics* 40:63–69, 1985.
2. Sirota DK: Thyroid function and dysfunction in the elderly: a brief review. *Mt Sinai J Med* 47:126–131, 1980.
3. Davis PJ: Endocrines and aging. *Hosp Pract* 12:113–128, 1977.
4. Simms JM, Talbot CH: Surgery for thyrotoxicosis. *Br J Surg* 70:581–583, 1983.
5. Beahrs OH, Sakulsky SB: Surgical thyroidectomy in the management of exophthalmic goiter. *Arch Surg* 96:512–516, 1968.
6. Katz AD, Bronson D: Total thyroidectomy in the

management of exophthalmic goiter. *Am J Surg* 136:450–454, 1978.
7. Clark OH, Greenspan FS, Dunphy FE: Hashimoto's thyroiditis and thyroid cancer: indications for operation. *Am J Surg* 140:65–71, 1980.
8. Woolner LB, McConahey WM, Beahrs OH: Struma lymphomatosa and related thyroidal disorders. *J Clin Endocrinol Metab* 19:53–83, 1959.
9. Thomas CG, Rutledge RG: Surgical intervention in chronic (Hashimoto's) thyroiditis. *Ann Surg* 193:769–774, 1981.
10. Mortenson JD, Bennett WA, Woolner LB: Incidence of

carcinoma in thyroid glands removed at 1,000 consecutive routine necropsies. *Surg Forum* 5:659–663, 1954.

11. Clark OH, Demling R: Management of thyroid nodules in the elderly. *Am J Surg* 132:616–619, 1976.

12. Hamburger JI: The presentation of thyroid malignancy in the geriatric patient. *Henry Ford Hosp Med J* 28:158–160, 1980.

13. Woolner LB, Beahrs OH, Black BM, McConahey WM, Keating FR: Thyroid carcinoma: general considerations and follow-up data on 1,181 cases. In Young S, Inman DR (eds): *Thyroid Neoplasia, Proceeding of the Second Imperial Cancer Research Fund Symposium.* London, Academic Press, 1968, pp 51–77.

14. Rossi RL, Cady B, Meissner WA, Wool MS, Sedgwick CE, Werber J: Nonfamilial medullary thyroid carcinoma. *Am J Surg* 139:554–558, 1980.

15. Brennan MF: Primary hyperparathyroidism. *Adv Surg* 16:25–47, 1983.

16. Block MA, Xavier A, Brush BE: Management of primary hyperparathyroidism in the elderly. *J Am Geriatr Soc* 23:385–389, 1975.

17. Paloyan E, Lawrence AM, Straus FH: *Hyperparathyroidism.* New York, Grune and Stratton, 1973.

18. Edis AJ, Beahrs OH, van Heerden JA, Akwari OG: Conservative versus liberal approach to parathyroid neck exploration. *Surgery* 83:466–473, 1977.

19. Lifschitz BM, Barzel US: Parathyroid surgery in the aged. *J Gerontol* 36:573–575, 1981.

20. Purnell DC, Smith LH, Scholz DA: Primary hyperparathyroidism: a prospective clinical study. *Am J Med* 50:670–678, 1971.

21. Satava RM, Beahrs OH, Scholz DA: Success rate of cervical exploration for hyperparathyroidism. *Arch Surg* 110:625–628, 1975.

22. van Heerden JA, Kent RB, Sizemore GW, Grant CS, ReMine WH: Primary hyperparathyroidism in patients with multiple endocrine neoplasia syndromes. *Arch Surg* 118:533–536, 1983.

23. Cohn KH, Silen WS: Lessons of parathyroid reoperations. *Am J Surg* 144:511–517, 1982.

24. Donaldson MD: Hyperparathyroidism in elderly disabled patients. *Med J Aust* 14:455, 1983.

25. Alveryd A, Bostrom H, Wengle B, Wester PO: Indications for surgery in the elderly patient with primary hyperparathyroidism. *Acta Chir Scand* 142:491–494, 1976.

Chapter 10

Plastic and Reconstructive Care in the Elderly

John B. Lynch, M.D., F.A.C.S., R. Bruce Shack, M.D., F.A.C.S.

Plastic and reconstructive surgical care in the elderly may be required for a wide variety of benign or malignant conditions and may be either aesthetic, reconstructive, or a combination of both. Because the major malignant conditions affecting the elderly, such as melanoma, parotid tumors, and other head and neck surgery, are amply covered in other sections of this book, this presentation will be limited to skin lesions and common benign and functional reconstruction required by elderly patients.

Age alone is never a contraindication to surgical therapy in and of itself (1), but we continue to see many patients with non-emergency conditions who have been discouraged from having elective surgical procedures by their primary physician when, in fact, the burden of their problem may be worse by virtue of their advancing years and the benefit to be achieved by an elective procedure is much greater. For example, one 75-year-old patient with symptomatic mammary hypertrophy had been discouraged for 10 years from undergoing surgical correction of this condition based on her age alone. Although this condition may be quite symptomatic in a younger patient, in this lady the symptoms were further aggravated by osteoarthritis of the cervical spine, and following reduction mammoplasty, the symptomatic improvement achieved was even greater than in an otherwise healthy, younger patient.

SKIN LESIONS

One of the most frequent reasons that patients seek plastic surgical consultation is for the evaluation of skin lesions. Many of these are benign

degenerative changes characterized by localized areas of hyperpigmentation. They may cause the patient to be concerned about melanoma. Although dozens of lesions, both benign and malignant, develop in the elderly patient, by far the most frequently encountered ones are cysts, seborrheic keratosis, actinic keratosis, basal cell carcinoma, and squamous cell carcinoma. A variety of lesions arising in the skin and mucosa, which are not in themselves neoplastic, give rise to carcinoma with sufficient frequency that they are properly termed precancerous. These include (1) the keratoses—actinic, localized (cutaneous horn), and arsenical; (2) occupational dermatosis (from tar products); (3) x-ray or radiation dermatitis; (4) xeroderma pigmentosum; and (5) leukoplakia.

Cysts

Cystic lesions of epithelial origin cause frequent tumor like formation in the skin, varying in size from a few millimeters to several centimeters. Within the cyst is a cheesy substance composed of keratinized material, desquamated partially cornified cells, and granular debris. The walls of the cyst are lined by epithelium, and these may have skin appendages as well. Once established these tend to enlarge slowly and are exposed to trauma and recurrent infection and always require total surgical removal for cure.

Seborrheic Keratosis

These pigmented type papillomas occur most commonly on the trunk, but also on the arms, neck, and face. Clinically the lesion is black or brown, is flat to polypoid in profile, and can be mistaken for melanoma. Microscopically the lesion consists of a thickened epidermis in which are cystic areas containing keratin. The cells in the lesion usually resemble basal cells, and the cysts appear to form from invaginations of the horny layer. Melanin present in the cells of the tumor give it its characteristic pigmentation. These lesions are quite superficial, involving only the epidermis. After a punch biopsy is done to establish the diagnosis, treatment is only for cosmetic purposes because these lesions have no malignant potential. Discrete lesions respond well to surgical excision. Because of the superficial nature, they also can be adequately treated by superficial cautery, curettement, or application of other destructive agents, such as liquid nitrogen, all with minimal scarring.

Actinic Keratosis

These precancerous lesions are characterized by hyperkeratosis and thickening of the outer cornified layers of the epithelium. Clinically these present as small plaque-like lesions that frequently tend to be ulcerated and produce itching and other minor symptoms. Often the hyperkeratinized plaque will peel off, and the lesion will appear to be healed, only to recur within a few weeks. Histologically, these lesions exhibit atrophy in the deeper portions of the skin, and a striking feature is the presence of atypia in the cells of the lower layers of the epidermis. Sunlight appears to be the primary causative factor, and if untreated, progression to carcinoma occurs in a high percentage of areas of actinic keratosis. Although localized lesions respond well to excisional biopsy, the extent of these skin changes in some patients may be so extensive and diffuse as to defy surgical treatment. In these patients with extensive disease, multiple biopsies are frequently required to establish the diagnosis of actinic keratosis, and then the application of topical 5-Fluorouracil on a daily basis for 3 to 6 weeks is an effective method of treatment. During the course of treatment, the reaction of the 5-Fluorouracil with the areas of abnormal skin is intense. It produces a marked degree of hyperemia, frequently with blistering and superficial ulceration, that is then followed by crusting and healing. When extensive areas are treated and some localized areas of abnormality persist

following treatment, repeat biopsy and surgical excision are indicated.

Basal Cell Carcinoma

Basal cell carcinoma is the most frequent type of skin cancer. It appears most commonly on the exposed surfaces of the body and is particularly frequent on the upper two-thirds of the face, about the nose and eyelids. Basal cell carcinoma is a tumor characterized by slow growth, and it rarely metastasizes. Clinically, the lesion presents as (1) nodular, (2) ulcerating, or (3) morphea form. The nodular form is a localized discrete lesion with sharp borders, is small in size in its early stages, and responds well to total surgical excision. As time goes by and the lesion enlarges, central ulceration occurs, the borders tend to become more irregular and indistinct, and wider excision is required. In the morphea form type of basal cell carcinoma, the lesion is characterized by the formation of fibrous tissue, which produces a serpiginous irregular lesion that exhibits multiple small ulcerations with very indistinct borders. In this type of tumor, the nests of tumor cells are interspersed in a dense fibrous stroma. Total surgical excision of these lesions may require resection of very extensive areas, and skin grafting or flaps may be required for coverage.

Although basal cell carcinomas are radiosensitive, the use of x-ray can require a protracted course of treatment and generally should be avoided because of the additional damage to the skin and surrounding tissue that may result from the irradiation. In certain recurrent lesions, particularly in important anatomic areas, such as the medial canthus of the eyelid where the borders of the lesion are clinically indistinct, the use of Mohs' chemosurgery (2) has been used increasingly in recent years. This technique involves either fixing the normal tissue in situ with zinc chloride or simply removing sections of the lesion for histologic examination and continuing to remove serial sections of the tissue until histologically clear margins have been obtained (3). By this technique, occasional difficult to evaluate tumors show much more extensive tissue involvement than can be appreciated clinically. This technique is extremely tedious and time consuming and often results in significant defects requiring plastic surgery closure. Although helpful in occasional cases, Mohs' chemosurgery should be reserved for the occasional lesion. It is most useful for recurrent lesions that have indistinct borders and cannot be clinically identified clearly and where excessive resection of tissue is undesirable. The overwhelming majority of basal cell carcinomas can be more expeditiously treated by total surgical excision and closure as required.

Squamous Cell Carcinoma

Squamous cell carcinoma, as is basal cell carcinoma, is most commonly seen in persons after the fifth decade. It is sometimes related to chronic injury or irritation. This tumor may present as a nodular mass or as an ulcerating lesion. Growth tends to be more rapid than in the basal cell carcinoma, and metastasis to regional lymph nodes will ultimately occur in inadequately treated lesions. Distant metastasis is rare and usually occurs as a terminal event in patients who have uncontrolled tumors. Following certain types of chronic irritation, such as burn scars, there can be demonstrated a progressive histologic change in the epidermis consisting of pseudoepitheliomatous hyperplasia that may imitate the appearance of squamous cell carcinoma, and differentiation may be difficult (4). In this reactive hyperplasia, the epidermal cells are usually limited by a definite membrane, and there is less irregularity of cells and arthitectural arrangement until invasive malignancy finally develops.

In early lesions, establishment of the diagnosis by incisional or excisional biopsy should be performed. After the diagnosis has been established, total surgical extirpation is the treatment of choice for early lesions. Because of the ultimate propensity for lymph node involvement if not totally removed, questionable surgical margins are always an indication for re-excision. In advanced lesions involving underlying muscles or bone, a combination of resection and irradiation may be the preferrable method of treatment. Regional node dissection is indicated when the regional lymph nodes become involved. The chemotherapeutic agents available for treatment of uncontrollable squamous cell carcinoma tend to produce irregular remissions of short duration and, until better drugs are developed, are of limited clinical usefulness at the present time.

Lentigo Maligna

This lesion is frequently seen in elderly patients, usually about the face (5). Clinically, it presents as an irregular pigmented lesion that varies in size from quite small to several centimeters in diameter. It tends to be smooth and flat and has irregular borders. The degree of pigmentation may vary from light brown to quite black. Histologically at this stage the lesion consists of intraepithelial melanoma in situ. Although the lesion may wax and wane, if untreated, the natural evolution is the development of melanoma within this lesion, and it should be totally extirpated (6, 7).

BREAST PROCEDURES

A variety of breast conditions in the elderly may require plastic surgical techniques. By far the most common indications are reconstruction of the breast following mastectomy and reduction mammoplasty.

Breast Reconstruction following Mastectomy

Breast cancer continues to be a disease of the older patient, but with increasing frequency it is being diagnosed earlier in younger patients. As a result, requests for breast reconstruction following mastectomy have increased exponentially in recent years. The objectives of breast reconstruction are (1) restoration of the breast mound to eliminate the need for an external prosthesis, (2) achievement of breast symmetry (usually requiring some modification of the remaining breast), and (3) reconstruction of the nipple-areolar complex if the patient desires. The current ablative techniques for treatment of breast cancer are more conservative with preservation of more skin and the pectoralis major and minor muscle. In patients where adequate skin is present, the insertion of a breast prosthesis, usually beneath the pectoralis muscle, and any required modification of the remaining breast, such as ptosis correction or reduction, are suffi-

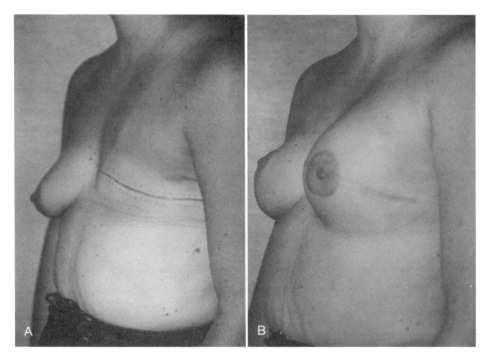

Figure 10.1. **A,** 58-year-old female with the typical sequelae of a left modified radical mastectomy. **B,** Result following left breast reconstruction with tissue expander technique, nipple areolar reconstruction, and mastopexy of the opposite breast for symmetry.

cient to achieve restoration of the breast mound and symmetry at the first procedure. After about 3 months any required adjustment to the breast reconstruction can be performed and reconstruction of the nipple-areolar complex accomplished (Fig. 10.1). In patients in whom the remaining skin is marginal, the use of a tissue expander has increased in recent years. This is an inflatable device that can be placed either beneath the skin or beneath the pectoralis major muscle. It contains a small valve or reservoir that can be injected percutaneously with intravenous saline at intervals of a few days until the desired degree of skin stretching has been achieved. The temporary device is then replaced with a permanent prosthesis and nipple areolar reconstruction performed.

In patients in whom the available skin is inadequate for reconstruction, because more extensive initial surgery was required, soft tissue replacement becomes a necessary part of the reconstruction. For this purpose, the latissimus dorsi musculocutaneous flap with an implant has

been extensively used (8–10). The texture of the skin from the back is thicker and stiffer than normal breast tissue and does not make an ideal skin replacement. In addition, the scar on the back is more objectionable to some patients. For this reason, there has been increasing use of the transverse rectus abdominus flap as a musculocutaneous tissue transfer, which provides adequate skin and soft tissue so that a prosthesis is usually not required (11–13).

Most breast reconstructions are performed in two stages at the present time. The morbidity is low, the complication rate is very acceptable, and these procedures are well tolerated by the elderly patient.

The timing of breast reconstruction is important because to defer reconstruction arbitrarily for a set period, such as 1 year, may deprive the patient of the benefit of reconstruction at the time that it is most important to her. After the mastectomy has been performed, the nodes have been evaluated for the presence of metastases that may dictate a need for chemotherapy, and the wound

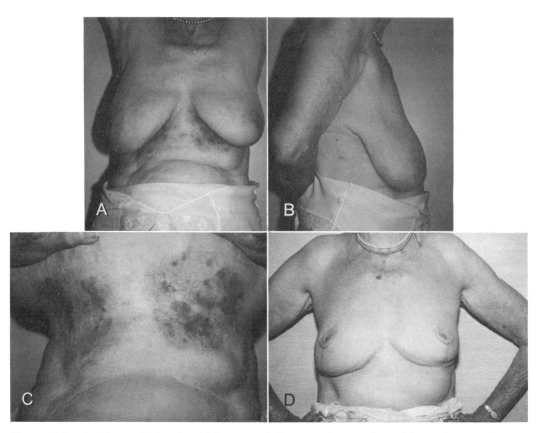

Figure 10.2. A, 76-year-old female with heavy ptotic breasts and severe intertriginous changes refractory to medical treatment for 4 years. **B,** Lateral view. **C,** Close-up of the severe intertrigo of the inframammary fold. **D,** Postoperative result showing complete resolution of the skin problem.

is well healed, there is no advantage for the surgeon or patient in deferring the reconstruction for an arbitrary period of time. The breast reconstruction techniques available do not interfere with subsequent chemotherapy or irradiation if this is indicated. A survey by the American Society of Plastic and Reconstructive Surgeons of its membership in the fall of 1985 indicated that 33% of patients undergo some initial reconstruction at the time of mastectomy and 66% of reconstructions are delayed until the wound is healed. In selected patients the insertion of a prosthesis or tissue expander at the time of initial mastectomy may have great psychological benefits.

Reduction Mammoplasty

Although mammary hypertrophy in an occasional patient may be associated with endocrine abnormalities, the overwhelming majority of patients develop this condition without any associated underlying pathology. In younger patients this can be a source of embarrassment and self-consciousness, as well as of physical symptoms. Depending upon the degree, mammary hypertrophy may produce symptoms of pressure and heaviness. In more advanced cases chronic pressure from the bra straps over the shoulder produces pain and discomfort in the shoulders, back, and neck, and brachial plexus symptoms can result from the continuous constriction of bra straps over the shoulder. Although many of these patients tend to be somewhat overweight, weight reduction alone does not have significant influence on the volume of the breast tissue itself. With advancing years, the nuisance and mild chronic symptoms may become more severe, particularly if aggravated by osteoporosis or osteoarthritis of the upper spine and shoulder. The

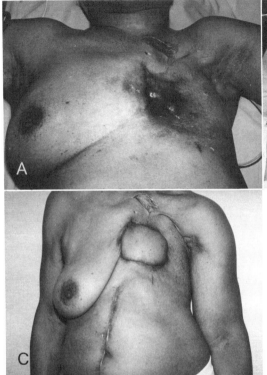
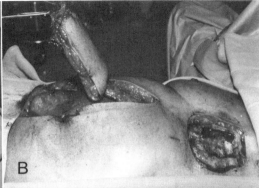

Figure 10.3. A, 82-year-old female following mastectomy and radiation with severe radiation ulcer of the anterior chest wall. **B,** Intraoperative photograph showing full thickness resection of the chest wall to remove the ulcer and elevation of a rectus abdominus musculocutaneous unit for reconstruction. **C,** Postoperative results showing stable, healed wound.

surgical procedures available for reduction mammoplasty are meticulous, tedious, and time consuming, but because no major cavities are entered and the normal body physiology is not disturbed, these procedures are well tolerated by elderly patients and the morbidity is minimal.

Most of the surgical techniques for reduction mammoplasty are based on designing a pattern of skin incisions that permits removal of excess skin and tissue to accomplish a satisfctory reduction of the breast while repositioning the nipple to a more normal superior position with the blood supply of the nipple based on a dermal pedicle (14, 15). An occasional patient is still seen for whom the most expeditious course, because of massive hypertrophy, may be partial amputation of the breast and transfer of the nipple as a free skin graft (16). The use of a vertical or inferiorly based dermal pedicle is more applicable to most patients, and the results are generally better. In properly selected patients the relief of symptoms achieved is so predictable that as a group these patients tend to have a high level of patient satisfaction (Fig. 10.2).

The complications that can result from this procedure include wound infection, hematoma or seroma formation, localized areas of delayed healing, areas of tissue necrosis that in extreme cases can include the nipple, and some temporary loss of sensation in the surgical area with a variable degree of recovery over time. The incidence of major complications of this type is very low, and the morbidity of the procedure is small compared with the symptomatic improvement achieved. One occurrence that must be kept in mind is that as a result of the extensive surgical dissection required, it is not uncommon for small localized areas of fat necrosis to develop, which may not be apparent until several weeks to a few months following the procedure. These areas of fat necrosis usually present as a localized area of tenderness and mild pain associated with a palpable, firm, hard nodule that is clinically suspicious of carcinoma. When this fat necrosis develops during the early postoperative period, if the mammogram shows no calcifications suggestive of malignancy and if the pathology report of the tissue removed at operation shows no

Table 10.1 Muscles Most Frequently Utilized for Muscle Flap or Musculocutaneous

Flap Reconstruction
Head and Neck
Temporalis
Sternocleidomastoid
Platysma
Trapezius
Pectoralis major
Latissimus dorsi
Trunk and Perinuem
Pectoralis major
Latissimus dorsi
Rectus abdominus
Gluteus maximus
Biceps femoris
Gracilis
Tensor fascia lata
Lower Extremity and Foot
Tensor fascia lata
Rectus femoris
Vastus lateralis
Vastus medialis
Gastrocnemius
Soleus
Extensor digitorum communis
Flexor digitorum brevis

proliferative or other precancerous changes, it is safe to defer biopsy and keep these patients under observation for a period of time with the expectation that the fat necrosis will resolve spontaneously.

One other complication that occurs occasionally is Mondor's disease. This is an inflammatory process of the veins in the anterior chest wall and inferior surface of the breast. It presents clinically as vertical, linear bands immediately beneath the breast or on the inferior surface of the breast. The exact etiology is unknown, but it can occur following any type of breast surgery. It is a completely benign, self-limiting condition that resolves spontaneously over a few weeks and requires only symptomatic treatment and patient reassurance.

Difficult Reconstructive Problems

In recent years reconstructive techniques have developed that enable one-stage correction of difficult problems that formerly required multiple stages over a prolonged period of time or for which no good solution was present. These in-clude the use of (1) muscle flap transfers on their vascular pedicle with application of skin grafts; (2) transfer of musculocutaneous flap units as a one-stage procedure on the muscles' vascular pedicle; and (3) free transfer of muscle, musculocutaneous flaps, or skin flaps as a free transfer utilizing microvascular anastomoses. A list of the more commonly utilized musculocutaneous flaps is shown in Table 10.1.

Despite the presence of associated medical disease, such as diabetes, and the increasing frequency of peripheral vascular arteriosclerotic disease in elderly patients, the muscle flap, musculocutaneous flap (Fig. 10.3), or free microvascular flaps (Fig. 10.4) offer the potential of one stage reconstruction with a minimum of morbidity and complications.

AESTHETIC SURGERY

In addition to functional reconstructive problems encountered in the elderly, one of the more frequent reasons for plastic surgical consultation by older patients is a request for aesthetic surgery. With our society's emphasis on physical appearance and physical fitness, many elderly patients are interested in achieving improvement in their appearance.

Preoperative evaluation of patients seeking cosmetic surgery is of paramount importance. In stable, well-adjusted individuals who are seeking some physical improvement in their appearance for their own satisfaction and who have anatomic defects that can be reasonably improved, the results are good and the patients tend to be very satisfied. If on the other hand, patients are seeking cosmetic surgery in an attempt to regain their lost youth from a sense of loss as they approach retirement or from a sense of uselessness following a loss of a spouse or retirement, great caution should be exercised. The most commonly requested procedures are for facelifts, eyelid surgery, and forehead or brow lift, but requests for evaluation include a wide variety of other procedures, such as rhinoplasty, chemical face peel, collagen injections, suction-assisted lipectomy, and correction of excess tissue folds about the arms, breast, abdomen, and thighs.

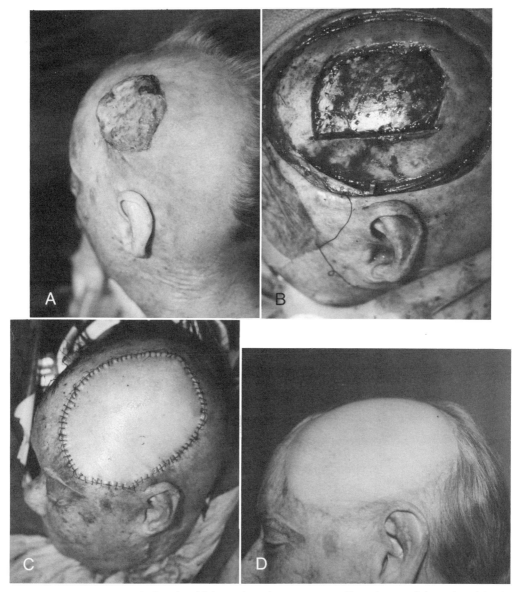

Figure 10.4. **A,** 73 year old female with large, invasive squamous cell carcinoma of the scalp arising in an old burn scar which is the result of a burn in infancy. **B,** Defect of the scalp and calvarium following full thickness resection down to dura. **C,** Immediate postoperative result following reconstruction of the defect with a free latissimus dorsi musculocutaneous flap. **D,** Healed, stable wound 6 months following ablation and reconstruction.

Facelift

Patients seeking consultation regarding facelifts are usually most concerned about tissue relaxation and sagging that involve the nasal labial crease, the jaw line, and the neck, with or without the presence of vertical bands. The surgical approach in suitable patients consists of an incision in the temple that extends down the preauricular area and behind the ear. Through this incision the skin flap of the face and neck is undermined, and the skin is advanced, trimmed, and sutured into position. A variety of ancillary procedures tailored to the individual patient's requirements are currently incorporated as part of the facelift procedure. These include plication, advancement, and other uses of tissue; flaps utilizing the superficial musculoaponeurotic system (SMAS) over the parotid and upper neck region; surgical correction of the vertical bands caused by the leading edge of the platysma; use of platysma flaps; and suction lipectomy of the submental area. This procedure can be performed under local anesthesia and is increasingly performed as an outpatient procedure. The morbidity includes bruising and swelling and temporary sensory changes in the undermined skin of the face and neck. Major complications of infection, hematoma, tissue necrosis, and nerve injury are infrequent and collectively are found in less than 5% of the patients undergoing this procedure.

Eyelids

Patients frequently seek correction of excessive fullness in the upper and lower eyelids or both. This fullness may be simply skin redundancy and, in the upper lid, can be sufficiently severe to exclude lateral vision partially. In addition to the skin redundancy, there is often bulging of the orbital fat to produce the characteristic baggy eyelids which tend to retain edema fluid and give a puffy appearance to the eyelid tissue. Careful preoperative evaluation in these patients is required, not only of visual acuity but also of associated problems of brow ptosis, ptosis of the lacrimal gland, atony of the lower eyelid that predisposes to postoperative ectropion, and other associated abnormalities. The most common

procedure for correction of upper or lower eyelid problems is a local anesthetic procedure usually performed as an outpatient; skin is removed from the upper eyelid, and the incision is deepened if necessary through the orbicularis muscle and the septum orbitale to remove the bulging fat pads that present in the middle of the lower eyelid and in the medial portion of the upper eyelid. In the lower eyelid the skin excision must be conservative to avoid overresection with resulting ectropion. Again the incision is deepened if required to remove the fat bulges in the lower eyelid, which are three in number as compared to two in number of the upper eyelid.

SUMMARY

In summary, all the procedures required for younger patients are equally applicable in the elderly age group. These include repair of all forms of trauma, such as wounds, lacerations, facial fractures, burns, etc. Precancerous and malignant lesions tend to be encountered more frequently in older patients, as are a variety of degenerative skin changes. Aesthetic surgical procedures have increasingly been requested by elderly patients, and the majority of these can be safely performed under local anesthesia as an outpatient with minimum morbidity and good results. In summary, all of the techniques utilized in aesthetic and reconstructive surgery in younger patients are equally applicable to the elderly patient, and the ones most frequently encountered in the elderly patient have been briefly reviewed.

REFERENCES

1. Brown LL: Anesthesia in the geriatric patient. *Clin Plast Surg* 12:51–60, 1985.
2. Mohs FE: Chemotherapy for microscopically controlled excision of skin cancer. *J Surg Oncol* 3:257-n-267, 1971.
3. Tromovitch TA, Stegman SJ: Microscopic-controlled excision of cutaneous tumors: chemosurgery, fresh tissue technique. *Cancer* 41:653–658, 1978.
4. Arons MS, Rodin AE, Lynch JB, Lewis S, Blocker TG: Scar tissue carcinoma—an experimental study with special reference to burn scar carcinoma. *Ann Surg* 163:445–460, 1966.
5. Davis J, Pack GT, Higgins GK: Melanotic freckle of Hutchinson. *Am J Surg* 113:457–463, 1967.
6. Franklin JD, Reynolds VH, Bowers DG, Lynch JB: Cutaneous melanoma of the head and neck. *Clin Plast Surg* 3:413–427, 1976.
7. Shelley WB, Shelley ED: The ten major problems of aging skin. *Geriatrics* 37:107–113, 1982.
8. Bostwick J: *Aesthetic and Reconstructive Breast Surgery.* St. Louis, CV Mosby Co, 1983.
9. Mathes SJ, Nahai F: *Clinical Applications for Muscle and Musculocutaneous Flaps.* St. Louis, CV Mosby Co, 1982.
10. McCraw JB, Penix JO, Baker JW: Repair of major defects of the chest wall and spine with the latissimus dorsi myocutaneous flap. *Plast Reconstr Surg* 62:197–206, 1978.
11. Robbins TH: Rectus abdominus myocutaneous flap for

breast reconstruction. *Aust NZ J Surg* 49:527–530, 1978.

12. Drever JM: Total breast reconstruction. *Ann Plast Surg* 7:54–61, 1981.

13. Hartrampf CR, Scheflan M, Black PW: Breast reconstruction with a transverse abdominal island flap. *Plast Reconstr Surg* 69:216–225, 1982.

14. Strombeck JO: Mammoplasty: report of a new technique based on the two-pedicle procedure. *Br J Plast Surg* 13:79–90, 1960.

15. McKissock PK: Reduction mammoplasty with a vertical dermal flap. *Plast Reconstr Surg* 49:245–252, 1972.

16. Conway H, Smith J: Breast plastic surgery: reduction mammoplasty, mastopexy, augmentation mammoplasty, and mammary construction: analysis of 245 cases. *Plast Reconstr Surg* 21:8–19, 1958.

Chapter 11

Cancer of the Head and Neck in the Elderly

Louis Rosenfeld, M.D., F.A.C.S., Riley S. Rees, M.D., F.A.C.S.

Malignant neoplasms of the head and neck occur with great frequency in persons in the older age group. Etiologic factors conducive to cancer in this anatomic area include excessive consumption of alcoholic beverages, excessive use of tobacco products, and excessive exposure to actinic rays of sunlight. The detrimental effects of these multiple carcinogenic agents do not show up as tumors that develop rapidly, but the effects accumulate progressively over many years and often are responsible for a malignant growth in the sixth, seventh, and even the eighth decade of life (1–4). These phenomena, plus the steadily increasing numbers of the population reaching these advanced years, result in a large percentage of the elderly requiring treatment for cancer that originates in the head and neck area (5). The over age 65 population increased 21.1% from 1950 to 1970, and a major medical risk to this group in the sixth decade or later is the development of cancer of the head and neck (6).

It has been believed by some that treating the aged is less satisfactory, less remunerative, and more likely to end in failure. Some follow the advice of the Roman physician, Alexander of Tralles (525–605 A.D.), who suggested that, "Care should be taken not to do harm to one's reputation by treating the aged where failure is to be expected." This negative attitude is not justified today. Caring for the elderly patient with head and neck cancer can now be quite satisfying to the surgeon, adequately remunerative, and need not end in failure.

Physicians serving these patients have a better opportunity to cure or offer palliation to them than the physician caring for patients with cancer arising in most other sites. They also have the opportunity to use their significant influence to teach their patients about the harmful effects of the substances mentioned above and to strongly encourage them to cease or at least to limit exposure to these agents. The opportunity for cancer surgeons and others in our profession to emphasize these hazards should not be overlooked or taken lightly. The vast majority of head and neck cancers arise from the surface squamous epithelium or from glandular tissue just beneath the surface. The presence of an abnormality in these easily accessible areas should therefore be recognized in its early stage. The mucous membrane of the oral cavity is usually quite sensitive to irritation. People look in a mirror daily and examine their mouths and throats when pain or soreness becomes evident. A nodule or fullness is easily noted intraorally, as well as it is on the face or the neck. One would expect that medical attention would be sought early in the course of any disease occurring in these locations, but unfortunately this is not so.

The physician is not always totally without blame for allowing these easily seen and felt lesions to go untreated for weeks, months, and sometimes even years. For example, the patient with a mass in the parotid may even be advised to ignore it, to avoid surgery, or to have x-ray treatment, because some physicians are fearful of damage to the seventh nerve if an operation is performed. A sore throat that persists may be blamed on infection for a long period before a biopsy is finally taken. An enlarged lymph node or a mass in the neck may be blamed on "inflammation." Such an assumption may sometimes be justified in an infant, a child, or even a teenager, but a nodule in the neck of an adult must always be presumed to be cancer until proven otherwise.

Improper or inadequate treatment of these curable lesions may also result from fear on the part of the patient: fear that a surgical approach to the problem will result in disfigurement and mutilation. This fear is unjustified. Surgical ablation of small lesions usually leaves no physiologic or cosmetic deficit. Radical excision of the more advanced lesions now obligates the modern head and neck surgeon to utilize accepted present day techniques for the restoration of function and appearance of the area. These newer techniques of reconstruction are well established and are highly successful. They are now part of the armamentarium of every well-trained and experienced head and neck surgeon. The final cosmetic and functional result of cancer ablation is now usually quite satisfactory.

Therapeutic Considerations

Salvage of life and long-term cure by surgical excision of cancer of the oral cavity, salivary glands, and of the head and neck in particular are generally good today, with the exception of those lesions that have been allowed to become far advanced by the time they are first seen (7, 8). Death from locally recurrent or persistent cancer of the head and neck is devastating, not only for the patient but for the family and attendants as well. The course of the disease is protracted. Ulceration, bleeding, and a foul putrid odor are inevitable. A tracheostomy is usually required for airway maintenance. When eating becomes impossible, feeding via a gastrostomy, a cervical esophagostomy, or a nasal feeding tube is necessary. Death is frequently secondary to rupture of a carotid artery by the tumor. In an attempt to avoid such a tragic situation a major surgical procedure, even if only for palliation, is often indicated (9). Temporizing in therapy is the easy path early in the course of the disease and may be chosen by both the patient and doctor. However, if radical surgical resection, even though only palliative, is successful the patient may not suffer the often-seen tragedy described above. The patient may die quite comfortably of organ failure due to distant metastatic disease or from some other complicating factors developing outside the area of the head and neck, which are usually less devastating to the patient and the family.

Jun, Strong, Saltzman, and Gerold in 1983 reported an interesting series of 159 patients aged 80 to 95 who were suffering from head and neck cancer (1). The oral cavity was the most common site of the lesion in this report, with larynx and pharynx next in order of frequency. The operative mortality from head and neck procedures in 133 of these elderly patients was only 5.3% in contrast to a 12% operative mortality from most general surgical procedures reported in this age group. No patients with stage I or II tumors died in the postoperative period, even though 77% of the 159 patients had associated major medical illnesses. One hundred nineteen (74.8%) were treated by surgical resection alone, with an average survival of 41 months. Twenty-three (14.4%) patients were treated by irradiation alone, and the average survival for this group was 33 months. When it was necessary to open into the pharynx the mortality rate of the operative group increased, as it also did if preoperative irradiation was given. In this group of patients of far advanced age the effectiveness of treatment is best measured by the absence of cancer during their remaining years. Only 10 of the 73 definitively treated patients died of recurrent cancer.

There are obvious contraindications to operations of great magnitude in the older age group. It is mandatory that the surgeon be able to extirpate the lesion with at least a minimally safe margin. Intractable heart disease with congestive failure that cannot be controlled or diminished pulmonary reserve that cannot be improved by preoperative pulmonary toilet and bronchial dilators are two of the most frequent obstacles. Distant metastases below the clavicles or direct extension of the tumor upward into the base of the skull may also obviate the possibility of a worthwhile surgical procedure (10).

It is not germaine to this discussion to state the proper place of irradiation and/or chemotherapy in treatment of all of these lesions. (See Chapter 6) It should suffice to say that, there should be complete rapport and cooperation among the surgeon, the radiotherapist, and the chemotherapist. There is no place for narrow-minded jealousies among these three specialties. The surgeon should employ adjuvant therapy when indicated, but should not become the technician for the whim of the other two specialists. New chemotherapeutic agents and radiation techniques are continually being tried in prospective studies, and the results from these modalities of treatment are promising for the future. The surgeon should remain the patient's principal physician throughout the therapeutic and postoperative phase.

Diagnostic Considerations

An accurate diagnosis is relatively easy to establish in patients with cancer about the head and neck. After the usual history and general physical examination have been carried out, biopsy of the suspicious area is necessary to obtain tissue for exact determination of the cell type of the neoplasm. Frequently this is a simple office procedure if the lesion is accessible. Local anesthesia and a small biting biopsy forceps or a scalpel are usually adequate for gingiva, buccal, floor of the mouth, tongue, palatal, and tonsillar lesions. Ulcerated lesions of these areas may require no local anesthesia for biopsy.

Needle biopsy is now becoming a technique of value for securing tissue from a neck nodule. A pathologist must be available who is comfortable with this method and who is competent in interpreting this type of material. Needle biopsy is not suited for the securing of tissue from salivary tissue, nor is it of much help in biopsy of intraoral lesions.

Adequate examination to find the primary lesion inside the mouth requires the use of a head mirror or head lamp to allow the examiner the use of both hands. Inspection of the area is important, but palpation is often equally rewarding. A glove or fingercot is used on at least one hand for this purpose. A metal tongue depressor is much superior to wooden blades. The use of a topical anesthetic spray or some other type of local anesthesia reduces the gag reflux. Laryngeal and nasopharyngeal mirrors are a must, and they should either be warmed or an effective antifog material applied. Frequently, squamous cell cancers arising in the upper aerodigestive tract are multicentric, and a complete examination should always be carried out to exclude a second primary neoplasm.

Prior to operation the hospitalized elderly patient with head and neck cancer requires an ECG, a chest x-ray, the usual urine and blood analyses, and also a battery of serum electrolytes and liver function studies. Depending on the site and extent of the lesion, special studies, such as CT scans, tomogram x-rays, and isotope uptake studies, may be indicated. In the elderly patient pulmonary function studies are necessary and are of great importance. Endoscopic investigation with the nasopharyngoscope, laryngoscope, bronchoscope, and esophagoscope are frequently indicated before a complete and final decision can be made about the operative procedure.

Two methods of classifying and staging cancers of the head and neck as to size and extent of disease have been developed (7). The use of these systems makes possible the proper comparison of results of different types of treatment. Classification should be done clinically preoperatively, and pathologic staging of the specimen must be done postoperatively. The TNM and the stage tables are as follows:

T =   Size, N=neck nodes, M=distant metastases
TIS =   In Situ
T1 =   Greatest diameter less than 2 cm
T2 =   Greatest diameter 2 to 4 cm
T3 =   Greatest diameter greater than 4 cm
T4 =   Massive tumor greater than 4 cm with deep invasion
N0 =   Negative nodes clinically
N1 =   Single ipsilateral node less than 3 cm
N2 =   Single ipsilateral nodes 3–6 cm (N2A) or multiple ipsilateral nodes less than 6 cm (N2B)
N3 =   Massive ipsilateral, bilateral, or contralateral nodes
M0 =   No evidence of distant metastases
M1 =   Distant metastases present

Stage of Disease
  Stage I =T1 N0 M0
  Stage II =T2 N0 M0
  Stage III =T3 N0 M0 *or* T2, T3 N1 M0
  Stage IV =T4 N0 or N1, any TN2 or N3, T any N with M1

CERVICAL NODULES AND MASSES

The presence of a neck nodule in an elderly patient, with the exception of a benign thyroid nodule or a soft lipoma-like mass, demands a presumptive clinical diagnosis of cancer, probably metastatic (11). The rule of 80 states that in an adult with enlarged cervical node or nodes the following generalizations hold: 80% of non-thyroid nodules are neoplastic; 80% of these nodules are malignant; 80% of the malignant lesions are metastatic from a primary site above the clavicles.

The more common benign neck masses, in addition to thyroid nodules, are lipomas, salivary gland tumors, and neurilemomas (12). The presence of the neck nodule may be the presenting symptom, or it may have been noted by the referring physician during an examination for an unrelated complaint. Investigation should go forward from that point to establish a primary diagnosis. The history elicited may simplify the search. Oral pain or bleeding, a sore throat lasting several weeks or longer, persistent earache, or hoarseness are all symptoms pointing to the upper aerodigestive tract as being the primary site of trouble. A history may be given that a skin lesion has been excised or removed by irradiation or cautery in the recent or even in the distant past. A fullness or nodule may have been noted for months or years in the parotid area, the inner cheek, the palate, or tongue without pain or ulceration. There may be no symptoms suggesting an oral, cheek, or pharyngolaryngeal lesion, but instead a complaint of chronic temperature elevation, malaise, and weight loss may be elicited and be suggestive of Hodgkin's disease or non-Hodgkin's lymphoma. A thyroid mass may be the presenting complaint, with a lateral neck nodule as an incidental finding.

In the search for the primary lesion, it is helpful to divide the neck in one's mind into upper, middle, and lower third zones (13). Cancer metastasizes primarily along lymphatic vessels via lymphatic fluid and thus lymph nodes will tend to contain metastatic deposits from primary lesions located more cephalad to the involved node.

In the upper neck, the "chief" node, so called because of its frequent involvement in trapping cancer cells, lies adjacent to the internal jugular vein just below the site at which the vein passes beneath the digastric muscle. This node is an close proximity to the bifurcation of the common carotid artery, and it may be confused with the carotid bulb or vice versa (14).

Lymph node enlargements in the middle third of the neck may contain metastases from primary lesions arising superiorly. They may also contain cancer from thyroid, larynx, esophagus, or skin or they may represent primary lymphoma or sarcoma (15).

In the lower third of the neck an additional dimension is added to the search for the primary site. Visceral cancers arising from the lungs, esophagus, stomach, liver, or pancreas may metastasize via the thoracic duct to the left neck and appear in a supraclavicular node (Virchow's) at the site of the duct's entry into the venous system. This is at the junction of the left subclavian and internal jugular veins. These lymph nodes are felt deep within the neck just above the clavicle and are usually fixed and immobile. In the vast majority of patients with a metastatic neck mass the primary cancer will be above the clavicles (16).

Biopsy and microscopic diagnosis of the primary cancer are mandatory before treatment can begin. A punch drill, or a biting forcep biopsy will often suffice to secure material from a skin or oral lesion. Aspiration biopsy of a neck nodule will frequently yield adequate material for definitive diagnosis if an experienced pathologist is available who is comfortable with and skilled at the interpretation of this type of specimen.

Before entering the neck surgically in an attempt to secure tissue for diagnosis, it is imperative that a diligent preoperative search has been carried out in an effort to locate the original site of the tumor. If this search is not done preoperatively and the neck mass proves to be squamous cell cancer, several unfortunate situations result:

1. The wound is closed, and a subsequent complete search is in order.
2. The opportunity is lost to make an incontinuity neck and primary site *en bloc* excision as one operation.
3. The anatomic tissue planes of the neck are violated; cancer cells may be spread, and the fascial planes, so beautiful in the virgin neck, become fused by scar from the surgical violation.
4. The patient is subjected to the added risk and expense of two operations.
5. The biopsy incision may be so placed as to interfere with the use of a subsequent reconstruction flap.

Isolated Radical Neck Dissection

If an adequate preoperative search for the

primary lesion has been made and has been fruitless and a squamous cell carcinoma is proven by frozen-tissue microscopic section, the surgeon must be prepared, able, and willing to proceed with an isolated radical neck dissection. If this is to be done it is necessary that the patient be mentally prepared and be in agreement with the plan preoperatively. Advanced age should not be a deterrent to this procedure. The morbidity and mortality of a neck dissection alone are minimal. The long-term success of this approach to the problem of the unknown primary lesion is good. In some 10% of these patients the primary lesion will never become evident (16). Careful follow-up and repeated search will often reveal the site of origin for the primary site months to years later. The pyriform sinuses and the posterior third of the tongue are the most frequent hidden sites, not the nasopharynx as previously thought (17). While waiting and watching for these lesions to become evident and biopsy proven, irradiation therapy should not be instituted. It would of necessity be a blind "shotgun" approach to the treatment of a large area. It is best to watch closely and to institute the indicated therapy in the precise area after the primary site becomes manifest.

Some normal structures in the neck at times may be mistaken for abnormal nodules or masses. Among these are the carotid bulb where the common carotid artery bifurcates, the lateral end of the second cervical transverse process, and the cornu of both hyoid and thyroid cartilages (18).

The posterior neck is rarely involved by metastatic cancer. This is fortunate because it is an area that lends itself poorly to a clean and complete en bloc dissection. An occasional melanoma of the scalp spreads to this area, usually with a fatal consequence.

Treatment Options

The treatment of a mass in the neck, when feasible, is with surgical extirpation by a radical or modified radical neck dissection (19). The modified neck dissection implies preserving the spinal accessory nerve, the internal jugular vein, and the sternocleidomastoid muscle. A neck dissection in contunuity with excision of the primary site of the cancer is desirable when feasible. Cancer of the larynx, the hypopharynx, the

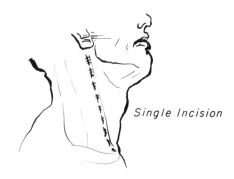

Figure 11.1. The single vertical incision along the anterior border of the sternocleidomastoid muscle allows exposure to the carotid, jugular, and anterior cervical triangular areas and is preferred for operations in the area that do not involve the thyroid, larynx, or posterior cervical triangular structures.

thyroid, the submaxillary, and parotid salivary glands, and lesions of the gingiva, buccal area, tongue, and floor of the month lend themselves to this en bloc operation (20). This procedure removes not only the primary cancer and metastatic deposits in the neck but also the intervening lymphatics as well. The complete description of the technique of these procedures is not within the scope of this discussion (21–23), although a few of the more commonly used skin incisions are illustrated. (Figs. 11.1–11.5) There are many articles discussing all phases of the radical neck dissection, beginning with the earliest paper by George Crile, Sr. published in the *Journal of the American Medical Association* in 1906 (24). Hayes Martin in his article entitled "The Treatment of Cervical Metastatic Cancer," which was published in the *Annals of Surgery* in 1941, popularized the procedure(25).

Infection, thanks to a liberal blood supply in this area, is uncommon. When infection or necrosis of or "floating" skin flaps occur they may result in wound dehiscence, which in turn may lead to the exposure of the carotid artery with its possible subsequent rupture and the patient's rapid exsanguination (26, 27). Transient lymphedema of the face and neck is not unusual, but should the edema subside and later recur, it is an ominous sign and probably denotes a recurrence of tumor. Preoperative irradiation increases the likelihood of skin flap necrosis, poor

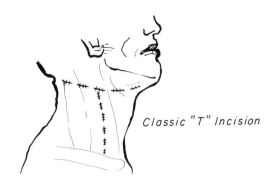

Classic "T" Incision

Figure 11.2. We will occasionally use some variation of the classic "T" incision when an extension into the upper third of the neck, floor of mouth, submental triangle, and supraomohyoid area is found to be necessary after a simpler operation is begun.

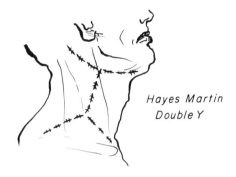

Hayes Martin
Double Y

Figure 11.3. The best exposure for all of the structures of the head and neck area is achieved by a Hayes Martin Double Y incision also called the champagne glass incision. This incision has the obvious disadvantage of poor healing because of multiple long flaps and corners.

healing, and infection and has largely been abandoned in favor of postoperative radiotherapy when radiation is indicated (28). There is a fourfold increase in some type of complication in the neck if as much as 6000 rads is given preoperatively.

It is difficult to make an accurate determination of the benefit of postoperative irradiation. Factors to consider are variable and numerous:

1. Failure to complete therapy;

2. Size and location of the primary cancer;
3. New disease in the neck;
4. Death from uncontrolled local disease or from distant metastases;
5. Complications of the irradiation therapy.

DeSanto, Holt, and co-workers from the Mayo Clinic analyzed 881 patients and concluded there was no benefit from combined surgical and radiation therapy in stage II disease (22). Surgeons at the M.D. Anderson Hospital in Houston

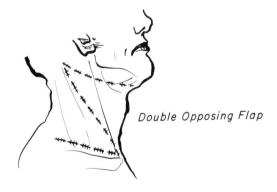

Double Opposing Flap

Figure 11.4. The double opposing flap incision is used when more than the classic "T" is necessary for exposure to the entire neck. It has the same obvious disadvantages as the Hayes Martin Double Y and is used only rarely when the single is found to be inadequate.

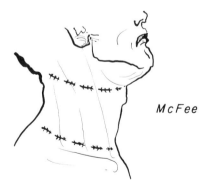

McFee

Figure 11.5. Because of relatively good exposure to the entire neck for procedures of any magnitude and because of the excellent cosmetic result and good healing, we prefer the McFee incision for most procedures about the head and neck.

reviewed the results of treatment of 210 patients who received both surgical and radiation treatment. They concluded that combined therapy in this group was beneficial (29). A recent study by O'Brien and his colleagues from Birmingham noted no increase in the longevity of their patients with combined treatment, but they did record a lesser tendency for neck lesion recurrence in that group (28). They noticed, therefore a greater number of those patients dying of distant metastases. This result might be considered beneficial as the previously described distress of the patient dying of local disease would this be avoided. McGuirt and McCabe surveyed the records of 714 patients requiring radical neck dissection, alone or composite, of whom 162 were over age 70 (30). The operative mortality of those patients aged 70–79 years was 4.6%, and of those over age 80 it was 19.4%. Thirty-seven elderly patients who had not had an elective neck dissection at the time of treatment of their primary cancer returned later with metastatic tumor in the neck when they were older and were a poorer operative risk. Thus, the case for elective neck dissection at the time of primary treatment is strong (23). In contrast, the argument against neck dissection when the neck is clinically negative for metastatic tumor is as follows:

1. The primary lesion may not be cured.
2. Metastases may occur in the contralateral neck.
3. Subsequent ipsilateral neck dissection may be equally beneficial if and when cervical metastasis does become evident.
4. Distant metastases may be present but undetected.
5. Radiation therapy is effective in destroying microscopic cancer in the neck that is clinically negative for metastatic cancer.

In spite of these possibilities most surgeons working in this field agree that the added risk of the prophylactic neck dissection is minimal and that the potential benefit derived from removing clinically undetectable metastatic deposits is great.

Bilateral radical neck dissection, either simultaneous or metachronous, is also a justified and feasible procedure (31). McGuirt reported bilateral dissections in 91 of 697 patients who had radical neck dissection with no operative

deaths and no greater number of complications than with unilateral dissections (30). If both internal jugular veins are sacrificed, temporary facial and neck edema ensues cephalad, thereby requiring that a nasotracheal tube be utilized for several days or else that a temporary tracheostomy be performed.

SALIVARY GLAND CANCER

Salivary gland neoplasms arise in the parotid, the submaxillary, and the sublingual glands, as well as from minor salivary tissue located in the lips, oral cavity, pharynx, palate, and larynx. The most common benign tumor is the pleomorphic adenoma, the so-called benign mixed tumor, and the parotid gland is the site of origin of the great majority of these. These benign tumors usually are seen in young to middle-age persons, whereas the malignant tumors have a predilection for older persons with a peak incidence of onset in the sixth decade (32). A previously benign pleomorphic adenoma that has been present and untreated for many years or following repeated incomplete and unsuccessful operations may in later years become malignant (33). When malignant change occurs, it is known as the carcinoma ex-mixed tumor.

Pathologic classification of malignant salivary tumors is as follows:

1. Adenocarcinoma;
2. Low-grade mucoepidermoid carcinoma;
3. Intermediate-grade mucoepidermoid carcinoma;
4. High-grade mucoepidermoid carcinoma;
5. Adenoid cystic carcinoma;
6. Infiltrative mixed tumor;
7. Carcinoma ex-mixed tumor;
8. Acinic cell carcinoma;
9. Squamous cell carcinoma;
10. Undifferentiated carcinoma.

This pathologic classification helps delineate the lesion and gives some indication of what to expect from the natural history of these neoplasms. It also assists the surgeon in appreciating the prognosis and in selecting the most advantageous form of treatment for each particular lesion. Articles in the current literature pertaining to salivary cancer now are of more value because all authors are comparing tumors of similar cell types.

The least aggressive salivary gland cancers are the acinic, the low and intermediate-grade mucoepidermoid carcinomas, and the two forms of malignant mixed tumors (33, 34). Acinic cell neoplasms are usually slow growing and formerly were considered to be benign tumors (35). Yet, Batsakis refutes this belief and states, "Would that the patients who have died of their acinic cell carcinomas could be so reassured," (36). Adenoid cystic carcinoma, the so-called cylindroma, is a remarkable tumor with a prolonged natural history characterized by a great propensity for local recurrence, for permeation along nerve sheaths, for metastases to the lungs, and for rare metastases to cervical lymph nodes (37). There is doubt whether patients with this cancer are ever completely cured though they may survive 20–25 years or longer. The long survival of many of these patients with "cylindroma," as well as the long survival of many patients with all other types of salivary cancer, especially the less aggressive group, require many years of follow-up before there can be accurate determination of the results of any form of treatment. Although the recurrence of most squamous cell cancers arising elsewhere will usually be evident in 2 to 3 years after treatment, salivary gland neoplasms require 5, 10, or even 15 or more years of follow-up before any degree of assurance of cure can be given.

Adenocarcinoma, undifferentiated carcinoma, squamous cell carcinoma, and high-grade mucoepidermoid carcinoma are the more virulent neoplasms (36, 38–40). They frequently metastasize to lymph nodes in the neck. Wider resection of those arising from the parotid gland with sacrifice of the seventh nerve may be necessary (41, 42). Exenteration of the area with resection of the entire gland, the nerve, the underlying masseter muscle, and the mandible may be required for tumors of these cell types. In contrast, the less aggressive cancers usually can be adequately treated by wide local excision. This local excision technique for the treatment of parotid cancers may require only a lateral or superficial lobectomy with dissection and preservation of the facial nerve.

When attacking a lesion of the hard palate, another common site for salivary gland cancer,

adequate local excision may vary from a small operation to resection of the maxilla. Approximately 25% of parotid tumors, 50% of submaxillary tumors, and 100% of sublingual salivary neoplasms are malignant (43). Minor salivary gland neoplasms of cheek, tongue, and elsewhere are usually cancerous. Spiro reported in 1973 a series of 493 neoplasms of minor salivary glands, of which only 11% were benign (44). Adenoid cystic carcinoma was the most common cell type of minor salivary gland cancers, comprising 35.4% of the series. The palate was the most common site involved. Patient ages ranged from 7 to 86 years, with 53 years being the median age for patients with minor salivary tumors. Others have reported a similar experience (45).

It is obvious that the surgeon is very dependent upon the pathologist for the staging and planning the extent of the operative procedure. A diagnosis must frequently be made intraoperatively on frozen microscopic sections. Needle biopsy is usually of little value in securing sufficient material from salivary gland lesions to allow for proper diagnosis and classification. The pathologist, even with a large piece or sometimes with the entire tumor in hand, may be sorely tested to supply the surgeon, using the frozen section technique, with the correct diagnosis. It may be impossible for the pathologist even to be able to inform the surgeon whether the lesion is benign or malignant.

Parotid tumors should not be biopsied preoperatively. The proper approach for their diagnosis is the removal of the lateral lobe, which will usually contain the growth. This should be done while striving to keep the plane of dissection well away from the tumor and at the same time dissecting and preserving the facial nerve (41, 46). It is best to dissect and identify the facial nerve's main trunk just after it exits from the stylomastoid foramen and before its first bifurcation. The entire specimen is then dissected from the nerve and submitted to the pathologist, and while awaiting the verdict the deep lobe, which is smaller and which lies medially beneath the seventh nerve and adjacent to the external carotid artery, can be excised easily. This approach to parotid neoplasms is proper for both the benign and most malignant lesions and diminishes the likelihood of local recurrence of either type of tumor. If enlarged lymph nodes are evident in the neck or if the cancer proves to be one of the highly aggressive types, an associated neck dissection is advisable (23, 47-49).

Surgical trauma of the magnitude just described is well tolerated by the elderly. In contrast to chest and abdominal operations, pain and discomfort are minimal. Cough and deep breathing are excellent, and ambulation is possible the day of the surgical procedure. Oral feeding need not be curtailed, even with maxillary gland resection. Postoperative complications are minimal, convalescence rapid, and the hospital stay usually relatively brief.

Cancer in the parotid gland may be due to secondary involvement from other primary sites either by metastatic spread to parotid lymph nodes or by direct penetration from an adjacent neoplasm. The primary site of origin of these lesions is most frequently from a nearby skin lesion. Either squamous cell cancer or melanoma, whose origin is in the scalp, the skin of the auricle, the forehead, or the cheek, may involve the parotid gland secondarily (50). The intraparotid lymph nodes are the first site of drainage and are primary barriers to the spread of cancer cells from much of this area. Jackson and Ballantyne in 1981 reported their experience with 169 patients with head and neck skin cancer, excluding melanoma, that involved the parotid gland (51). The age range was from 34 to 95 years, with an average of 65 years. One hundred fifty of the 169 patients were male, as would be anticipated due to the excessive exposure to sunlight experienced by males. Rees and co-workers in 1981 reported their experience with 52 secondary parotid tumors (50). Squamous cell cancer comprised 59.6% of this series of metastatic tumors, and melanoma accounted for 13.4%. Surgical ablation of the gland with these lesions yielded favorable results. At times the addition of a radical neck dissection was required. Preservation of the facial nerve was often possible. Postoperative radiotherapy was frequently employed, but it was not always without complications, such as mandibular osteonecrosis, trismus, severe chondritis of ear cartilages, and/or refractory otitis media.

GINGIVAL AND ALVEOLAR CARCINOMA

Carcinoma of the gingiva and alveolus is for all practical purposes exclusively squamous cell carcinoma in histologic type. In 1950 the incidence of these cancers was six times greater in males than females, whereas in 1980 this male:female ratio had changed to 2.4 to 1, apparently due to increased smoking by females. The heavy use of tobacco either in the form of cigarettes, cigars, chewing tobacco or snuff is considered the prime etiologic factor. Poor oral hygiene, carious teeth, and poorly fitting dentures have been blamed for causing gingival cancer, but without firm statistical confirmation (52). The average age at onset is 60 years.

These cancers are surface lesions and are frequently ulcerated when diagnosed. They may be verrucous in type and are often associated with leukoplakia of the oral mucosa. Biopsy is easily obtained with a biting forceps using local infiltration or topical anesthesia. A liberal amount of material should be secured for it may be difficult for the pathologist to differentiate between invasive cancer and non-invasive leukoplakia without adequate tissue. Verrucous carcinoma may be especially difficult to identify properly from a small biopsy speciman.

The treatment of gingival and alveolar carcinoma is surgical. The important and often the most difficult surgical decision is how to manage properly the underlying bone (53). Should the bony resection be an upper superficial margin or a full thickness bony segment? Imaging studies with x-ray photographs, bone scan, and CT scans, as well as clinical judgement, are all of much assistance (54). If appreciable bone destruction is evident a segmental resection of the mandible is indicated (55). In edentulous patients with resulting alveolar bone atrophy, the inferior dental nerve is near the crest of the jaw and presents an avenue for permeation of the cancer along the nerve and through the mandibular canal to the base of the skull. In the absence of proof of bone destruction or even with minimal erosion, a marginal resection may suffice. This procedure is especially worthwhile for treating lesions at or near the midline anteriorly. In the anterior portion near the area of the symphysis, the mandible is usually wider and thicker than in the region of the horizontal rami. This anterior area lends itself to the technique of resection of only the upper margin of bone in which a lower rim is left to maintain the dental arch.

This will obviate the ''Andy Gump'' deformity or the necessity for bone grafting (56).

An associated radical neck dissection is always indicated if enlarged lymph nodes are present in the neck, if the primary lesion is stage III or IV, or if a segmental resection of the mandible is done. When treating a patient with a smaller lesion and one in whom only a marginal mandibular resection is required, neck dissection is not always necessary, and if so only a supramohyoid neck dissection may suffice.

Proper reconstruction of the resected mandible is vital to enable the patient to return to both a functional and cosmetically acceptable state (57–59). To accomplish this reconstruction may require the transfer of bone and/or soft tissue from a distant site. Methods of reconstruction of a mandibular defect may be divided into four catagories: (1) free bone grafting, (2) use of alloplastic materials, (3) freeze-dried bone or irradiated bone allografts, and (4) vascularized bone grafts. Neither freeze-dried, irradiated bone, nor alloplastic materials have been extensively utilized to replace mandibular defects. Free bone grafts require a clean bed and a watertight closure of the oral mucous membrane. Immediate insertion of a free graft, even with a firm mucous membrane closure, is more prone to failure than if grafting is delayed until firm healing of the oral tissues has occurred. In all types of grafting of the lower jaw, the dental arch must be maintained in its normal position by external pins and bars (60). Iliac crest is the favored site from which to harvest both good cancellous and cortical bone. In recent years transfer of vascularized bone has become popular. One technique is microvascular anastamoses to obtain blood supply to nourish bone, muscle, and skin in their new site. Franklin and co-workers describe a successful technique for immediate repair of mandible, soft tissue, and skin defect in one stage by transferring iliac bone and soft tissues utilizing the deep circumflex iliac vessels (61). The artery is anastamosed to a branch of the external carotid artery and the vein to any available neck vein. Another method to transfer vascularized bone and soft tissue is the osteomyocutaneous pedicle graft (62). The pectoralis major muscle with a segment of rib or sternum incorporated is most frequently utilized (63). Other composite grafts utilize the sternocleidomastoid muscle with a section of clavicle included or the trapezius muscle with a segment of scapula. These vascularized grafts are less prone to infection and are promising for long term success with less atrophy of the transplanted bone.

CANCER OF BUCCAL MUCOSA

Carcinoma of the cheek mucosa is a disease of the elderly, and the incidence is recorded to be the greatest in the seventh decade of life (64). Tumors in this area are virtually all squamous cell carcinoma. They can be divided into exophytic, ulcero-infiltrative, and verrucous, as arranged by their frequency of occurence (65). This tumor is frequently associated with a ''leukoplakic patch,'' smokeless tobacco (66–68), or such irritants as betel nuts (69). Authors have observed these lesions in patients with malnutritution (70), and abnormalities of vitamin A metabolism have been reported in the tumor tissue (71).

Exophytic and ulcero-infiltrative lesions may begin in an area of a long-standing leukoplakic patch. They have been considered to be more aggressive because they locally invade cheek muscles or the pterygoid fossa early, producing trismus. Although orginally thought to be less aggressive because of their indolent appearence, verrucous carcinomas (20%) have been associated with multifocal areas of less well differentiated squamous cell carcinoma (72), which may account for their radioresistant nature (73). These tumors are typically discovered late in the clinical course of the disease in elderly patients who tend to ignore them because they may be painless and may have a benign appearance.

Survival rates vary according to the extent of the lesion and type of treatment. Experience in 121 patients from Memorial Hospital showed a 5-year overall survival of 42% (74). Obviously survival was better in lesions detected early (77%) and worse in advanced ones (18%). These survival rates have improved little in 30 years (69). Because these lesions tend to be refractory to radiotherapy, we prefer surgical therapy in all groups. Resection and reconstruction are well tolerated in the elderly (69). Reconstruction is easily accomplished by primary closure, skin grafts, or local flaps.

LIP CANCER

Cancer of the lip is the most frequent mucosal head and neck malignancy by anatomic site (75). The tumor is common in the elderly, but has another early peak incidence in patients under age 40 (76). It is particularly common in males (95%) who are prone to exposure to sun or tobacco, especially patients who smoke pipes (75). Although at times present in the upper lip as basal cell carcinoma, it typically presents as an ulcerative squamous cell carcinoma (95%) at the junction of the lateral and midline third of the lower lip. The lower lip lesions may be accompanied by long-standing pre-existing leukoplakia that is often dismissed by the clinician as "chapped lips" in its early phases (77).

Because the lesions are clinically accessible, the diagnosis can be made early by punch biopsy and treated effectively either with radiation or surgical resection (80%–95%). Resection is preferable to radiation treatment in the elderly (78) because it avoids lip atrophy and/or dryness in a lip already damaged by solar radiation. Surgical excision is accomplished by "wedge" or "shield" excisions, often with an associated lip shave (79). This procedure is done to avoid the likelihood of a second primary tumor developing in the remaining damaged lip vermilion. Reconstruction is accomplished by tissue advancement (80) or lip sharing techniques (81) that will precisely reconstruct the anatomy. If not done well, the reconstructed mouth will not admit dentures, or the dentures may not sit properly in the buccal sulcus. Basal cell carcinomas rarely involve the vermilion, and they can usually be excised and closed with local skin flaps.

Indications for an associated radical neck dissection and for supramohyoid dissection remain controversial. Clearly, if clinically positive nodes are present, the radical neck dissection is indicated. Some authors advocate a neck dissection for all larger lesions (greater than 2 cm) (29, 78). Equally good success is achievable with radiation if the neck is clinically negative for node enlargement (82).

CARCINOMA OF THE TONGUE

Carcinoma of the tongue appears to be a spectrum of illnesses that are influenced by age, anatomic location, and the extent of the disease. These tumors are virtually all squamous cell carcinomas (97%) and are slightly less common than all other malignant *intraoral* tumors combined (65). Traditionally, it has been suggested that alcohol and tobacco use and poor oral hygiene contribute to the development of this lesion. As with many head and neck tumors, frequency increases with age. The majority (greater than 75%) occur on the mobile, anterior two-thirds of the tongue. They characteristically appear as an ulcerative lesion on the lateral edge of the tongue (65). Most lesions are painful, and many are identified by dentists if the patients still have teeth. If the lesion is on the posterior one-third of the tongue, the diagnosis is usually made late in the course of the disease after the tumor has spread to the cervical nodes or into the pre-epiglottic space.

In the elderly patient, carcinoma of the tongue is a frustrating illness because the tongue contributes so heavily to swallowing and to speech. Although some authors (83–85) advocate primary radiotherapy, we and others (86–88) advocate surgical excision of lesions on the mobile tongue. Because the incidence of cervical lymph node metastasis is so common, treatment of the neck prophylactically with radiation (79) for microscopic disease in clinically negative necks or radical neck dissection for clinically palpable neck nodes is very necessary (86). Five-year survival rate for patients with tongue cancer is 65% in those with negative nodes, but falls to 21% if the nodes are positive (87).

Treatment of large lesions, recurrent lesions (89), or those of the posterior one-third of the tongue present special problems. Of concern to the head and neck surgeon is the observation that elderly patients tolerate near-total glossectomy very poorly. Extensive resections of the posterior tongue, tonsil, and larynx may leave the patient a significant oral cripple. After extensive resection, the patient is an incompetent speaker and requires supplemental gastrostomy feedings to maintain nutrition (90). Unless the patient is a candidate for a tongue prosthesis (91) or for a tracho-esophageal puncture (92) for voice restoration, oral rehabilitation is fruitless. Alternative forms of treatment using radiotherapy show promise, but currently they are ineffective in achieving local control (93) in large tumors.

CARCINOMA OF THE OROPHARYNX

The oropharynx is an anatomic area in the mouth that includes the tonsil, retromolar trigone, palate, and vallecula (65). The tumors of this area have been considered biologically more aggressive because of their propensity to metastasize earlier to regional lymph nodes than comparably sized tumors of the anterior oral cavity. By the time these tumors are discovered, the rich lymphatics of the nearby cervical nodes will already contain tumor in cases of palate (60%), tonsil (50%), and retromolar trigone (50%) tumors (94–96). Many times, bilateral or contralateral cervical lymph node enlargement from metastasis is the first sign of cancer in these patients (97).

Tumors of the Tonsil and Tonsillar Region

These tumors are virtually all squamous cell carcinomas and occur almost exclusively in elderly males after the fifth decade of life. Patients may present with sore throat, dysphagia, and weight loss that are frequently in association with ipsilateral ear pain. The gross clinical appearance of the lesion may be either velvety red overlying the tonsillar pillar or ulcero-infiltrative into the retromolar trigone region. Early tumors are often hidden in the tonsillar crypts, or they may appear as a small papilloma on the tonsil.

The management of this tumor is difficult in elderly patients. The extensive surgical resection or therapeutic radiation necessary to cure these lesions is tolerated very poorly in this anatomic area. Radiation therapy is associated with severe mucositis, radio-osteonecrosis, and failure to feed due to pain when eating. Unfortunately, surgical therapy, either for cure or palliation, can reduce the patient to a serious oral cripple. Disorders of oral pharyngeal swallowing occur because of denervation of the oropharynx, tongue resection, surgical scarring, or flap placement at the resection site.

Survival rates with surgical resection (40%–50%) or radiation (15%–40%) have been reported (98–102). However, survival is more dependent on the stage of the disease at the time of therapy than the modality of treatment. In our experience, we prefer a combination of resection with postoperative radiotherapy for large tumors because palliation cannot be achieved without debulking oropharyngeal tumors. Unfortunately, we must agree with the great head and neck surgeon, Hayes Martin, who pointed out that what the surgeon has to offer for carcinoma of the tonsil was "the worst for any operative procedure" and noted that it was "the surgery of despair" (74).

Tumors of the Palate

Palatal carcinoma occurs in the anatomic junction area between the oral cavity and the pharynx where functional unity is critical for speech and eating. Although lymphoma and minor salivary gland tumors occur in this area, most tumors of the palate are of squamous cell origin (74). These tumors must be recognized as another manifestation of the regional diathesis of carcinoma in the oropharynx. Many times, palatine tumors are multicentric or are associated with a synchronous tumor in the larynx or base of the tongue (102). These tumors can be treated either by surgical excision or with radiation therapy, and the choice of therapy depends on size, location, previous therapy, and stage of disease (102, 103). Surgical excision requires the postoperative use of palatal obturators to ensure that the patient can eat and speak effectively. Sometimes elderly patients tolerate these obturators very poorly. The proper use and dosage of radiation therapy are limited by the patient's tolerance for mucositis and poor nutrition during therapy. These problems are not easily solved in patients who are old and who may respond poorly to the stress of surgical resection or radiation therapy for these tumors.

NON-MELANOTIC SKIN CANCER IN THE HEAD AND NECK

Basal cell carcinoma arises in the epidermis or appendages of the skin (104) and is the most common malignant tumor of the head and neck, affecting 1.5% of females and 1.9% of males in the general population (105). It commonly affects the nose, medial canthus, nasolabial sulcus, auricular, and pre-auricular areas (106). Treatment of small head and neck basal cell carcinomas can be either surgical or radiologic. Recurrent, large, or sclerosing lesions pose a difficult challenge. The tumors are common in the elderly, particularly in the scalp, alar base, and auricular region. Traditional surgical excision or microscopic controlled excision (Mohs' chemosurgery) offer more effective treatment for these lesions. Mohs' chemosurgery has the advantage of resection under local anesthesia so that only the reconstruction need be done under general anesthesia (107). When the basal carcinoma spreads to regional lymph nodes, it has a grave prognosis. Metastatic disease, although exceedingly rare, does occur in lesions that are recurrent, large, or deeply invasive (107–109). These tumors are particularly difficult to treat because the proper reconstruction of the resultant defects requires healthy, vascular tissue, which is often unavailable in old patients.

Squamous cell carcinoma of the skin is very common in the elderly and is prone to early regional lymphatic spread or to aggressive local invasion if left untreated. Because of the duration of sun exposure with attendant actinic skin damage, squamous cell carcinoma commonly occurs in actinic keratosis or in areas of cutaneous horns (110). The older members of the population may also develop these lesions in longstanding burn scars, previously irradiated areas, or in chronic wounds. Early recognition makes feasible less radical treatment of these cutaneous lesions with their aggressive malignant potential and eliminates much of the morbidity that would follow extensive therapeutic procedures required to ablate more advanced lesions. The reported incidence of cervical metastasis in cutaneous squamous cell carcinoma is between 0.1%–11.0% depending on lesion size, degree of cellular differentiation, and previous therapy (111–113). If the parotid gland is involved with the tumor, then our experience and that of others (50, 114) suggest that the mortality is high (30%–40%). Combined surgical excision and postoperative radiation are necessary for local control.

SUMMARY

Older age alone should never be a deterring factor in the selection of surgical treatment as the method of choice for either early or even for some of the far advanced head and neck cancers. The opinion is commonly held that an elderly patient has so little time to live that radical surgical procedures should never be employed. There is a tendency for a lesser modality of therapy to be the first one to be used when the patient is 70 years of age or older. Six months or so later, a recurrence, or more correctly a persistence of the tumor, will often become evident. It is then that the proper extirpative procedure is requested by the patient, family, or physician. Then the definitive procedure must be carried out with the elderly patient perhaps even less capable of withstanding the surgical trauma than he or she would have been earlier. At this late date distant metastases may already be present. Whether for palliation or for potential cure of these devastating lesions, it is of extreme urgency not to procrastinate but to perform a proper surgical procedure early, in spite of the advanced years of the patient.

REFERENCES

1. Jun MY, Strong EW, Saltzman EL, Gerold FP: Head and neck cancer in elderly. *Head Neck Surgery* 5:376-n-382, 1983.
2. Trott JA, David DJ, Edwards RM, Experience with surgery for head and neck cancer in a geriatric population. *Aust NZ J Surg* 52:149–153, 1982.
3. McGuirt WF, Loevy S, McCabe BF, Krause CJ: The risk of major head and neck surgery in the aged population. *Laryngoscope* 87: 1378–1382, 1977.
4. Harrold CC, Jr. The surgical significance of chronic obstructive lung disease in the patient with head and neck cancer. *Am J Surg* 130: 383–389, 1975.
5. Vikram B: Changing patterns of failure in advanced head and neck cancer. *Arch Otolaryngol* 110: 564–565, 1984.
6. Cancer incidence and survival in patients 65 years of age and older. *CA* 36:26–42, 1986.
7. Beahrs OH, Myers MH: *Manual for Staging of Cancer,* ed 2. Philadelphia, JB Lippincott Co, 1983.
8. Martin H, Rasmussen LH, Perras C: Head and neck surgery in patients of the older age group. *Cancer:* 8:707–711, 1955.

9. Lore JM, Boulos EJ: Resection and reconstruction of the carotid artery in metastatic sqaumous cell carcinoma. *Am J Surg* 142:437- 442, 1981.

10. Papac RJ: Distant metastases from head and neck cancer. *Cancer* 53:342–345, 1984.

11. Rosenfeld L: The significance of a mass in the neck. *J TN Med Assoc* 51:5–7, 1958.

12. Rosenfeld L, Graves H, Lawrence R: Primary neurogenic tumors of the lateral neck. *Ann Surg* 167:847–855, 1968.

13. Martin H: *Surgery of Head and Neck Tumors.* New York, Paul B. Hoeber Inc, 1957, pp 119–126.

14. Martin CE, Rosenfeld L, McSwain B: Carotid body tumors—a 16 year followup of seven malignant cases. *South Med J* 66:1236–1243, 1973.

15. Gullane PJ, Gilbert RW, van Norstrand AW, Slinger RP: Malignant schwannoma in the head and neck. *J Otolaryngol* 14:171–175, 1985.

16. MacComb WS: Diagnosis and treatment of metastatic cervical cancerous nodes from an unknown primary site. *Am J Surg* 124:441–449, 1972.

17. Cunningham MJ, Johnson JT, Myers EN, Schramm VL, Thearle PB: Cervical lymph node metastasis after local excision of early sqaumous cell carcinoma of the oral cavity. *Am J Surg* 152:361–366, 1986.

18. Lore JM: *An Atlas of Head and Neck Surgery.* Philadelphia, WB Saunders, 1962, pp 309–319.

19. Jesse RH, Ballantyne AJ, Larsen D: Radical or modified neck dissection: a therapeutic dilemma. *Am J Surg* 136:516–519, 1978.

20. Lingeman RE, Helmus C, Stephens R, ULM J: Neck dissection: radical or conservative. *Ann Otol Rhinol Laryngol* 86:737–744, 1977.

21. Beahrs OH: Surgical anatomy and technique of radical neck dissection. *Surg Clin N Am* 57:663–700, 1977.

22. DeSanto LW, Holt JJ, Beahrs OH, O'Fallon WM: Neck dissection: is it worthwhile? *Laryngoscope* 92:502–509, 1982.

23. Ariyan S: Radical neck dissection. *Surg Clin N Am* 66:133–148, 1966.

24. Crile GW: Excision of cancer of the head and neck with special reference to the plan of dissection based on 132 operations. *JAMA* 47:1780–1786, 1906.

25. Martin H: The treatment of cervical metastatic cancer. *Ann Surg* 114:972–986, 1941.

26. Razack MS, Sako K: Carotid artery hemorrhage and ligation in head and neck cancer. *J Surg Oncol* 19:189–192, 1982.

27. Moore O, Baker HW: Carotid artery ligation in surgery of the head and neck. *Cancer* 8:712–726, 1955.

28. O'Brien CJ, Smith JW, Soong SJ, Urist MM, Maddox WA: Neck dissection with and without radiotherapy. *Am J Surg* 152:456–463, 1986.

29. Jesse RH, Perez CA, Fletcher GH: Cervical lymph node metastasis: Unknown primary cancer. *Cancer* 31:854–859, 1973.

30. McGuirt WF, McCabe BF: Bilateral radical neck dissections. *Arch Otolarygol* 106:427–429, 1980.

31. Rosenfeld L, Jacobs JK: Bilateral radical neck dissection. *Surgery* 49:359–364, 1961.

32. Hunter RM, Davis BW, Gray GF, Rosenfeld L: Primary malignant tumors of salivary gland origin—a 52 year review. *Am Surg* 44:82–89, 1983.

33. Spiro RH, Huvos AG, Strong EW: Malignant mixed tumors of salivary gland origin. *Am J Surg* 144:428–431, 1982.

34. Spiro RH, Huvos AG, Stong EW: Malignant mixed tumors of salivary origin—a clinicopathologic study of 146 cases. *Cancer* 39:388–396, 1977.

35. Spiro RH, Huvos AG, Strong EW: Acinic cell carcinoma of salivary origin. *Cancer* 41:924–935, 1978.

36. Tortoledo ME, Luna MA, Batsakis JG: Carcinoma expleomorphic adenoma and malignant mixed tumors. *Arch Otolaryngol* 110:172- 176, 1984.

37. Spiro RH, Huvos AG, Stong EW: Adenoid cystic carcinoma of salivary origin. *Am J Surg* 128:512–520, 1974.

38. Olsen KD, Devine KD, Weiland LH: Mucoepidermoid carcinoma of the oral cavity. *Otolaryngol Head Neck Surg* 89:783–791, 1981.

39. Saunders JR, Hirata RM, Jaques DA: Salivary glands. *Surg Clin N Am* 66:59–81, 1986.

40. Spiro FH, Huvos AG, Berk R, Strong EW: Mucoepidermoid carcinoma of salivary gland origin. *Am J Surg*

41. Rosenfeld L, Walker WE: The management of a mass in the parotid gland. *J TN Med Assoc* 65:1007–1009, 1972.

42. Lanier VC, McSwain B, Rosenfeld L: Mixed tumors of salivary glands. *South Med J* 65:1485–1488, 1972.

43. Spiro RH, Hajdu SI, Strong EW: Tumors of the submaxillary gland. *Am J Surg* 132:463–468, 1976.

44. Spiro RH, Koss LG, Hajdu SI, Strong EW: Tumors of minor salivary gland origin. 492 cases. *Cancer* 31:117–129, 1973.

45. Singer R, Bowers DG, Lynch JB: Intraoral cancer of the minor salivary glands. *Clin Plast Surg* 3:405–411, 1976.

46. Rosenfeld L: Experiences with vascular abnormalities about the parotid gland and upper neck. *Arch Surg* 79:553–566, 1959.

47. Wood JE, Chong GC, Beahrs OH: Experience with 1360 primary parotid tumors. *Am J Surg* 130:460–462, 1975.

48. Foote FW, Frazell EL: Tumors of the major salivary glands. *Cancer* 6:1065–1133, 1953.

49. Spiro RH, Huvos AG, Stong EW: Cancer of the parotid gland—a study of 288 primary cases. *Am J Surg* 130:452–459, 1977.

50. Rees R, Maples M, Lynch JB, Rosenfeld L: Malignant secondary parotid tumors. *South Med J* 74:1050–1052, 1981.

51. Jackson GL, Ballantyne AJ: Role of parotidectomy for skin cancer of the head and neck. *Am J Surg* 142:464–469, 1981.

52. Byers RM, Newman R, Russell N, Yue A: Results of treatment for squamous carcinoma of the lower gum. *Cancer* 47:2236–2238, 1981.

53. Gilbert S, Tzadik A, Leonard G, Farmington CT: Mandibular involvement by oral squamous cell carcinoma. *Laryngoscope* 96:96- 101, 1986.

54. Luyk NH, Laird EE, Ward-Booth P, Rankin D, Williams ED: The use of radionuclide bone scintography to determine local spread of oral squamous cell carcinoma to mandible. *J Maxillo Fac Surg* 14:93–98, 1986.

55. Marchetta FC, Sako K, Murphy JB: The periosteum of the mandible and intraoral cancer. *Am J Surg* 122:711–713, 1971.

56. Wald RM, Calceterra TC: Lower alveolar carcinoma. *Arch Otolaryngol* 109:578–582, 1983.

57. Kudo K, Miyasawa M, Fujioka Y, Sasaki J: Immediate repair of mandibular defects following surgery for carcinoma of lower alveolus and gingiva using a pectoralis major osteomyocutaneous flap. *J Maxillo Fac Surg* 13:116–120, 1985.

58. Cuono, CB, Ariyan S: Immediate reconstruction of a composite mandibular defect with a regional osteomusculocutaneous flap. *Plast Reconst Surg* 65:477–483, 1980.

59. Bergman SA, Elias EG, Didolker MS, Morris DM: Maintenance of function and esthetics after partial mandibulectomy without bone grafting. *J Oral Surg* 39:421–425, 1981.

60. Cohen M, Schultz RC: Mandibular reconstruction. *Clin Plast Surg* 12:411–422, 1985.

61. Franklin JD, Shack RB, Stone JD, Madden JJ, Lynch JB: Single stage reconstruction of mandibular and soft tissue defects using a free osteocutaneous groin flap. *Am J Surg* 140:492–498, 1980.

62. Pearlman NW, Albin RE, O'Donnell RS: Mandibular reconstruction in irradiated pateints utilizing myosseous cutaneous flaps. *Am J Surg* 146:474–477, 1983.

63. Robertson GA: The role of sternum in osteomyocutaneous reconstruction of major mandibular defects. *Am J Surg* 152:367–370, 1986.

64. O'Brien PH, Catlin D: Cancer of the cheek (mucosa). *Cancer* 181:392–1395, 1965.

65. Batsakis JG: Squamous cell carcinomas of the oral cavity and the oropharynx. In *Tumors of the Head and Neck,* ed 1. Baltimore, Williams & Wilkins, 1974, pp 89–90.

66. Rosenfeld L, Callaway J: Snuff dipper's cancer. *Am J Surgery* 106:840–844, 1963.

67. Moore GE, Bissinger LL, Proehl EC: Tobacco and intra-oral cancer. *Surg Forum* 3:685–688, 1952.

68. Moore GE, Bissinger LL, Proehl LL: Intraoral cancer and the use of chewing tobacco. *J Am Geriatr Soc* 1:497–506, 1953.

69. Paymaster JC: Cancer of the buccal mucosa. *Cancer* 9:431–435, 1985.

70. Gates RE, Rees RS: Altered vitamin A binding proteins in carcinoma of the head and neck. *Cancer* 56:2598–2604, 1985.

71. Medina JE, Dichtel W, Luna MA: Verrucous-squamous carcinomas of oral cavity: a clinicopathologic study. *Arch Otolaryngol* 110:437–440, 1984.

72. Burns HP, Van Nostrand AW, Palmer JA: Verrucous carcinoma of the oral cavity: management by radiotherapy and surgery. *Can J Surg* 23:19–21, 1980.

73. Bloom ND, Spiro RH: Carcinoma of the cheek mucosa: a retrospective analysis. *Am J Surg* 140:556–559, 1980.

74. Verbin RS, Bouquot JE, Guggenheimer J, Barnes L, Peel RL: Cancer of the oral cavity and Oropharynx. In Barnes L (ed): *Surgical Pathology of the Head and Neck,* ed 1. New York, Marcel Dekker, 1985, pp 337–343.

75. Bernier JL, Clark ML: Squamous cell carcinoma of the lip. *Milit Surg* 109:379–381, 1951.

76. Gibson LE, Perry HO: Skin lesion fron sun exposure: a treatment guide. *Geriatrics* 40:87–89, 1985.

77. Wurman LH, Adams GL, Meyerhoff WL: Carcinoma of the lip. *Am J Surg* 130:470–474, 1975.

78. Wilson JS, Walker EP: Reconstruction of the lower lip. *Head Neck Surg* 4:29–44, 1981.

79. Madden JJ, Erhardt WL, Franklin JD, Withers EH, Lynch JB: Reconstruction of upper and lower lip using a modified Bernard- Burrow technique. *Ann Plast Surg* 5:100–105, 1980.

80. Jababley ME, Clement RL, Orcutt TW: Myocutaneous flaps in lip reconstruction. *Plast Reconstr Surg* 59:680–688, 1976.

81. Marshall KA, Edgerton MT: Indications for neck dissection in carcinoma of the lip. *Am J Surg* 133:216–217, 1977.

82. Botstein C, Silver C, Ariaratnam L: Treatment of carcinoma of the oral tongue by radium needle implantation. *Am J Surg* 132:523–524, 1976.

83. Spiro RH, Strong EW: Epidermoid carcinoma of the mobile tongue. *Am J Surg* 122:707–710, 1971.

84. Lampe I, Fayos JV: Radiotherapeutic experience with squamous cell carcinoma of the oral part of the tongue. *J Univ Mich Med Ctr* 33:215–218, 1967.

85. Mendelson BC, Woods JE, Beahrs OH: Neck dissection in the treatment of carcinoma of the anterior two-thirds of the tongue. *Surg Gynecol Obstet* 14:375–80, 1976.

86. Spiro RH, Strong EW: Discontinuous partial glossectomy and radical neck dissection in selected patients with epidermoid carcinoma of the mobile tongue. *Am J Surg* 126:544–546, 1973.

87. Effron MZ, Johnson JT, Myers EN, Curtin H, Beery Q, Sigler B: Advanced carcinoma of the tongue: management to total glossectomy without laryngectomy. *Arch Otolaryngol* 107:694–697, 1981.

88. Gobbel WG, Adkins RB, Sawyers JL: Carcinoma of tongue. *Am Surg* 33:635–641, 1967.

89. Rees RS, Ivey GL, Shack RB, Franklin JD, Lynch JB: Pectoralis major musculocutaneous flaps: long term follow-up of hypopharyngeal reconstruction. *Plast Reconstr Surg* 77:586–590, 1986.

90. Ballard J, Kerner E, Tyson J, Ashford J, Rees RS: Adenocarcinoma of the tongue complicated by a hemimandibulectomy: soft tissue support for a tongue prosthesis edentulous glossectomee patient. *J Prosthet Dent* 5:6470–473, 1986.

91. Johns ME, Cantrell RW: Voice restoration of the total laryngectomy patient: the Singer-Blom technique. *Otolaryngol Head Neck Surg* 89:82–86.

92. Spanos WJ, Shukovsky LJ, Fletcher GH: Time dose and tumor volume relationships in irradiation of squamous cell carcinoma of the base of the tongue. *Cancer* 37:2591–2599, 1976.

93. Scanlon PW, Gee VR, Erich JB, Williams HL, Woolner LB: Carcinoma of the palatine tonsil. *Am J Rad Ther Nuc Med* 80:781–784, 1958.

94. Matthews J: Malignant tumors of the tonsil. *Larngoscope* 22:737- 752, 1912.

95. Petrovich Z, Kuisk H, Jose L, Barton R, Rice D: Advanced carcinoma of the tonsil. *Acta Radio Oncol* 19:452–431, 1980.

96. Feind CR, Cole RM: Contralateral spread of head and neck cancer. *Am J Surg* 118:660–665, 1969.

97. Fayos JV: Carcinoma of the oropharynx. *Radiology* 138:675–681, 1981.

98. Jesse RH, Sugarbaker EV: Squamous cell carcinoma of the oropharynx. *Am J Surg* 132:435–438, 1976.

99. Fleming PM, Matz GJ, Powell WI, Chen JA: Carcinoma of the tonsil. *Surg Clin N Am* 56:125–136, 1976.

100. Whicker JH, DeSanto LW, Devine KD: Surgical treatment of squamous cell carinoma of the tonsil. *Laryngoscope* 84:90–97, 1974.

101. Givens CD, Johns ME, Cantrell RW: Carcinoma of the tonsil. *Arch Otolaryngol* 107:730–734, 1981.

102. Healy GB, Strong MS, Uchmakli A, Vaughn CW, DiTroia JF: Carcinoma of the palatine arch: the rational treatment selection. *Am J Surg* 132:498–503, 1976.

103. Evans JF, Shah JP: Epidermoid carcinoma of the palate. *Am J Surg* 142:451–455, 1981.

104. Popkin GL, DeFeo CP: Basal cell epithelioma. In Andrade R, Gumport SL, Popkin GL, Rees TD (eds): *Cancer of the Skin,* ed 1. Philadelphia, WB Saunders, 1976, pp 821–844.

105. Gellin GA, Kopf AW, Garfinkel L: Basal cell epithelioma. *Arch Dermatol* 91:38–45, 1965.

106. Levine HL, Bailin PL: Basal cell carcinoma of the head and neck: identification of the high risk patient. *Laryngoscope* 90:955–961, 1980.

107. Tromovitch TA, Stegman SJ: Microscopic controlled excision of cutaneous tumors. *Cancer* 41:653–657, 1978.

108. Farmer ER, Helwig EB: Metastatic basal cell carcinoma: a clinicopathologic study of 17 cases. *Cancer* 46:749–757, 1980.

109. Constanza ME, Dayal Y, Binder S, Nathanson L: Metastatic basal cell carcinoma: review, report of case and chemotherapy. *Cancer* 34:230–235, 1974.

110. Sage HH, Casson PR: Squamous cell carcinoma of the scalp, face and neck. In Andrade R, Gumport SL, Popkin GL, Rees TD: *Cancer of the Skin,* ed 1. Philadelphia, WB Saunders, 1976, pp 899–915.

111. Binder SC, Catlin D: Epidermoid carcinoma of the skin of the nose. *Am J Surg* 117:506–509, 1968.

112. Ratzer ER, Strong EW: Squamous cell carcinoma of the scalp. *Am J Surg* 114:570–573, 1967.

113. Lund HZ: How often does squamous cell carcinoma of the skin metastasize? *Arch Dermatol* 92: 635–639, 1965.

114. Ridenhour CE, Spratt JS: Epidermoid carcinoma of the skin involving the partoid gland. *Am J Surg* 112:504–507, 1966.

Chapter 12

Surgical Care of Rhinolaryngologic Problems in the Elderly

James L. Netterville, M.D., Robert H. Ossoff, M.D., D.M.D., F.A.C.S.

The nasal and laryngeal regions are subjected to a great deal of wear and tear over 4-score years that results in an increased incidence of upper airway and communicative problems. Rather than providing a superficial overview of the numerous maladies in the elderly that affect this region, this chapter addresses selected common problems that relate to surgical care in sufficient detail to be useful to the reader.

FUNCTIONAL ANATOMY OF THE LARYNX

The larynx is divided into three anatomic subunits based on function and lymphatic drainage. The supraglottic portion of the larynx extends from the tip of the epiglottis down to and including the superior one-half of the ventricle separating the true and false vocal cords. The glottic region includes the lower one-half of the ventricle, the true vocal cords, the mucosa covering the vocal process of the arytenoid, the anterior and posterior commissure, and the mucosa that extends 10 mm below the free margin of true vocal cord. The subglottic region consists of the mucosa overlying the inner aspect of the cricoid cartridge.

The supraglottic region develops embryologically from the buccopharyngeal anlage. This region has a rich lymphatic drainage to both the contralateral and ipsilateral lymph nodes. The glottic and subglottic regions orginate from the laryngotracheal anlage. The true vocal cord, which has a sparse lymphatic network, drains through the ligament at the anterior commissure through the tracheal cartilage to the pretracheal "Delphan" lymph node. The subglottic region

164

has a richer lymphatic network and drains to the ipsilateral paratracheal nodes with extension toward the mediastinal nodes.

The true vocal cord is composed of five layers: the epithelium; the superficial, middle, and deep layers of the lamina propria; and the vocalis muscle. These layers glide over each other during normal phonation, allowing a near fluid-like motion of the epithelial layer that results in the pleasing quality of normal speech. Abnormalities of these layers, such as nodules, cysts, or tumor infiltration, as well as scarring from surgical procedures, can prevent this normal motion, resulting in hoarseness.

The intrinsic musculature of the larynx includes the posterior and lateral cricoarytenoids, transverse and oblique arytenoids, and the thyroarytenoids. These muscles, which are innervated by the recurrent laryngeal nerve, function conjointly in a complex fashion to control both the adduction and abduction of the true vocal cords. The extrinsic cricothyroid muscle, which is innervated by the external branch of the superior laryngeal nerve, extends from the anterior inferior border of the thyroid cartilage to the anterior surface of the cricocartilage. Contraction of the muscle tilts the laryngeal cartilage forward, producing increased tension of the true vocal cords. The internal branch of the superior laryngeal nerve passes through the thyrohyoid membrane and provides sensory innervation to the pyriform sinus and the supraglottic larynx.

FUNCTIONAL DISORDERS OF THE LARYNX

The primary function of the larynx is to act

as a sphincter, thus protecting the tracheobronchial tree. Secondarily the larynx serves as a sound source for voicing. Functional disorders can affect one or both of these functions. A complete discussion of these disorders is beyond the scope of this chapter, but it is appropriate to discuss several problems common in the geriatric population.

Aspiration

Chronic aspiration is a serious disorder with potential life-threatening sequelae. This problem most often occurs in the elderly as a result of brain stem cerebral vascular accidents. Other etiologic factors of neurologic origin include posterior fossa tumors, head injuries, myasthenia gravis, bulbar palsy, and amyotrophic lateral sclerosis. Anatomic alterations resulting from previous surgical procedures on the pharynx and hypopharynx, as well as neoplasms of the upper aerodigestive tract, also commonly produce chronic aspiration in the elderly. Other more readily treatable causes of aspiration include Zenker's diverticula, cricopharyngeal dysfunction, and gastroesophageal reflux.

When neuromuscular dysfunction is the cause of aspiration, the surgical therapy must be tailored to each patient based on the severity of the problem and the mental status of the patient. With unilateral vocal cord paralysis, the patient usually responds well to medialization of the paralyzed cord by injection into the paraglottic space with gelfoam for temporary weakness or Teflon for permanent paralysis. More recently, medialization of the paralyzed vocal cord has been accomplished with implants of Silastic placed between the inner table of the thyroid cartilage and the elevated perichondrium. This allows medialization of the vocal cord without instrumentation into the substance of that cord, as is done with Teflon injection.

Numerous methods have been proposed for isolation of the respiratory tree from the digestive tract in patients with chronic aspiration. The ideal procedure should be simple, reliable, and reversible. When planning a procedure to prevent chronic aspiration the relative importance of each of these criteria is based on the condition of that individual patient.

Tracheotomy utilizing a cuffed tube is used very successfully for short-term prevention of aspiration in the postoperative period, but it is a poor choice for treatment for chronic aspiration. It tethers the larynx and trachea to the skin, causing an increased tendency to aspirate with deglutition. Usually a reservoir of food and secretions collects above the cuff, filling the upper trachea and larynx. This collection leaks around the cuff with each cough or trach tube manipulation, as when suctioning, cleaning, or changing the tracheotomy tube. Therefore, tracheotomy has not proved to be a reliable treatment for patients with chronic aspiration.

Laryngeal closure can be accomplished with the endoscopic placement of a laryngeal stent. This stent is secured in place with transcutaneous permanent sutures tied over Silastic buttons, resulting in total obstruction of the supraglottic and glottic regions of the larynx. A recent innovative modification of this procedure utilizes a Montgomery Silastic T-tube with a duckbill valve placed on the superior end. This is inserted through a tracheotomy site into the superior trachea, ending in the supraglottic region of the larynx. This one-way valve prevents aspiration, but allows the patient to continue transoral communication.

Various methods of laryngeal closure have been described for debilitated patients with no ability to use verbal communication. Habal and Murray first described de-epithelialization of the free edge of the epiglottis, AE folds, and the arytenoid (1). These denuded edges were sutured together, resulting in a reversible closure of the supraglottic larynx. Montgomery through a midline laryngofissure approach de-epithelialized both the true and false vocal cords and performed a multilayer closure of the larynx (2). This method, which has an excellent success rate, is probably not reversible. Saski modified this procedure by placing the sternohyoid muscle into the ventricular dead space to further ensure successful obliteration of the larynx (3). Others have described transsecting the cervical trachea, creating a tracheostoma with a distal segment of trachea, and oversewing the proximal tracheal segment, creating a blind laryngeal pouch. Although this procedure prevents aspiration and is readily reversible the blind laryngeal pouch can act as a reservoir for collection of malodorous partially digested food.

Lindeman initially described the technique of

laryngeal diversion for treatment of chronic aspiration (4). In this procedure, after the trachea is divided at the third or fourth tracheal interspace, a tracheostoma is created with the distal trachea end. The proximal segment of the trachea is then either anastomosed using an end-to-side fashion into the anterior esophageal wall, or it is brought out and sutured to the skin of the neck. Both forms of this procedure work well for aspiration and are readily reversible. However, the neck diversion technique results in cutaneous salivary drainage that complicates the care of an already debilitated patient.

Total laryngectomy is the most definitive procedure for prevention of aspiration. However, it is usually a poor alternative for it is an extensive surgical procedure with high perioperative morbidity in elderly debilitated patients. Several of the techniques described above can be performed in a simpler, more efficient manner and are equally successful in the prevention of chronic aspiration.

Vocal Cord Paralysis

Paralysis of the true vocal cords, which can either be unilateral or bilateral, is more commonly seen with unilateral involvement. The primary cause of unilateral vocal cord paralysis is surgical trauma, which may occur in the chest, neck, or at the skull base. Other common causes of unilateral paralysis include neoplasms, inflammatory diseases, along with an idiopathic group. The most common cause of bilateral true vocal cord paralysis is trauma secondary to thyroidectomy and parathyroidectomy. In the elderly there is an increased incidence of bilateral true vocal cord paralysis of unknown etiology.

Most patients with gradual onset of unilateral paralysis compensate for it with increased motion of the normal contralateral vocal cord; very little voice change and little or no aspiration result. With acute loss of unilateral cord function as seen with surgical trauma, the patient usually has an acute change in voice quality, with mild to severe aspiration. The treatment of these symptoms depends on the integrity of the vagus and recurrent laryngeal nerves. With an intact nerve, implying the possibility of a slow reinnervation and laryngeal recovery, no permanent treatment should be undertaken. If the paralysis results in aspiration that is moderate to severe,

preventing oral intake, or resulting in inadequate communication secondary to poor voice, gelfoam can be injected into the paraglottic space for rapid resolution of these symptoms. This substance is slowly absorbed over a 4- to 5-week period, allowing the patient to compensate gradually for the paralysis.

If the vagus or recurrent laryngeal nerve is sacrificed during an operation or a patient with unilateral paralysis and an intact nerve is still symptomatic after 1 year with no functional recovery, then permanent vocal cord medialization is indicated. Two methods are available to aid in permanent glottic closure. First, one can inject Teflon, a non-absorbable substance, into the paraglottic space to add bulk to the vocal cord, thus moving the free edge of the vocal cord into the midline. Second, one can implant cartilage or a Silastic block between the inner table of the thyroid cartilage and its perichondrium. This results in moving the free edge of the vocal cord toward the midline without the potential side effects of an intracordal injection.

The treatment of bilateral vocal cord paralysis is a compromise between attempting to provide an adequate airway and leaving the patient with a useful voice and the ability to protect the airway. In acute bilateral paralysis tracheotomy is usually necessary in the early stages to maintain an adequate airway. To decannulate these patients successfully, one must lateralize either of the paralyzed true vocal cords to enlarge the airway. This is most commonly accomplished by either surgical removal or laser obliteration. Ossoff described a method of endoscopic laser obliteration of the arytenoid that allowed adequate lateralization of the true vocal cord with fair residual vocal quality and with very little surgical morbidity (5). This laser obliteration has become the standard at present for treatment of bilateral vocal paralysis.

LARYNGEAL NEOPLASMS

The vast majority of neoplasms arising in the larynx are squamous cell carcinomas. An in-depth discussion of the less common benign and malignant tumors is beyond the scope of this chapter. Thus, we will concentrate on the staging and treatment of squamous cell carcinoma of the larynx in the elderly.

The incidence of laryngeal cancer is still increasing and continues to present a major health risk to the geriatric population. Jun et al. found in a study of geriatric patients over the age of 80 that laryngeal carcinoma accounted for 15% of all head and neck malignancies (6).

The actual causes of malignant degeneration of laryngeal tissues are difficult to ascertain, but strong evidence links a combination of factors to the increased incidence of laryngeal carcinoma in certain population groups. The association between smoking tobacco products and laryngeal carcinoma is widely accepted. Wynder in 1956 first published data implicating smoking as a possible cause of laryngeal tumors that statistically demonstrated that these tumors rarely develop in nonsmoking males (7). Auerbach et al. in an evaluation of cadaveric larynges demonstrated a much greater degree of epithelial atypia in smoking males than in larynges of nonsmokers (8). Alcohol consumption in association with smoking increases the incidence of laryngeal carcinoma in all areas of the larynx, but particularly in the supraglottic region. Other factors implicated in laryngeal carcinoma include radiation exposure, industrial chemicals, chronic exposure to wood dust, asbestos exposure, and some types of dietary deficiencies.

Squamous cell carcinoma of the larynx can be classified as arising from four anatomic regions, which include the supraglottic, glottic, subglottic, and transglottic. Tumors arising in each of these areas behave individually with marked differences in their 5-year survival rates. This fact underlies the importance of this classification.

Supraglottic Tumors

A brief description of the anatomy and lymphatic drainage of the larynx was presented earlier. Small tumors of the supraglottic region metastasize early in the course of the disease via the ipsilateral thyrohyoid membrane along the course of the superior laryngeal vessels. The rich lymphatic network of the supraglottic region results in frequent bilateral metastasis with larger tumors. Two anatomic spaces also serve to direct tumor extension. The pre-epiglottic space is a fat-filled space located between the anterior surface of the epiglottic cartilage and the thyrohyoid membrane just inferior to the vallecula.

Table 12.1 Staging Of Supraglottic Squamous Cell Carcinoma

Tis	Carcinoma in situ
T1	Tumor confined to site of origin with normal mobility
T2	Tumor involves adjacent supraglottic site(s) or glottis without fixation
T3	Tumor limited to larynx with fixation or extension to involve postcricoid area, medial wall of pyriform sinus, or pre-epiglottic space
T4	Massive tumor extending beyond the larynx to involve the oropharynx, soft tissue of neck, or destruction of thyroid cartilage

Supraglottic tumors gain access to this region through small fenestra in the epiglottic cartilage. From this space tumor can readily spread to the neck through the thyrohyoid membrane or down to the anterior commissure and the paraglottic space laterally. The paraglottic space is located lateral to the quadrangular membrane and the conus elasticus on the deep surface of the false and true vocal cords, within the thyroid cartilage and pyriform sinus. Tumors involving this space rapidly become transglottic and extend into the neck and the thyroid gland through the cricothyroid membrane.

Two distinctive growth patterns have been observed in supraglottic tumors. Tumors with "pushing margins" are found more often in the supraglottic region. These tumors spread with raised, well-defined margins. The surrounding bulky margins encircle the raised exophytic tumor mass that resides superficially, usually without deep invasion. These lesions have a better prognosis than the apparently smaller, "infiltrating" lesions. The latter smaller, ulcerative-type lesion, which tends to be less differentiated than the former, presents with infiltrating obscure margins and a deeply penetrating central ulcer. These infiltrating lesions can rapidly invade the paraglottic and pre-epiglottic spaces with an apparently small tumor as it is seen at laryngoscopy. The classification of supraglottic tumors is shown in Table 12.1.

Patients with supraglottic tumors usually present in a later stage of their disease than those with glottic primaries. These tumors tend to be silent until they reach 2 to 3 cm in size, and by then, they usually involve structures outside the supraglottic region. Early symptoms include muffled voice, hoarseness, dysphagia, sore throat, otalgia, and, all too often, only a large neck mass. The symptom of otalgia that is often seen with supraglottic and pharyngeal tumors is caused by referred pain through the vagus nerve to the external auditory canal.

Treatment options for tumors of the supraglottic larynx include primary radiation therapy, laser excision of the small lesions, horizontal supraglottic laryngectomy, total laryngectomy, and chemotherapy.

With T1 lesions of the supraglottic larynx, treatment with primary radiation therapy or surgical resection has resulted in equal 5-year survival rates ranging from 65% to 85% in various studies (9, 10). Lymph node metastasis is rare in this group, but when it is present, surgical resection of the primary site with in continuity nodal dissection and possible postoperative radiotherapy would be the treatment of choice. Supraglottic T2N0 tumors may also be treated with radiation therapy or surgical resection. The 5-year survival rates range from 55% to 80% in various studies, with a slight increase in survival with treatment primarily with surgical resection (11, 12). Again, positive nodal disease would dictate surgical resection of the primary site with en bloc nodal dissections and probable postoperative radiotherapy for disease with extracapsular nodal spread. Supraglottic tumors that present in the clincial stage of T3 and T4 categories with no palpable neck metastasis still have a high likelihood of harboring occult metastatic disease in the jugular chain nodes. Therapeutic planning is required to address this occult disease. Primary radiation therapy has produced poor survival rates when compared to resection and also when compared to excision plus radiotherapy for these groups. The 5-year survival in one large study for patients treated with surgical resection and postoperative radiotherapy was 64% for T3 and 48% for T4 lesions. With radiotherapy only, this figure drops to 33% and 14% for 5-year survival, respectively (13).

Many have debated the efficacy of postoperative radiotherapy in T3 and T4 stage patients with stage N0 necks. Most feel that the likelihood of occult nodal metatasis necessitates some form of treatment directed toward this nodal disease.

If no nodal dissection is performed, then prophylactic radiotherapy is probably indicated. One can accurately stage the nodal disease by performing bilateral functional neck dissections. If no occult metastatic neoplasm is present or the neck is a pathologic stage N1 with no extracapsular nodal spread then the patient can be observed safely with no postoperative radiotherapy. The practice of performing a standard radical neck dissection to stage an apparent stage N0 neck should be condemned.

Surgical options for T1 and T2 lesions of the supraglottic larynx include laser excision of small epiglottic lesions, supraglottic laryngectomy, and total laryngectomy. In the younger population most supraglottic T1 and T2 lesions can be excised safely with a supraglottic laryngectomy. This procedure leaves the airway unguarded, presenting a formidable task for the patient to relearn swallowing without aspiration, especially in the early postoperative period. Very few patients over the age of 65 who have any degree of pulmonary disease can tolerate such an insult to the airway. Therefore, radiation therapy is the treatment of choice for T1 and T2 lesions in the elderly patient, reserving total laryngectomy for surgical treatment in patients with recurrent disease.

When the patient presents with a clinical stage T3 or T4 tumor of the supraglottic larynx, the lesion has extended beyond the supraglottic region and is no longer amenable to resection with the supraglottic technique. The treatment of choice for the elderly patient with this tumor is total laryngectomy. When these patients also present with N2 or N3 nodal disease of the neck, either a modified radical neck dissection sparing the spinal accessory nerve or a standard radical neck dissection is performed en bloc with the laryngectomy, depending on the involvement of nodal groups lying along the spinal accessory nerve. This treatment is usually followed by postoperative radiotherapy to decrease the incidence of local and regional recurrence.

Glottic Carcinoma

Glottic carcinoma is the most common laryngeal tumor and usually occurs as a well-differentiated form of squamous cell carcinoma. Patients with tumors of the glottic region present

Table 12.2 Staging Of Glottic Squamous Cell Carcinoma

Tis	Carcinoma in situ
T1	Tumor confined to vocal cord(s) with normal mobility (including involvement of anterior or posterior commissures)
T2	Supraglottic or subglottic extension of tumor with normal or impaired cord mobility
T3	Tumor confined to the larynx with cord fixation
T4	Massive tumor with thyroid cartilage destruction or extension beyond the confines of the larynx or both

early because of changes that occur in vocal quality even with very small lesions. The overall prognosis of glottic neoplasms therefore is excellent due to two factors: early detection and delayed metastasis. The vocal cords contain a very sparse lymphatic network that delays spread to regional lymph nodes until an advanced stage of tumor growth has been reached.

Treatment options for glottic tumors include primary radiotherapy, laser excision, cordectomy, vertical hemilaryngectomy, near-total laryngectomy, and total laryngectomy. The staging of glottic carcinoma is shown in Table 12.2. Primary radiation therapy has been the mainstay of treatment for T1 glottic lesions, resulting in a 5-year survival of greater than 95% with fair-to-good voice quality following treatment (13). Total cordectomy has been performed with equal survival rates, but with very poor postoperative vocal quality. Ossoff has demonstrated 5-year survival of 98% with endoscopic laser cordectomy with good postoperative voice (14).

With tumor extension to the vocal process of the arytenoid or to the anterior commissure, surgical therapy is a more effective option than radiotherapy in producing local control of tumor. Resection can be usually accomplished by either standard or extended vertical hemilaryngectomy. This procedure is tolerated very well in the geriatric patient unless the entire arytenoid cartilage has to be resected. Doing so leaves the laryngeal introitus unprotected, and aspiration occurs with extensive postoperative morbidity. The near-total laryngectomy as described by Pearson is the procedure of choice for extensive T1 lesions and early T2 lesions (15). With extensive T1 lesions, 5-year survivals drop to approximately 80%. Total laryngectomy is usually reserved for radiation failure recurrences in the

treatment of these early lesions.

With vertical tumor spread of a glottic lesion, the rich lymphatics of both the supraglottic and subglottic regions cause these tumors to have an increased chance of cervical metastasis. Subglottic extension of the tumor greater than 10 mm anteriorly or 5 mm posteriorly places the lesion over the cricothyroid membrane and the upper border of the coracoid cartilage. This subglottic extension reduces 3-year survival rates from greater than 90% for T1 lesions to 50% to 70%, depending on whether the anterior commissure is involved with tumor (16). An extended vertical hemilaryngectomy with resection of the upper border cricoid and/or the arytenoid cartilage can be used to resect lesions with less than 15 mm of subglottic spread, but this procedure leaves the larynx unprotected and is poorly tolerated in the elderly. Total laryngectomy or primary radiation therapy with total laryngectomy for surgical salvage is the most reasonable and most often used treatment plan for these lesions.

Supraglottic extension of glottic lesions to involve the false vocal cord opens the paraglottic space for possible tumor extension. These lesions are termed "transglottic" lesions. Partial laryngeal resection for transglottic lesions with vocal cord immobility is accompanied by a high rate of recurrence. There, total laryngectomy is the surgical treatment of choice for this lesion. In small transglottic lesions with normal cord mobility, primary radiation therapy with total laryngectomy reserved for surgical salvage has resulted in approximately 70% 5-year survival (17).

Tumor limited to the vocal cord with cord fixation, a clinical stage T3 lesion, is the result of deep invasion into the intrinsic muscles of the larynx. These lesions often spread rapidly to involve the laryngeal cartilages, resulting in a pathologic stage of T4. Radiotherapy treatment for the lesions has resulted in a poor 5-year survival, ranging from 20% to 30% (13). This figure can be raised to 50% when total laryngectomy is used for radiation failures. Surgical therapy consists of near-total laryngectomy or total laryngectomy. Hemilaryngectomy can be used in selected small lesions if the surgical margins are examined well at the time of the procedure and frozen sections are done to detect deep

Table 12.3 Staging Of Subglottic Squamous Cell Carcinoma

Tis	Carcinoma in situ
T1	Tumor confined to the subglottic region
T2	Tumor extension to vocal cords with normal or impaired cord mobility
T3	Tumor confined to larynx with cord fixation
T4	Massive tumor with cartilage destruction or extension beyond the confines of the larynx or both

occult extensions. Near-total laryngectomy as described by Pearson requires a permanent tracheotomy, but transoral vocal communication with normal deglutition is maintained (15). Survival in patients treated surgically ranges from 50% to 70% over a 5-year period.

Tumors that *invade* the laryngeal cartilages or *extend* outside the larynx are classified as a clinical T4 lesion; these extensions result in a marked drop in survival when treated with primary radiotherapy. Even with total laryngectomy and postoperative radiotherapy, the 5-year survival ranges from 25% to 50% for these lesions (18). With positive nodal disease, the 5-year survival drops to only 20% to 30% (18). These lesions must be treated aggressively with total laryngectomy and nodal dissection with postoperative radiation therapy.

Subglottic Carcinoma

Primary subglottc tumors are rare. Most subglottic tumors actually represent subglottic extension of tumors from a primary vocal cord lesion. The staging of subglottic tumors is shown in Table 12.3. Tumors in this region are very aggressive with early direct spread to the cricoid cartilage, cricothyroid membrane, and paraglottic space with vocal cord fixation. They also spread posteriorly over the cricoid cartilage to involve the postcricoid esophageal regions. Almost one-half of these lesions will spread to the paratracheal lymph nodes. Treatment should be aggressive with total laryngectomy and peritracheal nodal dissection. Even with this treatment survival is poor, with 40% to 60% 5-year survival rates reported (19).

VOCAL REHABILITATION

Since the first laryngectomy was performed aggressive efforts have been underway to find ways to rehabilitate the verbal communication of the laryngectomized patients. Although esophageal speech has only a 40% patient success rate, it was the main form of vocal rehabilitation in the first half of this century. In 1957, Bell Laboratories introduced the "electro-larynx", which opened the door to transoral communication for many patients who are unable to use esophageal speech successfully. Communication with the electro-larynx is adequate, but the mechanical monotone quality produced is often distracting in clinical use. Many surgical procedures have been described and used to reconstruct a one-way valve between the airway and the articulating oral cavity. Most of these have failed secondary to either salivary leakage or fistula stenosis.

A major breakthrough in this effort was made in 1979 with the introduction of the Blom-Singer prosthesis (20). This was shortly followed by the introduction of the Panje voice button (21). These devices provided a simple, fairly reliable way to shunt air from the trachea into the oral cavity without significant salivary leakage. Success rates utilizing these devices range from 65% to 90% (22–24). The critical factor in successful tracheoesophageal speech is not the age or the mental capability of the patient, but the efforts of a dedicated speech pathologist teamed with the surgeon who can motivate these patients and train them in the care and use of their stoma and prosthesis. Careful selection of the candidates is essential to prevent needless frustration to the patient and to the rehabilitative team. If the patient has limitations in dexterity, resulting in the inability to occlude the stoma with a finger, or if there is poor visual acuity that will prevent the patient from taking care of the prosthesis and the stoma, he or she is unlikely to become a successful tracheoesophageal speaker. Other relative contraindications include a small tracheostome, esophageal stenosis, tracheal hypersensitivity, general debility, and chronic alcoholism.

EPISTAXIS

Epistaxis has an increased incidence in the geriatric population. The incidence of most etiologic factors for nose bleeds in the elderly is increased because the atrophy of the nasal mucosa causes a predisposition toward desiccation and ulceration of the intranasal tissues. This thin, delicate, atrophic mucosa is also more prone to breakdown with local trauma to the nose. An increased incidence of hypertension, as well as atherosclerotic vascular disease, in this population further predisposes these patients to epistaxis. The more common predisposing factors in the elderly are infection, trauma, allergy, hypertension, atherosclerotic vascular disease, blood dyscrasias, tumors, and hereditary hemorrhagic telangiectasia. One can see that with advanced age the incidence of many of these factors would be increased because of the associated mucosal atrophy.

To treat epistaxis appropriately, the anatomy of the entire nose, as well as its vascular supply, must be well understood. The nasal mucosa derives its rich blood supply from both the internal and external carotid arteries. The two major sources of arterial supply are the internal maxillary artery and the facial artery, both branches from the external carotid artery. The internal maxillary artery ascends on the posterior wall of the maxillary sinus and branches into the sphenopalatine artery, the descending palatal arteries, and the infraorbital artery. The sphenopalatine artery passes through the sphenopalatine foramen to enter the nasal cavity at the posterior aspect of the middle turbinate. The artery then branches, sending a lateral branch to supply the middle and inferior turbinates and the medial wall of the ethmoid and maxillary sinuses. The second branch, the posterior septal artery, crosses over the roof of the posterior choanae and supplies the nasal septum. It anastomoses distally in the anterior aspect of the nasal septum with the incisive artery—the distal branch of the greater palatine artery—to give the very rich vascular supply to the anterior septum. The facial artery adds a portion of the blood supply to the anterior septum also through the septal branch of the superior labial artery. The internal carotid artery contributes to the nasal blood supply through two branches of the ophthalmic artery—the anterior and posterior ethmoidal arteries. Both of these arteries pass through the medial wall of the orbit into the superior aspect of the ethmoid sinuses. They continue along the cribriform plate to supply the superior aspect of both the septum and the lateral nasal wall, including the superior turbinate.

One can see from this anatomic discussion that two highly vascular regions of intranasal mucosa stand out as common sites for epistaxis. Primarily, the anterior nasal septum that derives its blood supply from the three major arterial branches, known as Little's or Kiesselbach's area, is the most common site for the origin of the anterior epistaxis. Second, where the sphenopalatine artery divides in the nasal mucosa at the posterior aspect within the mucosa of the middle turbinate is the most common site of posterior epistaxis. Although anterior epistaxis is more common in general, bleeding from the posterior aspect of the nasal cavity has a marked increase in frequency in the geriatric population.

The management of epistaxis can be broken down into three main steps: (1) the initial evaluation; (2) outpatient management, including medical therapy and intranasal packing; and (3) inpatient management, including surgical ligation or embolization of feeding arteries. Most epistaxis is handled by the patient and/or family with age-old remedies of digital pressure and ice packs, without the need for physician involvement. Those patients that do present to the physician with epistaxis usually have already bled sufficiently to cause marked anxiety to both the patient and surrounding family members.

The initial step in management of a patient with epistaxis is to calm the patient, allay his or her fears, and develop a rapport with both the patient and the family. After assessing the degree of urgency, including the patient's vital signs and hemoglobin concentration, one may then do an in-depth evaluation of the patient's medical history to discover any causes that might lead to this particular episode of epistaxis. Underlying medical causes, such as hypertension, should be rapidly addressed and treated as necessary. It is important to remember the assessment and protection of the airway in these patients. Rapid institution of intravenous fluid replacement is usually necessary, as well as providing intravenous access for sedating drugs and antihypertensive agents that may be needed.

In severe episodes of epistaxis with hemorrhage, unstable vital signs, and shock, one can institute rapid pressure on the site of bleeding by placing Foley catheters transnasally into both sides of the nasopharynx. After instilling 10 to

15 cc of fluid into each of the ports, the balloons are pulled forward snugly against the posterior choanae. At this point, tight anterior packing is placed bilaterally and left in place until the patient's vital signs are stabilized. Most emergency rooms have in stock commercially manufactured nasal packs that use a double-balloon catheter, with one balloon residing in the nasopharynx and another balloon residing in the nasal cavity. These nasal packs are excellent in emergency situations and allow one to place a marked amount of pressure on the intranasal and nasopharyngeal tissues that will stop life-threatening hemorrhages. However, these packs have little use in the chronic management of epistaxis or non-emergent epistaxis because of their potential for serious complications. A pack of this nature, when left inflated for 48 hours, can cause necrosis of the septal and turbinate tissues.

After stabilization of the patient and management of associated medical problems, one must progress to the physical examination of the nose and to the identification of the actual site of bleeding. One must have an excellent light source with a parallel light beam to the vision of the examining physician. Utilizing a Frazier suction catheter and a nasal speculum, both sides of the nasal cavity must be inspected during the acute bleeding episode in an attempt to identify bleeding that may be occurring from the anterior nasal septum. Nasal pledgets instilled with a topical agent that causes both constriction and anesthesia of the nasal mucosa are then placed into the nose. The most common agent for this is cocaine used in a 4% solution. To prevent catastrophic disasters from overdoses of cocaine, one should limit the use of this drug to 200 mg (i.e., only 5 cc of a 4% solution) for the evaluation of a patient with epistaxis. Upon removal of these pledgets one can inspect the nose with a headlight and nasal speculum and identify the exact site of anterior epistaxis without difficulty. If bleeding is coming from the posterior aspect, one may use a fiber optic nasopharyngoscope or rigid Hopkins nasal scope to allow inspection of the posterior nasal cavity and to identify discretely the site of epistaxis. If the site of epistaxis is identified, then using either electrocautery or silver nitrate topical cautery, one may accurately cauterize the bleeding site and the surrounding tissues to that area for approximately 3 mm. The

most common cause of failure to stop the bleeding with this coagulation technique is the inappropriate use of silver nitrate. It should always be held in place for 20 seconds against the bleeding mucosa. Application of silver nitrate to the blood vessel for only 5 to 10 seconds will inevitably result in rebleeding in a matter of minutes.

If the bleeding site cannot be discretely identified, intranasal packing is the next step in treatment. If bleeding is in the anterior nasal cavity, which extends from the nasal vestibule to an area near the posterior aspect of the turbinates, an anterior nasal pack is all that is needed. While preparing the pack, cocaine pledgets are replaced into the nose to increase the topical anesthesia and the vasoconstriction. The anterior pack is usually formed from 1/2" by 72" lengths of either plain gauze or Vasoline gauze instilled with antibiotic ointment. During placement of the pack, both ends of the packing are carefully monitored to prevent it from prolapsing through the posterior choanae into the hypopharyngeal region. The initial portion of the pack is placed into the superior nasal recess along the middle turbinate and superior turbinate. As one reaches the level of the superior aspect of the posterior choanae, the gauze is layered from front to back to prevent prolapse into the nasal pharynx. This pack should fill the intranasal cavity snugly. The anterior pack is left in place from 2 to 5 days depending on the seriousness of the bleeding and the difficulty of controlling the etiologic factors. With only an anterior pack in place, the patient may be discharged from the hospital setting and observed at home. During the period of intranasal packing, the patient should remain on oral antibiotics, as well as a decongestant antihistamine by mouth, to decrease the likelihood of developing paranasal sinusitis.

Upon removal of the packs, the patient should continue intranasal hygiene with a topical decongestant spray, such as Neosynephrine, for a 3-day period. For 2 weeks after the nasal packing is removed, the patient should continue to use an intranasal saline spray as frequently as each hour during the daytime to prevent desiccation and rebleeding from the healing nasal mucosa.

If the anterior packing fails to stop the nasal bleeding, one must then institute pressure both in the nasopharynx and the anterior nasal cavity. The posterior pack accomplishes two objectives: (a) It places pressure on the nasopharyngeal region and the posterior aspect of the turbinates, which may stop some posterior epistaxis, and (b) it forms a buttress with which one can better place the anterior pack, thereby allowing increased pack pressure in the posterior aspect of the nasal cavity.

A 16 French Foley catheter with a 30-cc balloon is placed through the side of major bleeding and into the nasal pharynx. After 10 to 15 mm of saline is placed into the balloon it is pulled snugly into the nasal pharynx against the posterior choanae. Anterior packing as previously described is placed around the Foley catheter passing through the nasal cavity. A piece of plastic tubing, either the flared end of the Foley catheter or a cut piece of endotracheal tube, can be placed around the catheter and pushed up against the intranasal pack prior to clamping the catheter tube against this plastic supplemental ring. This allows counter-tension to be applied to the intranasal pack and not against the alar rim. It should prevent necrosis of the alar rim from the pressure over the 2-to-3-day period that the pack may remain in place. Because of the abnormalities of respiration caused by the effect of the posterior nasal pack upon the nasopharyngeal pulmonary reflex, hypoxemia leading to cardiac arrhythmias and possibly cardiac arrest has been reported. In elderly patients with posterior packs, it is advisable to monitor these patients in the hospital and to use moist oxygen supplementation. To have a combination of anterior and posterior packs is quite an uncomfortable situation, and adequate analgesia must be provided to the patient. Prophylactic antibiotics, as well as decongestant antihistamines, are given to the patient while the packs remain in the nose. The anterior and posterior packs are removed in 2 to 5 days, depending on the severity of the bleeding and the the ability to control the etiologic factors that are causing the bleeding. In patients with marked thrombocytopenia or with coagulopathy, it is helpful to use an intranasal pack that will eventually dissolve, thus preventing the need for removal and further trauma to the nose. Such agents as oxidase cellulose, topical thrombin, or microfibrillar (Avatene) all work well in this situation.

Surgical Therapy for Epistaxis

When intranasal packing fails to control the epistaxis or the epistaxis rapidly recurs after removal of the packing, other techniques to control the bleeding must be instituted. These consist of (a) surgical ligation of feeding vessels, (b) angiographic arterial embolization, and (c) laser coagulation of the bleeding sites. When considering surgical ligation of the arterial bleeding, one must ascertain whether the bleeding is coming from the inferior posterior aspect of the nose and therefore the internal maxillary artery system, or from the superior anterior aspect to the nose in which case the bleeding is most likely caused by the ethmoid artery system. In recurrent epistaxis, early ligation of the feeding vessel is very efficacious and prevents multiple repacking of the already traumatized nasal mucosa.

The ethmoid arteries are usually the supplying vessels of recurrent bleeding from the superior nasal cavity. They are surgically approached through an incision halfway between the nasion and the medial canthus. The periosteum is elevated off of the medial canthal region and along the lamina papyracea until the anterior ethmoid artery is encountered. This artery is usually 2 cm from the anterior lacrimal crest. The artery is coagulated and ligated with either vascular clips or surgical ties. One must be careful to ligate the artery adequately to prevent it from retracting into the orbital floor area and causing retro-orbital hematoma. The posterior ethmoid artery is located 10 mm behind the anterior ethmoid artery and approximately 5 mm anterior to the optic nerve. Because of its proximity to the optic nerve, it is rarely ligated because of possible injury to the optic nerve, which could result in blindness. During this ligation procedure, one must carefully monitor the degree of pressure placed on the orbit and the globe to prevent ocular damage.

If the bleeding can be roughly identified in the posterior inferior aspect of the nasal cavity and it has failed to cease with nasal packing, ligation of the internal maxillary artery is the treatment of choice. With the patient under general anesthesia, an incision is made in the buccal mucosa identifying the anterior face of the maxilla. After removing the anterior wall, the posterior wall of the maxillary sinus is removed, leaving the posterior periosteum intact. After careful incision of this periosteum, the maxillary artery, and its branches, the infraorbital, and the sphenopalatine arteries can be identified under microscopic control. The vessels are then ligated with multiple vascular clips. An alternate method for ligation of the maxillary artery is through a buccal mucosal incision. The maxillary artery is identified proximally as it passes between the medial and lateral pterygoid muscles.

Routine ligation of the external carotid artery for prevention of posterior epistaxis as used in the past has fallen in disfavor because the collateral blood flow that feeds into the maxillary artery distal to the point of ligation sustains a high flow rate in the artery. This results in a high failure rate for this method. However, in life-threatening intranasal hemorrhage, rapid vascular control can be gained by either temporary or permanent ligation of the external carotid artery under local anesthesia.

One disease that should be specifically mentioned when discussing epistaxis is hereditary hemorrhagic telangiectasia (Rendu-Osler-Weber disease). This is a rare disease resulting from a congenital absence of the contractile elements in the walls of small vessels. It results in multiple telangiectasias, which are dilated venules and capillaries, presenting on most of the mucosal surfaces of the body. These patients usually suffer from recurrent epistaxis and gastrointestinal hemorrhage, resulting in the need for multiple blood transfusions. These telangiectasias are quite friable and bleed with minimal trauma to the lips, tongue, or intranasal region. Septal dermoplasty has been the primary treatment for this disease since it was described by Saunders in 1968. The anterior nasal septum, floor of the nose, and the medial portion of the inferior turbinate are stripped of their mucosa. This region is then resurfaced with a dermal graft. This has resulted in decreased epistaxis episodes in the anterior nasal region. Some reports have shown regrowth of the telangiectasias through the dermal graft. Recent reports utilizing the neodymium:yttrium aluminum garnet (Nd:YAG) laser to photocoagulate the telangiectasias have been encouraging. The larger more prominent telangiectasias in the anterior nasal region are photocoagulated, resulting in increased intervals between significant bleeding episodes. It is im-

possible to irradicate completely the telangiectasias from the intranasal region due to the inaccessibility of most of these lesions and their rapid recurrence after coagulation. Therefore, repeated treatments are performed in these patients as needed for epistaxis or prophylactically every 4 to 6 months.

REFERENCES

1. Habal MD, Murray JE: Surgical treatment of life-endangering chronic aspiration pneumonia. *Plast Reconstr Surg* 49:305-311, 1977.
2. Montgomery WW: Surgery to prevent aspiration. *Arch Otolaryngol* 101:679-682, 1975.
3. Sasaki CT, Milmoe G, Yanagisawa E, Berry K, Kirchner JA: Surgical closure of the larynx for intractable aspiration. *Arch Otolaryngol* 106:422-423, 1980.
4. Lindeman RC: Diverting the paralyzed larynx: a reversible procedure for intractable aspiration. *Laryngoscope* 85:157-180, 1975.
5. Ossoff RH, Sisson GA, Duncavage JA, Moselle HI, Andrews PE, McMillan WG: Endoscopic laser arytenoidectomy for the treatment of bilateral vocal cord paralysis. *Laryngoscope* 94:1293-1297, 1985.
6. Jun MY, Strong EW, Saltzman EI, Gerold FD: Head and neck cancer in the elderly. *Head Neck Surg* 5:376-n-382, 1983.
7. Wynder EL, Bross IJ, Day E: Epidemiological approach to etiology of cancer of the larynx. *JAMA* 160:1384-1391, 1956.
8. Auerbach O, Hammond EC, Garfinkel L: Histologic changes in relation to smoking habits. *Cancer* 25:92-104, 1970.
9. DeSanto LW: Cancer of the supraglottic larynx: a review of 260 patients. *Otolaryngol Head Neck Surg* 93:705-711, 1985.
10. Bocca E, Pignataro O, Oldini C: Supraglottic laryngectomy: 30 years of experience. *Am Otol Rhino Laryngol* 92:14-18, 1983.
11. Ogura JH, Sessions DG, Spector GJ: Conservative surgery for epidermoid carcinoma of the supraglottic larynx. *Laryngoscope* 85:1808-1815, 1975.
12. Fu KK, Eiesenberg L, Dedo HH, Phillips TL: Results of integrated managements of supraglottic carcinoma. *Cancer* 40:2874-2881, 1977.
13. Vermund H: Role of radiotherapy in cancer of the larynx as related to the TNM system of staging. A review. *Cancer* 25:485-504, 1970.
14. Ossoff RH, Sisson GA, Shapshay SM: Endoscopic management of selected early vocal carcinoma. *Ann Otol Rhinol Laryngol* 94:560-564, 1985.
15. Pearson BW. Subtotal laryngectomy. *Laryngoscope* 91:1904-1912, 1981.
16. Sessions DG, Maness GM, McSwain B: Laryngofissure in the treatment of carcinoma of the vocal cord: a report

of forty cases and a review of the literature. *Laryngoscope* 75:490–502, 1965.

17. Harwood AR, DeBoer G: Prognostic factors in T2 glottic cancer. *Cancer* 45:991–995, 1980.

18. Jesse RH: The evaluation of treatment of patients with extensive squamous cancer of the vocal cords. *Laryngoscope* 85:1424–1429, 1975.

19. Stell PM, Tobin KE: The behavior of cancer affecting the subglottic space. In Alberti PW, Bryce DP (eds): *Workshops from the Centennial Conference on Laryngeal Cancer.* New York, Appleton-Century-Crofts, 1976, p. 620.

20. Singer MI, Blom ED: Tracheoesophageal puncture: a surgical prosthetic method for postlaryngectomy speech restoration. Third International Symposium on Plastic and Reconstructive Surgery of the Head and Neck, New Orleans, LA, 1979.

21. Panje WR: Prosthetic vocal rehabilitation following laryngectomy, the Voice Button. *Ann Otol Rhinol Laryngol* 90:116–120, 1981.

22. Singer MI, Blom ED, Hamaker RC: Further experience with voice restoration after total laryngectomy. *Ann Otol Rhinol Laryngol* 90:498–502, 1981.

23. John ME, Cantrell RW: Voice restoration of the total laryngectomy patient: the Singer-Blom technique. *Otolaryngol Head Neck Surg* 89:82–26, 1981.

24. Wetmore SJ, Krueger K, Wesson K: The Singer-Blom speech rehabilitation procedure. *Laryngoscope* 91:1109–1117, 1981.

Chapter 13

Otology in the Elderly

Michael E. Glasscock, III, M.D., F.A.C.S., Michael H. Fritsch, M.D., Eva A. Dimitrov, M.D.

Currently there are more than 25 million people in the United States over the age of 65, and this number is steadily increasing. As this trend continues, the physician is more frequently faced with otologic problems in the elderly patient. Some of these problems are managed the same in older patients as they would be in a younger individual. Usually, however, there are some changes in management plans that are necessary because of the physiology and psychology of aging.

The physician must deal with any medical problems that have, in the course of a long life, accumulated to cause various degrees of dysfunction (1, 2). The cardiovascular system will usually have some degree of decreased cardiac output and some of the effects of atherosclerosis. Pulmonary oxygen diffusion is decreased, and tissue oxygenation is less efficient. The ability to cough is decreased, and a predisposition to pneumonia is encountered. Changes in kidney function develop with decreased renal blood flow and glomerular filtration rate, and the dosage for urinary excreted medications is affected. Arthritic conditions of the neck, shoulders, and back may impede surgical positioning. Thus, the organ systems in the elderly patient may not tolerate procedures of large surgical or anesthetic magnitude. Multistaged procedures likewise may be less applicable. Good judgement must be exercised when weighing the natural history of the disease against life expectancy. The quality of life after surgical therapy must also be considered.

Within surgical otology there are major subcategories of pathology to be considered: chronic ear disease. Ménière's disease and vestibular dysfunctions, cerebellopontine angle tumors, paragangliomas of the jugulo-tympanic area, middle ear disease, and external ear disease.

THE EXTERNAL EAR

This section will discuss disease processes of the ear canal, including problems with pruritus and cerumen, infection, and tumors. Specific problems related to the aging process in the ear canal stem primarily from anatomic and biochemical changes in the skin and its adnexa (3). These changes leave the skin atrophic and create significant changes in the character of cerumen and hair (4, 5).

A brief review of anatomy will assist in understanding these changes. The external canal extends from the tragus (or conchal cartilage) laterally to the tympanic membrane medially. It is about 2.5 cm in length in the adult. The lateral 30% to 40% of the canal is cartilaginous. The skin in this area has well-developed dermal and subcutaneous layers and contains numerous hair follicles, and sebaceous and ceruminal glands. The skin is thus thicker here and has a diameter of 0.5 to 1.0 mm. The thinner skin overlying the bony portion of the canal is quite thin (.2 mm) and contains no subcutaneous elements, although small hairs and sebaceous glands can occasionally be seen.

The hairs found in the external canal are of two types—the fine vellus hairs and the tragi that are large and found more laterally, as well as on the tragus. These tragi are found in adult males and tend to become coarser, longer, and more noticeable starting in the fourth decade of life.

The numerous sebaceous glands in the lateral portion of the canal secrete a material that lubricates the skin and hairs. Secretion from these glands is subject to androgen control, and therefore a significant decline in secretion is noted in women over 50 years of age as the significant decrease in gonadal activity occurs after menopause. There is only a slight decrease in men over 50 years.

Ceruminal glands are also affected by aging (as are all apocrine sweat glands) as glands atrophy and decrease in activity. Therefore, cerumen has a tendency to become much drier in older people.

Problems with Pruritus and Cerumen

The thin aging skin of the ear canal that has also become dry and itchy can be plagued with dry accumulations of cerumen. Cerumen impactions seem to be more common in males and may be due to the large tragi that trap the dried cerumen. Removal of these impactions must be done carefully. Attempts with "Q-tips" can lead to traumatization of the thin skin, which can then become secondarily infected. Vigorous water or peroxide irrigations or use of "Water Piks" can drive water through an unseen tympanic membrane perforation or even cause a perforation if done too vigorously.

Prevention of impaction is a valuable tool here. Mineral oil (or sweet oil) can provide needed lubrication that is lacking in the elderly, and it will soften dry cerumen. Two drops twice a week is a good starting routine. The individual with intact tympanic membranes can use gentle irrigation once monthly with warm water in a bulb syringe while in the shower. Alcohol should in general be avoided, but can be used in combination with acetic acid to displace water in the ear canal before symptoms of swimmer's ear occur. Strong soap or shampoo can aggravate the pruritus and dryness. Hydrocortisone cream instilled at the meatus can also provide relief for dry, itchy ears.

Infections

Otitis externa is not solely a disease of the elderly. It becomes a problem, however, when one considers the predisposing factors that were mentioned in the previous section. Even though hearing aids are well tolerated by most (and these are not worn only by the elderly), some people are more susceptible to the development of problems that are not easily explained by a poor fit or an occlusive mold.

Bacterial otitis externa is a common infection in all age groups. Numerous contributory factors to its development include maceration of the skin from prolonged water exposure or high humidity (environmental or secondary to hearing aid occlusion of the canal), obstruction of glands by keratin debris or secretions, trauma or contamination, induced implantation of exogenous organisms, and absence of an effective protective layer of cerumen in the canal (because of repeated washing or cleaning of the canal of normal cerumen).

Management of infection of the ear canal is based on frequent thorough cleansing of the canal. Either acetic acid irrigations or manual suctioning under binocular vision is helpful. Providing topical antibiotics in sensible amounts, systemic antibiotics when needed, supportive care of associated symptoms, and advice for general ear care and prevention of infection all should be done.

Chronic conditions may require months of frequent follow-up to resolve thoroughly. Time must be allowed for regrowth of the normal protective mechanisms of the ear canal skin. Rarely is surgical treatment necessary to remove chronically thickened skin, to enlarge the bony canal, and to resurface the canal with skin grafts.

Mycotic infections occur in approximately 10% of symptomatic ear canal infections (6, 7). They occur more frequently in tropical or subtropical climates, but should not be overlooked even in areas where climate is not a factor. They are especially more common in patients with open cavity mastoidectomies or in those who use hearing aids with occlusive molds. *Candida, Aspergillus,* and *Actinomyces* are the most common pathogens. Management includes thorough cleansing of all debris with instruments and suction. Irrigation may be used if the tympanic membrane is intact. Otic drops are not effective against otomycosis. The most effective medications are Cresylate, merthiolate, nystatin (Mycolog®), and Lotrimin®. Cresylate and merthiolate can be painted on the ear canal or may be used to soak a wick that is placed in the ear canal. They should not be used if the tympanic membrane is perforated as middle and inner ear toxicity is not known. Nystatin or Lotrimin® can be instilled to fill the ear canal under direct vision using a syringe and blunt needle or angiocath.

The key to treatment is frequent follow-up for cleansing and reapplication of medication. An excellent irrigating solution (even with a perforated tympanic membrane) is a 1:1 mixture of sterile distilled water and white vinegar, or a 1.5% acetic acid mixture, warmed to body temperature. The patient can use this in a bulb syringe to flush out debris effectively.

A particularly dangerous type of infection should also be mentioned here. Malignant external otitis is an infection originating in the external ear canal and progressing as a necrotizing process to involve tissues of the skull base, including cortical bone, bone marrow, veins and blood vessels, cranial nerves, middle ear, pneumatized spaces of the temporal bone, meninges, and brain (8, 9). Susceptible individuals tend to be elderly and diabetic or otherwise immune-compromised patients. The responsible organism, *Pseudomonas aeruginosa,* is the most common causative agent in the majority of those infectious processes in the external canal. In the elderly diabetic, however, this gram-negative organism can invade blood vessels, nerves, and even bone and produce an intense inflammatory process. The resulting bone destruction, neural dissolution, vessel thrombosis, and tissue necrosis begin in an insidious fashion and fail to respond to the usual treatment for external otitis. Subsequent hearing loss, persistent purulent drainage, and severe constant pain widely involving the temporal region also characterize this infection at its worst.

The diagnosis of malignant external otitis should be made cautiously and not on the basis of a single examination. Common findings include marked ear pain, suppuration unresponsive to the usual medical treatment, and the presence of granulation tissue particularly at the bony-cartilaginous junction on the floor of the ear canal. Granulation tissue may also arise from dehiscences anteriorly and posteriorly. There may be considerable swelling of the temporomandibular joint with trismus and pain on chewing. Abscess formation may occur in the soft tissues of the skull base or parotid gland. Mastoiditis can also occur.

Even though malignant external otitis begins as a relatively minor process, the diagnosis should not be made until the process is shown to be unresponsive to local treatment (debridement and topical antibiotics) and even systemic antibiotics. If no change is seen after 2 weeks, a culture should be performed to determine the organism and its antibiotic sensitivities. Treatment requires intravenous antibiotics for a minimum of 3 weeks and sometimes as long as 2 to 3 months, depending on the extent of disease and its response to treatment. Surgical debridement may be helpful, but generally local curettage and removal of bony and cartilaginous sequestrations can be accomplished with local anesthetic. Extensive surgical debridement is rarely indicated. Radiographic studies are variably useful. A gallium scan or bone scan can be most helpful in assessing the extent of the disease and the response to treatment. Close monitoring of blood glucose, urea-nitrogen, creatinine, and drug levels is important. A baseline audiogram must be obtained, as possible ototoxicity from the antibiotics should be monitored biweekly. Aminoglycosides at the level required here can also cause vestibular side effects with instability and ataxia.

The most important antibiotics have been ticarcillin combined with an aminoglycoside. Pipericillin is also used, and combinations thereof with third-generation cephalosporins are also effective. No extensive studies of the treatment of malignant external otitis with these newer drugs have been done yet, but early clinical trials indicate excellent response.

Length of treatment is determined by the inspection of the ear canal and assessment of symptoms, as well as by changes seen on gallium or bone scan. Generally, antibiotics are continued for an additional 7 days after the ear returns to normal and there is no pain. Cases of recurrence are not uncommon nor is bilateral disease.

Although it is a relatively rare entity, failure to recognize this condition can result in disaster for the patient.

Tumors

Tumors of the external canal cannot be considered a manifestation of the aging process even though a number of reported series indicate a higher prevalence in elderly individuals. They span all age groups, but will be mentioned here as a reminder that we must consider tumors in all patients complaining of chronic otalgia, especially if it is associated with otorrhea or cranial nerve symptoms. Also, lesions in the ear canal that persist or grow or expose bone are serious indicators. The majority of tumors of the ear (including ear canal and pinna) are squamous cell carcinoma (60%), basal cell carcinoma (30%), and ceruminomas. Ten to 25% of these tumors present initially in the ear canal. There are four types of ceruminomas: adenomas, pleomorphic adenomas, adenoid cystic carcinoma, and adenocarcinoma (10–14).

Prolonged chronic otorrhea has been considered to lead to a susceptibility for the development of carcinoma in the external or middle ear. It is unclear if the drainage represents the cause or the effect of the carcinoma. There is also speculation on the carcinogenic effect of toxins produced by some of the flora (especially aspergillus) encountered in chronic otorrhea.

THE MIDDLE EAR

Problems affecting the middle ear are included in this section. They are eustachian tube dysfunction, infection, and conductive hearing loss.

The aging process in the non-diseased ear has been studied histologically. The ossicular articulations have been shown to develop arthritic changes even to the point of calcification of the joint capsule. These changes progress with increasing age. However, corresponding audiometric data do not show any effect on sound transmission so these arthritic changes appear to be of no consequence (15, 16).

Eustachian Tube

The eustachian tube performs three functions: the regulation of middle ear pressure, drainage of middle ear secretions (also guarding the middle ear against nasopharyngeal secretions), and the protection of the inner ear against intense sound.

The ventilatory function of the eustachian tube is affected by body position and changes in a surface tension-reducing substance that enables rapid, short-duration dilation. The tube does not dilate with every swallow. It becomes less efficient the more horizontally the body is positioned.

The mucociliary system of the eustachian tube is continuous with that of the middle ear. At rest, the tube remains closed, preventing retrograde passage of secretions from the nasopharynx. It also blocks sound waves and thus protects the

middle and inner ear structures from infection and acoustic damage.

The two muscles felt to be directly involved with tubal function are the tensor veli palatini and levator veli palatini. Studies of human temporal bones have shown atrophy of the muscle fibers with advancing age predominantly in the tensor muscle. This would suggest that the function of opening of the eustachian tube performed by the tensor probably deteriorates with age (17).

Tubal dysfunction in the elderly may be contributed to by these muscle changes, as well as by changes in the mucociliary action. The bedridden patient has poor opening due to body position, which may lead to venous engorgement. Thus, serous otitis media can become a recurring problem in the elderly and may require placement of ventilating tubes. One must remember, however, to rule out mechanical obstruction as a cause of the otitis, especially in cases with unilateral serous effusions. Tumor can exist either primarily in the nasopharynx or by extending from the oropharynx. A thorough examination for these lesions is mandatory. The diagnosis may be established by using a CT scan or MRI. Examination under anesthesia with biopsy may be indicated in certain cases. Unilateral serous otitis media without other aural reasons is considered to be tumor in the nasopharynx until proven otherwise. Mention should also be made here that otalgia may be *referred* pain from the hypopharynx.

Infection

Acute middle ear infections are rare in this population group when compared to the pediatric age group. Most infections will involve a tympanic membrane perforation and therefore a draining ear. Considerations for etiology and treatment are no different from that of any other age group. The success of medical treatment is determined by the clearing of the infection without drainage. Topical treatment includes cleaning of debris, prevention of water introduction into the ear, leaving the hearing aid out of the ear, and provision of systemic antibiotics. Patient compliance may be a problem. The coexistence of medical problems, such as diabetes, steroid use, absence of eustachian tube function, sinus disease, and the presence of bilateral tympanic perforations, may make the patient more susceptible to poor healing. Surgical success is also related to these underlying factors and *not* to age.

Medical disease may prevent the use of general anesthesia, but simple tympanoplasty can be performed under local anesthesia if necessary. Tympanoplasty should be considered in patients who have recurrent drainage that can clear with treatment, but is a recurrent nuisance that may prevent normal hearing aid use. Mastoidectomy may be necessary in ears that do not clear with medical measures. Elective tympanoplasty can be performed to improve hearing loss in some cases.

In elderly, bedridden patients who are unable to communicate specific symptoms, the draining ear can be the instigator of serious complications. Temporal bone infections are rare complications, but they may go unrecognized in these patients. The draining ear should be irrigated with acetic acid solution (1.5% mixture described previously) to clean out debris and allow for inspection. Most ear drainage can be adequately treated with irrigations, antibiotic drops, and systemic antibiotics. Those that are not cured will require further evaluation and consultation.

The following classification of complications combines those of Mason, Schuknecht, and Neely (4, 17–20):

I. Aural Complications
    a. Ossicular and tympanic membrane destruction;
    b. Mastoiditis with bone destruction;
    c. Subperiosteal abscess;
    d. Petrositis with bone destruction;
    e. Facial paralysis;
    f. Labyrinthitis (serous, suppurative, or chronic).
II. Intracranial Complications
    a. Extradural abscess;
    b. Lateral sinus thrombophlebitis or thrombosis;
    c. Subdural abscess;
    d. Meningitis;
    e. Brain abscess;
    f. Otitic hydrocephalus.

This list serves primarily as a reminder to the reader. No attempt will be made here to go into detail as to recognition and treatment of each specific entity.

In addition to considering possible complications of the chronically draining ear, it must be remembered that several more generalized disease entities can closely mimic the symptoms of chronic suppurative otitis media. Those that might be encountered in the elderly population include Wegener's granulomatosis, tuberculosis, autoimmune inner ear disease, relapsing polychondritis, polyarteritis nodosa, sarcoidosis, and syphilis (17, 21–23).

Wegener's may present with an upper respiratory infection of the nose and sinuses that commonly involves the ear. Granulomas may cause obstruction of the eustachian tube and result in a serous otitis media. There is often an associated sensorineural hearing loss.

Autoimmune inner ear disease can produce middle ear abnormalities, including erythema of the tympanic membrane, serosanguinous effusion, and even granulation tissue. Occasionally this may be seen in the periauricular tissues. Relapsing polychondritis is an autoimmune disease that involves painless swelling of the cartilaginous structures of the head and neck and upper respiratory tract. The pinna is a frequent anatomic location of relapsing polychondritis. Sensorineural hearing loss may also be found.

Polyarteritis nodosa may produce conductive and sensorineural hearing loss and facial nerve paralysis.

Sarcoidosis may involve the auditory, vestibular, and facial nerves, and granulomas can be found in the temporal bone.

Syphilis may affect the middle ear by rarefying osteitis with leukocytic infiltrations of the ossicles and mastoid. Gumma may occur in the ear canal or middle ear. Superinfection can result in chronic otitis media.

Otosclerosis and Other Causes of Conductive Hearing Loss

This section will discuss conductive hearing loss in general, recurrent hearing loss after previous correction, the role of revisional procedures, and the role of hearing amplification, as well as associated inner ear conditions.

Histologically, otosclerosis is uncommon in the elderly. It is a process of unknown etiology that is confined to the temporal bone and is manifested as a conductive hearing loss (24). Usually, the stapes bone is fixed from movement by bony union at the oval window. This produces a conductive hearing loss. Using clinical criteria, hearing loss usually becomes apparent between puberty and 30 years and is bilateral in more than 90% of those seeking therapy. Many patients with unilateral disease are never evaluated. There is a positive family history in 50% of otosclerosis patients. Most patients seek treatment within 5 years of the onset of noticeable hearing loss. Otosclerosis is discussed here as a reminder that it is a surgically treatable cause of hearing loss that can be overlooked in the elderly.

The hearing loss of otosclerosis is gradually progressive, generally reaching a maximum loss within a few years and then stabilizing. The conductive loss is rarely greater than 50 dB. In stapedial otosclerosis, there may also be coexisting cochlear otosclerosis, producing a sensorineural component to the hearing loss that may be so severe as to prevent amplification. Otosclerosis can also coexist with congenital middle ear abnormalities in which case the patient with a stable conductive loss at birth or recognized in early childhood may develop a progressive loss later in life. Other causes of conductive hearing loss should be considered in the differential diagnosis. A primary attic cholesteatoma can be overlooked if the disease process is high in the attic and the drum has remained intact preventing visualization. The conductive loss is rapid (occurring in 1 to 2 weeks) and usually 40 to 60 dB of loss. Progressive conductive hearing loss in patients 60 years or older can also be the result of malleus fixation. This can sometimes be diagnosed by observing lack of movement of the manubrium during pneumatic otoscopy (11, 25).

There are few contraindications for the surgical correction of stapes fixation. It must be remembered that the treatment is elective (17, 26, 27). However, some studies done on the unoperated ear in cases of bilateral otosclerosis indicate that a more rapid sensorineural hearing loss occurs in the opposite ear than occurs in the ear that was operated on in the same patient (28). Age is not a contraindication as long as there is sufficent cochlear reserve to provide a useful increase in auditory acuity and speech discrimination. Even severely deaf patients can gain much benefit from surgical correction if their hearing can be restored to a level that is useful with amplification. Without surgical correction, the severity of hearing loss could preclude the use of a hearing aid.

Two specific conditions, however, contraindicate stapedectomy procedures. These are *active* chronic lymphocytic leukemia and active endolymphatic hydrops (17). Patients in both of these groups, if operated on for stapes fixation, are at high risk to develop total sensorineural hearing loss. It is thought that the inner ear membranes in both instances are much more susceptible to injury either from toxins or manipulation. If the chronic lymphocytic leukemia is in remission, the patient does not seem to have the same risk. It must be mentioned here that one must not confuse the momentary positional disequilibrium frequently experienced by patients with otosclerosis with the more severe spinning vertigo of endolymphatic hydrops.

Conductive hearing loss can recur after surgical repair and can be a result of shifting of position of the prosthesis, regrowth of otosclerotic foci, malpositioning of the prosthesis allowing for loosening of the wire, or formation of scar tissue (26, 29). Surgical revision can be performed, but the incidence of sensorineural hearing loss is 5% as opposed to 2% to 3% with the primary procedure. Closure of the air-bone gap to within 30 dB is somewhat less than 90% effective compared to 98% with the initial procedure.

In general, conductive hearing loss in the elderly should be considered no different from that of a younger population. Careful history will help to elucidate the cause. There are few contraindications to surgical correction, especially as local anesthesia with intravenous sedation is actually preferred and is quite safe for the elderly. It should always be remembered, however, that this is *elective* surgical treatment. A hearing aid is often entirely satisfactory for the patient, and it should always be offered. Age has no bearing on the success of surgical treatment.

THE INNER EAR

Presbycusis

According to national health surveys, at least 40% of all Americans 65 and older suffer some degree of hearing loss. In simple terms, presbycusis is a gradually progressive decline in hearing acuity due to the aging process, which is otherwise unexplained (30, 31). Other forms of pathology must first be excluded. Common examples would be head trauma, ototoxic drugs, ear disease, noise exposure, postoperative sequela, and a family history of hearing loss (32, 33). General criteria that suggest presbycusis are bilaterally symmetric hearing loss, a conductive loss less than 10 dB, and age greater than 65 years (34).

Histologically, four different types of degenerative changes have been identified; each has a typical audiologic correlate. These are strial, neural, sensory, and cochlear presbycusis. These individual types of degenerative patterns can be identified clinically, but in many cases there appear to be combinations. The two most easily indentified sites of inner ear dysfunction causing presbycusis are the stria vascularis and the organ of Corti (2, 35, 36).

Audiologic tests used for the evaluation of hearing loss must include more than an evaluation of thresholds for pure tones, which reflects the activity of only a few auditory nerve fibers. As many as 75% of nerve fibers can be lost without a change occurring in the pure tone threshold (37). The ability to hear and understand phonetically balanced monosyllablic words adds further information to the evaluation and is termed "speech discrimination". Evaluation of central auditory dysfunction should include acoustic reflexes, speech with competing noise or reverberation, frequency selectivity, and other detailed tests (38). Acoustic reflex thresholds for broad-band noise are elevated in normal hearing elderly adults when compared to young adults. This may then be a sensitive measure for identification of central auditory dysfunction (39, 40). More detailed information about these specialized tests is available in published audiologic texts (36).

Rehabilitation of presbycusis focuses on amplification with a hearing aid, which compensates for loss of sensitivity (41–43). A trial period of hearing aid use is essential. Counseling of the patient and family and evaluation of eyesight are invaluable tools in reducing the overall communication handicap. Dexterity and other health problems must also be assessed as they may affect the ability to use and adjust the hearing aid (44).

Other communication problems involve the use of a telephone, radio, or television and may require special instruments other than a hearing aid. Lip reading can also be of assistance. Special devices are available through different outlets and suppliers to deal appropriately with the given problem. Most audiologists or otologists can be of assistance in locating sources of these devices and determining patients' needs.

Ménière's Disease and Vestibular Disequilibria

Dizziness, lightheadedness, falling, and fainting are very common complaints in the elderly patient. The potential causes are diverse, and the key to diagnosis is to apply a systematic clinical approach (45). Initially, a large diagnostic dichotomy exists between "provoked" and "unprovoked" dizziness. The differential diagnosis in provoked dizzy spells includes positional vertigo, postural hypotension, cough-syncope, and micturition-syncope. Unprovoked episodes may be due to Ménière's disease, cerebellar hemorrhage, infarctions of the cerebellum or brain stem, cardio-cerebro-vascular disease, subdural hematoma, and metabolic disease.

In the characterization of the patient's complaint one should always document whether vertigo, the hallucinatory sense of rotational movement, is occurring, or if the dizziness is in actuality a lightheadedness, faintness, or "wooziness." Generally, motion is associated with vestibular disorders. If tinnitus, hearing impairment, and "ear-pressure" symptoms are present, then inner ear dysfunction may be suspected. Nausea and vomiting may also indicate vestibular disease. Vertigo that was initiated at the time of a Valsalva maneuver, such as lifting or straining, or with direct head trauma, such as a motor vehicle accident or slap to the ear, may indicate a perilymph fistula. Onset of symptoms associated with neck movements, particularly neck extension, points toward a vertebro-basilar type of vascular problem. Upper respiratory tract infection for several days prior to the sudden onset of vertigo is suggestive of a viral labyrinthitis. Vestibular neuronitis or viral labyrinthitis is relatively uncommon in the elderly.

Deafness, hemifacial paresthesias, and unilateral limb ataxia suggest cerebellopontine angle (CPA) pathology. Accompanying headaches, difficulty in standing and walking, and limb ataxia suggest a cerebellar lesion. Bilateral facial and limb paresthesias or paresis, dysarthrias, and diplopia indicate brain stem involvement. If amnesia, hemisensory symptoms, and automatisms are present, temporal lobe seizures should be suspected. Behavioral changes and dementia also may indicate a frontal lobe disorder. Palpitations, pallor, sweating, and fainting suggest cardiogenic disease or postural hypotension. A drug history may be helpful, as many elderly patients take several medications concurrently. By far the most common cause of recurrent dizziness and falls in the elderly is postural hypotension. After several falls, postconcussive vertigo and subdural hematoma may overlie the primary etiology.

A number of tests are available to evaluate the dizzy patient. Audiometric examination is used initially to screen for hearing acuity and speech discrimination. Perilymph fistula, a surgically correctable cause of vertigo, is diagnosed by a special test. The test may be conducted with a pneumatic otoscope with gentle bulb insufflation or by placing a finger on the tragus of the ear and pressing it briskly into the canal. A positive test produces vertigo and nystagmus. These tests may be formally performed and recorded on the electronystagmogram (ENG). It should be noted that approximately 30% of Ménière's patients have a positive fistula test. Also, patients who have a fistula may not show a positive test. Another test, the "Hallpike's maneuver," is useful for diagnosis of positional vertigo. The patient is placed in a sitting position with the head turned 45° to one side and then placed into a laying, head-hanging position. The positional change may elicit vertigo and nystagmus. The test must be performed for each side with the ear turned downward.

ENG may also help differentiate between peripheral or central vertigo, and it may characterize and document nystagmus that is not clinically apparent. Drugs affecting the vestibular system should be withheld for 72 hours prior to this test. Ice-water testing is sometimes used to diagnose end-organ vestibular disease, especially in patients in whom routine ENG reveals absent vestibular response. Auditory brain-stem response (ABR) measures auditory tract electrical response to sound similar to an EEG. The ABR is sensitive to retrocochlear lesions, such as acoustic neuromas, but is normal in Ménière's disease and other vestibular diseases. Head CT x-ray imaging is an important test to help differentiate vestibular from central problems. However, it should be noted that subacute subdural hematomas and acoustic neuromas may be isodense with the brain, and therefore, contrast infusion should be used. Additionally, care must be taken to visualize both internal auditory canals during this test. Magnetic resonance imaging (MRI) is a useful adjunctive test for delineation of soft tissue problems. Intricacies of the MRI are still being delineated. Cardiovascular examination to document valvular or arterial stenoses, postural hypotension, or arrhythmias should be completed; neurologic examination for cranial nerves and cerebellar testing are also important.

Positional Vertigo

Positional vertigo is divided into two categories: vestibular and central. Characteristically, the vestibular vertigo and nystagmus have a slight delay of onset and are very prominent. The duration of the nystagmus is less than a minute and is undirectional. Fatigability of vertigo on repeated Hallpike-positional testing is evident. The usual causes for positional vertigo are posttraumatic and idiopathic or aging related. Central positional vertigo has changing directions of nystagmus, mild or absent vertigo, and nonfatigability on testing and may be secondary to cerebellar or cerebellopontine angle tumors.

The condition of benign positional vertigo (BPV) is seen after degeneration of one or more of the sense organs supplied by the vestibular nerves. The insult to the labyrinth may be by head trauma, stapedectomy, chronic otitis media, or occlusion of the vestibular artery. An idiopathic form is also seen. The degenerative effect, seen histopathologically, reveals degeneration of the utricle, and it is hypothesized that this degeneration unleashes otoconia that became embedded in the posterior canal crista. These deposits cause the cupula of the posterior canal to become sensitive to gravitational change. Therefore, change in the head position elicits the cupula to move, promptly causing vertigo (46, 47).

The management of BPV is conservative. Cawthorne head exercises are recommended. This method entails provocation of symptoms by head tilting until the vertiginous response completely fatigues. The procedure is repeated every 6 to 8 hours during waking hours. Antivertiginous drugs are usually not highly effective because the episodes are momentary, but treatment for nausea is usually recommended. Another treatment for this problem is by singular neurectomy (46). A high risk of sensorineural hearing loss is the major disadvantage to this procedure. The procedure is reserved for severe recurrent episodes of approximately 9 months or more duration. The natural history of the disease in the vast majority of patients is self-limiting.

Ménière's Disease

Prosper Ménière's described a symptom complex in 1861 of episodic vertigo, fluctuant hearing loss, roaring tinnitus, and aural fullness (48). In 1938, Hallpike and Cairns described histologically the characteristic distention of the endolymphatic system with minimal effects on auditory and vestibular neuroepithelia (49). Since then, investigations into endolymphatic hydrops have been undertaken in basic research and clinical studies. The actual causes are yet unclear and appear to be multifactorial.

The diagnosis of Ménière's disease is primarily dependent on the history. The predominant symptoms are vertigo, fluctuant hearing loss, tinnitus, and aural pressure or fullness. Other symptoms include sound distortion and occipital headaches. A high salt diet and emotional stress are the primary risk factors. The patient classically describes unilateral problems; however, bilateral cases may present in 15% of individuals. Additionally, it should be noted that atypical forms of Ménière's disease exist that may show more limited manifestations of the classic symptoms. Audiometric testing reveals a predominantly low tone and fluctuating sensorineural hearing loss; later a flat audiometric curve is more characteristic. Improvement in fluctuating hearing through the use of osmotic agents, such as 95% glycerol, may occur. ENG usually shows the caloric response on the affected side to be diminished, and occasionally it may be absent. The differential diagnosis includes postural vertigo, serous labyrinthitis, and cerebellopontine angle tumor.

The mainstay of treatment is medical. Initially, patients are placed on a 2-gram/day sodium diet.

They are asked to reduce caffeine, alcohol, and nicotine consumption and, if possible, to modify their lifestyle to reduce stress. After an initial therapeutic trial of this strategy, medications may be added. Alone or in combination, the most effective medications for Ménière's disease are diuretics, Diazepam-type drugs, and an anticholinergic drug (50). Almost 85% of patients may be brought to an acceptable therapeutic status on this regime. That, however, leaves 15% of patients with incapacitating symptoms to some degree.

In these patients, various surgical interventions may be offered (51, 52). The three predominant current surgical therapies are the endolymphatic mastoid shunt, the vestibular nerve section, and labyrinthectomy. In recent years, questions of efficacy of the endolymphatic mastoid shunt have been raised. Studies of this procedure are ongoing. At the current time, therefore, vestibular nerve section and labyrinthectomy have emerged as the most useful of surgical treatment modalities. The vestibular nerve section procedure allows for the possibility of preserving hearing and facial nerve function while totally interrupting aberrant vestibular signals to the brain stem. The approach is through a small suboccipital craniotomy with subsequent exposure of the eighth nerve complex, followed by selective neurectomy. Labyrinthectomy is usually reserved for the patient with marked loss of hearing with no fluctuation, as is seen in the later disease stages. Labyrinthectomy may be performed in a number of ways, but the preferred method is a transmastoid complete removal of the bony and membranous labyrinth. Transcanal labyrinthectomy with streptomycin packing of the vestibule may incompletely destroy the neuroepithelium and result in residual vertigo. Transcanal cochleovestibular neurectomy may endanger the facial nerve as the visualization of the internal auditory canal is difficult from this exposure. There is a possibility of hearing deterioration and loss following endolymphatic sac operations and neurectomy. These procedures should probably not be performed in the only hearing ear.

Streptomycin, a powerful vestibulotoxic drug, may be given for bilateral Ménière's until both vestibular responses have ceased. Careful titration is necessary to ensure continued cochlear function as streptomycin at a higher dosage is cochleotoxic (53).

Of concern with both selective neurectomy and surgical destruction of the vestibular apparatus is the elderly patient's ability to compensate after the procedure. The initial clinical changes involve disequilibrium. The acute stage lasts approximately 6 weeks and is characterized by central inhibition of the contralateral vestibular nucleus to allow realignment to a new lower baseline activity level. During the chronic stage, cerebellar suppression of the vestibular nucleus decreases, and accommodation of the resulting increased activity follows. In younger individuals, this equalization process may take up to 3 years. Elderly patients may never reach equilibrium. Indeed, 25% of patients over age 75 will have persistant disequilibrium after labyrinthectomy. The decision to operate may commit the patient to accepting lifelong disequilibrium in exchange for relief from incapacitating vertiginous episodes.

A problem arises with streptomycin ablation of bilateral vestibular systems: Dandy's syndrome. This situation arises when limiting the normal triad of the balance system to only proprioceptive and visual functions. It also occurs after loss or ablation of one vestibule with malfunctioning of the contralateral side. Compounding the problem in the elderly is the age-related degeneration of the remaining vision and proprioception. Darkness is completely incapacitating. Oscillopsia is often encountered. Maximization of visual and proprioceptive functions is achieved by use of a cane or walker, good overhead lighting, and removal of soft carpets.

ACOUSTIC NEURILEMMOMA

The most frequent lesion of the cerebellopontine angle is the eighth nerve acoustic neurilemmoma. Charles Bell clearly described this lesion in 1930 though the first observed tumor at autopsy was found in 1777 by Sandifort. Since then, many surgeons have advanced knowledge in this field, most notably Cushing, Dandy, and House (54).

The tumor is a benign, encapsulated, Schwann cell tumor of the eighth nerve, arising predominantly on the superior vestibular division. These tumors may present in as many as 2.4%

of the population and are twice as frequent in women as in men (55, 56).

The diagnosis of an intracranial tumor in the elderly patient may be confusing. Symptoms are all too easily attributed to a dementing or cerebrovascular disease. Ataxia and cerebellar signs, together with intellectual deterioration and headache, are very common symptoms of posterior fossa tumors in this age group. Thus, the typical clinical picture in the elderly person may be indistinct (57). Acoustic tumor diagnosis through symptomatology is difficult, because it is a slow-growing tumor that is dependent on its eighth nerve location for producing symptoms (58). If the tumor is lateral on the eighth nerve, in the "blind-pouch" internal auditory canal, symptoms may be produced early in its course due to pressure phenomena. If the tumor is medial on the eighth nerve, in the cerebellopontine angle (CPA), prolonged asymptomatic or mildly progressive clinical course may result until the tumor is quite large. The main symptoms are tinnitus; loss of speech understanding in the ear, such as when speaking and listening through a telephone; imbalance; and occipital headaches. Sudden hearing loss is the presenting symptom in 15% of the cases. Physical examination is usually normal. Very large tumors, however, may produce facial numbness, aberrant taste sensation, twitching of the face, and numbness of the sensory portion of the seventh nerve to the posterior ear canal. The differential diagnosis of the acoustic neurilemmoma includes meningioma, congenital cholesteatoma, and neuromas of other cranial nerves (56).

Objective laboratory studies are most helpful. The audiometric studies may show a pure tone sensorineural hearing loss, especially marked in the high tones. Speech discrimination scores are usually disproportionately low. ENG testing usually shows a reduction in vestibular response. Retrocochlear tests, such as tone decay and alternate binaural loudness balance (ABLB), may be abnormal. The auditory brain-stem response (ABR) test has proven to be highly reliable for the detection of acoustic neuroma. The tumor causes pressure upon the eighth nerve resulting in delay of electrical impulses as measured by the ABR. Additionally, CT scan with and without contrast, with attention placed upon visualization of both internal auditory canals, is helpful, especially if decreased hearing precludes auditory testing. In the last several years, the MRI scan has emerged as a useful adjunct in initial detection. Its ultimate status, however, has yet to be determined.

Treatment of the acoustic tumor is either through watchful follow-up or through surgical removal. Pivotal to the decision of vigilance versus surgical treatment is knowledge of tumor growth rate. Clearly, if the tumor is enlarging very slowly and morbidity has not been inflicted, the patient may ultimately live out his or her full life without handicap by any tumor effects. The natural biology of the tumor is of relatively slow growth. Surgical intervention implies possible complications of injury to the facial, trigeminal, and other adjacent nerves. More seriously, irreversible brain stem injury or meningitis may occur. Further, disequilibrium and rehabilitative problems may produce incapacitating results.

What exactly is the rate of tumor growth in an individual older than 65 years? Within the literature, several attempts have been made to quantify growth rate. The range for the growth rate annually is from .05 to .69 centimeters (59). Other studies have shown the mean growth rate at .55 centimeters per year and at .2 centimeters per year (60). Unfortunately, great variability exists among tumors, and for this reason approximately 26% of patients eventually come to tumor resection out of vital necessity (59). Surgical results clearly favor earlier removal. Preferably, surgical therapy should be undertaken at a very early time, as hearing and facial nerve function can thus be best preserved. There is currently no way to differentiate slow- from fast-growing tumors other than by serial measurement through CT or MRI scan. The usual regimen is repeated scans at 3-months to 1-year intervals (61).

Chemotherapy and radiotherapy are of no proven value in these tumors. High-dose steroid treatment is less likely to produce a shrinkage of tumor with these types of tumors than in grossly malignant tumors. Thus, non-surgical treatment amounts to careful observation only.

If it is determined that a rapid growth is in fact characteristic of a particular tumor, then surgical intervention may be necessary (62). The classic approach to this tumor is through the translabyrinthine route. Virtually all tumors may be removed through this route (63). However, if significant hearing remains, then a hearing conservation procedure may be attempted (64). Significant hearing implies at least 50% speech discrimination and less than 50 dB hearing loss. The middle cranial fossa route is reserved for patients younger than 60 years with tumors that have remained in the internal auditory canal. Suboccipital and retrolabyrinthine approaches are useful for small tumors in the medial portion of the internal auditory canal (IAC) of patients with salvageable hearing. If an extemely large tumor is encountered, a combined approach utilizing the translabyrinthine and the suboccipital routes may be necessary (65, 66).

If a surgical approach is attempted in an elderly individual, the surgeon may opt to remove the tumor completely or to remove it partially. Tumor growth after debulking may occur at a slower rate or not at all (67). The decompression offered through subtotal removal has a major advantage in some tumors of not necessitating brain stem, neural, or vascular manipulation. Thus, the length of the procedure may be shortened dramatically, and complications may be minimized.

Once fraught with high complication rates and severe morbidity, translabyrinthine removal of acoustic neuromas has now evolved and minimal problems are the rule. Individualization of treatment is increasingly possible.

FACIAL NERVE SURGERY

The facial nerve proceeds through the constraints of the longest bony canal of any nerve in the body and thus is paralyzed more often than any other nerve (68). Facial nerve innervation of the facial musculature is important for eye protection from drying, mastication without drooling, and also facial expression. If there is a paralysis of the facial nerve, the etiology can be traced to the intratemporal portion of the nerve in the great majority of cases. Throughout life a number of palsy pathologic conditions may occur. When a patient presents with a facial nerve paralysis, a systematic evaluation is needed before idiopathic or "Bell's palsy" can be diagnosed. In the elderly patient, the facial nerve is involved with two main pathologies: traumatic injuries and tumor.

Initial evaluation can be quite revealing (68). A central unilateral facial paralysis usually involves only the lower face as the upper facial fibers receive crossed and uncrossed brain input. Bilateral simultaneous paralysis is a central sign. Progressive and recurrent palsies or no recovery after the palsy within 6 months may be of neoplastic origin. Vesicles on the ear, hearing loss, and dizziness may accompany the viral Ramsay-Hunt syndrome. Synkinesis of the face is demonstrative of previous paralysis as reinnervation occurs no faster than 4 months for recovery from facial paralysis.

For treatment purposes, determination of the level of injury is important. Confirmation of taste impairment and the presence of stapedial reflex and the Schirmer's test for lacrimal secretion are undertaken. Status of neural integrity and progress of regeneration can be ascertained through electromyography and nerve excitability testing. Ancillary tests appropriate for the particular circumstance should be ordered, such as a CT scan with bone windows in a traumatic nerve palsy.

Treatment is specific for each type of injury (68, 69). Primary traumatic or iatrogenic nerve disruptions need to be explored surgically and repaired. Because the nerve has a long course through a complex anatomic canal, various surgical approaches are usually necessary to gain access to the nerve. The surgeon must be prepared to operate on all segments of the nerve throughout its bony course. Indeed, a surgical approach that at first appears to involve a relatively distal segment of the nerve in the middle ear or mastoid region may eventually need to be traced into the internal auditory canal or the brain stem.

Ramsey-Hunt syndrome has been treated with acyclovir intravenously. Primary facial nerve tumors may be treated surgically with possible nerve grafting as needed. Treatment of secondary involvement by tumor is tumor-type specific and must follow oncologic principles. In proven idiopathic or Bell's palsy, the nerve is not actively treated in the great majority of cases as spontaneous regeneration usually occurs.

Care of the eye is of paramount importance in the management of facial paralysis. With loss of facial function, the blink reflex is not complete, and moisture is not distributed over the cornea. In some cases, the eye desiccation may be compounded by loss of tearing function. If untreated, exposure keratitis is possible. Several types of treatment are necessary. After evaluation of tearing function by the Schirmer test, lubrication drops, ointments, and a moisture chamber are placed on the eye. If rapid recovery of facial function over several weeks is anticipated, this treatment may be all that is necessary. If a prolonged recovery is foreseen, a reversible lateral canthoplasty is useful to retain eye protection without the constant need for a moisture chamber or repetitive drop application.

For facial rehabilitation, the facial musculature may be reinnervated by cranial nerve crossover procedures. The most common anastomosis is the seven to twelve anastomosis. Synkinesis of facial movement invariably occurs with this procedure. At 1 year's time, however, good facial tone and spontaneous and voluntary movement of some degree are usually present. Muscle and facial slings are other options. Elevation of the drooping mouth by Z-plasty techniques may be useful.

PARAGANGLIOMAS OF THE EAR

Glomus tumors of the temporal bone present a wide spectrum of different clinical problems. The tumor may present as a small lesion on the middle ear promontory or as a widely spread lesion of the skull base (70). Each of these tumors has a common denominator—vascularity. A number of problematic variations are frequently encountered: catecholamine secretion, cranial nerve involvement, major vessel involvement, and intracranial extension. Serious treatment complications include CSF leakage and meningitis, problems associated with cranial nerve loss, and catecholamine-induced cardiovascular manifestations. Thus, these skull base lesions must be evaluated and treated in a systematic fashion to minimize complications and enhance surgical results.

The most frequent presenting symptoms and signs include pulsatile tinnitus and conductive or sensorineural hearing loss followed by a mass visualized in the middle ear. Vertigo and seventh cranial nerve involvement are also seen. Other symptoms, such as dysphagia, aural pressure or pain, tenth and eleventh nerve involvement, and less commonly bleeding from the ear, may occur. These later findings must make the clinician especially suspicious of a skull base lesion (71).

Diagnostic evaluation starts with a careful examination of cranial nerves and the ear and a baseline audiogram. Most importantly, however, will be radiologic diagnosis. Currently, the initial diagnostic examination of choice is the CT scan with contrast. The glomus tumors are very vascular and therefore enhance very well. MRI scan is very helpful with defining the extent of soft tissue masses, including extension into the neck and intracranially. Indeed, although the CT scan is clearly superior for delineation of bony defects, the MRI has shown marked clarity of soft tissue evaluation. Usually, a lobulated tumor mass in close relation to the jugular bulb is found. In the glomus tympanicum, this mass will variably extend from the hypotympanum superiorly to the middle ear or mastoid or anteriorly to the carotid artery. The glomus jugulare tumors may extend into the neck or the hypotympanum and have intracranial extension. Lastly, the radiologic evaluation may include arteriovenography. This is helpful in delineating tumor blood supply that confirms cerebral blood cross-over flow and also patency of the jugular vein itself and sigmoid sinus. Carotid resection may be necessary, and it is important to ascertain contralateral circulatory status. Bilateral head and neck evaluation and an abdominal CT scan to evaluate the adrenal glands are useful as multicentricity of glomus tumors is as high as 15%.

Another important aspect of the glomus pathology is secretion of vasoactive catecholamines by approximately 3% to 6% of tumors (72). Serum catecholamine levels fifty-fold higher than normal have been seen. Symptoms of tachycardia, profuse sweating, high blood pressure, headache, episodic diarrhea, and tremor may all be due to secretion of these compounds. Some patients initially present with this condition, having been placed on high blood pressure medication for some time prior to diagnosis of the glomus tumors. This catecholamine secretion needs to be pharmacologically managed by alpha and beta blockade prior to surgical intervention. Turbulent operative and postoperative vasoactive phenomena can occur.

In exercising judgement regarding therapy, it is necessary first to classify accurately and to map the full extent of the lesion (73). This allows the surgical team of the neuro-otologist, head and neck surgeon, and neurosurgeon to come to grips adequately with the extent of the disease.

Therapeutic options for glomus tumor management can be divided into palliative or definitive types. Palliation includes radiation therapy, embolization, or a combination thereof. Definitive treatment includes surgical removal, combinations of resection and radiation, or embolization followed by resection.

Radiotherapy for jugulotympanic paraganglionoma has been documented in the past (74–76). A total radiation dose to the tumor between 5000 and 6500 rads may produce significant palliation and slowing of growth. Radiotherapy has, however, failed to eradicate tumor cells and does cause significant long-term complications. Preradiation embolization may reduce oxygen saturation in the tumor and therefore lower the efficacy of radiation. Additionally, dosimetry adjustments for protection of vital brain stem structures may cause incomplete dosage at the most medial extensions of the lesion. With intracranial extension, radiotherapy cannot be given in dosages sufficient to be curative. Following high doses of irradiation, residual tumor vascularity with probably viable tumor is often still present. In the elderly or debilitated patient, therefore, radiotherapy may slow tumor growth, but not be curative.

Surgical treatment for glomus tympanicum tumors includes a transcanal approach for type I tumors and transmastoid-extended facial recess approaches for types II, III, and IV (71). Glomus jugulare tumors are all dealt with by modified infratemporal fossa approaches (77–79). If there is an associated lesion, the secondary lesion is often treated at a later time. Treatment with surgical infratemporal fossa approaches entails formidable surgical challenges. These procedures may involve major arteries, cranial nerves, and brain stem structures and thus give rise to significant complications. Individuals in good health may tolerate these problems and their remedies, but an individual in a debilitated state is likely to suffer severe and enduring incapacitation. Generally, these procedures are not recommended in patients older than 60 years.

Treatment planning for glomus tumors that are found to be malignant in type has not been well established. Emphasis when possible is placed upon preservation of the tenth cranial nerve and laryngeal competency. The cough reflex and capacity are reduced in the elderly, and aspiration pneumonia may ensue. The problems of aspiration and pneumonias are prevented by initial placement of a nasogastric tube for decompression of the stomach contents. This tube may be placed for a prolonged period and, after bowel function has been reestablished, may be used initially to bypass the larynx while feeding is done enterally. Tracheostomy placement has been found to be helpful in controlling the airway initially. Early vocal cord injection with Teflon to bolster vocal cord size and help the contralateral cord to compensate is advocated. Management of cerebrospinal fluid leakage is by free fat graft, fascia-lata, lyophilized dura reconstructions, temporalis rotation flaps, possible free flap transfer and decompression of the CSF by indwelling lumbar catheters, atrioventricular shunts, or repeated lumbar punctures. In dealing with the seventh nerve, mobilization or selective severance with reanastomosis and nerve grafting is useful.

REFERENCES

1. Kinney RA (ed): *Physiology of Aging: A Synopsis.* Chicago, Year Book, 1982.
2. Schuknecht HF: *Pathology of the Ear.* Cambridge, MA, Harvard University Press, 1974.
3. Waisman M: A clinical look at the aging skin. *Postgrad Med* 66:87-93, 1979.
4. Meyerhoff W, Kim D, Paparella M: Pathology of chronic otitis media. *Ann Otol Rhinol Laryngol* 87:749-760, 1978.
5. Senturia BH, Marcus MD, Lucente FE: *Disease of the External Ear,* ed 2. New York, Grune & Stratton, 1980.
6. Muglistan T, O'Donoghue G: Otomycosis: a continuing problem. *J Laryngol Otol* 99:327-333, 1985.
7. Saunders WH: Otomycosis. In Gates G (ed): *Current Therapy in Otolaryngology Head and Neck Surgery* St. Louis, CV Mosby, 1984-1985, pp 1-2.
8. Chandler JR: Malignant external otitis. *Laryngoscope* 78:1257-1294, 1968.
9. Chandler JR: Malignant external otitis: further considerations. *Ann Otol Rhinol Laryngol* 86:417-428, 1977.
10. Crabtree JA, Britton BH, Pierce MK: Carcinoma of the external auditory canal. *Laryngoscope* 86:405-415, 1976.
11. Cummings CW, Fredrickson JM, Harker LA, Schuller DE (eds): *Otolaryngology—Head and Neck Surgery* St. Louis, CV Mosby, 1986.
12. Deher LP, Chen KT: Primary tumors of the external and middle ear. *Arch Otolaryngol* 106:13-19, 1980.
13. Eden AR, Pincus RL, Parisier SC, Som PM: Primary adenomatous neoplasms of the middle ear. *Laryngoscope* 94:63-67, 1984.
14. Lewis JS: Cancer of the ear: a report of 150 cases. *Laryngoscope* 70:551-579, 1960.
15. Etholm B, Belal A: Senile changes in the middle ear joints. *Ann Otol Rhinol Laryngol* 83:49-54, 1974.
16. Wolff D, Bellucci RJ: The human ossicular ligaments. *Ann Otol Rhinol Laryngol* 65:895-910, 1956.
17. Tomoda K, Morii S, Yamashita T, Kumazawa T: Histology of human eustachian tube muscles: effect of aging. *Ann Otol Rhinol Laryngol* 93:17-24, 1984.
18. Gower D, McGuirt WF: Intracranial complications of acute and chronic infectious ear disease: a problem still with us. *Laryngoscope* 93:1028-1033, 1983.
19. Neely JG: *Complications of suppurative otitis media. Part I. Aural Complications (Self-Instructional Package).* Washington, DC, American Academy of Otolaryngology, 1978.
20. Neely JG: *Complications of suppurative otitis media. Part II. Intracranial Complications (Self-Instructional Package).* Washington, DC, American Academy of Otolaryngology, 1979.
21. Blatt IM, Seltzer HS, Rubin P, Furstenberg AC, Maxwell JH, Schull WJ: Fatal granulomatosis of the respiratory tract (lethal midline granuloma—Wegener's granulomatosis). *Arch Otolaryngol* 70:707-717, 1959.
22. Hybels RL, Rice DH: Neuro-otologic manifestations of sarcoidosis. *Laryngoscope* 86:1873-1878, 1976.
23. McCabe BF: Autoimmune sensorineural hearing loss. *Ann J Otol* 88:585-589, 1979.
24. Schuknecht HF: *Pathology of the Ear.* Cambridge, MA, Harvard University Press, 1974.
25. McGee TM: Stapedial otosclerosis: a continuing problem. In Gates G (ed): *Current Therapy in Otolaryngology Head and Neck Surgery.* St. Louis, CV Mosby, 1984-1985, pp 31-36.
26. Causse JR, Causse JB: Eighteen year report on problems of stapedial fixation. *Clin Otolaryngol* 5:49-59, 1980.
27. Moon CN, Hahn MJ: Partial versus total footplate removal in stapedectomy: a comparative study. *Laryngoscope* 94:912-915, 1984.
28. Karjalainen S, Karja J, Harma R, Vartiainen E: Hearing in otosclerotic ears not subjected to operation. *J Laryngol Otol* 98:255-257, 1984.
29. Sheehy JL, Nelson RA, House HP: Revision stapedectomy: a view of 258 cases. *Laryngoscope* 92:43-51, 1981.
30. Gilad O, Glorig A: Presbycusis: the aging ear. *J Am Audiol Soc* 4:195-206, 1979.
31. Maurer JF, Rupp RR: *Hearing and Aging.* New York, Grune and Stratton, 1979.

32. Catlin FI: Prevention of hearing impairment from infection and ototoxic drugs. *Arch Otol* 111:377–384, 1985.

33. Lebo CP, Reddell RC: The presbycusic component in occupational hearing loss. *Laryngoscope* 82:1399–1409, 1972. Correction: *Laryngoscope* 83:2050–2051, 1973.

34. Sataloff J, Vassallo L, Menduke H: Presbycusis: air and bone conduction thresholds. *Laryngoscope* 75:889–901, 1965.

35. Hawkins JE, Johnson LG: Otopathological changes associated with presbycusis. *Semin Hearing* 6:115–133, 1985.

36. Northern JL (ed): *Hearing Disorders*. Boston, Little, Brown and Co, 1984.

37. Schuknecht HF, Woellner RC: Hearing losses following partial section of the cochlear nerve. *Laryngoscope* 63:441–465, 1953.

38. Duquesnoy AJ, Plomp R: Effect of reverberation and noise on the intelligibility of sentences in cases of presbycusis. *J Acoust Soc Am* 68:537–544, 1980.

39. Grimes AM, Grady CL, Foster NL, Sunderland T, Patronas NJ: Central auditory function in Alzheimer's disease. *Neurology* 35:352–358, 1985.

40. Thompson DJ, Sills JA, Recke KS, Bui DC: Acoustic reflex growth in the aging adult. *J Speech Hear Res* 23:405–418, 1980.

41. Cashman M, Corbin H, Riko K, Rossman R: Effect of recent hearing aid improvements on management of the hearing impaired. *J Otolaryngol* 13:227–231, 1984.

42. Corso JF: Presbycusis, hearing aids and aging. *Audiology* 16:146–163, 1977.

43. McCandless GA, Parkin JL: Hearing aid performance relative to site of lesion. *Otolaryngol Head Neck Surg* 87:871–875, 1979.

44. Hayes D, Jerger J: Aging and the use of hearing aids. *Scand Audiol* 8:33–34, 1979.

45. Venna N: Dizziness, falling, and fainting: differential diagnoses in the aged. *Geriatrics* 41:30–42, 1986.

46. Gacek RR: Cupulolithiasis. *Adv Otol Rhinol Laryngol* 28:80–85, 1982.

47. Tumerkin L: Otolithic catastrophy: a new syndrome. *Br Med J* 2:175–177, 1936.

48. Meniere MP: "Maladies de L'oreille Interne" *Gaz Med Paris* 16:55, 1861.

49. Hallpike CS, Cairns H: Observations on the pathology of Meniere's syndrome. *J Laryngol Otol* 53:625–655, 1938.

50. Jackson CG, Glasscock ME, Davis WE, Hughes GB, Sismanis A: Medical management of Meniere's disease. *Ann Otol Rhinol Laryngol* 90:142–147, 1981.

51. Stupp H: Advantages and disadvantages in the surgical treatment of Meniere's disease. In Vosteen KH, Schuknecht H, Pfalpz CR, Wersall J, Kimura RS, Morgenstern C, Juhn SK (eds): *Meniere's Disease: Pathogenesis, Diagnosi and Treatment*. New York, G.Thieme Verlag, 1981.

52. Glasscock ME, Kveton JF, Christiansen SG: Current status of surgery for Meniere's disease. *Otolaryngol Head Neck Surg* 92:67–72, 1984.

53. Graham MD, Kemink JL: Titration streptomycin therapy for bilateral Meniere's disease: a progress report. *Am J Otol* 5:534–535, 1984.

54. Hoogland GA: Some historical remarks on acoustic neuroma. *Adv Otol Rhinol Laryngol* 34:3–7, 1984.

55. Tos M, Thompson J: Epidemiology of acoustic neuromas. *J Laryngol Otol* 98:685–692, 1984.

56. Slooff JL: Pathological anatomical findings in the cerebellopontine angle: a review. *Adv Otol Rhinol Laryngol* 34:89–103, 1984.

57. Godfrey JB, Caird FI: Intracranial tumors in the elderly: diagnosis and treatment. *Age Aging* 13:152–158, 1984.

58. Cremers CWRJ: Evaluation of diagnostic routine in cerebellopontine angle pathology. *Adv Otol Rhinol Laryngol* 34:104–109, 1984.

59. Nedzelski JM, Canter RJ, Kassel EE, Rowed DW, Tator CH: Is no treatment good treatment in the management of acoustic neuromas in the elderly? *Laryngoscope* 96:825–829, 1986.

60. Wazen J, Silverstein H, Norrell H, Besse B: Preoperative and postoperative growth rates in acoustic neuromas documented with CT scanning. *Otolaryngol Head Neck Surg* 93:151–155, 1985.

61. Clark WC, Mortz WH, Acker JD, Gardner LG, Eggers F, Robertson JH: Nonsurgical management of small and intracanalicular acoustic tumors. *Neurosurgery* 16:801–803, 1985.

62. Morrison AW, King TT: Space-occupying lesions of the internal auditory meatus and cerebellopontine angle. *Adv Otol Rhinol Laryngol* 34:121–142, 1984.

63. Sterkers JM, Desgeorges M, Sterkers O, Corlieu P: Our present approach to acoustic neuroma surgery. *Adv Otol Rhinol Laryngol* 34:160–163, 1984.

64. Sterkers JM, Sterkers O, Maudelonde C, Corlieu P: Preservation of hearing by retrosigmoid approach in acoustic neuroma surgery. *Adv Otol Rhinol Laryngol* 34:187–192, 1984.

65. Glasscock ME, Hays JW, Jackson CG, Steenerson RL: One-stage combined approach for the management of large cerebellopontine angle tumors. *Laryngoscope* 88:1563–1576, 1978.

66. Hughes GB, Sismanis A, Glasscock ME, Hayes JW, Jackson CG: Management of bilateral acoustic tumors. *Laryngoscope* 92:1351–1359, 1982.

67. Silverstein H, McDaniel A, Norrell H, Wazen J: Conservative management of the acoustic neuroma in the elderly patient. *Laryngoscope* 95:766–770, 1985.

68. Shambaugh GE, Glasscock ME: Facial nerve decompression and repair. In *Surgery of the Ear*, ed 3. Philadelphia, WB Saunders, 1980, pp 519–557.

69. Stennert E: Indications for facial nerve surgery. *Adv Otol Rhinol Laryngol* 34:214–226, 1984.

70. Van Huijzen C: Anatomy of the skull base and infratemporal fossa. *Adv Otol Rhinol Laryngol* 34:242–253, 1984.

71. Jackson CJ, Glasscock ME, Harris PF: Glomus tumors: diagnosis, classification, and management of large lesions. *Arch Otolaryngol* 108:401–406, 1982.

72. Schwaber MK, Glasscock ME, Wissen AJ, Jackson CG, Smith PG: Diagnosis and management of catecholamine secreting glomus tumors. *Laryngoscope* 94:1008–1015, 1984.

73. Wiet RJ: Skull base mapping. *Laryngoscope* 92:515–523, 1982.

74. Maruyama Y: Radiotherapy of tympanojugular chemodectomas. *Radiology* 105:659–663, 1972.

75. Spector GJ, Compagno J, Perez CA, Maisel RH, Ogura JH: Glomus jugulare tumors: effects of radiotherapy. *Cancer* 35:1316–1321, 1975.

76. Sharma PD, Johnson AP, Whitten AC: Radiotherapy for jugulo- tympanic paragangliomas. *J Laryngol Otol* 98:621–629, 1984.

77. Jenkins HA, Fisch U: Glomus tumors of the temporal region. *Arch Otolaryngol* 107:209–214, 1981.

78. Gardner G, Cocke EW, Robertson JT, Trumbull ML, Palmer RE: Glomus jugulare tumors—combined treatment, Part I. *J Laryngol Otol* 95:437–454, 1981.

79. Jenkins HA, Fisch U: Glomus tumors of the temporal region. *Arch Otolaryngol* 107:209–214, 1981.

Chapter 14

Breast Disease in Elderly Women

R. Benton Adkins, Jr., M.D., F.A.C.S.

The female breast is a dynamic organ that gradually changes over the course of a woman's lifetime. Following embryologic development of a mammary ductal system, the glandular changes begin with puberty, continue during the childbearing years with menstruation and lactation, and are seen to regress in later years as mammary involution occurs. We are concerned here with the changes and diseases of the involutional period.

Mammary involution begins with the termination of ovarian function. Two separate phases of this process have been described. The first phase of involution occurs in women aged 35 to 45. They experience a moderate decrease in glandular mammary epithelium combined with a gradual disappearance of acinar and lobular tissue, along with some loss of elasticity of the supporting connective tissue. Between the ages of 45 and 75 and especially during menopause, the second phase occurs. There is a further reduction of glandular tissue along with a simultaneous increase in fat deposition. The amount of connective tissue increases, which is most evident in this second phase. The loss of glandular elements, both lobular and alveolar structures, toward the end of this phase is striking. The remaining ducts gradually regress until finally only small islands of epithelial parenchyma remain. These ductal remnants are surrounded by a hard, fibrous connective tissue, stroma, and fat (1).

BENIGN BREAST DISEASE

The incidence of benign breast disease in older women is lower than that of breast cancer. Women who have fibrocystic breast disease should be followed by their physician from youth into old age with careful attention to the potential for development of breast cancer. Occasionally, the older woman will experience other benign disorders, such as abscess, mastodynia, fat necrosis, and benign tumors. In most instances, her treatment should be identical to that given to a younger person with the necessary attention to concomitant disease and with a high index of suspicion for cancer at all times.

CANCER OF THE BREAST

Incidence

Older women seek treatment for and are actually found to have the diagnosis of carcinoma of the breast more often than that of any other breast disease. Cancer of the female breast is a common disease and accounts for more deaths of American women than any other malignancy (2). In 1981, breast cancer was the leading cause of death from malignancy in women aged 55 to 74 years and the second leading cause of death from malignancy in women over 75 years of age. It has been estimated that in 1985, 119,000 new cases of female breast cancer would be reported and that there would be 38,400 deaths from the disease (3). As the expected longevity continues to increase each year in this country, it is reasonable to expect that more and more older women will require treatment for carcinoma of the breast. The probability of developing breast cancer within the next 10 or 20 years is higher for the female aged 65 and older than for the 55-year-old. An 85-year-old woman is twice as likely to develop breast cancer as a 50-year-old woman (4). The question for the clinician is, "Should the treatment of an older women with breast cancer differ substantially from that treatment which would have been offered to her at a younger age?"

Characteristics of Breast Cancer in the Elderly Female

The elderly woman with breast cancer is characteristically different in her presentation from her younger counterparts. For instance, most observers have noticed a substantial delay in seeking treatment and in making a diagnosis among elderly women. In a series of 94 patients 65 years of age and older, Hunt et al. (5) found an average delay of 18 months between the time the patient discovered the disease and the time she sought medical advice and treatment. In a review of 60 patients aged 75 years and older, we found that 23% had delayed seeking treatment from 1 to 8 years (mean 3.7 years) (6). Robins and Lee (7) found that one-third of their older patients delayed seeking medical advice for breast masses for more than 6 months. Other investigators have reported similar findings (8–10). We also suspect that a definitive medical recommendation after a mass is discovered by or reported to the family physician is also delayed in the more advanced age group.

Because of this delay, many older patients present to the surgeon with relatively large tumors. Rosen et al. (11) have also noticed a tendency for older women to have medial and central tumors more often than younger women. The elderly patient, then, will most likely present with what may at first appear to be far-advanced disease. In spite of this delay and the large tumor size, the disease in many of these cases is not as widespread and hopeless as it first appears. Because of large size, many of these tumors in older patients must be classified as stage II, III, and IV disease by the use of the TNM classification system (12), thereby indicating fairly advanced disease. They are usually classed as a more advanced stage solely on the basis of the size of the lesion, rather than because of the presence of node metastases. In our experience, we have found this to be true. Forty-eight of our older patients had stage II, III, or IV disease, but only 23 of them had nodal metastases and only

4 were considered unresectable (6). Hunt and his colleagues (5) found that 55 of 58 elderly patients with stage II lesions were classified as such based upon the size and fixation of the lesion to muscle alone, rather than because of regional nodal metastases.

Even in elderly women with large, often fixed lesions and with axillary lymph node involvement, the extent of tumor spread to regional nodes is often surprisingly minimal. Seventy-three percent of the total number of older patients reported by Davis et al. (13) had less than three involved nodes. Veronesi et al. (14) reviewed 1,119 patients of all ages with breast cancer, all of whom had extended mastectomy. They found that internal mammary chain metastases occurred in only 15.6% of patients greater than 51 years of age compared to 27.6% of those less than 41 years of age. Most observers agree that older patients present with larger tumors but that nodal spread tends to be delayed.

In spite of these seemingly favorable signs related to metastasis, there is widespread agreement that elderly women with breast cancer require aggressive surgical treatment to prevent more local, nodal, and distant spread and to prolong survival. The larger, fixed tumors will require standard radical or extended modified radical mastectomies to remove local and nodal involvement.

Estrogen Receptor Status and Age

Jensen et al. (15) reported in 1971 the importance of the level of cytosolic estrogen receptor sites as a predictor of the clinical response to endocrine treatment of breast cancer. This determination has been widely utilized in treatment planning since that time. Several authors have observed that breast carcinoma in elderly patients is more often responsive to hormonal manipulation than it is in younger women (16–19). Some investigators have concluded that patients who are postmenopausal are more likely to have estrogen receptor positive tumors than premenopausal women. Raynaud (16), Hawkins (20), and Allegra (21) have all found that estrogen receptor levels of the tumor have a significant correlation to the menopausal status of the patient. Others, however, have determined that a more significant relationship exists between es-

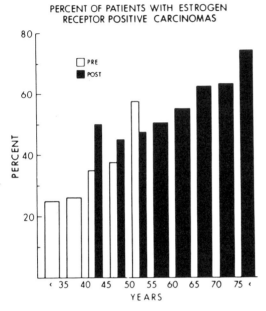

Figure 14.1. Percentage of patients with estrogen receptor values less than 10 fmole/mg protein are shown for each 5-year increment. Premenopausal patients-*open bars;* postmenopausal patients-*solid bars.* (Reprinted by permission from McCarty KS, et al: Relationship of age and menopausal status to estrogen receptor content in primary carcinoma of the breast. *Ann Surg* 197:123–127, 1983.)

trogen receptor levels and age (19, 22). McCarty and his co-workers (19) at Duke University studied 1037 primary mammary carcinomas and found that cytosolic estrogen receptor activity steadily increases with age from the third through the tenth decade. (Figure 14.1) They found that age further correlates with estrogen receptor levels even after menstrual status has been considered. Their report supports the earlier work of Elwood et al. (22) that proposed the notion that there is a very close correlation between estrogen receptor status and age and that this relationship is statistically more significant than the association between estrogen receptor levels and the patients' menopausal status. Rochman et al. (23) have reported similar findings. They found that one-sixth of patients below age 29 had estrogen receptor positive tumors, 27% of patients aged 40 to 49, 46% of patients aged 70 to 79, and 62% of patients 80 years or older.

The explanation for the age/estrogen receptor relationship is probably multifactorial. Theve et al. (24) and Nagai et al. (25) suggest an inverse

relationship between the *serum* estrogen levels and the estrogen receptor levels in the developing and growing breast carcinoma. Another suggested theory is that the cyclic levels of serum progesterone in premenopausal women inhibit or limit the formation of estrogen receptor sites in the tumor (26). Indeed, variations of estrogen receptor levels have been shown to occur that were found to be affected by the menstrual cycle in normal human endometrium (27, 28) and in the normal human breast (19). Hormonally dependent tumors are likely to behave in a manner similar to normal breast and endometrium. Finally, the pituitary-ovarian axis also is linked to age (29). As the reciprocal influence of the aging ovary upon the pituitary is diminished and lost, perhaps the breast tumor is stimulated by the uninhibited pituitary to develop more estrogen receptor sites. The elderly woman, in whom cyclic ovarian function no longer exists, may have consistent levels of adrenal and ovarian androgen that can be converted to estrogens peripherally. It is likely that a combination of all of these factors results in the increased likelihood of estrogen receptor positive tumors developing in older patients. If this is the case, one would expect that the older the patient, the more likely the tumor will be receptor positive.

Estrogen Receptors and Degree of Differentiation of Breast Tumors

Estrogen receptor status also has been studied in terms of its relationship to the other pathologic characteristics of breast carcinoma. It has been found that tumors with high degree of nuclear content and low histologic grades, absence of necrosis, and presence of marked tumor elastosis and tumors in older patients are all significantly associated with increased levels of positive estrogen receptor sites. Statistical analysis also has shown that those tumors that are well differentiated are more frequently associated with positive estrogen receptor status in older women than are similar tumors found in younger women (2).

Chabon et al. (30) studied 350 cases of breast cancer to investigate the interrelationships among histopathologic characteristics, estrogen receptor status, and age of the patient. They determined that three variables—estrogen receptor positivity, nuclear grade, and lymphocytic infiltration—are interdependent in their function. When the level of lymphocytic infiltration was intermediate, there appeared to be a steady percentage of estrogen receptor positivity regardless of the nuclear grade. When lymphocytic infiltration was at a minimum, however, estrogen receptor positivity increased with the worsening of the nuclear grade. In the women over 50, the percentage of estrogen receptor positive cases decreased very gradually as the nuclear features approached normal. Among the elderly, they found a high percentage of estrogen receptor positive cases regardless of the degree of nuclear atypia when the degree of lymphocytic infiltration was at a low level.

Relationship between the Histopathology of Breast Cancer and Age

Invasive Ductal Carcinoma

Approximately 70% to 75% of cases of breast cancer in all age groups are classified by pathologists as invasive ductal carcinoma (31). Schottenfeld and Robbins (9) found this to be true in the population of women aged 65 and older as well. Clinically, these tumors are hard to palpation and are usually poorly circumscribed. Grossly, they often have yellowish, chalky streaks on the cut surface that represent sclerotic elastic tissue. Generally, these tumors do not grow to a large size before lymph node metastases are present. Microscopically, there are strands and columns of various sizes of tumor cells growing in an abundant, densely collagenous stroma. The size and shape of the tumor cells are not uniform, and glandular formation varies with the degree of differentiation of the tumor. Areas of necrosis are seen in approximately 60% of these lesions. Multiple foci of origin in these kinds of tumors are more common in younger women than in older patients. The prognosis for patients with these tumors is the least favorable of all types of breast cancer (31).

Intraductal Carcinoma

True intraductal carcinoma is not frequently seen in any age group. In these in situ lesions, the tumor cells are confined to the ducts and are not invasive. The incidence of multicentricity in these lesions is relatively high, whereas bilaterality is unusual (31). They are likely to be centrally located in the breast. Three common patterns of cell growth have been identified: solid, papillary, and cribriform (31, 32). These types are generally clinically occult and rarely, if ever, associated with nodal metastases.

In contrast, a usually clinically palpable, more aggressive type of intraductal carcinoma has been aptly named "comedo carcinoma." The gross appearance of these tumors is characterized by thick-walled ducts, and often, worm-like necrotic substance extrudes from the cut surface of the tumor. Microscopically, the involved ducts are distended with proliferating cells that are much more atypical than those found in papillary or cribriform carcinomas. Areas of necrosis are common within the ducts. Haagensen has found that rare nodal metastases with intraductal carcinoma occurred in the comedo carcinoma type (32). The importance of intraductal and lobular carcinoma in situ lies in the increased risk of subsequent invasive cancer.

Lobular Carcinoma

Lobular carcinoma comprises 6% to 14% of breast cancer occurring in all age groups (31). Schottenfeld and Robbins (9) found a comparable incidence of 7% in older women, whereas in Rosen's (33) experience, lobular carcinoma occurred largely in the elderly. Lobular carcinoma arises from the lobules and terminal ducts of the breast and may evolve from lobular carcinoma in situ, which is commonly multifocal and bilateral. Although in situ lobular carcinoma is seen occasionally in younger women, it is very rare in women aged 65 and older. In lobular carcinoma, the breast lobules are filled and expanding with cells that are uniform in size and shape and are minimally atypical. Infiltration is characterized by the haphazard cell growth that is most often in "Indian file" arrangements. Alternatively, infiltrative lobular carcinomas can form nests of cells with or without single filing. Lobular carcinoma is widely accepted as an aggressive form of cancer and should be treated as such in all age groups (31).

Epidermoid Cancer

Epidermoid carcinoma occurs almost solely in

elderly women, but it is rare even among the aged. The gross appearance is not characteristically different from other breast carcinomas. Microscopically, areas of squamous metaplasia occur in what must be assumed to be long-standing ductal adenocarcinoma. Malignant squamous foci are also sometimes found in the lining of the wall of an area of cyst formation within an adenocarcinoma. Within the areas of squamous carcinoma, intercellular bridges are often seen, and the stroma may be abundant. The prognosis is similar to that of ductal adenocarcinoma without squamoid areas (31).

Inflammatory Carcinoma

Inflammatory carcinoma is characterized by a reddened, warm, and edematous breast. These lesions are usually undifferentiated carcinomas with widespread involvement of the dermal lymphatic vessels. These tumors are associated with a poor prognosis (2, 31). In a recent report from the Mayo Clinic, Knight et al. (34) support modified radical mastectomy after irradiation and chemotherapy to reduce residual tumor burden. Of 18 patients treated by this protocol, 3 are alive without evidence of disease 19 to 21 months after onset of symptoms.

Paget's Disease

Paget's disease of the breast occurs in 1% to 4% of all patients with breast cancer (2). In these cases, a crusted lesion of the nipple is usually the presenting sign, but an underlying carcinoma is always present. Other nipple changes, such as bleeding and itching, have usually been present for some time. Microscopically, there is involvement of the nipple's epidermis, hair shafts, and sweat glands by numerous large tumor cells with clear cytoplasm and atypical nuclei. A connection between the nipple lesion and the underlying lesion can be found in most cases. The management and prognosis of these lesions depend largely on the nature of the underlying carcinoma (2, 31).

Medullary Carcinoma

Medullary carcinoma comprises 5% to 7% of reported breast cancers, but are more uncommon in older women. Patients are usually under age 50, and only 2% to 3% of women 65 and older who have cancer of the breast will have medullary carcinoma (31). These lesions are well circumscribed and can grow to be quite large with low-grade histologic qualities. The cells of a medullary tumor are large and pleomorphic with numerous mitotic figures. Glands are not usually formed. A prominent infiltration of small lymphocytes is a usual characteristic. The prognosis for patients of all ages with this tumor is better than for most other breast cancers (31). Ridolfi et al. (35) found that 84% of their patients with these tumors who had adequate treatment survived at least 10 years.

Papillary Carcinoma

Papillary carcinoma is found more commonly in the older age groups than is medullary carcinoma. Schottenfeld and Robbins (9) found papillary carcinoma in 3% to 5% of older women with breast cancer. Papillary carcinomas arise from the duct epithelium or from pre-existing intraductal papillomata and can present as a well-circumscribed mass or involve an entire segment of breast tissue. In contrast to benign papillary lesions that may have numerous cellular variations, the cells of a papillary carcinoma are usually quite uniform in size and shape. The nuclei are elongated and are usually perpendicular to the duct lumen. A cribriform growth pattern with little stroma is usually indicative of malignancy. These lesions tend to be estrogen receptor positive and are not associated with a high incidence of lymph node metastases (33). If completely excised, survival for patients of all age groups with these malignant breast tumors can be expected to reach 100% (9).

Mucinous Carcinoma

Schottenfeld and Robbins (9) found mucinous carcinoma in 3% of older women with breast cancer. These tumors present as well-circumscribed lesions that are occasionally crepitant or fluctuant to palpation. These tumors are often referred to as "colloid" tumors, which is a misnomer as the tumors are filled with mucin, rather than colloid. Grossly, they appear as a jelly-like mass with delicate connective tissue support. Hemorrhage into the mass is not uncommon. Microscopically, mucin is the prominent feature. Islands of tumor cells appear to be floating in a sea of mucin, and the tumor cells usually form well-defined acini. The prognosis for patients with these tumors is good, but recurrences can occur many years after primary treatment. This is in contrast to the mucinous tumors that occur in the gastrointestinal tract, which usually portend a more dismal outcome than other gastrointestinal tract tumors. Mucoid breast tumors reportedly occur most often in older women and rarely metastasize (31). Recent observers have found that many mucinous tumors contain argyrophilic cells and neurosecretory granules, leading one to wonder if these tumors somehow may be related to the rare primary carcinoid tumors found in the breast (31).

Tubular Carcinoma

Tubular carcinomas are favorable lesions. These tumors are grossly suggestive of carcinoma because of their poorly circumscribed margins and hard consistency. Microscopically, however, they are very well differentiated and resemble sclerosing adenosis. Necrosis, mitotic figures, and cytologic atypia are generally absent. The diagnostic features are those of neoplastic cells forming well-defined tubular gland structures, a stellate growth pattern, and isomorphic nuclei. There is usually minimal, if any, lymph node involvement. The prognosis for patients with this lesion is excellent. They occur about equally in all age groups.

Lymphoma and Sarcoma

Lymphoma and sarcoma of the breast are rare, but occur more often in postmenopausal women than in the younger age groups. Malignant lymphoma grows rapidly, although it does not produce skin changes. The tumors are soft and occur in the right breast more often than in the left. Sarcomatous tumors are large, firm, and often necrotic. In young women, the most commonly occurring lesion of this type is cystosarcoma phyllodes. Lymphosarcoma is more usual in the elderly woman. Microscopically, breast sarcomas lack an epithelial component, and most have the characteristic features of fibrosarcoma. The prognosis for older women with either of these lesions is thought to be better than that for young women with similar tumors (36–39). Excision of the lesion is the only effective treatment regardless of tumor size (40).

Treatment of Breast Cancer in the Elderly Patient

In earlier years, breast cancer was considered to be a much less deadly disease in older women than it was in younger women. It was thought that an elderly woman would likely die of another disease before the breast cancer could invade or metastasize to a lethal degree and cause her death. Therefore, the elderly patient was often "spared the trauma" of an aggressive surgical approach to the treatment of the breast cancer. Moreover, because some of these patients were quite elderly, they were often considered to be poor operative risks based upon age alone, regardless of their general health status or the extent of the tumor, and they were denied the treatment considerations that would have been given to younger women.

Reluctance to engage in aggressive treatment of the elderly is gradually being replaced both in the medical and surgical community by a more positive approach to the older woman with breast cancer. As early as 1962, Kraft and Block (10) reported their experience with 75 patients aged 75 and older who were treated for breast cancer. They found that the more aggressive, more complete procedures (i.e., mastectomy with lymph node dissection) increased the opportunity for long-term survival two-fold over less adequate procedures, i.e., simple mastectomy or lumpectomy. The operative mortality in their series was only 4.5%, suggesting that older patients could tolerate the appropriate operation and were not as frail as they had once been thought to be.

In Canada, Crosby (41) echoed these findings of Kraft and his co-workers (10) in 1971. He and his colleagues presented results that suggested that surgical treatment must always be tailored to suit the patient's ability to tolerate a procedure regardless of age and that older patients require and deserve as adequate a form of treatment for breast cancer as younger patients. They also maintained that each patient's potential survival period should be considered when planning her treatment.

A more recent report from Canada indicates that this attitude remains strong and continues to grow in that country as it does in the United States (7). In 1985, Robins and Lee (7) reported a series of 152 women treated for breast cancer who were 80 years of age or older. They suggested that an aggressive surgical treatment for breast cancer was justified even in the advanced age group. Because of the recent considerable increase in the expected longevity, which would otherwise allow most elderly patients to outlive their malignant disease by many years, they are convinced that this approach is justified. One-third of the patients and/or physicians in their series of elderly women delayed seeking surgical treatment until the disease was far advanced. The authors call for both patient and doctor education regarding the seriousness of a breast mass in an elderly woman. They, like others, noted that the majority of deaths in their series of elderly women who had the diagnosis of breast cancer were from the breast cancer itself, rather than from some intercurrent, chronic disease of the patient.

Mueller et al. (42) have suggested that breast cancer is perhaps *more* lethal in older women than in younger women. They analyzed 3,558 women by age groups, and using life-table analysis they determined that improperly treated breast cancer is a more lethal disease and is more rapidly fatal in the older age groups than it is in younger women. Eighty-eight percent of all deaths in their study of all women with breast cancer, regardless of age, were due to breast cancer. The survival times became progressively shorter as age increased, but the cause of death was still breast cancer, not some other chronic disease. (Figure 14.2) In spite of somewhat better histology, positive estrogen receptor status, slow growth, and delayed metastasis in the older patient with breast cancer, once lymph node metastasis has occurred, its lethal potential is at least as ominous as in the younger woman. It has been suggested that this paradox may be due to the weakened immune defense in older patients (43). The work of Black et al. (44) supports this notion. In their experience, they found that a lymphoid infiltrate, lymph node sinus histiocytosis, and a high degree of nuclear differentiation associated with a breast tumor in all age groups have a positive effect on survival. The presence of a significant lymphoid response appeared to improve 10-year survival by about 10%. In older patients, in whom the defense mechanisms are suboptimal or lacking, breast tumors may be allowed to progress unopposed even when the more favorable histologic features

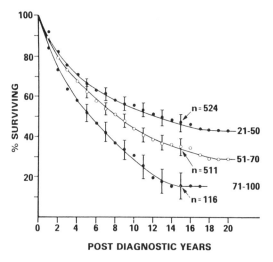

Figure 14.2. Life-table analysis of three age groups computed for deaths due to breast cancer only. Confidence limits at the 0.95 level are shown and the effective number at risk at 15 years is calculated according to Cutler, SJ: Maximum utilization of the life table in analysing survival. *J Chronic Dis* 22:485, 1969. (Reprinted by permission from Mueller CV, Ames F, Anderson GD: Breast cancer in 3,558 women, age as a significant determinant in the rate of dying and causes of death. *Surgery* 83:123–132, 1978.)

and other aspects of the tumors are present.

Schottenfeld and Robbins (9) agree that breast cancer is very malignant in older patients. They reviewed 1,277 patients aged 65 and older and 5,976 younger patients with breast cancer. They found that the 5-year adjusted survival rate was significantly better in the younger patients with breast cancer than in the older patients who had similar lesions. Adami and his co-workers (45) also report a decline in relative survival after age 49 among women who have breast cancer. Women older than 75 had the worst relative survival rate in their series. This has also been our experience.

For years Haagensen (32) has argued that breast cancer is not a less lethal disease in the old. When deaths from intercurrent diseases were excluded in his series, he found that 10-year survival in his experience was poorer in patients 65 and older than for younger patients who were treated identically. In his personal series, 109 patients aged 65 and older were all treated by standard radical mastectomy. There were no operative deaths and no serious postoperative complications in these older patients.

The current literature is filled with increasing numbers of reports of and recommendations for a more aggressive surgical treatment for breast cancer in older women. In 1975, Cortese and Cornell (46) reported a series of 142 women with breast cancer who were 75 years of age or older. Fifty-eight of these patients had a radical mastectomy with no operative mortality. Fifty-one percent of these patients lived longer than 5 years. At the end of 5 years, 49% of their patients who had had radical mastectomy were still alive and cancer free compared to 35% of those who had had only a simple mastectomy. Thirty-three of the 58 patients who had radical mastectomy had lymph node metastasis, and 12 of that subgroup were alive and cancer free at 5 years. The authors ask, "Would these patients have survived with simple mastectomy alone?" They concluded that radical mastectomy remains the treatment that offers the best chance for long-term survival. It is now known that age alone would not have protected these older patients from dying from their breast cancer. It is becoming increasingly clear that the disease is not less lethal in the elderly, and we, like most observers, would now recommend a modified radical mastectomy in most instances.

Herbsman et al. (47) reported in 1981 the treatment of 138 patients aged 70 or greater with an operative mortality of 0%. They also contend that breast cancer in the elderly should be treated by the same surgical methods that will offer a woman of any age the best opportunity for cure. They point out that 90% of patients aged 70, 73% of those aged 75, and 63% of those aged 80 are now expected to survive at least 5 years. Breast cancer left untreated or poorly treated will obviously decrease that life expectancy.

There is sometimes a hesitancy to use chemotherapeutic agents in elderly women because of the fear of excessive toxicity. Recent reports, however, have not been supportive of this notion (48, 49). In a double-blind comparison of tamoxifen with placebo in elderly women with stage II breast cancer, tamoxifen improved the disease-free interval without significant toxicity. They found no increase in survival, however, in the patients who were treated with tamoxifen (49).

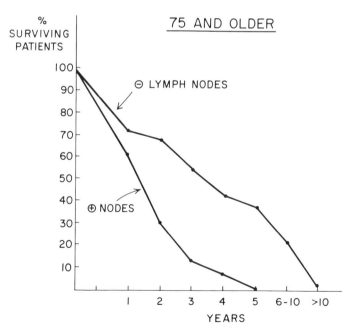

Figure 14.3. Comparison of survival in group of elderly patients who had negative lymph nodes at time of initial treatment with those who had axillary metastases shows ominous implications of this positive finding. (Reprinted by permission from Adkins RB, Whiteneck JM, Woltering E; Carcinoma of the breast in the extremes of age. *South Med J* 77:553-559, 1984.)

For a detailed discussion of the use of chemotherapy in elderly women who have breast cancer, see Chapter 6.

CONCLUSIONS AND RECOMMENDATIONS

The experience of this author is much the same as those discussed above (6). In a study comparing the behavior of breast cancer in the young patients to that seen in very old patients with the same disease, it was apparent to us that the presence of lymph node metastasis was much more indicative of the lethal behavior of the disease than the length of time between symptoms and treatment, the size of the tumor, or the age of the patient. (Figure 14.3) Estrogen receptor status appears to be another strong prognostic factor. Perhaps this has become even more evident as the longevity of North American women has increased over the past few years, and we are now able to follow them into older ages and for longer postoperative periods. We therefore have concluded from our own experience and from that of others that an aggressive surgical approach that involves dissection of the axilla, as well as adequate, total removal of the primary lesion, is the most appropriate treatment for breast cancer for all patients, regardless of age. We also maintain that breast reconstruction is a reasonable consideration if the patient of any age desires the procedure and if her condition permits.

Recently, many clinicians have considered performing "lumpectomies" and segmental resections as the initial treatment for patients with breast cancer more often than in years past. We would agree that there is a definite place for "lumpectomy," segmental resection, subcutaneous mastectomy, and even radiation in the treatment of some selected cases of breast cancer. The determining factors for the selection of this mode of treatment should be the well-differentiated histologic type and overall malignant potential of the tumor, the small tumor size, the convenient tumor location within the breast, and other such favorable clinical considerations, rather than the age of the patient or an overzealous tendency to conform to unproven, trendy attitudes of the public. It may be true that a good number of tumors that fit the indications for some of the less aggressive surgical procedures will be found in the elderly, especially if we can begin to diagnose and treat them earlier. The elderly female with breast cancer deserves an approach to her disease that is at least as thoughtful and aggressive as that which would be offered to her younger sisters.

REFERENCES

1. Reyniak JV: Physiology of the Breast. In Gallager HS, Leis HP, Snyderman RK, Urban JA (eds): *The Breast.* St. Louis, CV Mosby, 1978, pp 23–32.
2. Hellman S, Harris JR, Canellos GP, Fisher B: Cancer of the breast. In DeVita VT, Hellman S, Rosenberg SA (eds): *Cancer: Principles and Practice of Oncology.* Philadelphia, JB Lippincott, 1982, pp 914–970.
3. Holleb AI (ed): *Ca-A Cancer Journal for Clinicians.* American Cancer Society 35:19–56, 1985.
4. Holmes FF: Aging and cancer. *Rec Results Can Res* 87:9–13, 1983.
5. Hunt KE, Fry DE, Bland KI: Breast carcinoma in the elderly patient, an assessment of operative risk, morbidity, and mortality. *Am J Surg* 140:339–342, 1980.
6. Adkins RB, Whiteneck JM, Woltering E: Carcinoma of the breast in the extremes of age. *South Med J* 77:553–559, 1984.
7. Robins RE, Lee D: Carcinoma of the breast in women 80 years of age and older, still a lethal disease. *Am J Surg* 149:606–609, 1985.
8. Kesseler HJ, Seton JZ: The treatment of operable breast cancer in the elderly female. *Am J Surg* 135:664–666, 1976.
9. Schottenfeld D, Robbins GF: Breast cancer in elderly women. *Geriatrics* 26:121–131, 1971.
10. Kraft RO, Block GE: Mammary carcinoma in the aged patient. *Ann Surg* 156:981–985, 1962.
11. Rosen PP, Lesser ML, Kinne DW: Breast carcinoma at the extremes of age: a comparison of patients younger than 35 years and older than 75 years. *J Surg Onc* 28:90–96, 1985.
12. Beahrs OH, Myers MH (eds): *Manual for Staging of Cancer,* ed 2. American Joint Committee on Cancer, Philadelphia, JB Lippincott, 1983, pp 127–133.
13. Davis SJ, Karrer FW, Moor BJ, Rose SG, Eakins G: Characteristics of breast cancer in women over 80 years of age. *Am J Surg* 150:655–657, 1985.
14. Veronesi U, Cascinelli N, Greco M, Bufalino R, Morabito A, Galluzzo D, Conti R, De Lellis R, Donne VD, Piotti P, Sacchini V, Clemente C, Salvadori B: Prognosis of breast cancer patients after mastectomy and dissection of internal mammary nodes. *Ann Surg* 202:702–707, 1985.
15. Jensen EV, Block GE, Smith S, DeSombre E: Estrogen receptors and breast cancer response to adrenalec-

tomy. *National Cancer Institute Monograph* 34:55–70, 1971.

16. Raynaud JP, Ojasoo T, Delarue JC, Magdelenat H, Martin P, Philibert D: Estrogen and progestin receptors in human breast cancer. In McGuire WL, Raynaud JP, Baulieu EE (eds): *Progesterone Receptors in Normal and Neoplastic Tissue.* New York, Raven Press, 1977, pp 171–191.

17. Kleinfeld G, Haagensen CD, Cooley E: Age and menstrual status as prognostic factors in carcinoma of the breast. Ann Surg 157:600- 605, 1963.

18. Block GE, Jensen EV, Polley TZ: The prediction of hormonal dependence of mammary cancer. *Ann Surg* 182:342–352, 1975.

19. McCarty KS, Silva JS, Cox EB, Leight GS, Wells SA, McCarty KS: Relationship of age and menopausal status to estrogen receptor content in primary carcinoma of the breast. *Ann Surg* 197:123–127, 1983.

20. Hawkins RA, Roberts MM, Forrest APM: Oestrogen receptors and breast cancer, current status. *Br J Surg* 67:153–169, 1980.

21. Allegra JC, Lippman ME, Thompson EB, Simon R, Barlock A, Green L, Huff KK, Do HMT, Aitken SC: Distribution, frequency, and quantitative analysis of estrogen, progesterone, androgen, and glucocorticoid receptors in human breast cancer. *Cancer Res* 39:1447–1454, 1979.

22. Elwood JM, Godolphin W: Oestrogen receptors in breast tumours, associations with age, menopausal status, and epidemiological and clinical features in 735 patients. *Br J Cancer* 42:635–644, 1980.

23. Rochman H, Conniff ES, Kuk-Nagle KT: Age and incidence of estrogen receptor positive breast tumors. *Ann Clin Lab Sci* 15:106- 108, 1985.

24. Theve NO, Carlstrom K, Gustafsson JA, Gustafsson S, Nordenskjold B, Skoldefors H, Wrange O: Oestrogen receptors and peripheral serum levels of oestradiol-17 beta in patients with mammary carcinoma. *Eur J Cancer* 14:1337–1340, 1978.

25. Nagai R, Kataoka M, Kobayashi S, Ishihara K, Tobioka N, Nakashima K, Naruse M, Saito K, Sakuma S: Estrogen and progesterone receptors in human breast cancer with concomitant assay of plasma 17 B-Estradiol, progesterone, and prolactin levels. *Cancer Res* 39:1835–1840, 1979.

26. Saez S, Martin PM, Chouvet CD: Estradiol and progesterone receptor levels in human breast adenocarcinoma in relation to plasma estrogen and progesterone levels. *Cancer Res* 38:3468–3473, 1978.

27. Levy C, Robel P, Gautray JP DeBrux J, Verma U, Descomps B, Baulieu E: Estradiol and progesterone receptors in human endometrium, normal and abnormal menstrual cycles and early pregnancy. *Am J Obstet Gynecol* 136:646–651, 1980.

28. Pollow K, Schmidt-Gollwitzer M, Nevinny-Stickel J: Progesterone receptors in normal human endometrium and endometrial carcinoma. In McGuire WL, Raynaud JP, Baulieu EE (eds.): *Progesterone Receptors in Nor-*

mal and Neoplastic Tissues. New York, Raven Press, 1977, pp 313–338.

29. Baird DT, Guevara A: Concentration of unconjugated estrone and estradiol in peripheral plasma in nonpregnant women throughout the menstrual cycle, castrate and postmenopausal women and in men. *J Clin Endocrinol* 29:149–156, 1969.

30. Chabon AB, Goldberg JD, Venet L: Carcinoma of the breast. *Hum Pathol* 14:368–372, 1983.

31. Rosai J (ed): *Ackerman's Surgical Pathology,* ed 6. St. Louis, CV Mosby, 1981, pp 1087–1149.

32. Haagensen CD: The clinical classification of carcinoma of the breast and the choice of treatment. In *Diseases of the Breast,* ed 2. Philadelphia, WB Saunders, 1971, pp 617–668.

33. Rosen PP, Lesser ML, Senie RT, Duthie K: Epidemiology of breast carcinoma IV. Age and histologic tumor type. *J Surg Oncol* 19:44–47, 1982.

34. Knight CD, Martin JK, Welch JS, Ingle JN, Gaffey TA, Martinez A: Surgical considerations after chemotherapy and radiation therapy for inflammatory breast cancer. *Surgery* 99:385–391, 1986.

35. Ridolfi RL, Rosen PP, Port A, Kinne D, Mike V: Medullary carcinoma of the breast, a clinicopathologic study with 10 year follow-up. *Cancer* 40:1365–1385, 1977.

36. Sonnenblick M, Abraham AS: Primary lymphosarcoma of the breast: review of the literature on occurrence in elderly patients. *J Am Geriatr Soc* 24:225–227, 1976.

37. Lawler MR, Richie RE: Reticulum cell sarcoma of the breast. *Cancer* 20:1438–1444, 1967.

38. Lattes R: Sarcoma of the breast. *JAMA* 201:531–532, 1967.

39. Yoshida Y: Reticulum cell sarcoma of the breast. *Cancer* 26:94–99, 1970.

40. Case TC: Bilateral lymphosarcoma of the breast. *J Am Geriatr Soc* 23:330–332, 1975.

41. Crosby CH, Barclay THC: Carcinoma of the breast, surgical management of patients with special conditions. *Cancer* 28:1628- 1636, 1971.

42. Mueller CV, Ames F, Anderson GD: Breast cancer in 3,558 women, age as a significant determinant in the rate of dying and causes of death. *Surgery* 83:123–132, 1978.

43. Vorherr H: Pathobiology of breast cancer. In *Breast Cancer.* Baltimore, Urban & Schwarzenberg, 1980, pp 347–373.

44. Black MM, Barclay TH, Hankey BF: Prognosis in breast cancer utilizing histologic characteristics of the primary tumor. *Cancer* 36:2048–2055, 1975.

45. Adami HO, Malker B, Holmberg L, Persson I, Stone B: The relation between survival and age at diagnosis in breast cancer. *N Engl J Med* 315:559–563, 1986.

46. Cortese AF, Cornell CN: Radical mastectomy in the aged female. *J Am Geriatr Soc* 23:337–342, 1975.

47. Herbsman H, Feldman J, Seldera J, Gardner B, Alfonso AE: Survival following breast cancer surgery in the elderly. *Cancer* 47:2358–2363, 1981.

48. Begg CB, Carbone PP: Clinical trials and drug toxicity

in the elderly: the experience of the Eastern Cooperative Oncology Group. *Cancer* 52:1986–1992, 1983.

49. Cummings FJ, Gray R, Davis TE, Tormey DC, Harris JE, Falkson G, Arseneau J: Adjuvant tamoxifen treatment of elderly women with stage II breast cancer. *Ann Intern Med* 103:324-329, 1985.

Chapter 15

Cardiac Surgery in the Elderly

Duncan A. Killen, M.D., F.A.C.S.

Cardiac disease is the leading cause of death in the industrialized countries. In 1983, in the United States, heart disease was the cause of death in 39.6% of residents dying at age 65 to 74, 43% of those dying at age 75 to 84, and 48.4% of those dying at age 85 and beyond (1). There has been a modest but significant reduction in age-adjusted cardiac mortality rates during recent years (1). This change is primarily due to a decreasing risk for coronary artery disease mortality, but also probably has been influenced by the decreasing incidence of rheumatic heart disease, as well as other factors. In spite of this beneficial trend in cardiac mortality rates, the demographic realities of an increasing proportion of elderly individuals in the general population will make cardiac disease the continuing dominant cause of death in the foreseeable future (2).

Decreased cardiac functional capacity and reserve is a normal consequence of the aging process. This trend is evident in middle age and becomes accentuated in the elderly. Although it is normal to have a decreased cardiorespiratory capacity with aging, it is abnormal to have such a severely decreased capacity that the individual cannot continue to do nonstrenuous activities. It is, however, obvious that any superimposed pathologic condition that may cause further deterioration in cardiac reserve makes elderly individuals more susceptible to limitations of their physical activities and to the occurrence of cardiac decompensation.

CARDIAC PATHOLOGY IN THE ELDERLY

The most frequent clinically significant cardiac pathologic changes seen in the elderly are those of coronary artery atherosclerosis (3). Coronary artery atherosclerosis does not always accompany aging; however, there is an increasing incidence with age, which, in fact, is the most significant identified risk factor for the occurrence of coronary artery occlusive disease (4). The clinical presentation of elderly patients with coronary disease differs somewhat from that of younger individuals who have the disease and who most frequently have angina of exertion as the presenting symptom. As a group the elderly patients present with further advanced (three vessel coronary artery obstruction, left main coronary artery obstruction, myocardial scarring, etc.) disease. Unexpected sudden death, acute myocardial infarction, and/or congestive heart failure therefore are relatively more frequent as the presenting symptom in elderly individuals (4).

Elderly individuals who suffer an acute myocardial infarction exhibit an increased tendency for left ventricular rupture (3). Especially is this true in elderly females and individuals of either sex who are experiencing their first infarction (3). Rupture (disruption) of the left ventricular free wall is most frequent, and disruptions of the interventricular septum and papillary muscles occur less frequently.

Because of the decreased myocardial reserve in the elderly, healed myocardial infarctions often result in clinically significant congestive failure. The resulting left ventricular scars and/or aneurysm may be localized or of a more diffuse distribution. In addition to discrete myocardial scarring, obviously the result of a healed acute infarction, long-standing coronary artery disease may be associated with scattered focal degeneration and/or scarring throughout the myocardium in the elderly. Patients with diffuse scattered focal damage may present with an "ischemic cardiomyopathy" and resultant congestive heart failure and/or arrhythmias. Ischemic cardiomyopathy, as well as cardiomyopathies of unknown or poorly understood etiologies, often first reach clinical significance in the elderly (3).

Myxomatous degeneration of the connective tissue of the cardiac valves occurs with aging. There is stretching and enlargement of all valves but especially the mitral leaflets, as well as elongation and thinning of the chordae tendineae. Myxomatous degeneration of the cardiac valves is present at autopsy in 5% to 7% of all individuals greater than 60 years of age (3). These changes lead to mitral valve prolapse that may eventually result in mitral regurgitation. The "mitral valve prolapse syndrome" is often found in younger females; as these individuals grow older the added myxomatous degeneration that occurs with aging accentuates the pathologic changes in the mitral valve leaflets and chordae tendineae. Rupture of the chordae tendineae is a common complication of myxomatous degeneration and occurs with increased frequency in older individuals (3). Also, there seems to be an increased incidence of unexpected sudden death in patients with mitral valve prolapse (3). Similar myxomatous degeneration of the valves and the cardiac fibrous skeleton is seen in association with Marfan's syndrome in younger individuals; however, those changes encountered in the elderly cannot be correlated with any of the other clinicopathologic findings characteristic of Marfan's syndrome.

Any degenerative and/or inflammatory changes in the cardiac valves may lead to scarring and in some instances eventually to calcification. This is particularly true following episodes of acute or subacute inflammation of the cardiac valves of the left side of the heart as seen in patients with rheumatic fever. This postrheumatic scarring, especially of the mitral valve, results in progressive thickening, distortion, fusion, and contracture of the leaflets and chordae tendineae. There is associated increasing valvular calcification as the individual ages.

Calcifications of the aortic and mitral valves occur in the elderly even in the absence of any prior acute inflammation. This is especially true for calcification of the aortic valve, particularly a congenitally bicuspid aortic valve, which results in valvular stenosis in the elderly (3). Although a bicuspid aortic valve is of a congenital origin, the clinical significance is often not apparent until an older age when secondary scarring and calcification occur that result in stiffening of the abnormal valve with resultant stenosis. Isolated mitral valve annulus calcification is usually found only in older individuals, especially females (3, 5). It usually involves the posterior region of the mitral valve annulus and is not a consequence of postrheumatic scarring. When the calcification is severe it may lead to mitral regurgitation and rarely can be obstructive, resulting in mitral stenosis.

There is progressive degeneration of the collagenous fibers of the cardiac fibrous skeleton with aging. Senile cardiac amyloidosis, a form of primary amyloidosis, is a connective tissue degenerative process associated with aging (5). There is an increasing prevalence in patients more than 70 years of age. Histologic changes of senile cardiac amyloidosis in an incidence as high as 84% have been reported to be found in necropsies of individuals older than 90 years of age (3).

Isolated dilatation of the aortic valve annulus (annuloaortic ectasia) is sometimes a consequence of aging of the cardiac fibrous skeleton. This entity is most often idiopathic, but it may be associated with nonspecific aortitis, atherosclerosis, and/or long-standing hypertensive cardiovascular disease (6, 7). As the aortic annulus enlarges, the aortic valve becomes incompetent, although the leaflets themselves may remain anatomically normal. The usual presentation in these patients is that of progressive aortic regurgitation and heart failure at an older age. Annuloaortic ectasia also may be associated with a similar dilatation of the ascending thoracic aorta, resulting in aneurysm formation. Cystic medial degeneration and atherosclerosis of the aortic wall may result in aneurysm formation in the ascending aorta without aortic valve involvement.

Acute aortic dissection is especially prone to occur in those patients with myxomatous or cystic medial degeneration of the aorta. The dissection usually starts in the ascending aorta and extends proximally to involve the aortic valve and possibly the coronary artery ostia, as well as distally for a variable distance; however, it may involve the entire aorta. If untreated, death most often occurs as the result of rupture of the aorta into the pericardial space, left pleural space, or into the mediastinum (8, 9).

Another consequence of aging of the cardiac fibrous skeleton is damage to the specialized conducting system of the heart. Although the conducting tissue is muscular, these myocardial bundles pass through normally present defects in the cardiac fibrous skeleton, particularly at the atrioventricular level. At this level, the conducting system is particularly vulnerable to scarring and/or calcification of the cardiac fibrous skeleton that may cause interruption of the conduction pathway that results in atrioventricular "heart block" (10). In fact, the occurrence of third degree heart block can be better correlated with "aging" than with the presence of coronary artery disease or with any other specific cardiac disease process (10).

OVERVIEW OF CARDIAC SURGERY ON THE ELDERLY

The majority of the cardiac pathologic changes and diseases occurring in the elderly do not lead to clinical situations that could be best treated surgically. However, those patients with coronary artery occlusive disease, certain complications of acute myocardial infarction, severe valvular dysfunction, some types of malignant arrhythmias, and other rare conditions may be candidates for surgical therapy with expectant symptomatic improvements. In some instances, surgical intervention may be immediately life saving and/or increase the long-term survival in the elderly. Cardiac surgical procedures, particularly "open heart" procedures, in elderly patients carry a high risk for morbidity and mortality. In each particular situation, the risk/benefit ratio of surgical intervention versus alternative nonsurgical management must be weighed carefully.

The marked calcification in the proximal coronary arteries and the ascending thoracic aorta presents a particular technical problem in elderly patients. Operative manipulation of such ascending aortas is thought to cause an increased incidence of cerebral embolism resulting in postoperative neurologic deficits. The intra-aortic balloon pump, usually well tolerated in younger individuals, is sometimes impossible to insert or, if used, may compromise the leg circulation because of pre-existing iliofemoral atherosclerosis in the elderly. Sternotomy is well tolerated in younger individuals, but many elderly patients have marked sternal osteoporosis, and a high incidence of postoperative sternal dehiscence is encountered. The dehiscence results when the sternal wires cut through the soft bone, and a stable closure by secondary repair is often difficult to accomplish. Pre-existing pulmonary, urinary, gastrointestinal, and/or musculoskeletal disease often complicate postoperative management of the elderly.

Often, elderly patients, especially those who present with coronary artery disease, have associated atherosclerotic involvement of the peripheral and cerebral arteries. The presence of concomitant extracardiac vascular pathology often dictates that these lesions also be treated either by staged procedures or concomitantly with the cardiac procedure. This is particularly true of potentially life-threatening conditions, such as abdominal aortic aneurysm and cerebrovascular insufficiency. Although controversy exists, in general, staging of such procedures is preferable in the elderly.

The use of more sophisticated intraoperative and postoperative monitoring, the evolution of improved cardiopulmonary bypass systems, and the realization of better myocardial protection through cold cardioplegia have, in recent years, contributed to safer cardiac surgical procedures in the elderly. The complex and sophisticated care, often involving specialists from multiple disciplines, associated with cardiac procedures in the elderly is very expensive. Recently, cardiac surgery in the elderly has come under some criticism, especially when public resources are consumed to treat such patients. The increasing trend toward rationing of third party funding, on the one hand, and the increasing expense of medical care for the elderly, on the other hand, are definitely on a collision course. In the future the application of cardiac surgical care to elderly patients as discussed in this chapter may be subjected to more stringent scrutiny by our peers and/or the governmental bureaucracy.

The following descriptions of cardiac procedures and their outcome in the elderly are primarily based on analysis of certain subsets of the experience accrued since 1971 at the Mid America Heart Institute of the Saint Luke's Hospital, Kansas City, Missouri. Analysis has been arbitrarily limited to those patients age 70 years and older and, with few exceptions, to those whose operation required the use of the pump oxygenator. No case was excluded because of its emergency status or for any other extenuating circumstance. In addition to this local experience, the surgical literature has been reviewed and cited in some instances. The subject matter has been segregated into rather broad categories as follows: (1) coronary artery bypass, (2) surgery for complications of acute myocardial infarction, (3) valvular surgery, and (4) miscellaneous cardiac and juxtacardiac great vessel surgery. Permanent pacemaker implantation might well have been included as another category of cardiac surgery. However, in this country there has been a recent trend for cardiologists to assume complete responsibility for implantation and management of permanent pacemakers. Implantation of pacemakers will be discussed only as it relates to the treatment of heart block as a complication of acute myocardial infarction.

Operative techniques have not been described in detail because they are, in general, modified little from those utilized in any adult. Although much has been written about heart operations in the elderly, there has been a paucity of reported late follow-up data. Here, an attempt has been made to accentuate the late follow-up data because the actual, as well as potential, survival is an important consideration in the application of such complex and expensive care in elderly patients.

CORONARY ARTERY BYPASS

During a 15-year period ending December, 1985, 1156 isolated coronary artery bypass procedures were performed in patients aged 70 to 89 yrs (mean 74.0 yrs). There was an increasing frequency of operation and an increasing median age at operation in these elderly individuals over this 15-year period. Although women make up approximately 15% of patients of all ages un-

Table 15.1 Post-CAB[a] Hospital Stay and Mortality by Age

Age	Number of Patients	Hospital Stay[b] days	Operative Mortality %
70–74	817	13.6	6.1
75–79	279	14.2	6.5
80–84	52	14.5	5.8
85–89	8	18.1	12.5

[a]Coronary artery bypass.
[b]Mean number of postoperative days in survivors.

dergoing coronary artery bypass, they accounted for 29.2% of these older individuals (11). The incidence of three vessel coronary artery disease in coronary artery bypass patients of all ages is approximately 50%, but it was 80% in patients aged 70 years and older (11). The incidence of left main coronary artery occlusive disease is approximately 10% in all ages, but was 27.1% in this elderly group. The overall operative mortality (30 day) of 6.2% is significantly greater than the 1% mortality in patients under 70 years of age operated upon at the same institution (11). However, within the group of elderly patients the operative mortality did not appear to increase significantly with increasing age. (Table 15.1) Although there was no significant correlation between the increasing age of the elderly and operative mortality, there was a correlation between increasing age and hospital stay. Increased age, female preponderance, and the presence of three vessel or left main coronary artery disease, all prevalent in this group of patients, have been documented to result in a more complicated, prolonged postoperative recovery and a higher operative mortality in patients subjected to coronary artery bypass (12–15). However, the precise causes of increased mortality were not always clearly indentified, but often were multifactoral and related to the diminished reserve of the various organ systems in the elderly.

Beginning in 1980, percutaneous transluminal coronary angioplasty (PTCA) has been applied with increasing aggressiveness at the Mid America Heart Institute, especially in older individuals (16). Ninety-seven patients (8.4% of the total experience) underwent coronary artery bypass following PTCA failure. The operative mortal-

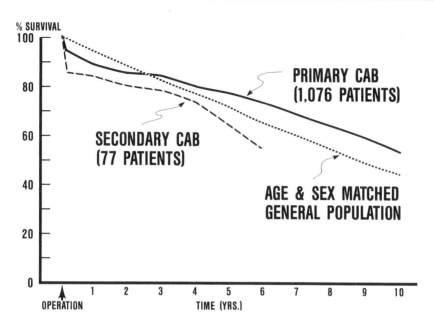

Figure 15.1. Survival following primary *(solid line)* and secondary *(broken line)* isolated coronary artery bypass. Dotted line represents survival of age- and sex-matched general population.

ity in this group was 12.4%, which is significantly more ($p=0.01$) than the mortality (5.7%) in those elderly patients not undergoing a previous PTCA. Coronary artery bypass done as an emergency following PTCA failure in the elderly had an associated operative mortality of 20%!

The 10-year survival following *primary* coronary artery bypass in 1076 elderly patients was assessed on the basis of 5870 patient-years of follow-up. The survival curve, at least through the first 10 postoperative years, is comparable to that expected in an age- and sex-matched general population. (Figure 15.1) The great majority of these patients were symptomatically improved for prolonged periods; 63% of survivors were angina free 5 years postoperatively, and 50% were angina free 10 years postoperatively. Unfortunately, the leading causes of late death continued to be cardiac in nature; of all late deaths, 53.7% were due to congestive heart failure, acute myocardial infarction, unexpected sudden (arrhythmia?) death, or repeat coronary artery bypass.

During the same period (1971–1985) 77 patients aged 70 to 83 years (mean 74.0 year) underwent a *secondary* isolated coronary artery bypass procedure. Repeat coronary bypass procedures resulted in a significantly higher

($p=0.02$) operative mortality (12.5%) than did the initial or primary coronary artery bypass (5.8%). The 5-year survival was 63.6% for all patients undergoing secondary bypass, and 71.4% of survivors were angina free 5 years postoperatively (see Figure 15.1). There were, in addition, three elderly individuals who underwent a *tertiary* coronary artery bypass procedure. All three patients survived the operative procedure. One patient died suddenly and unexpectedly 9 months postoperatively. The other two patients are surviving 1 year 2 months (Class III angina) and 5 years 3 months (Class I) postoperatively.

Comment

Comparable results for coronary artery bypass in the elderly have been published by others (13, 14, 17, 18). From those data and the series reviewed above it can be concluded that coronary artery bypass is appropriate in many elderly patients with symptomatic severe coronary artery disease. The operative mortality is increased in this older group, but the long-term symptomatic improvement and survival, which approximate that of an age- and sex-matched population, support a liberal attitude toward

Table 15.2 Postinfarctional Rupture Interventricular Septum

Patient	Age-Sex	Location of AMI	Clinical Presentation	Time[a] of Operation	Postoperative Complications	Operative Outcome	Follow-Up
T.S.	71 M	Anterior	LCOS	35 hrs	None	Survival	Alive without symptoms (8 yr 9 mo)
R.R.	72 F	Anterior	LCOS	38 hrs	Recurrent VSD	Survival	Alive without symptoms (7 yr 3 mo)
V.A.	77 F	Anterior	LCOS	2 days	LCOS	Death (POD 1)	—
E.H.	79 F	Anterior	LCOS	3 days	LCOS	Death (OR)	—
H.M.	70 F	Anterior	LCOS	4 days	LCOS, V-tachycardia, resp insuff, sepsis,CVA,DIC	Death (POD 28)	—
K.C.	72 M	Anterior	LCOS	4 days	None	Survival	Asymptomatic until death (5 yr 6 mo)
A.P.	72 F	Anterior	LCOS	5 days	LCOS, recurrent VSD, empyema	Survival	Class II angina until sudden death (6 yr 3 mo)
F.M.	84 M	Inferior	LCOS	8 days	LCOS, resp insuff renal failure UGI bleed	Death (POD 1)	—
D.E.	71 M	Anterior	CHF	15 days	CVA	Survival	Death due to CVA (2 mo)
H.C.	72 F	Anterior	CHF	35 days	None	Survival	Alive without symptoms (9 yr 9 mo)

[a]Time after acute myocardial infarction.

LCOS=low cardiac output syndrome
CHF=congestive heart failure
CVA=cerebrovascular accident
UGI=upper gastrointestinal

DCI=disseminated intravascular coagulopathy
VSD=ventricular septal defect
POD=postoperative day
OR=operating room

operative treatment. A secondary or even a tertiary coronary artery bypass procedure in the elderly seems appropriate in some instances.

Over the last 15 years, there has been a progressive change in physician attitude wherein a more aggressive approach has been taken toward evaluating elderly patients for myocardial revascularization. In recent years this trend has sharply increased because the myocardium can potentially be revascularized by balloon angioplasty (PTCA), a relatively noninvasive technique. This new therapeutic modality has extended revascularization to many elderly patients who formerly would not have been considered candidates for coronary artery bypass. However, there are complications that may occur during a PTCA procedure, making high-risk emergency coronary artery bypass mandatory (16).

Although the intraoperative and postoperative care undoubtedly have improved over the last 15 years, the overall increase in the numbers of "high risk" cases has resulted in an increased operative mortality. In our experience, the operative mortality during 1971 to 1975 was 4.8%.

This increased to 5.7% during the interval from 1976 to 1980 and to 6.7% during the period of 1981 to 1985. The conclusion that higher-risk patients are now being operated upon is borne out by the fact that only 751 (64.9% of the total) elderly patients underwent coronary artery bypass during 1981 to 1985, whereas during the same period 64 (80%) of the 80 patients undergoing secondary or tertiary procedures, 87 (89.7%) of the 97 patients having had a previous PTCA, and 56 (93.3%) of the 60 patients aged 80 years or older were operated upon.

SURGERY FOR COMPLICATIONS OF ACUTE MYOCARDIAL INFARCTION

Acute myocardial infarction complications that necessitate surgical interventions can in general be categorized as (1) *left ventricular disruptions* (free wall, septal, or papillary), (2) *left ventricular dyskinesia* (acute infarct, scar, or aneurysm), (3) *"nonflail" mitral regurgitation* (resulting from left ventricular dysfunction and/or dilatation), (4) *arrhythmias* (recurrent ventricular tachyarrhythmias or atrioventricular "heart block"), and (5) *systematic arterial embolism* (from an intracardiac mural thrombus). Although specific surgical procedures must be performed in the treatment of these complications, often concomitant myocardial revascularizations by coronary artery bypass are an integral component of the operation. The surgical treatment for arterial embolism as a complication of an acute myocardial infarction is not described here (see Chapter 29).

Left ventricular disruptions usually present as dire emergencies. In most instances these patients follow a rapidly fatal course. The most frequent site of rupture is the left ventricular free wall. Unfortunately, this complication is usually immediately fatal so that surgical treatment is not feasible. In a minority of instances, however, the rupture (leak) is limited so that the patient develops cardiac tamponade and shock, but survives long enough for diagnosis and the initiation of surgical therapy. At the Mid America Heart Institute attempts at surgical treatment have been made overall in eight such patients of whom two were 70 years of age or older. The experience in these two cases has been disappointing, with no operative survivors.

The next most frequent site of left ventricular disruption is the interventricular septum. This tends to occur in older individuals, especially those without a history of a previous acute myocardial infarction (4, 19). Without surgical treatment, only approximately 15% of patients with this complication will survive longer than 2 months (19). During a 9-year period ending December 1979, ten patients, 70 to 84 years of age, underwent surgical therapy for postinfarctional septal rupture. Because of cardiogenic shock, eight of these patients underwent repair within 8 days of their myocardial infarction; five patients were operated upon within 24 hours of occurrence of the ventricular septal defect (VSD). Only four of the emergency group of patients survived. Two other patients presenting with congestive heart failure underwent delayed (15 day and 35 days postinfarction) repair, and both survived. The appropriate data from these ten cases are summarized in Table 15.2. Five of the ten patients have survived beyond 5 years postoperatively.

The third type of left ventricular disruption, papillary muscle rupture, results in a flail mitral valve and massive regurgitation. This complication is usually rapidly fatal, and 70% of such patients will succumb within 24 hours and 90% within 2 months if not treated surgically (20). Sixteen patients, of whom three were elderly (70 to 79 years), underwent surgical therapy for ruptured papillary muscle during a 9-year period ending December, 1979 (20). The pertinent clinical data in these three cases are shown in Table 15.3. It is encouraging that each patient has been a long-term survivor.

Mitral regurgitation secondary to left ventric-

Table 15.3 Surgical Treatment of Ruptured Papillary Muscle

Patient	Age-Sex	Clinical Presentation	Time[a] of Operation	Operative Procedure	Postoperative Complications	Follow-Up
E.C.	78 F	LCOS and pulmonary edema	2 days	MVR and closure PFO	LOCS and hemiparesis	Alive Class I, 9 yr 11 mo
T.K.	72 M	CHF	5 weeks	MVR and CAB × 1	None	AMI, 2 yr now Alive Class II, 9 yr 3 mo
J.B.	76 M	LCOS	1 day	MVR	None	Alive Class I 8 yr 2 mo

[a]Time after occurrence of papillary muscle rupture.

MVR=mitral valve replacement (Bjork prosthesis)
PFO=patent foramen ovale
CAB=coronary artery bypass
(See also Key, Table 15.2)

Table 15.4 Resection of Left Ventricular Scar or Aneurysm

Patient	Age-Sex	Concomitant Procedure	Operative Outcome	Follow-Up
R.W.	71 M	CAB × 2	Death (POD 1)	—
E.H.	72 M	CAB × 2	Survival	Death due to CHF, 9 yr 4 mo
N.C.	71 M	CAB × 1	Survival	Death due to lung cancer, 5 yr 11 mo
N.N.	76 F	CAB × 1	Survival	Death due to CVA, 7 yr 2 mo
E.R.	71 F	CAB × 1	Death (POD 8)	—
I.W.	72 M	None	Survival	Death due to CVA, 9 yr 4 mo
V.H.	72 F	None	Survival	Death due to AMI, 1 yr 5 mo
W.A.	74 M	None	Survival	Alive, Class I, 10 yr 10 mo
T.F.	71 M	MVR + CAB × 1	Death (OR)	—
P.F.	70 M	None	Survival	Death due to CHF, 9 yr 2 mo
F.M.	77 M	CAB × 3	Survival	Alive, Class I, 8 yr 6 mo
V.W.	73 M	CAB × 2	Survival	Death due to lung cancer, 5 yr 6 mo
R.T.	70 F	CAB × 1	Survival	Alive, Class I, 7 yr 11 mo

AMI = acute myocardial infarction
See also Key, Tables 15.2 and 15.3.

ular dysfunction (left ventricular infarction, scar, ischemic cardiomyopathy, papillary muscle dysfunction, and/or mitral annular dilation) is a frequent complication of acute myocardial infarction. However, only a few such patients become candidates for surgical treatment for their mitral insufficiency. There is a high mortality associated with such operations. It is often difficult to clearly identify this subset of mitral valve repair patients based on clinical grounds only; however; that group of patients undergoing mitral valve replacement or annuloplasty for left ventricular dysfunction is composed primarily of such patients as described below under valvular surgery. (See Tables 15.7 and 15.8)

Acute infarction may cause severe left ventricular free wall akinesis or dyskinesis, which in spite of supportive medical therapy and even the use of the intra-aortic balloon pump, results in unrelenting cardiogenic shock or intractable congestive heart failure. Such patients usually do not survive. Rarely, resection of an acute left ventricular infarction (so-called acute left ventricular aneurysm) is performed in hopes of increasing the effectiveness of the remaining viable left ventricular muscle. Our experience in elderly patients over a 9-year period ending in 1979 was limited to only one such patient who underwent left ventricular wall resection within 30 days of an acute myocardial infarction. He was a 72-year-old male who suffered progressive heart failure, low cardiac output, and decreasing renal function in spite of inotropic support and use of the intra-aortic balloon pump.

Resection of the infarction and single coronary artery bypass were performed 15 days after a large anterior acute myocardial infarction, but he succumbed with continued low cardiac output on the second postoperative day.

Patients who survive the early phase of an acute myocardial infarction may have as a residium a large scar or aneurysm of the left ventricle. These patients most often present late after myocardial infarction. In some instances, the scar thins and enlarges, producing a progressively dyskinetic scar (aneurysm) so that cardiac failure may first occur months or even years after the acute myocardial infarction. Many of these patients are candidates for resection of the left ventricular scar or aneurysm. During an 8-year (1971 to 1978) period, 13 such patients, aged 70 to 77 years, underwent resection of a left ventricular scar or aneurysm. In nine patients concomitant coronary artery bypass was performed; one patient also had concomitant mitral valve replacement. These cases are summarized in Table 15.4. The operative mortality was 23%, but 69.2% survived beyond the fifth postoperative year.

Recurrent ventricular tachyarrhythmias sometimes result from an irritable focus in or adjacent to a healing or healed myocardial infarction. In some instances such episodes, especially if there is ventricular fibrillation, lead to sudden death. Often, sustained ventricular tachycardia is compatible with adequate survival to permit emergency resuscitation. If observation and electrophysiologic studies show that such episodes

Table 15.5 Electrophysiologic Mapping and Resection of Ventricular Subendocardial Scar

Patient	Age-Sex	Symptoms and Signs	Ancillary Operative Procedures	Follow-Up
W.S.	76 M	LV scar, recurrent V-tachycardia	Resection LV scar and CAB × 4	One episode V-tachycardia early postop, sudden death (11 mo)
J.H.	73 M	LV aneurysm, recurrent V-tachycardia	Resection LV aneurysm and CAB × 1	V-tachycardia, LCOS, and death (POD 1)
D.D.	78 M	LV aneurysm, recurrent V-tachycardia	Resection LV aneurysm and MVR	No V-tachycardia, CHF (Class III) alive (2 yr 7 mo)
M.H.	70 M	LV aneurysm, recurrent V-tachycardia	Resection LV aneurysm and CAB × 1	No V-tachycardia, alive (2 yr 4 mo)
G.S.	77 M	LV aneurysm, recurrent V-tachycardia	Resection LV aneurysm and CAB × 2	No V-tachycardia; alive (2 yr 3 mo)

LV = left ventricular
V = ventricular
See also Key, Tables 15.2, 15.3, and 15.4.

do in fact recur, or are likely to recur in spite of optimal medical management, these patients may be candidates for elective surgical intervention. Surgical therapy is aimed at destroying the focus of origin of the tachyarrhythmia (21).

Attempts to localize intraoperatively and specifically ablate these foci have been made at the Mid America Heart Institute beginning in 1980. Intraoperative ventricular epicardial and/or left ventricular endocardial electrocardiographic mapping for localization and resection of a focus of origin of recurrent ventricular tachycardia have been performed in five patients aged 70 years or older. In each of these patients, the mapping was performed in association with resection of a left ventricular scar or aneurysm. In addition to left ventricular wall resection, the irritable focus was localized and ablated by resection of a specific area of endocardial fibrosis. The results obtained in these five cases are summarized in Table 15.5. Recently, another surgical procedure, the implantation of a self-contained cardioverter/defibrillator, has been introduced with successful treatment of recurrent ventricular tachyarrhythmias (22). We have treated two elderly patients by this method. Although the follow-up period is short, both currently survive.

Atrioventricular heart block, which occurs as a complication of an acute myocardial infarction, is almost always managed initially by the cardiologist. If there is only first- or second-degree heart block, drug therapy is often adequate. On other occasions, however, emergency placement of a temporary pacing electrode and external pacing are mandatory. The need for an implantable permanent pacemaker is often determined only after a period of observation with temporary pacing.

Heart block associated with *inferior* myocardial infarctions is usually secondary to involvement of the internodal conduction pathways and/or the atrioventricular node, and often the heart block exhibits gradual progressive onset and/or a varying severity. Even when there is complete heart block, a *junctional* escape rhythm with a rate of 40 to 60 beats per minute is present. In general, the severity of heart block is less catastrophic, there is usually functional recovery of the conduction system, and permanent pacing is not required with acute inferior wall infarctions.

On the other hand, *anterior* myocardial infarction that results in heart block carries a much worse prognosis. Heart block in such patients is usually present only if there has been a massive myocardial infarction involving much of the interventricular septum. The mechanism of production of the heart block is usually ischemic injury and/or necrosis of the bundle of His. Characteristically, the onset of heart block is sudden and complete, and the resultant idioventricular rhythm is very slow (20–40 beats per minute) and unstable, often deteriorating into ventricular fibrillation. Such patients develop sudden profound shock often with loss of consciousness, and they must be resuscitated immediately by emergency ventricular pacing. Even if resuscitated successfully, anterior acute myocardial infarction complicated by complete heart block is usually fatal because of the massive size of the infarction. In those few patients who become potential long-term survivors, the heart block is

Table 15.6 Aortic Valve Replacement

Concomitant Procedures	Number of Patients	Operative Deaths
None	56	1
CAB	20	1
Resection HSS	4	0
Mitral valvotomy	3[a]	0
Resection ATA	2[a]	0
Totals	85	2 (2.4%)

[a]One patient also had coronary artery bypass.

CAB = coronary artery bypass
HSS = hypertrophic subaortic stenosis
ATA = ascending thoracic aorta

usually permanent, and permanent pacemaker implantation is indicated. Such patients who survive have poor cardiac reserve, and if possible a dual chamber (atrial and ventricular) pacemaker should be used in order to optimize the cardiac output. To minimize operative risk the pacemaker and transvenous electrodes should be implanted under local anesthesia.

Comment

Surgical treatment of the catastrophic complications of acute myocardial infarction is associated with a high mortality, especially in the elderly. Nevertheless, in most instances, these complications are immediately life threatening, are of a mechanical nature, and can be resolved only by a surgical approach. The physicians and cardiologists caring for such elderly patients often have a tendency to temporize. Usually they have exhausted their armamentarium of medical regimens and mechanical supportive measures (intra-aortic balloon pump, etc.) before surgical intervention is considered. Such continued efforts are usually futile and, in fact, may allow the patient to worsen and become even a poorer candidate for definitive treatment. The continued low cardiac output syndrome, oliguria, supervening lactic acidosis, and multiple organ system failure then decrease the chances for the patient's survival with surgical intervention (19). Reports of others have strongly suggested that earlier surgical intervention will result in a greater salvage in these deathly ill patients (23).

On the contrary, the late complications of acute myocardial infarction, such as left ventricular aneurysm and recurrent ventricular tachyarrhythmias, often present a dilemma in the choice of surgical or medical therapy. The recent addition of new inotropic drugs and afterload reducing agents has improved the ability to manage patients medically with severe congestive heart failure. The possible occurrence of arterial thromboembolism or rupture of left ventricular aneurysms, is in general, not an indication for surgical intervention. Currently, more sophisticated electrophysiologic evaluation, newer antiarrhythmic agents, and percutaneous ablation of irritable ventricular endocardial foci offer an alternative to the direct surgical treatment of many patients with postinfarctional recurrent ventricular tachyarrhythmias.

VALVULAR SURGERY

During the period from 1971 to 1978, 85 patients aged 70 to 84 years (mean 74.5 years) underwent aortic valve replacement. The operative mortality (30 day) was 2.4%. The hemodyamic lesion necessitating aortic valve replacement was aortic stenosis in 76 patients. In three instances, aortic stenosis was the result of rheumatic heart disease; in the remainder it was due to nonspecific "senile" aortic valve calcification. In at least seven instances, the aortic valve affected by senile calcification was a congenitally bicuspid valve. Eight patients underwent aortic valve replacement for aortic regurgitation. Annuloaortic ectasia was the etiology in seven patients. One patient had aortic regurgitation resulting from dissection of the ascending thoracic aorta. In the remaining patient, an aortic valve prosthesis was replaced because of severe prosthetic-related hemolysis. In 29 of the entire group of 85 patients, concomitant cardiac procedures were performed at the time of aortic valve replacement (Table 15.6). The operative mortality (30 day) was 1.8% in the 56 patients with isolated aortic valve replacement and 3.4% in those patients in whom aortic valve replacement was combined with other procedures. Postoperative survival following aortic valve replacement (all patients) was 62% at 5 years and 43.8% at 8 years.

Aortic valvoplasty can sometimes be utilized as an alternative to aortic valve replacement for calcific aortic stenosis in the elderly (24, 25). This is particularly applicable when there is pure aortic stenosis, the valve is tricuspid, there is no or limited commissural fusion, and the calcifi-

Table 15.7 Mitral Valve Replacement in Elderly by Etiology and Concomitant Operative Procedures

Etiology of Mitral Valve Disease	None	Concomitant Operative Procedures + +			
		CAB	Other Valve[a]	Resection LVA[b] & CAB	Totals[c]
Left ventricular dysfunction[d]	8	9	1	1	19 (7)
Rheumatic heart disease	11	1	3	0	15 (1)
Ruptured chordae tendineae[e]	9	3	1	0	13 (2)
Floppy valve syndrome[e]	3	2	0	0	5 (1)
Ruptured papillary muscle	2	1	0	0	3
Endocarditis	1	0	0	0	1
Calcification mitral annulus	0	1	0	0	1
Totals	34	17	5	1	57 (11)

[a]Tricuspid and/or aortic valvotomy or valvoplasty.
[b]LVA = left ventricular aneurysm.
[c]Operative (30-day) deaths in parentheses.
[d]Due to ischemic cardiomyopathy, papillary muscle dysfunction, or left ventricular/mitral annular dilatation.
[e]Most patients had associated myxomatous degeneration of mitral valve.

cation primarily involves the distal or aortic surface of the leaflets. This procedure is especially applicable when concomitant cardiac procedures are to be performed and it is desirous to keep the myocardial ischemic time to a minimum, for valve debridement requires less time than valve replacement. Also, there is no necessity for long-term anticoagulation if a valvoplasty is performed.

Aortic valvoplasty by mechanical decalcification was performed (1971 to 1985) in 63 patients aged 70 to 80 years who presented with senile calcific aortic stenosis. In 30 instances, a concomitant aortic commissurotomy was performed. Aortic valvoplasty was performed in combination with other cardiac procedure (coronary artery bypass and/or resection of subaortic muscular stenosis) in 26 instances. The overall operative mortality (30 day) was 7.9%. The 5-year survival was 56.3%. During a total follow-up of 140.5 patient years, five patients required aortic valve replacement.

Mitral valve replacement was performed (1971 to 1978) in 57 patients aged 70 to 86 years (mean 74.6 year) with an operative mortality (30 day) of 19.3%. The etiology of the mitral valve disease and its relationship to operative mortality are shown in Table 15.7. There was a particularly high operative mortality (36.8%) in those patients operated upon for mitral regurgitation secondary to left ventricular dysfunction. In the majority of these patients ischemic (acute or chronic) cardiomyopathy was felt to be the etiology of the valvular insufficiency. In all other patients with mitral valve replacement, either isolated or in combination with other cardiac procedures, the operative mortality was only 10.5%. The overall survival after mitral valve replacement was 44.7% at 5 years and only 24.8% at 7 years postoperatively.

In recent years (1980 to 1983), mitral valve annuloplasty and/or valvoplasty, in lieu of mitral valve replacement, was performed for mitral regurgitation in five elderly patients. In four instances, concomitant cardiac procedures were performed, and the fifth patient had previously undergone coronary artery bypass for multivessel coronary artery disease (Table 15.8). All five patients had mitral regurgitation secondary to left ventricular dysfunction. There were two operative deaths, and two patients currently survive. In addition, to the annuloplasty/valvoplasty patients listed in Table 15.8, one elderly patient (71-year-old male) underwent repair of a mitral periprosthetic leak and is alive 5 years, 10 months postoperatively.

Mitral valvotomy is occasionally utilized in elderly patients who suffer from postrheumatic mitral stenosis. Mitral valvotomy was performed (1971 to 1983) as an isolated operation in nine patients and in combination with some other cardiac procedures in six patients. There were no operative deaths, and no patient required mitral valve replacement in the follow-up period. The 5-year survival was 70.9% (Table 15.9).

Double-valve replacement was performed (1971 to 1983) in 14 patients aged 70 to 85 years. In 12 instances, the aortic and mitral valves were replaced; in the remaining two patients the mitral and tricuspid valves were replaced. Concomitant

Table 15.8 Mitral Annuloplasty/Valvoplasty

Patient	Age-Sex	Concomitant Procedures	Follow-Up
H.B.	75 M	CAB × 3	Death due to pneumonia, 3 yr 10 mo
E.J.	75 F	Closure ASD	Death, POD 25
K.R.	73 M	CAB × 3	Death, POD 2
G.S.	74 F	AV-Plasty and CAB × 4	Alive, 4 yr 3 mo
S.R.	74 F	None[a]	Alive, 3 yr 10 mo

[a]Previous CAB procedure.
ASD = atrial septal defect
AV = aortic valve

procedures were performed in six instances (Table 15.10). There were four operative deaths (28.6%), and the 5-year survival was only 50%.

In recent years (1981 to 1983) tricuspid annuloplasty/valvoplasty for tricuspid regurgitation was performed as a concomitant procedure to mitral, aortic, or multiple valve replacement in three elderly patients. The patient with double-valve replacement did not survive the early postoperative period, and only one of the three survived longer than the fourth postoperative month, but she is currently (3 years, 11 months) alive.

Pulmonic valvotomy for congenital stenosis was performed in conjunction with aortic valvoplasty in one patient, a 74-year-old female. Two years postoperatively she died following resection of a left ventricular aneurysm and aortic valve replacement.

Comment

It is evident that mitral valve and/or multiple valve replacement in the elderly, especially in patients with left ventricular dysfunction, is associated with a high operative mortality (26–28). More recently, mitral and tricuspid valve reconstructions (annuloplasty/valvoplasty) have become more popular in the treatment of patients with ventriculoatrial valvular regurgitation (29). There is some evidence to suggest that leaving the mitral valve apparatus in situ helps to preserve left ventricular contractility and overall cardiac efficiency (30). This is especially true

Table 15.9 Mitral Valvotomy in the Elderly

Patient	Age-Sex	Concomitant Procedure	Follow-Up
J.M.	71 F	None	Death due to malignancy, 11 yr 11 mo
N.S.	70 F	None	Alive, 10 yr
N.S.	73 F	None	Death due to CVA, 3 yr 1 mo
I.G.	75 F	None	Death due to ventricular fibrillation, 7 yr 11 mo
M.H.	71 F	None	Death, sudden, 2 yr 6 mo
M.P.	73 F	None	Death due to CHF, 6 yr 10 mo
L.D.	73 F	None	Alive, 8 yr 5 mo
M.K.	72 F	AVR	Death, 9 yr 8 mo
M.T.	70 F	Closure ASD and CAB	Death, sudden, 4 yr 5 mo
S.I.	70 F	AVR	Alive, 10 yr
J.P.	75 M	AVR and CAB	Alive, 9 yr 1 mo
M.C.	74 F	None	Death, sudden, 2 yr 4 mo
T.R.	72 F	AVR	Alive, 6 yr 1 mo
M.A.	70 F	None	Alive, 4 yr 6 mo
M.D.	71 F	CAB × 4	Alive, 3 yr 7 mo

AVR = aortic valve replacement   CVA = cerebrovascular accident
ASD = atrial septal defect   CHF = congestive heart failure
CAB = coronary artery bypass

Table 15.10 Double Valve Replacement

Patient	Age-Sex		Operative Procedures	Operative Outcome	Follow Up
N.R.	75	M	AVR and MVR	Death POD 17	—
L.G.	71	F	AVR and MVR	Survival	Death due to CHF, 3 yr 8 mo
R.E.	73	M	AVR and MVR	Survival	Death due to CHF, 5 yr 6 mo
C.M.	70	M	AVR and MVR	Survival	Death due to leukemia, 5 yr 8 mo
N.M.	76	M	AVR and MVR	Survival	Alive, 9 yr 7 mo
R.P.	72	M	MVR and TVR	Death POD 7	—
C.F.	72	M	AVR and MVR	Survival	Alive, 8 yr 7 mo
H.E.	76	M	AVR, MVR and CAB × 1	Survival	Death due to CHF, 7 yr 5 mo
C.L.	70	M	AVR, MVR and CAB × 1	Survival	Death due to lung cancer, 5 yr 10 mo
D.B.	70	F	AVR and MVR	Survival	Death due to CHF, 3 yr 6 mo
A.W.	71	F	AVR, MVR and TV-Plasty	Death in OR	—
W.B.	73	F	AVR, MVR and resection ATA	Survival	Alive, 4 yr
W.C.	74	M	AVR, MVR and AV-Plasty	Death POD 19	—
N.R.	85	F	AVR, MVR and CAB × 1	Survival	Death due to cancer, 1 yr 10 mo

AVR = aortic valve replacement
MVR = mitral valve replacement
TVR = tricuspid valve replacement
TV-Plasty = tricuspid annuloplasty/valvoplasty
ATA = ascending thoracic aorta
Also see Keys, Tables 15.2 and 15.3.

for patients in whom the valve itself is normal, but the regurgitation is secondary to left ventricular dysfunction and/or annular dilatation. Also, utilization of valve reconstructive techniques is desirable in the elderly because late valvular prosthetic and anticoagulant related complications can be avoided. However, we have not clearly experienced a reduction in operative mortality by using these reconstructive procedures.

The use of a bioprosthesis, rather than a mechanical valve prosthesis, should be given due consideration in valve replacement in the elderly. Use of a "central flow" bioprosthesis results in near-physiologic function and minimizes, or eliminates, the need for long-term anticoagulation. Bioprostheses tend to deteriorate over time; however, the expected shorter survival of the elderly is such that deterioration to the point of requiring a late replacement of the bioprosthe-sis occurs relatively infrequently. The majority of valves implanted in the elderly have been bioprostheses in recent years.

MISCELLANEOUS CARDIAC AND JUXTACARDIAC GREAT VESSEL PROCEDURES

Idiopathic hypertrophic subaortic stenosis usually presents in young adults, but rarely is encountered in the elderly (31). Secondary hypertropic subaortic stenosis may occasionally require resection at the time of aortic valve replacement in the elderly. Resection of subaortic hypertropic muscular stenosis was performed (1971 to 1978) in eight elderly patients. In each instance, resection was performed in combination with some other cardiac procedure (Table 15.11). In seven patients, a ventricular myomec-

Table 15.11 Resection Hypertrophic Subaortic Stenosis

Patient	Age-Sex		Associated Procedure	Follow-Up
F.S.	72	F	AVR	Death, sudden, 6 yr 3 mo
W.A.	72	M	AV-Plasty	Death, sudden, 2 yr 5 mo
L.G.	76	F	AVR	Alive, 1 yr 8 mo
B.O.	72	M	AV-Plasty and CAB × 1	Death, sudden, 6 yr 2 mo
F.E.	77	F	AVR	Death due to cancer, 8 mo
M.S.	74	F	CAB × 2	Death due to CHF, 5 yr 11 mo
C.U.	71	F	AVR	Alive, 8 yr 1 mo
L.P.	78	F	AV-Plasty and CAB × 2	Death due to CHF, 6 yr 8 mo

See Keys, Tables 15.8 and 15.10.

Table 15.12 Closure Atrial Septal Defect

Patient	Age-Sex	Associated Procedure	Follow-Up
I.S.	70 F	None	Alive, 11 yr 9 mo
M.T.	70 F	Mitral valvotomy and CAB × 1	Death, sudden, 4 yr 5 mo
B.K.	78 F	None	Death due to sepsis, 8 yr 7 mo
C.S.	73 F	None	Death, sudden, 3 mo
E.J.	75 F	MV-Plasty	Death, POD 25
R.R.	71 M	None	Alive, 5 yr 8 mo
Z.W.	76 F	None	Alive, 4 yr 2 mo

tomy was performed in association with an aortic valve procedure. There were no operative deaths. Six (75%) patients survived longer than 5 years.

During 1971 to 1982, seven elderly patients, of whom six were female, underwent closure of an ostium secundum interatrial septal defect (Table 15.12). In one patient, mitral valvotomy and single coronary artery bypass were combined with closure of the defect. The only operative death was in a patient in whom mitral annuloplasty, for mitral regurgitation secondary to left ventricular dysfunction, was done in association with closure of a small atrial septal defect. The 5-year survival was 53.8%.

Cardiac myxoma is an entity that occurs rarely in the elderly (32, 33). During a 16-year period, (1971 to 1986) at the Mid America Heart Institute, only eleven cardiac myxomas were removed, of which two were removed from elderly patients. One patient, a 70-year-old male with a left atrial myxoma, presented after progressive neurologic deterioration. The left atrial myxoma was removed, the postoperative course was uncomplicated, and he was discharged from the hospital on the 11th postoperative day. He suddenly and unexpectedly died 3 days later at home. The second patient, a 72-year-old male with a left atrial myxoma, underwent removal of the tumor and concomitant single coronary artery bypass. He survives without any cardiac symptoms 2 years 8 months postoperatively.

One patient, a 71-year-old male with late bacterial endocarditis following implantation of a transvenous pacemaker, underwent removal of a right atrial mass. The patient presented with persistent sepsis and was cured by removal of the mass (vegetations) with the incorporated pacing electrode. He survives 3 years 3 months postoperatively.

Acute aortic dissection involving the ascending thoracic aorta (Debakey Types I and II) is usually a lethal disease (8, 9, 34). The mode of death is most often rupture of the aorta into the pericardial space. The natural history of this disease is such that the mortality is approximately 50% within 2 to 3 days, and only 5% will survive beyond 2 months (8). Medical treatment improves survival somewhat, but the only definitive treatment is surgical (Figure 15.2). The dissection may extend distally throughout the entire aorta and usually proceeds retrograde to involve the aortic sinuses, making concomitant repair or replacement of the aortic valve necessary. In elderly patients there is often associated coronary artery disease. During a 9-year period (1971 to 1979), there were nine elderly patients who underwent reconstruction of the ascending aorta for aortic dissection (Table 15.13). In seven instances, the dissection was acute (less than 2 weeks old) at the time of repair. In addition to the aortic reconstruction, concomitant resuspension of the detached aortic valve commissures (four patients), aortic valve replacement (one patient), coronary artery bypass (three patients), and saphenous vein graft reconstruction (one patient) were performed in seven patients. Three of the seven patients with acute aortic dissection and one of the two patients with chronic aortic dissection did not survive the early postoperative period. Two additional patients died within the first 5 postoperative years. Three patients have survived beyond 8 years.

During a 13-year period (1971 to 1983), seven elderly patients underwent resection of an aneurysm (not associated with aortic dissection) of the ascending aorta. In each instance, there was aortic insufficiency on the basis of annular dilatation that required concomitant aortic valve replacement. A composite (prefabricated aortic

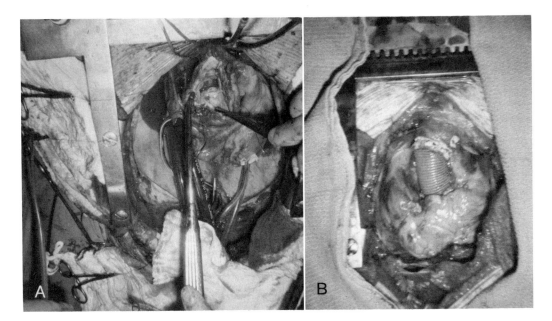

Figure 15.2. Acute aortic dissection of ascending thoracic aorta (head of patient at top). **A,** Opened aorta revealing transverse intimal tear and aortic dissection. **B,** Same view following aortic resection and graft replacement.

Table 15.13 Dissection of the Ascending Aorta

Patient	Age-Sex	Type of Dissection and Associated Pathology	Operative Procedure Aortic	Cardiac	Operative Outcome	Follow-Up
C.P.	71 F	Acute, type I and CAD	Circumferential suture and patch aortoplasty	CAB × 3	Death, POD 6	—
E.A.	70 F	Chronic, type I	Tube graft replacement	None	Survival	Alive, 12 yr 4 mo
R.M.	72 M	Acute, type I	Tube graft replacement	Suspension AV commissures	Survival	Alive, 11 yr 8 mo
W.B.	72 F	Acute, type I and CAD	Circumferential suture	AVR and CAB × 1	Survival	Death, sudden, 3 yr 11 mo
H.H.	72 M	Chronic, type I and CAD	Circumferential suture and patch aortoplasty	Suspension AV Commissure and CAB × 2	Death, POD3	—
J.S.	81 M	Acute, type II	Tube graft replacement	Suspension AV commissure	Survival	Death, due to lymphoma, 4 yr 7 mo
G.K.	73 M	Acute, type I	Circumferential suture	Reconstruction SVG	Death, OR	—
L.A.	71 M	Acute, type I	Circumferential suture	Resuspension AV commissure	Death, POD 18	—
E.P.	72 M	Acute, type I and CAD	Tube graft replacement	None	Survival	Alive, 8 yr

CAD=coronary artery disease
SVG=Saphenous vein graft to coronary artery

Table 15.14 Aneurysm (Nondissecting) of the Ascending Thoracic Aorta

Patient	Age-Sex	Etiology of Aneurysm	Operative Procedure	Operative Outcome	Follow-Up
I.H.	73 M	Cystic medial necrosis	Graft replacement and AVR	Survival	Alive, 9 yr 11 mo
F.P.	71 F	Atherosclerosis and annuloaortic ectasia	Graft replacement and AVR (Composite)	Death, POD 24	—
M.V.	72 F	Atherosclerosis and annuloaortic ectasia	Graft replacement and AVR (Composite)	Death, POD 1	—
J.D.	76 M	Atherosclerosis and annuloaortic ectasia	Graft replacement and AVR (Composite)	Survival	Death, due to CVA, 6 yr 3 mo
R.C.	72 M	Atherosclerosis and annuloaortic ectasia	Eliptical resection and AVR and CAB × 1	Death, POD 17	—
D.B.	70 M	Annuloaortic ectasia	Graft replacement and AVR (Composite)	Death, POD 3	—
W.B.	73 F	Atherosclerosis and annuloaortic ectasia	Graft replacement, AVR and MVR	Survival	Alive, 4 yr

and aortic valve prosthesis) graft was utilized in four patients. One patient required a concomitant coronary artery bypass and another mitral valve replacement. Four patients survived the operation and were long-term survivors (Table 15.14).

One elderly patient (73-year-old female) underwent resection of an aneurysm of the ascending and transverse thoracic aorta. The aneurysm was caused by myxomatous degeneration. The procedure was performed at 20° C with separate lines for arterial perfusion of the innominate and left carotid arteries. Concomitant aortic valve replacement and single coronary artery bypass were performed. She survived with no neurologic injury and is symptom free 5 years 7 months postoperatively.

Pulmonary embolism is a frequent complication in elderly individuals who are bedridden and/or physically debilitated. Most such emboli are best treated by anticoagulation or, more recently, by thrombolysis. Fatal pulmonary embolus usually results in sudden death so that surgical intervention is not possible. Rarely, there is a patient with a lethal pulmonary embolism, but the time course is such than surgical intervention is possible. We have performed embolectomy in one such elderly patient, an 85-year-old female who, 10 days previously, had undergone emergency coronary artery bypass for an evolving acute infarction that complicated an attempted percutaneous transluminal coronary angioplasty. She suddenly exhibited cardiovascular collapse, but was temporarily resuscitated by external cardiac massage. On massive in-

otropic infusions, she exhibited progressively severe shock over a 2-hour period at which time operation was undertaken with only the clinical diagnosis of pulmonary embolus. She indeed had a massive embolus. Embolectomy was performed. Her postoperative course was prolonged and difficult; however, she recovered completely. She is asymptomatic 1 year 6 months postoperatively.

A 71-year-old male presented with partial anomalous right pulmonary venous drainage to the superior cavoatrial junction. There was associated coronary artery disease. He underwent single coronary artery bypass and creation of an interatrial septal defect and (by construction of an intra-atrial baffle) diversion of the anomalous pulmonary venous return to the left atrium. He died of unknown causes 2 years 3 months postoperatively.

One patient, a 71-year-old female, underwent closure of a patent ductus arteriosus at the time of aortic valve replacement and coronary embolectomy. The ductus was closed via an opened pulmonary artery. She died suddenly 1 year 8 months postoperatively.

Comment

In this section are included the less frequently encountered cardiac surgical conditions in the elderly. In general, surgical treatment of hypertrophic subaortic stenosis, cardiac myxoma, and atrial septal defect can be applied with a low mortality and good long term survival. On the contrary, juxtacardiac great vessel procedures in the elderly are associated with a poorer prognosis. A high mortality is associated with resections of the ascending aorta, especially in the presence of acute aortic dissection. Other juxtacardiac procedures, such as pulmonary embolectomy, rerouting of anomalous pulmonary venous drainage, and closure of a patent ductus arteriosus, are only rarely applicable in the elderly.

ACKNOWLEDGMENTS. Appreciation is extended to the many colleagues, residents, nurses, and other individuals who have participated in the care of the patients treated at the Mid America Heart Institute. Particular acknowledgment is made to my surgical associates, William A Reed, M.D., William R. Hamaker, M.D., and Jeffrey M. Piehler, M.D. whose patients are included in this clinical review. Last, but not least, my thanks go to Mrs. Barbara Jolly whose diligence and perseverance made possible the obtaining of current patient follow-up information, as well as the preparation of the manuscript for this chapter.

REFERENCES

1. Advance report of final mortality statistics, 1983. *Monthly Vital Statistics Report: National Center of Health Statistics,* 34(suppl 2):6, 1985.
2. Somers AR, Fabian DR: *The Geriatric Imperative.* New York, Appleton-Century-Crofts, 1981, pp 3–6.
3. Pomerance A: Cardiac pathology in the elderly. In *Geriatric Cardiology: Cardiovascular Clinics,* vol 12, no 1. Philadelphia, FA Davis, 1981, pp 9–53.
4. Fleg JL: Alterations in cardiovascular structure and function with advancing age, *Am J Cardiol* 57:33C-44C, 1986.
5. Waller BF, Bloch T, Barker BG, Roe SJ, Hawley DA, Pless JC, Eble JN: The old-age heart: aging changes of the normal elderly heart and cardiovascular disease in 12 necropsy patients aged 91 to 101 years. *Cardiol Clinics* 2:753–779, 1984.
6. Selzer A, Pasternak RC: Congenital and valvular hear disease. In *Geriatric Cardiology: Cardiovascular Clinics,* vol 12, no 1. Philadelphia, FA Davis, 1981, pp 164–198.
7. Olson LJ, Subramanian R, Edwards WD: Surgical pathology of pure aortic insufficiency: a study of 225 cases. *Mayo Clin Proc* 59:835–841, 1984.
8. Hirst AE Jr, Johns VJ Jr, Kime SW Jr: Dissecting aneurysms of the aorta: a review of 505 cases. *Medicine* 37:217, 1958.
9. Miller DC, Stinson EB, Oyer PE, Rossiter SJ, Reitz BA, Griepp RB, Shumway NE: Operative treatment of aortic dissections, experience with 125 patients over a sixteen year period. *J Thorac Cardiovasc Surg* 78:353–382, 1979.
10. Bhat PK, Watanabe K, Roa DB, Luisada AA: Conduction defects in the aging heart. *J Amer Geriatr Soc* 22:517–520, 1974.
11. Killen DA, Reed WA, Wathanacharoen S, Beauchamp

12. Mac Arthur AE, Hall RJ, Gray AG, Mathur VS, Cooley DA: Coronary revascularization in the elderly patient. *J Am Coll Cardiol* 3:1398–1402, 1984.
13. Gersh BJ, Kronmal RA, Frye RL, Schaff HV, Ryan TJ, Gosselin AJ, Kaiser GC, Killip T III: Coronary arteriography and coronary artery bypass surgery: morbidity and mortality in pateint ages 65 years or older. *Circulation* 67:483–491, 1983.
14. Faro RS, Golden MD, Hushang J, Serry C, DeLaria GA, Monson D, Weinberg M, Hunter JA, Najafi H: Coronary revascularization in septuagenarians. *J Thorac Cardiovasc Surg* 86:616–620, 1983.
15. Loop FD, Golding LR, MacMillar JP, Cosgove DM, Lytle BW, Sheldon WC: Coronary artery surgery in women compared with men: analysis of risks and long-term results. *J Am Coll Cardiol* 1:383–390, 1980.
16. Killen DA, Hamaker WR, Reed WA: Coronary artery bypass following percutaneous transluminal coronary antioplasty. *Ann Thorac Surg* 40:133–137, 1985.
17. Meyer J, Wukasch DC, Seybold-Epting W, Ciariello L, Reul GJ, Sandiford FM, Hallman GL, Cooley DA: Coronary artery bypass in patients over 70 years of age; indications and results. *Amer J Cardiol* 36:342–345, 1975.
18. Jeffrey DL, Vijayanger RR, Bognolo DA, Eckstein PF: Results of coronary artery bypass surgery in elderly women. *Ann Thorac Surg* 42:550–553, 1986.
19. Killen DA, Reed WA, Wathanacharoen S, McCallister BD, Bell HH: Postinfarctional rupture of the interventricular septum. *J Cardiovasc Surg* 22:113–116, 1981.
20. Killen DA, Reed WA, Wathanacharoen S, Beauchamp G, Rutherford B: Surgical treatment of papillary muscle rupture. *Ann Thorac Surg* 35:243–248, 1982.
21. Josephson ME, Harken AH, Horwitz LN: Endocardial excision: a new surgical technique for the treatment of recurrent ventricular tachycardia. *Circulation* 60:1430–1439, 1979.
22. Thurer RJ, Luceri RM, Bolooki H: Automatic implantable cardioverter-defibrillator; techniques of implantation and results. *Ann Thorac Surg* 42:143–147, 1986.
23. Weintraub RM, Thurer RL, Wei J, Aroesty JM: Repair of postinfarction ventricular septal defect in the elderly. *J Thorac Cardiovasc Surg* 85:191–196,1983.
24. Weinstein GS, Reed WA, Killen DA: Aortic valvuloplasty for calcific aortic stenosis in the adult. *J Cardiovas Surg* 21:675–680, 1980.
25. King RM, Pluth JR, Giuliana ER, Piehler JM: Mechanical decalcification of the aortic valve. *Ann Thorac Surg* 42:269–272, 1986.
26. Jamieson WRE, Dooner J, Munro I, Janusz MT, Burgess JJ, Miyagishima RR, Gerien AN, Allen P: Cardiac valve replacement in the elderly: a review of 320 consecutive cases. *Circulation* 64 (suppl II):177–183, 1981.
27. Nicolaou N, Kinsley RH: Mitral valve replacement in the elderly. *SA Med J* 65:598–600, 1984.

G, McConahay DR, Arnold M: Normal survival curve after coronary artery bypass. *South Med J* 75:906–912, 1982.

28. Tsai TP, Matloff JM, Chaux A, Kass RM, Lee ME, Czer LSC, DeRobertis MA, Gray RJ: Combined valve and coronary artery bypass procedures in septuagenarians and octogenarians: result in 120 patients. *Ann Thorac Surg* 42:681–684, 1986.

29. Murphy JP, Sweeney MS, Cooley DA: The puig-massana-shiley annuloplasty ring for mitral valve repair: experience in 126 patients. *Ann Thorac Surg* 43:52–58, 1987.

30. Hansen DE, Cahill PD, Derby GC, Miller DC: Relative contributions of the anterior and posterior mitral choradae tendineae to canine global left ventricular systolic function. *J Thorac Cardiovasc Surg* 93:45–55, 1987.

31. Koch JP, Maron BJ, Epstein SE, Morrow AG: Results of operation for obstructive hypertrophic cardiomyopathy in the elderly. *Am J Cardiol* 46:963–966, 1980.

32. Guillet P, Baconnet C, LaBrousse A, Aigueperse I, Andre A, Grosgogeat Y, Laurenceau JL, Temkine J, Vanette A: Left atrial myxoma in the elderly: diagnosis by m-mode and bidemensional echocardiography. *J Am Geriatr Soc* 29:453–459, 1981.

33. Davison ET, Mumford D. Zaman Q, Horowitz R: Left atrial myxoma in the elderly. *J Am Geriatr Soc* 34:229–233, 1986.

34. Stephens DB, Killen DA, Reed WA: Operative experience with 50 thoracic aortic dissections. *South Med J* 75:1467–1470, 1982.

Chapter 16

Pulmonary Disease and Mediastinal Surgery for the Elderly

Richard M. Peters, M.D., F.A.C.S.

In this chapter we will address the disorders of the lungs and the mediastinum and those non-vascular cardiac diseases that occur in the mediastinum. Aging has important effects on the function of the lungs and the chest cage both of which compromise the ability of elderly patients to breathe and to tolerate surgical procedures. These common effects of aging are severely aggravated by the prolonged exposure to many deleterious noxious agents, such as smoking, asbestos, and other environmental pollutants. The integrity of the lungs in the elderly has often been compromised by past infections that leave residual damage to the lungs. These include such diseases as tuberculosis, bronchiectasis, and other pulmonary infections that may lead to fibrosis and destruction of lung tissue.

Conditions in the elderly for which surgical management may be indicated are carcinoma of the lung, asbestosis and mesothelioma, lymphoma, empyema, lung abscess, destruction of lung by infection, and emphysema and its complications, pneumothorax. In the elderly age group, metastatic carcinoma to the chest, which is often complicated by malignant pleural effusions, is not uncommon. Unfortunately, the elderly are also victims of trauma, particularly vehicular injury, which results in fractured ribs, pneumothoraces, and hemothoraces. Among the common pulmonary complications that can come about because of other diseases is aspiration from loss of control of the swallowing mechanism. This can lead to lung abscesses, pneumonia, and, in turn, their complications—pleural effusion and empyema.

The most common disease of the elderly that needs surgical management is carcinoma of the lung. This used to be predominantly a disease of males, but with the marked increase in cigarette smoking by women during and since World War II, the incidence of carcinoma in the lung in women has been rising, until now in much of the United States it is a more common female cancer than carcinoma of the breast. The incidence of chronic infection, such as tuberculosis, has declined and is now seen most commonly in patients who have compromised immune function. It is also seen occasionally in those unfortunate elderly people who have been released from institutions or who have been abandoned by their families to forage for themselves in the streets of our cities. Because carcinoma of the lung is the most common pulmonary disease seen in the elderly patients, it will be used in this chapter to illustrate many of the problems encountered during the surgical treatment of any intrathoracic disease in the elderly. The surgical treatment of carcinoma of the lung requires resection of the lung. It is important to understand the effects of aging on the chest cage and lung prior to thoracotomy.

EFFECTS OF AGING ON CHEST CAGE AND LUNG

With aging, there is a decrease in height due to some narrowing of the invertebral spaces and "wedging" of the vertebral bodies, which usually lead to a degree of progressive kyphosis. The change in the geometry of the chest wall is associated with a decrease in the chest wall compliance. The chest wall becomes stiffer. In emphysema, where the lungs have experienced a breakdown of the elastic tissue, the inward pull of the lungs is decreased, and the chest wall tends to expand, so the elderly patient has a larger AP diameter than a 20-year-old. As the elastic elements of the lung deteriorate (1–3), the actual number of alveoli decreases, which leads to a decrease in the capillaries. In addition, there is an increase of thickness in the small pulmonary arteries, which results in increased pulmonary artery pressure and increased pulmonary vascular resistance (4).

These structural changes are associated with a decrease in the vital capacity and the expiratory reserve volume. At the same time, the functional residual volume is increased from 30% of the total lung capacity at age 20 to levels as high as 55% of the total lung capacity at age 70. The closing volume, or that volume at which the small airways are collapsed, is increased so that, at functional residual volume, a number of small airways, particularly in the bottom of the lungs, may be closed. The consequence of this change is an increasing mismatch between ventilation and perfusion and an inefficiency of the lungs as gas exchangers. The ventilation-perfusion mismatch results in a decline in arterial PO_2 from 95 at age 20 to 75 at age 70, and it reflects an increase in the physiologic shunt from about 5%

at 20 to as high as 15% by age 70. In terms of the patient's total ability to respond to stress, the maximal oxygen consumption falls as much as 35% between ages 20 and 70.

There have been in the past and continue to be many efforts to develop accurate ways of predicting the pulmonary reserve required for a particular patient to tolerate safely a pulmonary resection. These efforts have not met with complete success because the gas exchange is dependent upon three elements: (a) the heart and circulation, (b) the lungs, and (c) the chest cage. (Figure 16.1) These integrated functions must be tested. If one is to use criteria for the adequate function of only one of these three systems, the prediction may be inaccurate. A patient with coronary artery disease or other cardiac problem is going to need to have better lung function, and a patient with compromised lung function will be less tolerant of further compromise of the function of the chest cage and heart. The interaction of these three systems means that it is important to evaluate all of them in the process of predicting the outcome of an operative procedure and also in designing safe and effective postoperative care for patients undergoing thoracic surgical procedures.

The two most commonly used methods for assessing the adequacy of pulmonary reserve are spirometry and arterial blood gases. Accurate

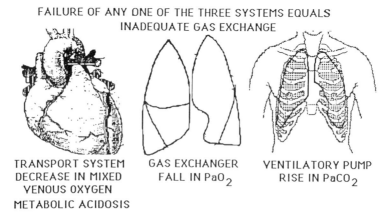

FAILURE OF ANY ONE OF THE THREE SYSTEMS EQUALS
INADEQUATE GAS EXCHANGE

TRANSPORT SYSTEM
DECREASE IN MIXED
VENOUS OXYGEN
METABOLIC ACIDOSIS

GAS EXCHANGER
FALL IN PaO_2

VENTILATORY PUMP
RISE IN $PaCO_2$

Figure 16.1. This figure depicts the three elements necessary for gas exchange—heart and circulation, the lungs, the ventilatory pump, the chest cage and its muscles. The surgeon must appraise both their individual and integrated function. The laboratory data most specific to failure of each component are listed. (Reprinted with permission from Peters RM: Routine respiratory care and support. In Hardy JD (ed): *Hardy's Textbook of Surgery,* ed 2. Philadelphia, JB Lippincott, in press.)

and meaningful spirometry depends on the patient's being able to cooperate and perform at a maximum to test their reserve. A well-done study includes a slow vital capacity to measure the maximum amount of air that the patient can breathe, and a forced vital capacity where the patient makes a maximum effort to expel air as fast as possible after a maximum inspiration. These two simple studies represent the major useful pulmonary measurements. In patients who have interstitial lung disease, such as sarcoidosis, some additional information may be gained by measuring diffusion capacity. The first-second forced expired volume (FEV_1) of the lungs is a measure of the speed with which the patient can force air out. FEV_1 and forced vital capacity both decrease with age. This decrease in the FEV_1 is due to the changes in the lung and also probably due to a decrease in muscle strength of the repiratory muscles as patients age.

Spirometry results should include the absolute value for each measurement and the percentage of the predicted value. The predicted normal values for spirometry are related both to the size and age of the individual. The unwary surgeon may make serious errors when dealing with elderly patients because, as age increases, calculations of normal values predict a decrease in FEV_1 and forced vital capacity. If only the percentage of normal is used to assess operability as the patient ages, the progressively smaller reserve will be missed.

Unfortunately, as people age, they do not necessarily need less reserve to function, nor is it easier for them to have a pulmonary resection. Therefore, in patients, particularly in the eighth decade of life or older, one must not use prediction formulas to decide whether the functional reserve is adequate, but one must look at the absolute figures. Perhaps more useful would be to use an age-45 predicted normal value, regardless of the age of the patient. Table 16.1 gives some of the values that have been put forward for setting the limits for pulmonary resection. For the patient undergoing pulmonary resection, the amount of function that would be left after resection is critical. To provide this essential information, it was necessary to develop a methodology that would allow the prediction of function remaining after pulmonary resection.

Spirometry should always be interpreted in association with evaluation of a chest x-ray, as illustrated in the clinical examples to follow. By assessing what segments of the lung need to be removed, the portion of lung that will remain can be predicted from figures of normal percentage of total tissue in each segment (5). However, this type of prediction may overestimate the decrease in function if the diseased portion of the lung to be removed is essentially nonfunctional, as it might be in a patient with central carcinoma obstructing the bronchus.

A more sophisticated way of predicting postpulmonary resection function is to perform a quantitative ventilation-perfusion scan. With such a scan, one can predict how much of the actual function is performed by the portions of the lung to be resected. By simple calculation, subtracting that percentage from the total gives one the prediction of the remaining function (6). An accepted rule of thumb is that a patient needs an FEV_1 of 800 ml. However, the 800 ml FEV_1 is a rough approximation that should not be used as an absolute criterion.

Table 16.1 Risk for Pulmonary Resection[a]

Test	High Risk	Moderate Risk	Low Risk
Vital capacity (VC) (L)	<1.85	1.85–3.0	>4.0
First-second forced expired volume (FEV_1)	<1.2	1.2–3.0	>3.2
Maximum voluntary ventilation (MVV) (L/min)	<28	>30 <80	>80
Maximum midexpiratory flow (FEF) (L/sec)	<1.0	>1.0 <2.0	>2.0

[a]Adapted with permission from Table 14.1 in Peters RM: The lung. In Peters RM, Peacock EE Jr, Benfield JR (eds): *The Scientific Management of Surgical Patients.* Boston, Little, Brown and Co, 1983.

Recent studies have suggested, as one might expect because the function of gas exchange involves the heart and the lung and chest cage, that the best predictor of pulmonary reserve would be exercise testing and measurement of the maximum oxygen uptake. However, this particular method of testing is not so useful in patients who have intermittent claudication or skeletal disease that limits their exercise capacity. A study done in Sweden showed that exercise testing was a superior predictor because it integrates the function of all three critical function components: the chest wall, the heart, and the lungs. They studied 82 patients over 70 years old and found the maximum oxygen consumption was reached at a mean level of 83 watts of exercise during 6 minutes (7). Patients whose work capacity fell below 83 watts had an operative mortality of 22%; those above it had none. This study supports the important principle: the risk factors defined by spirometry must not be considered alone, but in conjunction with the assessment of the general health of the patient. The factors most important to evaluate are (1) evidence of muscle wasting, (2) the activity level they have been able to achieve prior to their acute illness, (3) if the patient is continuing smoking, (4) evidence of chronic bronchitis and whether it has been maximally treated with a full and carefully planned medical regimen, (5) if the patient is overweight.

In patients who show evidence of compromised pulmonary function, preoperative blood gases are important. If the patient has a PCO_2 above 45, it is evidence that the patient already has ventilatory insufficiency. The patient with these values is not a candidate for pulmonary resection unless there is clear evidence that, at operation, something can be done that will improve function.

The significance of change in PO_2 is more difficult to predict. Resection of an atelectatic perfused area of the lung may improve PO_2. No set figure for the lower limit on PO_2 is appropriate. The PO_2 must be evaluated in terms of the abnormality of the lung to be resected.

A history of angina requires a careful workup in order to evaluate the degree of cardiac abnormality that occurs with exercise testing and with isotope studies. If these tests are positive, one must define the coronary anatomy with coronary angiograms. For patients who have significant coronary artery disease, the critical decision is the feasibility of a coronary bypass, which can be followed usually at a later date by the pulmonary resection (8). The final and important consideration when dealing with elderly patients who are going to require a thoracotomy is their mental status. Patients who are unable to cooperate postoperatively, cannot cough effectively, are hard to mobilize, and are likely to pull out chest tubes are poor operative risks. They will have a significantly increased morbidity and mortality. The increased morbidity and mortality must be considered in deciding the social and ethical issues that are inherent in advising operation on patients who cannot cooperate.

With the exception that one does not have to anticipate the effects of the lungs being removed, the same set of criteria is applicable to patients requiring other forms of intrathoracic operations.

CHARACTERISTICS OF CARCINOMA OF THE LUNG IN THE ELDERLY

Thirty percent of all cancer of the lung is squamous cell carcinoma, 30% is adenocarcinoma, 20% is small cell carcinoma, and about 20% is large cell undifferentiated carcinoma (9). Squamous carcinoma is more often proximal, occurs in the larger bronchi, and is therefore more likely to produce bronchial obstruction. It tends to metastasize late. Adenocarcinoma is usually present as a peripheral coin lesion and is more likely to have blood-borne metastases than the squamous cell type. Small cell carcinoma is more commonly proximal or central in location. It tends to metastasize early, and it can produce hormones that result in many types of endocrine abnormalities. Large cell undifferentiated carcinomas tend to be large, often with central necrosis. Fifty percent of patients at the time the diagnosis of carcinoma of the lung is made will have stage 3 tumor, which is not amenable to resection.

Carcinoma of the lung in the elderly age group behaves differently than in the younger age group (10–12). A number of these studies have shown that older patients are more likely to have earlier stages of carcinoma of the lung. Huang (13) suggests that older patients have a lower DNA protein content in their tumors, which may explain slower tumor growth and less frequent metastases. In contrast to virtually every other site of carcinoma, there is an inverse relationship between age and stage at diagnosis in carcinoma of the lung. The incidence of carcinoma is greater in older patients, but it is also more likely to be confined to lung at the time of diagnosis. Carcinoma of the lung is associated with a short time course in all age groups if it is not effectively treated. In most cases, survival for 2 and 3 years after surgical treatment signifies confidence for a cure. Five-year survival often indicates that permanant cure has been achieved. This is in constrast to breast or colon cancer, where recurrences may occur in significant numbers at 5 and 10 years. There are those who have written off the 70-year age group as candidates for pulmonary resection. Both the biological nature and the effectiveness of modern thoracic surgery make this attitude unsupportable.

An important problem to consider in carcinoma of the lung is that the carcinogen that induces the carcinoma, whether cigarette smoke or other pollutants, affects the entire lung parenchyma. Therefore, if one is successful in treating a first carcinoma of the lung and the patient survives, the incidence of second carcinomas increases. The thoracic surgeon must keep in mind the possibility of a second carcinoma of the lung when planning any lung resection. Removal of more lung than is absolutely essential for a first carcinoma may preclude the successful surgical treatment of the second carcinoma. This is particularly important in the elderly patient, where carcinomas are likely to be local and resection of a second cancer can be successful later on if the pulmonary reserve is still adequate. Patients who have had a carcinoma of the head and neck are very likely to have either synchronous or metachronous carcinoma of the lung (14). These patients can also present difficult clinical decisions.

Early diagnosis and treatment of carcinoma of the lung are often thwarted by asymptomatic cancers and also by symptomatic cancers for which the patient seeks help, but for which an incomplete workup leads to a failure to diagnose. Central carcinomas that cause bronchial obstruction that causes hemoptysis and pneumonia are most likely to produce symptoms. In caring for all patients who develop a pneumonia, and particularly for smokers over 45, the physician should be certain that the pneumonia is not a complication of bronchial obstruction from a tumor. Three to 4 weeks following treatment for the pneumonia, the physician should always obtain an x-ray to be sure that there is complete resolution. If resolution is not complete, the patient needs further study, in particular bronchoscopy, to be certain that there is no obstructing lesion. Hemoptysis is always an indication for bronchoscopy at the earliest possible time. The hemoptysis that is caused by a central carcinoma usually occurs at the time of a respiratory infection, when cough is increased and vigorous. The patients with lung cancer usually have only blood streaking in their sputum; they do not cough up significant amounts of blood. Cytologic examination of sputa with blood streaking is useful.

Peripheral lesions are more often picked up in the early stages by the routine chest film. In high-risk patients, people with history of heavy smoking, and/or toxic chemical exposures, it may be appropriate to obtain periodic chest films. This is a controversial subject that concerns the question of cost benefits that is so popular at this time. Cytology on sputums for discovery of early carcinoma of the lung is also not cost effective.

In a patient suspected of having carcinoma of the lung, either peripheral or central, it is our practice at the earliest possible time to carry out fiberoptic bronchoscopy. In the central cancers, the lesion will be easily viewed, and direct biopsy or brushings will provide a cytologic diagnosis. For peripheral lesions, fluoroscopic-directed brushing and transthoracic fine needle biopsy should be done to obtain cells for cytologic diagnosis. Bronchoscopy provides other information. If the cancer is central, bronchoscopy allows one to evaluate whether resection is feasible and how much lung will have to be taken out to encompass the tumor. If the carina is widened and blunted, then there is a strong suggestion that there is metastasis to the subcarinal nodes. Transcarinal needle biopsy is a useful method of verifying the involvement of subcarinal nodes (15).

Some comment is in order about the value of transthoracic needle biopsy. In a patient with a coin lesion, if the needle biopsy is negative, thoracotomy and excisional biopsy may still be required to be certain that the carcinoma is not missed. It is our experience that, in 95% of our patients, with the use of transbronchial biopsy and fine needle biopsy we obtain a preoperative diagnosis. Having a preoperative diagnosis shortens and simplifies the operative procedure and allows us to emphasize to the patient the importance of undertaking the risk of thoracotomy. We have found the morbidity of fine needle biopsy to be very low and the mortality negligible. The major morbidity is the pneumothorax, and in most circumstances the pneumothorax responds to the placement of a small catheter for closed suction drainage, if any treatment at all is needed.

When the cytologic diagnosis is established, it is essential to determine the extent of the tumor. Studies of ours and those of others have shown the futility of obtaining bone, liver, and brain radionucleotide scans to assess the extent of tumor in patients who have no neurologic symptoms, have a normal alkaline phosphatase, and have no evidence of bone pain (16, 17). The evidence is unclear about whether routine head computed tomography (CT) scans might pick up a significant number of patients with silent brain metastasis. Less is known about the study that should be the most accurate test, a magnetic resonance imaging (MRI) scan. In 1987, the CT scan and ultrasound have replaced the radionucleotide scan for evaluating the liver.

For assessment of the extent of tumor in the chest, we have used the CT scan (18). CT scan evidence of mediastinal lymph nodes larger than 1 cm in size is an indication for a mediastinoscopy. If the nodes are less than 1 cm in size, we proceed with a thoracotomy without mediastinoscopy. Because some patients with CT scan nodes less than 1 cm will have intranodal disease, in a poor-risk patient, we are much more inclined to do a mediastinoscopy regardless of the finding of the CT scan. It is extremely important to point out that nodes greater than 1 cm in size may not be carcinoma. The false-positive rate is over 20%. If there is node enlargement, a mediastinoscopy is mandatory to ascertain whether the nodes are involved with carcinoma.

Carcinomas are best staged by the anatomic TNM system: T=tumor size; N=nodal involvement; M=distant metastases. Precision of TNM staging is an essential part of the workup of a patient with carcinoma of the lung. At present, stages 1, 2, and 3 correlate the anatomic system with outcome. The classifications are being questioned because presence or absence of lymph node metastases has become a major determinant of survival (19). The size of the tumor, the location of lymph nodes, and the presence of distal metastases are individually identified. Using a lymph node map based on the anatomic structures within the mediastinum provides not only more accurate but also extra information. We use the map effectively for two purposes: (1) as an anatomic guide to very accurate nodal mediastinoscopy (20) and (2) to identify the location of the excised nodes to permit correlation of positive nodes of various locations to the prognosis of disease.

Differential diagnosis of coin lesions always raises the question of whether the tumor is primary in the lung or whether it might be metastatic from colon, breast, or another area. In the older age group, the overwhelming likelihood is that the tumor is primary in the lung. However, it is important to make some simple clinical tests to minimize the chance of missing a metastatic lesion. These include, of course, carefully obtaining the history of any prior carcinomas and the evaluation of the likelihood of a metastatic lesion. Careful examination of the breast, search for evidence of melanoma or other obvious surface carcinomas, and evaluation of the important source of metastatic disease, the colon, are always done. We always obtain a complete history of change in bowel function and ascertain that the patient has no occult blood in the stools.

Surgical Treatment of Carcinoma of the Lung

As pointed out above, the important part of the workup is to determine whether the carcinoma is likely to be controlled by surgical resection. Determining the stage of disease, particularly whether the patient has distant metastases or mediastinal node involvement, is more important than size of tumor in predicting its resectability. Equally important is determining whether the patient can tolerate the removal of a portion of the lung or lung and adjacent chest cage that could be essential to the complete removal of all of the cancer.

Until the early 1950s, the accepted treatment for all patients with carcinoma of the lung was a total pneumonectomy. Because not all patients could withstand this extensive resection, a number of patients received lesser resections. A classic paper by Dr. Churchill, presenting results of lobectomy for cancer of lung, evoked one of the most interesting discussions by all of the pioneers of cardiothoracic surgery (21). They complimented Dr. Churchill on his presentation and then declared their convictions that pneumonectomy, if possible, was the treatment for carcinoma of the lung of any size. However, following this presentation by Dr. Churchill, there was a progressive change, and the accepted form of treatment for cancer of the lung became a lobectomy where possible and pneumonectomy only if the tumor could not be resected by a lobectomy. With the change to lobectomy as the standard operation, surgeons started to operate on patients who could not tolerate lobectomy and did lesser resections.

There have now been a number of reports that begin to compare the experience with lobectomy versus lesser resections (22–24). When one hears the discussants of these reports, one is faced with the realization that a strange thing has occurred in our approach to science. This is the statement that the standard for which all treatment of carcinoma of the lung must be measured is now a lobectomy, a form of therapy that has never been subjected to any control studies that would justify this argument. There now are a number of studies of series of patients that show that limited resection gives very acceptable results and, most importantly, lowers the operative mortality and immediate operative morbidity (22–24). The problem that occurs with evaluating these various methods is that a rational basis of comparing the effects of various resections has not been worked out. There are no good studies of the incidence of local recurrence; the effects of operative mortality on group survival are also disregarded. The quality of life, namely how short of breath the patient is and whether he or she is able to do the activities that make life enjoyable, is also completely neglected. Finally, no consideration is given in these studies to the fact that the incidence of a second carcinoma is increasing as treatment success occurs. The more conservative the primary resection, the greater the chance of being able to treat a second carcinoma.

In this author's opinion, time will shortly bring us to the conclusion that the purpose of pulmonary resection is to remove the tumor in toto with the smallest amount of the lung possible. It is essential to provide an adequate margin to encompass all of the tumor. There is now one randomized prospective study underway that is designed to determine the incidence of local recurrence with limited resection versus recurrence with lobectomy. All thoracic surgeons should carefully collect prospective data on their patients and evaluate whether limited resections have smaller operative mortality and morbidity rates than lobectomy and a recurrence rate that is acceptable. At present, we use wedge or segmental resections to preserve function in a large portion of our elderly patients with limited pulmonary functions. In elderly patients with T3 tumors and chest wall invasion that would require a pulmonary resection and chest cage resection, the risks are very high. Wilcox, in a study of pulmonary resections in patients over 70 years of age, reached the conclusion that combined pulmonary and chest wall resection carried a very high risk (25). Also, as patients pass the 70th year, the risks of pneumonectomy begin to escalate logarithmically with age.

In patients with carcinoma of the lung, there should not be just one operative approach—pneumonectomy, lobectomy, or wedge resection. Both the amount of lung removed and the surgical incision used for this resection should be carefully tailored to meet the patient's needs. Unfortunately, most surgeons still use the complete posterolateral thoracotomy incision for all pulmonary resections. The major cause of morbidity of a patient having a pulmonary resection is not the operation on the lung but the effects of the operation on the chest cage. Procedures that limit damage to the chest cage can improve the prognosis of patients significantly. For wedge resections, a short thoracotomy that is carefully designed to overlie the area of lung to be removed permits minimal opening of the rib spreader, sparing the patient the disruption of the chest cage. In patients who require a lobectomy, we usually use a posterolateral thoracotomy, but leave the serratus anterior intact. The group in Chicago under Drs. Faber and Jensik has advocated the axillary incision without division of the latissimus or the serratus (26). More recently, Urschel and others have advocated in selected patients the use of a midline thoracotomy incision (27). The midline thoracotomy is the least painful and the least disruptive to the chest wall unless the rib spreader or sternal spreader has been markedly elevated and posterior ribs have been fractured. When the sternum is reapproximated and is immobile, the point of incision does not have to move so the pain is far less. With an incision in the posterolateral chest, with every cough and every breath the muscles tend to pull the closure apart. If a double-lumen tube is used to ventilate the patient and the retractor is carefully positioned, all lobes, except perhaps the left lower lobe, can be resected through a median sternotomy without great difficulty. It is not appropriate or feasible to go into the details of these various incisions in this chapter, but we urge the thoracic surgeon who is doing thoracotomies on the elderly to recognize that the posterolateral thoracotomy incision is only one of the many methods that may be used when entering the chest.

APPROPRIATE ANESTHESIA AND PERIOPERATIVE CARE OF ELDERLY PATIENTS REQUIRING THORACOTOMY

A major factor responsible for increasing the safety of thoracotomy and pulmonary resection in elderly patients has been the progress in anesthesiology. This has been accompanied by such technical improvements as one-lung anesthesia and by the cardiac anesthetic techniques used for patients requiring coronary artery bypass. The most common cause of death following pulmonary resection is a coronary occlusion. This might be expected because patients who have carcinoma of the lung also have all of the risk factors for coronary artery disease—heavy smoking, often little exercise, and not the most exemplary lifestyle. The safety of thoracotomies can be enhanced by careful, controlled anesthesia that avoids transient hypo- or hypertension and compromise of cardiac function. Prevention of periods of hypo- and hypertension also requires careful control of perioperative fluids, anesthetics, and analgesics.

We have found that the use of the double-lumen tube has a number of very real advantages. The double-lumen tube allows collapse of the lung undergoing resection and enables the surgeon to do the resection through a smaller incision or through an incision that gives less exposure, such as the sternal splitting incision. The double-lumen tube is necessary in some instances to prevent spillage into the good lung in patients who have abscesses, empyemas, or bleeding. It is important for anesthesiologists to obtain experience with one-lung anesthesia so that it is not used only at times of crisis. In addition to the classic tubes, there are now available tubes in which the full lumen for the size of a single-lumen endotracheal tube is available. A balloon attached to the tube is positioned with a fiberoptic bronchoscope in the major bronchus of the lung to be operated on. This avoids the shortcomings of the classical double-lumen tube, which is a stiff endotracheal tube with a small internal diameter.

Fluid Therapy

In the preoperative preparation, it is important to make sure that elderly patients, particularly those with emphysema, are not taken to the operating room in a dehydrated state. Patients placed on nothing by month at midnight usually receive nothing by mouth after they go to sleep on the evening before operation. If they are not operated on early in the morning, they will continue to be without fluids until the time of the operation. This may represent 14 to 18 hours of no fluid intake. In elderly patients with emphysema and bronchitis, this results in thickening of the secretions, and they are unable to cough up their sputum. The dehydration also results in a patient who arrives at the operating room relatively hypovolemic. The induction of anesthesia frequently leads to hypotension that the anesthesiologist tries to correct with the infusion of balanced salt solution. This in turn leads to the problem of excessive intraoperative fluid infusion. A much safer regimen is to give patients a liter of intravenous 5% glucose in water early in the morning the day of the operation to keep their hydration normal when they go to the operating room.

During the induction of anesthesia and throughout the operative procedure, fluid and blood loss should be replaced by precise administration of adequate but not excessive amounts of fluid. Pulmonary resections rarely require transfusions. Careful opening of the chest with a meticulous hemostasis and precise dissection usually can limit the blood loss to less than 500 cc or 700 cc at the most. These are amounts that do not in the non-anemic patient warrant a transfusion. If crystalloid or colloid solutions are infused in adequate quantities to maintain blood volume, a hematocrit above 25 is usually adequate. In patients with coronary disease, some drop in hematocrit decreases blood viscosity, increasing blood flow to areas of myocardium served by narrowed vessels (28). A lower hematocrit may also act to lower the incidence of pulmonary emboli. The use of unneccessary transfusions adds all the other known risks, particularly those of non-A, non-B hepatitis and, what is now becoming a real possibility, induction of the AIDS virus.

It is essential to recognize that patients following pulmonary resection have a decrease in the pulmonary vascular bed. To maintain the same preoperative cardiac output, an increase in the blood flow through the remaining capillary bed is necessary. Increase in flow in any capillary bed results in increase in fluid filtration. Fluid filtered in the remaining lung is dependent on the pulmonary lymphatics for its removal. When a portion of the lung is removed, lymphatics are removed also. The patient following pulmonary resection has a greater fluid filtration through the remaining lung with a lower lymph pump capacity. He or she is more vulnerable to postoperative pulmonary edema. In our laboratories, we have made some studies of this problem (29). Pulmonary edema's occurrence is best correlated with excessive intraoperative fluid infusion, which usually results in a large urine output in the immediate postoperative period.

It is important for the surgeon to check carefully to determine how much intraoperative fluid was given. Patients who receive a large amount of intraoperative salt solution and have high urine output are vulnerable to postpulmonary resection pulmonary edema. The pulmonary edema becomes clinically manifest after the first 24 hours, usually 36 to 48 hours postoperatively. From the time of lung removal, the lymphatic pump is progressively falling behind until clinical edema manifests itself. The accumulation of fluid within the interstitium of the lungs overflows into the alveoli to produce clinical pulmonary edema. In individuals who are found by careful postoperative evaluation to be at risk of getting pulmonary edema, it is essential to induce early diuresis. If they show any evidence of respiratory difficulty, intubate them early and maintain intubation and ventilation until their pulmonary function is clearly back to normal and pulmonary congestion has resolved. The complication of postpneumonectomy pulmonary edema is usually lethal. Aggressive diuresis and ventilatory support are essential.

A patient, following a pulmonary resection, increases minute ventilation, which, in turn, increases insensible water losses. In the postoperative period, care should begin to be taken not to overhydrate, but also to avoid underhydration. It is an error to stop all intravenous fluids in the morning following the operation and then disappear for the day and come back in the evening to find the patient dehydrated. It is better to give a modest amount of intravenous fluid throughout the first day until the patients have shown that they can sustain an oral intake adequate to avoid postoperative dehydration and to avoid thick secretions that cannot be coughed up. Patients should continue to have a minimum of 1200 to 1400 cc of free water (5% glucose in water) in the first and second postoperative days to replace their insensible and renal water losses.

Postoperative Pain Control

The most common type of postoperative complication for all patients is respiratory. Thoracotomy amplifies the incidence and severity of postoperative pulmonary complications. The pulmonary complications are not initiated by difficulties with the lung, but by malfunction of the chest bellows that is principally the result of pain. The usual manner of controlling this pain is to adminster morphine compounds, but in the elderly patients, the level of morphine necessary for control of pain frequently results in central respiratory depression and underventilation. Most of these patients have emphysema and so have inefficient lungs. When one adds an inefficient chest bellows to inefficent lungs, ventilatory insufficiency is common. The use of a ventilator increases the risk of disruption of bronchial closure and weakening of ventilatory muscles by disuse. It is important to use an analgesia technique that allows early spontaneous breathing, deep breaths and cough, and early getting out of bed. The goals of postoperative care depend on a method of controlling pain that does not require systemic narcosis (30). We have found it most useful to introduce an epidural catheter in the high lumbar area or the thoracic region and use continuous infusion of fentanyl anesthesia, a short-acting narcotic.

The protocol that we use for this infusion is as follows: The epidural catheter is put in just prior to or just following the thoracotomy. The catheter is inserted and in a routine manner is carried all the way up the back, taped along the spine, and the entry port for injection is taped at the shoulder. The catheter and the connection should be well secured. Strict sterile procedure is essential. After the anesthesiologists put in the epidural catheter, they give a test dose of xylocaine to ensure that the placement is adequate. The fentanyl solution contains 1250 mcg in 250 ml of normal saline (5 ug/ml) and is administered with an infusion pump at the rate of 10 to 20 ml/hr. It is imperative that *no sedatives or narcotics other than specifically ordered fentanyl infusion* run into the epidural catheter. Absolutely no other narcotics are to be given to the patient by any route, and the infusion should be discontinued immediately if the patient develops any side effects from the epidural fentanyl. These might include itching, urinary retention, nausea, and respiratory depression. If the dressing becomes loose or wet or the catheter becomes disconnected, the anesthesiologist checks the system immediately. The epidural catheter fluid pathway must be handled with strict sterile technique. If the patient exhibits profound respiratory depression (respiratory rate less than 6), oxygen by mask should be administered at 6 L/min and Narcan 0.2 mg IV given. The patient should be encouraged to breathe deeply.

We have administered this range of fentanyl without difficulty in the intensive care unit (ICU) and also after the patients are discharged from the ICU. We usually continue the epidural fentanyl for 2 or 3 days although in some cases we have continued for considerably longer, in one case as long as 2 weeks. We consider it critically important that the patients not receive other narcotics while the fentanyl is being given, except after in-person evaluation by the physician. There is a risk of cumulative effect of epidural narcotics leading to acute respiratory depression if the two forms of therapy are being administered simultaneously.

Patients who have had this form of analgesia have moderate euphoria at the very low dose of fentanyl and a concomitant superior pain control. They cough effectively. To control pain in this manner for these few days reduces the need for narcotics later on. If it appears that the acute immediate perioperative pain is well handled with the epidural analgesia, the mobility and cough are maintained with just moderate use of oral narcotics or analgesics. The result is quick re-expansion of the lungs, early oral fluids, and low incidence of atelectasis. It is hard to overemphasize the salutary effect of this form of control of postoperative pain. Its value is most apparent in the elderly or patients who have evidence of emphysema.

Care of Chest Drainage

A few words should be given about the care of chest tubes in these elderly patients. For lobectomy, segmental resection, or wedge resection of lung, a right angle chest tube is inserted through the fifth or sixth interspace in the posterior line, placed down into the posterior gutter, and a short anterior tube is inserted through the third or fourth interspace in the midaxilla, positioned up into the apex of the chest. The tubes are connected to closed drainage and 20 cm of water suction until the air leak is small, at which time they are put on gravity drainage. Most patients are gotten out of bed the night of the operation if the operation was done in the morning. They first sit on the side of the bed and then in a chair next to the bed and progress to walking by the end of 36 hours. The chest tube devices are placed in a small cart, usually the type that is used for laundry bags, so the patient can wheel the cart about and ambulate not later than 48 hours following operation. For ambulation, it is reasonable to disconnect the chest tube suction for a short time even if the patient still has an air leak. If the air leak stops and fluid effusion is less than 80 to 100 cc per day, it is our practice to remove the chest tubes. It is important not to leave chest tubes in for fear that leak may recur. Chest tubes have a negative effect as well as a therapeutic effect and should only be left in as long as they are essential. They decrease the patient's mobility and cause pain, which inhibit cough. A limited apical air cap that is not increasing is a benign space that will usually absorb itself within the first 3 postoperative weeks.

Arrhythmias

One of the not uncommon complications of thoracotomy and pulmonary resection is a supraventricular tachycardia, atrial fibrillation, or atrial flutter. This is usually adequately treated by digitalization to increase the AV block, but if the high ventricular rate is poorly tolerated, one of the calcium blockers should be given to control the heart rate. Digitalis should be maintained for 6 to 8 weeks to produce an adequate AV block to control tachycardia should the atrial fibrillation or flutter recur. There is a great difference of opinion about the advisability in all patients over age 60 of preoperative digitalization. With more skill in the handling of cardiac drugs by cardiothoracic surgeons, the indications for preoperative digitalis have decreased. We now confine its use to those patients for whom digitalis is indicated on the basis of pre-existing heart disease. With a regimen of double-lumen tube, careful control of fluids, epidural anesthesia, early effective cough, and early ambulation, the duration of chest tube insertion and hospitalization has decreased for patients requiring thoracotomy.

INFECTIONS

Surgical therapy is never a primary treatment for infections. Rather, it is the treatment of the complications of infections. The complications can be divided into those that occur in the pleura, those that occur within the lungs and by etiologic agent, those due to pyogenic bacteria, and those due to fungus and tuberculous infections. The pyogenic infections occur as complications of pneumonia, lung abscesses, trauma, and operations within the chest.

The most common infections within the chest are infections of the pleura—empyema. An empyema is an abscess of the pleural cavity. The diagnosis of empyema is made by an appropriately placed thoracentesis and a well-done culture to identify organisms. As do all abscesses, it requires drainage. The difference in the treatment of pleural infections compared to infections in other areas of the body is that open drainage will lead to collapse of the lung and a sucking chest wound. Until such a time as the lung is adherent to the parietal pleura, the primary treatment of an intrapleural infection is early closed chest drainage (31). Particularly in the elderly, for an infected pleural effusion greater than 150 or 200 cc, it is advisable to put in a chest tube to avoid the complications of a chronic empyema. Of course, simultaneously, the patient should have appropriate antibiotics. If drainage fails to remove all the fluid, one must determine whether the fluid is loculated and another procedure is necessary. In a healthy, vigorous individual with a loculated empyema and available effective antibiotics to control the spread of infection, one choice is to do an open thoracotomy and decortication and evacuate the empyema. In most elderly patients, this more radical form of therapy is not indicated. A safer and more appropriate therapy is open thoracostomy drainage in which the loculation is broken down. Open drainage can, if necessary, be done under local anesthesia with resection of one rib, preferably in the dependent portion of the empyema, usually the sixth or seventh interspace in the posterior axillary line.

To determine whether the patient will withstand open drainage, two methods are available. One way is to look at the type of drainage. If fluid sedimentation is more than 50% cellular mass, open drainage will almost certainly be tolerated because the lung will be stuck to the chest wall. The second method is to open the chest, and if it is found that the lung tends to collapse, a large tube can be placed and attached to water seal until such time as the lung does stick and open drainage becomes safe.

If prior to any tap there is any air fluid level, one knows that there is a bronchopleural fistula. It is very urgent to drain these patients because the bronchopleural fistula provides a route for the infected pus to flood the tracheobronchial tree and flood the good dependent lung. When doing this drainage, it is important not to put the healthy lung in the dependent position during the operation. Set the patient up or use a well-placed double lumen tube before laying the patient with a good lung down.

The pyogenic lung abscesses occasionally require surgical therapy. Pyogenic lung abscesses are principally the result of aspiration and therefore appear in the posterior portions of the lungs, the superior segment of the lower lobe, and the posterior segment of the upper lobe. These abscesses should be treated by vigorous antibiotic therapy, usually large doses of penicillin, and the patient should be bronchoscoped to remove any aspirated material and ascertain whether the abscess is actually a complication of an endobronchial tumor. With appropriate antibiotic therapy and postural drainage, most lung abscesses will resolve. Many of them are complicated by pleural effusions, and occasionally the abscess ruptures into the pleural cavity, a complication that demands immediate pleural drainage to prevent flooding of the tracheobronchial tree with pleural fluid.

Abscesses that persist in a sick patient may require drainage or removal. If the patient is toxic, with modern interventional radiology, a small drainage catheter can be introduced under radiologic control into the abscess. This is often a successful and definitive method of drainage. If a small catheter drainage is not effective in the elderly, very sick patient, surgical drainage may be necessary. Drainage is best done by localizing the area on the chest wall where the cavity abuts the parietal pleura and resecting a portion of rib right over the area. Usually with a chronic lung abscess, the area over the abscess will be adherent to the pleura so that the abscess can be entered and drained without contaminating the pleural cavity. If there are no adhesions, then it is best to pack the wound for a few days and allow some adhesions to develop before draining the cavity. It must be remembered that one of the problems of pyogenic abscesses such as this is hemorrhage. Therefore, hard tubes that might erode a vessel should not be put into the lung. If the patient is a good risk, resection of the cavity may be warranted.

Other infections of the lung in the elderly that occasionally require resection are the infections that occur as a result of complications of tuberculosis or fungus or a combination of these two. With modern chemotherapy for tuberculosis, it is rare that the elderly patient will be a candidate for resection. Tuberculosis is a benign disease. Most types of chronic pulmonary disease that in this day warrant resection are far advanced, for which resection is rarely indicated in the elderly patient (32). One would reserve surgical treatment for life-threatening complications, such as hemorrhage. One of the common combinations that leads to hemorrhage in the patient with tuberculous cavities is the colonization of the cavity with aspergilla organisms. These patients develop a fungus tumor within the cavity, which then erodes vessels and results in significant hemorrhage (33). Complications of chronic pulmonary cavities can present difficult therapeutic problems of balancing the threat of exsanguinating hemorrhage against the usually very compromised pulmonary function. If hemorrhage is uncontrollable, conservative methods may be the most appropriate. These can include the introduction of a Fogarty catheter into the bronchus of the bleeding area and blowing the balloon up to occlude the bronchus and tamponade hemorrhage in this manner. Some advocate interventional radiology to embolize the bronchial arteries, which usually gives only temporary respite. Particularly in the elderly, embolization carries the risk of some of the material blocking vessels to the spinal cord and producing neurologic damage.

It is impossible to outline a scenario for elderly patients with this complication. The surgeon must make the difficult judgment of what pulmonary function the patient will have left after resection. In patients with chronic abscess and bleeding, it is essential to use a double-lumen tube or some method to isolate and tamponade the bleeding area of the lung. The destroyed area of lungs usually has dense adhesions to the chest and mediastinum, and it is a slow and difficult dissection to reach the hilar vessels. In the elderly, the principal caveat in the treatment of the complications of pulmonary infections is conservatism. Be certain that the proposed surgery is going to improve the patient's condition, not threaten his or her life.

MEDIASTINAL TUMORS

Mediastinal tumors are often diagnosed by routine chest film or occasionally when a chest film is taken for symptoms as diverse as vague discomfort to severe pain and the effects of superior vena caval obstructions. A preoperative

CT scan of the chest is then essential. In most instances, a good indication of the type of mediastinal tumor present can be obtained with CT scanning. Histologic diagnosis of mediastinal tumors in most instances requires a generous biopsy. To make a differential diagnosis among lymphoma, thymoma, or germ cell tumor taxes a pathologist even with a generous biopsy. A mediastinal tumor that looks like lymphoma on CT scan may actually be one of the other tumors. To provide modern specific treatment requires a generous amount of tissue for precise definition using both cytologic and immunologic techniques.

THYMOMA AND MYASTHENIA GRAVIS

Thymoma is more frequently associated with myasthenia gravis in the elderly (34). Two peaks in the incidence of non-thymoma myasthenia gravis are between 10 and 30 years of age and again at 60 to 70 years. Following resection of the thymus, the remission rates are the same for both elderly and young patients. The remission rate gradually increases for all age groups over at least 3 years to become between 50% to 60%.

Elderly patients undergoing thymectomy for myasthenia gravis should have the same preparation as used in younger patients: optimum drug control of the myasthenia gravis, including, if necessary, steroids. Two approaches to operation are presently advocated for thymectomy without tumor for myasthenia gravis: a cervical incision without the opening of the sternum (35, 36) or a sternal splitting incision. This transcervical method is criticized by some because it is likely that portions of the thymus will be left in the mediastinum. Sternal splitting incision is mandatory in the patient with a tumor of the thymus. Determination of whether a thymoma is malignant or benign depends on the surgeon identifying whether the tumor has remained within the capsule or has invaded outside the capsule of the gland. Attempts should be made to remove all the tumor even if it requires resection of the pericardium. In elderly patients, resection of a phrenic nerve is almost certainly unwarranted because they will be unable to sustain ventilation with a total phrenic paralysis.

PLEURAL NEOPLASMS

Pleural malignancies have two principal etiologies: the mesotheliomas and metastatic malignancies to the pleura. For half a century, asbestos has been a widely spread pollutant of construction industries and foretells a long period of consequences. Over the next few decades, many elderly people will fall victim to this tragic carelessness. Asbestos exposure can cause the relatively benign disease, abestosis, which manifests as fibrotic changes within the lung and pleural plaques that inhibit pulmonary function without surgical implications. The surgeon must not confuse asbestosis with malignant disease. Benign mesotheliomas are usually pedunculated tumors that arise from visceral pleura often in an interlobar fissure. They are not associated with asbestos exposure. Usually they are picked up on routine chest x-ray.

Malignant mesotheliomas may be localized or diffuse with effusion and encasement of the lung (37). The most common symptoms are pain and dyspnea. The peak incidence is between the ages of 70 to 79. The malignant form can have two cytologic patterns: fibrosarcomatous or epithelial. The localized form is usually fibrosarcomatous and appears as a mass on x-ray. The diffuse form is more often epithelial. The fibrosarcomatous form is less common, but should be excised with adequate margin. The role of surgery in the diffuse form is more controversial. Eighty-five percent will have pleural effusion on presentation. Unfortunately, the problem of mesotheliomas, whether benign or malignant, is that the pathologic diagnosis is difficult. Without a large tissue biopsy, their histologic characteristics make a definitive diagnosis difficult. Cytology is usually nonproductive.

However, the x-ray and clinical picture of mesothelioma—pleural effusions and intrapleural sheets of tumor—is quite distinctive. In most cases the diagnosis can be made with this x-ray picture alone. To satisfy our demands for a definitive diagnosis and often for medico-legal reasons, it is often necessary to obtain a tissue biopsy in these patients. This should be done with as conservative a thoracotomy as possible and a large—at least 2 cm × 2 cm—piece of tissue should be taken for pathologic study.

Therapy of diffuse mesotheliomas is controversial; some consider all types of resection to be in vain. Pleurectomy and radical extrapleural pneumonectomy are avoided. En bloc resection of tumor in the lung together with the diaphragm has been unrewarding even in young patients and has no justification in the elderly. Pleurectomy as part of the resection is justified in good-risk patients. The better survival usually reported in this group of good-risk patients may be due to treatment of earlier stage disease. One of the major complications of mesothelioma is pleural effusion. This responds only marginally well to chest drainage. Mesothelioma results in progressive restrictive pulmonary disease with pain and dyspnea due to tumor within the chest and extension to surrounding chest wall, diaphragms, and mediastinum. Unfortunately, the treatment of mesothelioma is purely symptomatic, consisting of drainage of pleural effusion and pain control.

Pleural effusion from metastatic malignancy is most commonly seen in association with carcinoma of the colon or the breast. If the effusion is compromising the patient's pulmonary reserve, closed chest drainage is advisable. In perhaps 50% of patients, effective closed chest drainage will lead to obliteration of pleural space and to continued control of the effusion. If the effusion is large, it is important not to try to drain the fluid all at once. It is best to let the fluid out in increments of 500 to 1000 cc, stopping when the patient has any symptoms of cough. If a patient's lung does not expand rapidly, the mediastinum will be displaced toward the side of the effusion, and the patient will develop severe cough and difficulty in inflating the contralateral lung due to its overexpansion. In some patients, the lung will be so involved with the carcinoma that re-expansion is not possible. In these patients, drainage will have little effect. Whether or not to introduce sclerosing agents at the first drainage to increase the likelihood of pleural symphysis is controversial. The most commonly used sclerosing agent is tetracycline, a very alkaline drug that produces an inflammatory process in the pleura to obliterate the pleural space. Some people advocate the use of talc and other irritating agents. These unfortunately often lead to a very painful pleurisy, which is not a very happy outcome for a palliative procedure.

PNEUMOTHORAX

In the elderly patient with emphysema, pneumothorax is a dreaded and, unfortunately, not uncommon problem. In the elderly, it is best treated by the introduction of a large-bore chest tube. We usually put the chest tube in either the second anterior interspace or high in the axilla, just below the axillary hair. The chest drainage is connected to 20 cm of suction. It is important to manage the chest tubes for the spontaneous pneumothorax patient just as one does the postresection patient: Control the pain and get the patient out of bed and coughing. If the leak is not too big, at times the patient can be disconnected from suction and made to ambulate. When the leak is large, long pieces of tubing can be used to connect the chest drainage to the suction. This is maintained while the patients wander around their room. Confining such patients to bed leads to chronic leak. They need to expand the lung so it can stick to the parietal pleura, which requires coughing and moving, as well as suction.

In a young individual with pneumothorax, if a leak persists for 3 days, we would advise open repair. This is usually unwise in elderly patients. They have emphysematous lungs that are limited in function, and leaks are usually not confined to lung that responds well to stapling therapy.

In the elderly patient with emphysema, we would continue tube drainage for long periods, and in some cases we have sent the patient home with a Heimlich-type valve for control of small pneumothorax. Some advocate the use of strong sclerosing agents in these patients. It should be pointed out that sclerosing agents used in a patient with pneumothorax result in far more pain than in a patient with an already inflamed pleura from the effusion. If sclerosing agents are to be used in these elderly patients, we would advise that they have epidural analgesia. If the sclerosing agents obliterate the space, the leak will seal and further pneumothoraces will be prevented. In this elderly group of patients, some advocate the use of talc. The pleural pain associated with its use is so severe that we believe it is rarely justified.

SUMMARY

To summarize the important factors in general thoracic surgery for the elderly patient, one should carefully assess the patient's heart, lungs, chest cage function, and general health to ascertain that the operation chosen is appropriate to his or her anatomic and physiologic reserves. There are no absolute figures or rules that can be used because the pulmonary reserves are dictated by the integrated cardiac function, lung function, chest wall function, central nervous system function, and even functions of the organs within the abdominal cavity. Carcinoma of the lung is the most common surgical disease of the elderly and one that can have both synchronous involvement of different parts of the lung and, as treatment is successful, is likely to have metachronous cancers. The likelihood of second cancers of the lung dictates that lung resection of each cancer should conserve as must function as possible. Aging in itself reduces reserve. The etiologic agents producing carcinoma of the lung and mesothelioma restrict lung function, as do acute and chronic infection. Elderly patients who are candidates for thoracic surgery have limited respiratory reserve and will have even less postoperatively. The criterion for a well-conceived intrathoracic operation is conservation of as much normally functioning lung as possible. In the perioperative period, control of pain and early mobilization are essential to avoid pulmonary complications and deep venous thrombosis.

REFERENCES

1. Levitzky MG: Effects of aging on the respiratory system. *Physiologist* 27:102–107, 1984.
2. Peters TM: The lung. In Peters RM, Peacock EE Jr., Benfield JR (eds): *The Scientific Management of Surgical Patients.* Boston, Little, Brown and Co, 1983, pp 349–385.
3. Campbell JC: Detecting and correcting pulmonary risk factors before operation. *Geriatrics* 32:54–57, 1977.
4. Mackay EH, Banks J, Sykes B, Lee G: Structural basis for the changing physical properties of human pulmonary vessels with age. *Thorax* 33:335–344, 1978.
5. Nakahara K, Monden Y, Ohno K, Miyoshi S, Maeda H, Kawashima Y: A method for predicting postoperative lung function and its relation to postoperative complications in patient with lung cancer. *Ann Thorac Surg* 39:260–265, 1985.
6. Tisi GM: *Pulmonary Physiology in Clinical Medicine,* ed 2. Baltimore, Williams & Wilkins, 1983.
7. Berggren H, Ekroth R, Malmberg R, Naucler J, William-Olsson G: Hospital mortality and long-term survival in relation to preoperative function in elderly patients with bronchogenic carcinoma. *Ann Thorac Surg* 38:633–636, 1984.
8. Peters RM, Swain JA: Management of the patient with emphysema, coronary artery disease, and lung cancer. *Am J Surg* 143:710–705, 1982.
9. Matthay RA, Balmes JR: Lung cancer: A persistent challenge. *Geriatrics* 37:109–112, 1982.
10. Holmes FF: Aging and cancer. *Recent Results Cancer Res,* 87:1–75, 1983.
11. Holmes FF, Hearne EM: Cancer stage-to-stage relationship: implications for cancer screening in the elderly. *J Am Geriatr Soc* 29:55–57, 1981.
12. Ershler WB, Socinski MA, Greene CJ: Bronchogenic cancer, metastases, and aging. *J Am Geriatr Soc* 31:673–676, 1983.
13. Huang M-S, Kato H, Knoaka C, Nishimiya K, et al.: Quantitative cytochemical differences between young and old patients with lung cancer. *Chest* 88:864–869, 1985.
14. Shankar PS: Laryngeal carcinoma with synchronous or metachronous bronchogenic carcinoma. *J Am Geriatr Soc* 29:370–372, 1981.
15. Shure D, Fedullo P: The role of transcarinal needle aspiration in the staging of bronchogenic carcinoma. *Chest* 86:693–696, 1984.
16. Ramsdell JW, Peters RM, Taylor AT Jr., Alazraki NP, Tisi GM: Multiorgan scans for staging lung cancer: correlation with clinical evaluation. *J Thorac Cardiovasc Surg* 73:653–659, 1977.
17. Gutierrez AC, Vincent RG, Bakshi MD, Takita H: Radioisotope scans in the evaluation of metastatic bronchogenic carcinoma. *J Thorac Cardiovasc Surg* 69:934–941, 1975.
18. Friedman PJ, Feigin DS, Liston SE, Alazraki NP, Haghigh P, Young JA, Peters RM: Sensitivity of chest radiography, computed tomography and gallium scanning to metastasis of lung carcinoma. *Cancer* 54:1300–1306, 1984.
19. Mountain CF: A new international staging system for lung cancer. *Chest* 89 (suppl 4):225S–233S, 1986.
20. Tisi GM, Friedman PJ, Peters RM, Pearson G, Carr D, Lee RE, Selawry O: Clinical staging of primary lung cancer. *Am Rev Respir Dis* 127:659–664, 1983.
21. Churchill ED, Sweet RH, Soutter L, Scannell JG: The surgical management of carcinoma of the lung. *J Thorac Surg* 20:349–365, 1950.
22. Hoffmann TH, Ransdell HT: Comparison of lobectomy and wedge resection for carcinomas of the lung. *J Thorac Cardiovasc Surg* 79:211–217, 1980.
23. Jensik RJ, Faber LP, Kittle CF: Segmental resection for bronchogenic carcinoma. *Ann Thorac Surg* 28:475, 1973.
24. Stair JM, Womble J, Schaefer RF, Read RC: Segmen-

tal pulmonary resection for cancer. *Am J Surg* 150:659–664, 1985.

25. Keagy BA, Pharr WF, Bowes DE, Wilcox BR: A review of morbidity and mortality in elderly patients undergoing pulmonary resection. *Am Surg* 50:213–216, 1984.

26. Breyer RH, Zippe C, Pharr WF, Jensik RJ, Kittle CF, Faber LP: Thoracotomy in patients over the age seventy years. *J Thorac Cardiovasc Surg* 81:187–193, 1981.

27. Urschel HC Jr., Razzuk MA: Median sternotomy as a standard approach for pulmonary resection. *Ann Thorac Surg* 41:130–134, 1986.

28. Shah DM, Gottlieb ME, Rahm RL, Stratton HH, Barie PS, PaLoski WH, Newell JC: Failure of red blood cell transfusion to increase oxygen transport or mixed venous PO2 in injured patients. *J Trauma* 22:741–746, 1982.

29. Zeldin RA, Normandin D, Landtwing D, Peters RM: Postpneumonectomy pulmonary edema. *J Thorac Cardiovasc Surg* 87:359–365, 1984.

30. Staren ED, Cullen ML: Epidural catheter analgesia for the management of postoperative pain. *Surg Gynecol Obstet* 162:389–404, 1986.

31. Bell RC, Andrews AP: Pleural effusions: meeting the diagnostic challenge. *Geriatrics* 40:101–108, 1985.

32. Nagami PH, Yoshikawa TT: Tuberculosis in the geriatric patient. *J Am Geriatr Soc* 31:356–363, 1983.

33. Daly RC, Pairolero PC, Piehler JM, Trastek VF, Payne WS, Bernatz PE: Pulmonary aspergilloma. *J Thorac Cardiovasc Surg* 92:981–988, 1986.

34. Monden Y, Nakahara K, Fujii Y, Hashimoto J, Ohno K, Masaoke A, Kwashima Y: Myasthenia gravis in elderly patients. *Ann Thorac Surg* 39:433–436, 1985.

35. Slater G, Papatestas AE, Kornfeld P, Genkins G: Transcervical thymectomy for thymoma in myasthenia gravis. *Am J Surg* 144:254–256, 1982.

36. Miller JI, Mansour KA, Hatcher CR Jr.: Median sternotomy T incision for thymectomy in myasthenia gravis. *Ann Thorac Surg* 34:473–474, 1982.

37. Martini N, McCormack PM, Bains MS, Kaiser LR, Burt ME, Hilaris BS: Pleural mesothelioma. *Ann Thorac Surg* 43:113–120, 1987.

Chapter 17

Surgical Diseases of the Esophagus in the Elderly

Raymond W. Postlethwait, M.D., F.A.C.S.

The elderly are subject to the same diseases of the esophagus as the general population with the obvious exception of most of the congenital disorders. Certain lesions, predominantly carcinoma, are, of course, more frequent in the older age groups. Basically, the diagnosis and treatment of esophageal disease are not influenced by the age of the patient. The appropriate modifications of treatment for the elderly are usually selected because of concomitant disease, most often cardiovascular or pulmonary, rather than the age per se. The increasing numbers of the elderly in our population, as well as their greater longevity, indicates the need for better appreciation of the physical problems of the elderly, including those involving the esophagus.

The past two or three decades has seen a remarkable increase in publications (both articles and books) concerning esophageal disease. In these, a table or graph may show the age groups for the lesion being described, but unfortunately no information is provided specifically related to the older patients. A few articles do relate directly to the elderly, but certainly more specific numbers and results about older patients are needed.

Space does not permit detailed discussion of all esophageal disease that might require operation. This chapter will, therefore, be devoted to motility disorders, diverticula, perforation, benign stricture, benign tumors, malignant tumors, and brief notes of several miscellaneous disorders.

MOTILITY DISORDERS

Achalasia is the most frequently encountered esophageal motility disorder in the elderly. Presbyesophagus and diffuse spasm are of significant interest and should be discussed. An excellent review of these lesions in the elderly is provided by Pelemans and Vantrappen (1).

Presbyesophagus

Although surgical treatment has not been required, the clinical significance of these manometric changes in the elderly have probably been overemphasized. Presbyesophagus was originally defined as the manometric findings that are usually associated with a high incidence of absent peristalsis and frequent non-peristaltic contractions. The study of Khan et al. (2) added their observation that an inadequate lower sphincter response also occurs with significant frequency in normal subjects over the age of 60 years. Hollis and Castell (3), however, in a study group of men aged 70 to 87, found decreased amplitude of contractions only in those over 80 but no other associated abnormalities. The most important observation has been that most all of the subjects who have presbyesophagus are asymptomatic.

Diffuse Spasm

This disturbance has no predilection for the elderly; for example, the ages of the patients in the series reported by McGiffen et al. (4) range from 20 to 73 years, with a mean of 53 years. The manometric findings of this condition most clearly define diffuse spasm as simultaneous and repetitive contractions of abnormally high amplitude. The cause is unknown. Muscle hypertrophy is a consistent finding, but whether it is the cause or an effect is yet undetermined. Severe substernal pain, the major symptom, may occur spontaneously, but usually follows eating or drinking. The pain may radiate and suggest the diagnosis of angina pectoris. Dysphagia and regurgitation may also occur. Radiologic changes seen with barium swallow may indicate the diagnosis, but more confidence may be placed in the manometric studies. Medical treatment includes long-acting nitrates, nifedipine, and dilatation. In severe cases, a long myotomy, sparing the lower sphincter, will be necessary. Good results with surgical correction can be anticipated in about 80% of the patients.

Achalasia

This disease is manifested by failure of the lower esophageal sphincter to open in coordination with swallowing, uncoordinated peristalsis of the lower two-thirds of the esophagus, dilatation of the esophagus, and an abnormal response to parasympathomimetic drugs.

The author collected 826 cases from various reports (5). The largest percentage of 19.6% was in patients aged 30 to 39, but in the older patients, the frequency was as follows: age 50–59, 13.6%; age 60–69, 8.4%; age 70–79, 3.6%; and age 80–89, 1.2%. An interesting report by Lock and Ellis (6) emphasized that dysphagia in the elderly does not necessarily indicate the presence of carcinoma. Their patients with achalasia, all but one with recent onset of symptoms, were aged 73, 81, 83, 85, and 88 years. Myotomy was followed by one death and good results in the others.

The cause of achalasia has not been determined despite extensive experimental studies, including those that have investigated the effects of neurochemicals upon the esophagus. Inconsistent changes have been found at various sites in the nervous system, from central nuclei to the vagus nerves. Changes in Auerbach's plexus, ranging from a slight decrease in number to a total absence of ganglion cells, have repeatedly been described. This is the one alteration upon which there is a consensus. In Chagas' disease of Latin America, the changes in Auerbach's plexus are considered to be due to neurotoxins from the trypanosoma organisms, but in other patients no definite cause has ever been established.

The gross pathology shows a "narrow" segment that anatomically corresponds with the physiologic lower esophageal sphincter. Proximal to this, the esophagus is dilated to a variable degree and extent. The lower two-thirds are invariably involved, and infrequently the entire esophagus is dilated. The dilatation, elongation, and tortuosity of the esophagus vary, as noted, and a classification, such as flask, fusiform, or sigmoid, has been suggested to describe the gross configuration. The longitudinal and circular muscle layers are both thickened. The mucosal changes are usually not severe, but do develop due to the retention of food.

The physiologic alterations of the esophagus

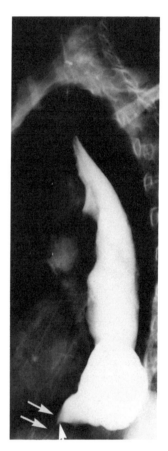

Figure 17.1. Typical appearance of achalasia with a narrowed lower esophageal segment before a smooth symmetrical "bird-beak" ending to the dilated segments in an elderly man. Notice the sacular dilatation of the lower third and the fusiform dilatation of the middle third of the esophagus. Twelve years of symptoms from the malady were relieved by esophagomyotomy and Nissen fundoplication.

are demonstrated by radiologic and manometric examinations. The radiologic changes were well described by Templeton (7). The primary peristaltic wave fades at about the suprasternal notch. The remaining esophagus shows purposeless, shallow segmental contractions with, at times, a generalized clonic contraction. In the early stages, a peristaltic wave may occur, but in the advanced state, peristalsis is absent. The retained barium, in the upright position, reaches a variable height, usually 8 to 10 cm. The distal end shows a characteristic, symmetrical, "birdbeak" configuration. (See Figure 17.1) Kramer and Ingelfinger (8) described in 1948 the manometric changes that have subsequently been extended with the use of improved techniques. Briefly, the upper sphincter and usually the upper third of the esophagus are normal. In the lower part, peristalsis is rare or absent, being replaced by the segmental, erratic contractions noted above. The lower esophageal sphincter shows an increased resting pressure, but more importantly, fails to relax in coordination with swallowing. Methacholine causes a massive and sustained tonic contraction.

The major symptoms of achalasia are dysphagia, regurgitation, substernal discomfort or pain, and weight loss. The duration of symptoms varies widely. The onset is usually insidious, with symptoms being intermittent and slowly progressive. Regurgitation may cause aspiration with the resultant pulmonary symptoms masking those of the esophageal disease. Pain may be severe enough to suggest angina pectoris.

Except in the very early stages of the disease, diagnosis is rarely a problem when radiologic and manometric studies are used. A scintiscan may be helpful. Esophagoscopy is a necessity to exclude other esophageal lesions and carcinoma of the cardia. In the latter case, passage of a bougie may be of help as a large bougie will pass with achalasia but not carcinoma. This test does not, however, exclude the requirement of biopsy in appropriate cases.

Pulmonary complications are the most frequent associated problems. The alleged frequent association of epiphrenic diverticula has not been confirmed by review of several reported large series. The increased risk of squamous cell carcinoma of the esophagus is always present in patients with achalasia. The frequency, however, is difficult to determine, with reports ranging from less than 1% to 10%. Parenthetically, myotomy provides no protection from this threat. Heiss et al. (9), in reporting on a 67-year-old woman who had a successful myotomy 23 years before developing carcinoma, found reports of 24 other cases who had their myotomy from 2 to 10 years earlier.

The treatment of achalasia is dilatation or myotomy of the lower esophageal sphincter, although recent studies suggest calcium antagonists, such as nifedipine, may be of value. Bortolotti and Labo (10) reported success in 17 out of 20 patients treated with this medication.

Dilatation should stretch the "narrow" lower segment so that the normal hydrostatic pressure of swallowing may more easily overcome the resistance to the passage of food and liquids. A number of instruments, using either pneumatic or hydrostatic pressure, are available. Vantrappen and Janssens (11) recently described pneumatic dilators consisting of bags of increasing diameter from 3.0 to 4.5 cm. Using these for progressively larger dilatation, they report good or excellent results in 76.9% of 403 patients. In most series, good results have been reported in 60% to 70% of patients treated by dilatation. In the author's collected reports of 1560 patients, good or excellent results were obtained in 72.3% (5). The major complication of esophageal dilatation is perforation, which was reported in 3% of 1851 patients. (See Figure 17.2a–c)

In an editorial, Orringer (12) has suggested that dilatation be tried first and that the failures be treated by myotomy. Certainly this is wise counsel for the frail elderly. Operation, however, should be considered (1) for a huge dilated esophagus, (2) with associated esophageal disease, (3) with pulmonary complications due to aspiration, (4) when carcinoma cannot be excluded, and (5) refusal of or failure of dilatation.

The fascinating history of surgery for achalasia has been reviewed by Ochsner and DeBakey (13); by Steichen, Heller, and Ravitch (14); and in the classical monograph by Ellis and Olsen (15). Currently, the accepted operation is myotomy, as first described by Heller in 1913 (16) and modified by Zaaijer in 1923 (17). The basic principle is division of the circular muscle layers over the narrow segment and into the dilated portion. The details of operation will not be

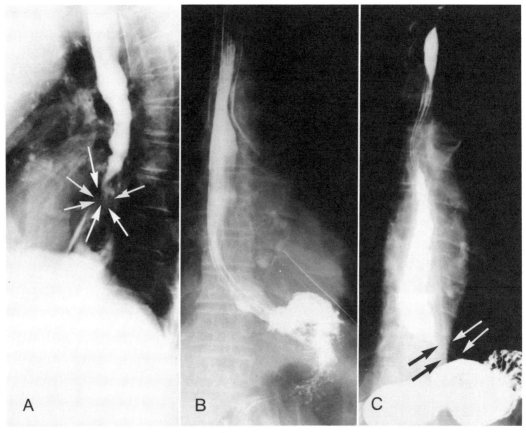

Figure 17.2. **A,** ·This 83-year-old man with a history of achalasia for several years had been managed by repeated episodes of dilitation. One of us (HWS, ed) was called upon to treat him after perforation occurred as shown in **A. B,** Postoperatively, a barium swallow showed no leak and the effects of a generous myotomy and a fundoplication. **C,** When last seen 4 years postoperatively, this patient remained symptom free, with an upper gastrointestinal series showing the effects of the myotomy and the Nissen fundoplication.

repeated here as these have frequently been described, but three points of possible disagreement merit mention. The operative approach may be abdominal or thoracic. Most surgeons, including the author, prefer a thoracic incision, mainly because of the excellence of the exposure obtained. Opinions differ as to the amount of extension of the myotomy onto the stomach. As advised by Ellis and Olsen (15), the incision should extend only to the esophagogastric junction, as this will decrease the possibility of reflux. Finally, a number of surgeons utilize an antireflux procedure after myotomy, usually some form of fundoplication. A problem with this procedure is the risk of the creation of a segment of possible increased resistance below an aperistaltic esophagus, a reason that prompts the

author to avoid this additional component of the operation. Perhaps the advice of Murray et al. (18) is most reasonable: An antireflux operation should be added only in selected patients with definite indications.

The results of the Heller myotomy may be illustrated by reports collected by the author including 2118 patients, with results as follows: excellent 74.8%; good 8.8%; fair 4.0%; poor 12.4% (5). The reason for the poor result was not always stated; 5.9% or 124 patients had a hernia, reflux, esophagitis, or stricture, however. Early failure usually means an incomplete myotomy; later failure indicates probably healing or scarring of the myotomy.

A caveat concerns interpretation of results. Even with correction at the lower esophageal sphincter, the body of the esophagus still has abnormal or no peristalsis so that completely normal swallowing can hardly be expected.

DIVERTICULA

The most common diverticula of the esophagus are classified on the basis of location as (1) pharyngoesophageal (Zenker's) posteriorly at the junction of the hypopharynx and esophagus, (2) parabronchial near the tracheal bifurcation, and (3) epiphrenic in the lower third of the esophagus. The Zenker's is pulsion in type, the parabronchial usually traction, and the epiphrenic either type but usually pulsion. In the author's collected series of 2016 cases, the Zenker's accounted for 62.0%, parabronchial 17.2%, and epiphrenic 20.8% (5).

Zenker's Diverticulum

These most often occur in older men, with the male to female ratio being about 3.4:1. In the author's collected series, two-thirds of patients were over 60 years of age (5).

The diverticulum develops in the midline posteriorly between the oblique fibers of the inferior pharyngeal constrictor and the transverse fibers of the cricopharyngeus (Killian's triangle). The pathogenesis described by Zenker and von Ziemssen (19) over a century ago remains valid. Briefly, with swallowing, the pressure generated by the pharyngeal constrictors forces the food bolus downward, and when a weak area of support exists, a mucosal bulge will develop. Repeated swallowing then slowly enlarges the diverticulum. Why this area is weak in some persons is not evident, although a congenital basis has been suggested. Logically, a disorder of the upper esophageal sphincter could be a causative factor. Manometric studies, however, are not in agreement, although incoordination of the sphincter is strongly supported by several reports.

The symptoms are largely dependent on the size of the diverticulum. With a small bulge of the mucosa through the weak area, only an annoying feeling of food catching in the throat may be experienced. As the diverticulum enlarges, the dependent portion extends downward. Food and liquids are now retained, which leads to regurgitation. This may occur after eating, drinking, bending over, or lying down. Occasionally, nocturnal regurgitation and aspiration predominate, and pulmonary complications develop. With a further increase in size, the opening of the diverticulum lies in the direct axis of the esophageal lumen, so that dysphagia becomes a major symptom both due to this factor and also because of compression of the esophagus by the distended diverticulum. Various other symptoms may occur, including noisy deglutition, halitosis, anorexia, nausea, hoarseness, or mass in the neck.

Diagnosis is not difficult and is by radiologic examination. Emphasis should be placed on the lateral views of the barium column, not only to demonstrate the diverticulum but also to aid in exclusion of other lesions, such as stricture or carcinoma. Esophagoscopy, because of the danger of perforation, is not always performed, but should be done if a complicating lesion is suspected.

The treatment for Zenker's diverticulum is operation. Myotomy inferior to the diverticulum has become a fairly standard procedure and may be all that is needed for a small pouch. The larger diverticula will require either excision or suspension. With excision, care must be taken not to remove excessive mucosa as stricture will result. For diverticulopexy, the tip of the diverticulum is attached superiorly to the prevertebral fascia.

Postoperatively, the most frequent complications are fistula formation and recurrent nerve injury. Both are usually temporary; the fistula will close and the hoarseness will improve if the nerve is intact. Postoperatively, mortality was reported in 1.1% of the author's collected series of 1848 patients (5). Symptomatic recurrence is infrequent, developing in less than 3.0% of the patients.

Parabronchial Diverticulum

These pouches usually extend anteriorly, to the right, and pass either horizontally or slightly upward. They, therefore, empty easily, are seldom symptomatic, and for this reason do not require surgical treatment. Complications have been reported that include fistula, bleeding, and carcinoma that will need operation.

Epiphrenic Diverticulum

The cause of these lesions cannot always be

determined; a congenital weakness has been suggested. In more recent years, some abnormality distal to the diverticulum, such as spasm or stricture, has been found. In some patients, a disorder of the sphincter and a hiatal hernia may be present. (See Figure 17.3)

The epiphrenic diverticulum may be asymptomatic, but because emptying may be impaired and distal disease present, symptoms are usually present. These include dysphagia, epigastric pain, vomiting or regurgitation, substernal discomfort, anorexia, belching, bloating, heartburn, and weight loss. Diagnosis by radiologic examination seldom presents any problem, although other lesions must be excluded. Manometric studies are advisable because of the frequency of associated disorders.

In the larger reported series, operation has been necessary in from 12% to 25% of these patients. This is best accomplished through a left thoracotomy although the diverticulum usually extends to the right, as the concomitant myotomy is more easily performed from the left. After the diverticulum has been excised and the esophagus closed, the myotomy is made on the opposite esophageal wall. (See Figure 17.4) The extent of the myotomy will depend on the preoperative findings (diffuse spasm, achalasia, sphincter dysfunction), as well as those findings at operation (muscle hypertrophy). It should be noted that most authors emphasize that any such associated esophageal disease must be corrected.

The recurrence rate is approximately 5% and is frequently due to untreated associated esophageal disease.

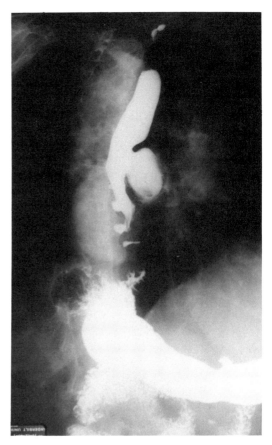

Figure 17.3. Barium swallow obtained in a 72-year-old patient of one of us (RBA, ed) who had dysphagia, substernal pain, heartburn, and regurgitation. The large diverticulum was located above an area of diffuse spasm, moderate achalasia, and an associated hiatal hernia. Symptoms at the time of this study had persisted and worsened over the past 2 years.

PERFORATION AND RUPTURE

Perforation and rupture of the esophagus are potentially disastrous because of the virulent infection that rapidly develops in the periesophageal tissues. Prompt recognition and appropriate treatment are necessary to prevent death. Occasionally a perforation or rupture may be contained, have minimal systemic manifestations, and may be treated expectantly under careful observation, but the majority need immediate active treatment.

In the author's survey of 1204 reported patients, the most frequent causes were iatrogenic, 58.1%; spontaneous, 19.1%; trauma, 15.8%;

and foreign body, 7.0% (5). Although a number of other causes may be seen, this discussion will be confined to these four.

Factors influencing treatment and results include (1) age and physical condition; (2) clinical response to the incident; (3) presence of other esophageal disease; (4) site and size of the disruption; (5) degree of involvement of mediastinum, pleura, etc.; (6) cause of the perforation or rupture; and (7) perhaps most importantly, the time interval from the incident to the diagnosis and treatment.

The principles of treatment are (1) secure closure of the disruption with or without reinforcement, (2) adequate drainage of the infected

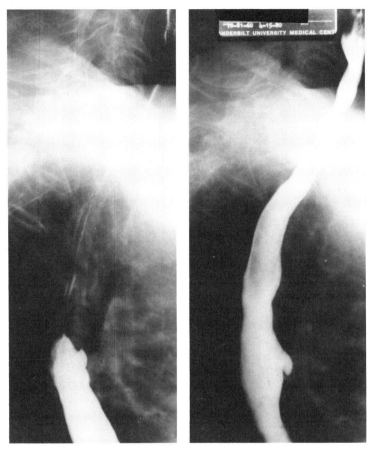

Figure 17.4. Postoperative barium swallow from patient in Figure 17.3 following excision of large diverticulum, myotomy of lower two-thirds of esophagus, and repair of hiatal hernia. She remains asymptomatic at age 79.

areas, (3) administration of appropriate antibiotics, and (4) provision for maintaining nutrition. If closure is impossible, exclusion or resection of the area of perforation should be considered.

Iatrogenic Perforation

The major causes of iatrogenic perforation are endoscopy, dilatation, and removal of foreign body. Based on the data provided by the surveys of Katz (20) and of Silvis et al. (21), the chances of various procedures causing perforation are approximately as follows: rigid esophagoscopy, 1 per 900; fiberoptic endoscopy, 1 per 3000; mercury bougie dilatation, 1 per 1000; metal olive dilatation, 1 per 200; and pneumatic dilatation, 1 per 90. Foreign body removal was not included in this list, but it accounts for about 5% of all

of the iatrogenic group.

Endoscopic perforation is most likely to occur in the region of the cricopharyngeus when the true esophageal orifice may not be recognized or is forcefully passed. The posterior esophageal wall may be compressed against the cervical spine. In the elderly, the endoscopist should be aware of the possibility of a prominent arthritic spur on the cervical spine that increases the danger of perforation. During dilatation, perforation usually occurs at or just above the stricture. Deep biopsy may, of course, transverse the esophageal wall.

Symptoms are dependent upon the site and size of the perforation, but pain predominates. In the cervical perforations, pain may be accentuated by swallowing or moving the head. Voice changes and subcutaneous emphysema may occur. In the thoracic esophageal perforations, pain is also the major symptom and is either substernal, in the back, or both. Odynophagia is common. Cardiovascular and respiratory symptoms depend on the degree of involvement of the mediastinum and pleural cavities.

Diagnosis will seldom present difficulty if the perforation is suspected. Plain x-ray films may show air in the mediastinum or soft tissues, but a contrast swallow is necessary in nearly all patients, as this not only will show the site but should also give some indication of the size of the perforation.

Treatment of iatrogenic perforations generally will be discussed later, but a special note should be made of this group of patients. If endoscopy or dilatation is performed, a number of them will have other esophageal disease. Closure alone may not suffice, for example, if the perforation is located above a severe stricture because healing will be unlikely. A carcinoma perforated by biopsy may be resectable, and if so, resection should be done at the time of operation for the perforation. With achalasia, closure and myotomy may be combined. Briefly, the associated disease of the esophagus must be considered for appropriate treatment at the time of the repair of the perforation.

Ancona et al. (22) published an extensive collective review of nearly 1000 patients with iatrogenic perforation and found an overall mortality of 24.3%.

Spontaneous Rupture

The Boerhaave syndrome is such a dramatic event that it has attracted the interest of numerous authors. The rupture is seldom truly spontaneous, but occurs during vomiting and retching. In this situation an excessively high intragastric pressure develops. If released suddenly into the esophagus against a closed cricopharyngeus or an area of esophageal spasm below this, the full force of the pressure is trapped and exerted on the esophageal wall. As this pressure exceeds the tensile strength of the wall, rupture results.

The longitudinal rupture is in the lower third of the esophagus in 85% of the patients and to the left side in 80%. The length of the defect is usually from 1 to 10 cm, and the edges may be clean and sharp in the early period or ragged and necrotic if treatment is delayed. The extravasation may be confined to the mediastinum or extend into the pleural cavity, usually the left. The severe mediastinitis is at first chemical and then followed by bacterial invasion. If penetration is through the pleura and into the pleural space, a hydropneumothorax can be anticipated, to be followed by empyema.

This mishap is of importance in the elderly, as in the author's collected series, 69.3% were over the age of 50 and 38.3% were over 60 years (5). In addition, the mortality rate has almost a linear increase in relationship to age.

Typically, the abrupt onset of symptoms is with excruciating pain, either substernal or epigastric. Radiation may occur to the back, chest, shoulders, or most frequently the abdomen. Additional symptoms depend in part on involvement of the pleural cavity and mediastinum. Dyspnea and circulatory collapse may follow.

Physical findings in addition to the possible dyspnea and shock include crepitus in the neck in about half the patients. A mediastinal crunch may be heard. The chest may show signs of fluid, pneumothorax, or hydropneumothorax. Abdominal findings are variable, but frequently suggest a perforated peptic ulcer. It has been estimated that 20% of these patients will have a laparotomy first with this diagnosis. The differential diagnosis includes a long list of other diseases, including coronary occlusion.

Diagnosis is not difficult if spontaneous rupture of the esophagus is considered and suspected. The radiologic findings include (1) air in the mediastinum and neck; (2) hydrothorax, pneumothorax, or hydropneumothorax; and (3) extravasation of contrast material from the esophagus. Esophagoscopy is usually unnecessary.

The treatment for the patient who is diagnosed early is thoracotomy for closure of the rupture. The late, undiagnosed, or neglected patient may best be treated first by a large empyema tube thoracostomy, with the adjuncts of gastric drainage, antibiotics, and intravenous feeding in the hope that stabilization will provide the opportunity for definitive operation and repair.

Mortality is dependent upon a number of factors, most importantly the treatment and time from rupture to treatment. This is well illustrated by the collected series of Blichert-Toft (23). He found that operation within 12 hours of rupture resulted in a mortality of 22%; within the next 12 hours, 36%, and beyond 24 hours, 64%. Treatment by primary closure in 106 patients gave a mortality of 34%, in 43 by intercostal tube drainage, 54%; in 25 other non-operative treatment, 60%; and in 47 with no treatment, 100%. The author in a more recent survey found the mortality after closure to be 16.6% (5).

Traumatic Perforation

Only brief note will be made of this group of patients. Traumatic perforation most often is reported in younger age groups, and is usually the result of knife or gunshot wounds. Because of concomitant injury to adjacent organs, diagnostic studies may have to be restricted and the perforation identified only during the operation.

Foreign Body Perforation

Most foreign body perforations are found in children, whose tendency to swallow various objects is well known. At least two factors should be noted concerning the elderly. They are more likely to wear dentures that will impair their ability to recognize such an object as bone in the food being masticated. As a result, a bolus of meat, poultry, or seafood containing a bone may be swallowed, lodge in the esophagus, and cause perforation. Perhaps because of the dentures, the size of a bolus of meat or poultry is also difficult to determine. The bolus is arrested in the esophagus, frequently above an asymptomatic stricture; rigid esophagoscopy is usually necessary for its removal. The numerous passes of the forceps required to remove a large bolus greatly increases the possibility of instrumental perforation.

Treatment

The principles of treatment have been noted, with emphasis on early operation and closure. Reinforcement of the closure may be accomplished by several methods: gastric wall, diaphragm, adjacent lung or muscle, and an intercostal bundle. Grillo and Wilkins (24) described the development of a pleural flap of appropriate size that is sutured over the defect for perforations recognized late.

When closure is impossible or marked drainage persists and in some cases is treated too late, temporary or permanent exclusion of the esophagus should be considered, providing that all infected areas are adequately drained. Cervical esophagostomy may be necessary, gastrostomy may be performed for decompression of the stomach, and possibly a jejunostomy may be done to provide nutritional access. Occasionally, ligation or division of the esophagus at the esophagogastric junction may be needed. In the favorable case, later decortication of the pleural cavity and closure of the perforation may be possible. In many cases, reconstruction, such as substernal colon interposition, will provide the only means of restoring the ability to swallow.

BENIGN STRICTURE

A number of causes of benign esophageal stricture have been recorded, but by far the most frequent etiology, especially in the elderly, is gastroesophageal reflux. As reflux is discussed in chapter 18, only stricture will be considered here.

The cause of reflux stricture is obviously the fibrous tissue formation in the wall of the esophagus secondary to prolonged esophagitis. An unanswered question is why some of these patients develop a stricture, whereas many others with an equivalent degree of esophagitis do not. Another problem that needs study is why a number of the patients present with an established stricture with no history suggesting esophagitis. Other common causes are the severe strictures that may follow nasogastric intubation, accompany scleroderma, and, more frequently in recent years, follow irradiation and chemotherapy.

Diagnosis is seldom a problem. Dysphagia, the predominant symptom, may be slowly progressive, or it may develop rapidly. In a few patients, acute obstruction is the first symptom. Radiographic examination will show the site, length, and severity of the stricture. Esophagoscopy is mandatory, not only to determine the extent of esophagitis but also to exclude malignancy. Adenocarcinoma of the cardia and squamous cell carcinoma of the lower esophagus may closely resemble the radiographic appearance of a reflux stricture.

The treatment options depend upon a number of factors, but of particular importance are the rigidity of the stricture and the age and general condition of the patient. A simple division of types into soft and hard strictures may be made. The soft stricture responds promptly to dilatation, and an antireflux operation is then performed to prevent recurrence. The hard stricture requires repeated dilatation or resection.

In the author's experience, an appreciable number of these patients will be elderly and have coexisting disease, usually cardiovascular, pulmonary, or both; the safest treatment in these patients is dilatation, even if this procedure must be repeated at intervals. A satisfactory functional result nearly always will be obtained. A mercury-filled bougie, Hurst or Maloney, commonly is employed. With a tight rigid stricture, the Eder-Puestow method may first be used. More recently, balloon dilatation has been utilized. As far as can be determined, London et al. (25) first used Gruntzig balloon catheters to dilate tight strictures, and reports of subsequent successes have been impressive. For example, Taub et al. (26) dilated severe strictures in 13 patients. All were improved, allowing subsequent passage of a 34 to 42F Maloney bougie. The cited advantages of balloon dilatation were that the dilating force is confined to the stricture and that it can be controlled by the patient reaction. The risk of esophageal perforation is less because of (1) the technique employed, (2) the balloon has low compliance and will burst if forced beyond maximum diameter, and (3) there is no longitudinal stretching force as with other methods because the balloon acts radially, using the stricture itself as a lever during inflation.

In addition to the well-known antireflux operations, a number of procedures have been described for the surgical treatment of strictures. When operation is being considered, two associated possibilities should be remembered. Acquired shortening of the esophagus may be present, which may be suspected if not identified by barium swallow examination. Second, panmural esophagitis can cause severe periesophageal inflammatory reaction, and no reliable means of determining this condition preoperatively has been described.

Intraoperative dilatation combined with an antireflux operation has been used successfully in many patients. For example, Mercer and Hill (27) reported 90% good results with this technique using a posterior gastropexy in 107 patients who had only one preoperative dilatation. Results were less satisfactory in their remaining 53 patients who had required multiple dilatations or had prior esophageal surgical procedures. Their emphasis was on prompt operation for these patients.

Because of shortening of the esophagus in many cases, gastroplasty has been used to allow placement of the reconstruction within the abdomen. Fundoplication is placed around the lesser curvature gastric tube to prevent further reflux.

Resection is seldom required, but it may be necessary for a tight unyielding stricture and, of course, for perforation. Rarely, carcinoma cannot be excluded and is the reason for resection of a stricture. Reconstruction may utilize the stomach, but is better accomplished by replacement with a short colon segment as continued reflux is less likely following that procedure.

The results in the author's collected series of peptic stricture treated by dilatation alone were satisfactory in 78.9% of 883 patients (these authors report in the same period 277 operations or 23.9% of 1160 patients) (5). The length of follow-up and the criteria of evaluation ranged widely. Intraoperative dilatation and some type of antireflux operation gave good results in 85.7% of 509 patients. Gastroplasty and fundoplication in 1571 patients gave 91.9% good results, although most series are compromised by including some patients without stricture. Resection produced good results in 91.7% of 678 patients followed (postoperative mortality was 5%). Colon interposition gave 93.5% good results and esophagogastrostomy, 84.5%.

Schatzki Ring

This unique form of stricture should be noted briefly. It is a narrow annular stricture that radiographically appears as a circumferential membrane or web consisting only of mucosa and submucosa, which projects into the lumen at a right angle to the long axis of the lower part of the esophagus, usually with a concentric opening. The author believes, based on histologic studies, that the ring is due to reflux.

The major symptom is acute obstruction to a large food bolus. This nearly always occurs with an opening of 13 mm or less, but it may occur with a larger opening.

Adjustment of diet and dilatation usually afford relief. With symptomatic reflux, an antireflux procedure may be required during which the ring can be dilated or incised. Rarely, a thick ring may require excision of mucosa and submucosa only as the muscle is not involved.

BENIGN TUMORS

These lesions are found very infrequently and have no predilection for the elderly, except for the esophageal polyp. Leiomyoma is the most common benign esophageal tumor in all age groups.

Leiomyoma

These are found less frequently in the esophagus than the stomach or small intestine. Usually found in the lower two-thirds of the esophagus, the leiomyoma is round or oval and from 5 to 10 cm in diameter, although multiple lesions and bizarre configurations are occasionally noted.

The symptoms are usually vague, including dysphagia and substernal discomfort, and in many patients, the leiomyoma is found incidentally during routine upper gastrointestinal x-ray series. Esophagoscopy should be performed to exclude other lesions, but biopsy of the intact mucosa is to be avoided. The treatment is enucleation through a thoracotomy incision.

Polyp

Although rare, a polyp occurs most often in men over the age of 60 years (27% in a collected series) (5). Fibrous and adipose tissues are usually the main components. The site of origin is commonly in the cervical region, and peristalsis will mold the mucosal polyp into an elongated structure. Although dysphagia usually occurs, about one-fourth of the patients will regurgitate the polyp into the mouth. The potential for laryngeal obstruction and asphyxia is obvious. The lesion may be missed by x-ray examination, with the dilated esophagus suggesting achalasia. Endoscopy may show only normal mucosa, but needs to be done because of the frequency of polypoid malignant tumors. If the pedicle can be identified, endoscopic removal may be utilized; otherwise, esophagotomy and resection are required.

MALIGNANT TUMORS

Squamous cell carcinoma is the most frequent malignant tumor of the esophagus, occurring in 96.3% of 7336 patients of reported series in which the histology was stated. The lesion is most common in men by a ratio of about 3:1 and in black men especially. The age adjusted mortality rate in this country from 1950 through 1981 shows the incidence in white men and women not to have changed, being about 5 and 2 per 100,000, respectively. In black women, a slight increase from 3 to 4 per 100,000 has occurred, whereas in black men the increase has been from 7 to 16 per 100,000.

The mean age is usually stated to be about 62 years; the range is shown in Table 17.1. In the collected series, 55% were over age 60. At the Duke-VA Medical Centers, the mean age was lower because of the number of black patients who develop the carcinoma earlier; the mean age for black men was 58.2 and for black women 55.7 years.

The site of the carcinoma is approximately 15% in the upper third, 50% in the middle third, and 35% in the lower third of the esophagus.

Etiology

The cause is, of course, unknown, but three conditions do predispose to the development of

Table 17.1 Carcinoma of Esophagus Age Distribution

Age	Collected Series 13,523 patients	Duke-VA Series 983 patients
20–29	22 (0.2%)	2 (0.2%)
30–39	308 (2.3%)	17 (1.7%)
40–49	1554 (11.5%)	156 (15.9%)
50–59	4166 (30.8%)	339 (34.5%)
60–69	4506 (33.3%)	313 (31.8%)
70–79	2481 (18.3%)	129 (13.1%)
80+	490 (3.6%)	27 (2.7%)

carcinoma: chemical burns, achalasia, and tylosis. The Plummer-Vinson syndrome, as well as irradiation, has also been implicated.

High incidence areas (Caspian Littoral of Iran, the Transkei in South Africa, and the Linksien province in China) have provided the opportunity for many epidemiologic studies with suggestive but not definitive findings. Tobacco and alcohol have been incriminated, but the available studies again are suggestive but not conclusive.

Pathology

The typical squamous cell carcinoma is an ulcerated lesion with a shaggy, irregular floor and elevated edges. Impingement on the lumen depends on the bulk of the tumor, as well as circumferential invasion with contraction of the walls. Longitudinal extent of the tumor in the earlier lesions will exceed its transverse dimension. In some carcinomas, the ulceration is less pronounced, but the wall is then invaded and the lumen severely constricted. Rarely, circumferential invasion is accompanied by very little loss of lumen. Occasionally, the tumor remains very superficial even with invasion of the wall. Bulky tumors do occur, and a verrucose type, resembling varices on the barium x-ray study, has been seen infrequently. Microscopic invasion of the wall and submucosa beyond the gross edges of the tumor is common, as attested by the frequency of a positive margin reported after resection.

Microscopically, these tumors are noted for their extremely varied appearance with all degrees of differentiation. The oat cell carcinoma is probably best called undifferentiated carcinoma, according to Stout and Lattes (28). Studies of grading, usually with Broders' method, have not been of significant value in the prognosis of rate of growth, metastases, radiosensitivity, or ultimate outcome.

Uniform staging would be of considerable value, particularly to compare treatment methods and prognosis. The two major systems and several modifications that are used only indicate the need for a universally accepted classification. Local invasion and distant metastases are unfortunately common in squamous cell carcinoma of the esophagus, as will be shown below. The anatomic position of the esophagus in the neck and mediastinum places it adjacent to important, if not vital, structures. In the cervical region, intramural spread may extend to the hypopharynx and larynx. Anteriorly, the trachea may be invaded; laterally, the thyroid gland and carotid sheath; and posteriorly, the prevertebral fascia. The latter may be involved at any point in the course of the esophagus. In the upper part of the thorax, the trachea or main stem bronchi, usually the left, is frequently invaded, as well as the left recurrent nerve. Invasion or dense adherence to the aorta may occur. In the lower third, the pleura, pericardium, or aorta may be involved, as well as the diaphragm. Extension of an esophageal cancer into the stomach occurs less frequently than invasion of carcinoma of the cardia of the stomach into the lower esophagus.

The lymphatic drainage of the esophagus is not segmented, and although adjacent nodes are usually first involved, metastases may extend widely to mediastinal nodes, to nodes in the neck, and to nodes along the lesser curvature of the stomach and around the celiac axis. The pattern of spread is rather unpredictable, as lower-third lesions may metastasize to neck nodes and middle-third lesions to celiac nodes. Blood-borne metastases most frequently spread to lung, liver, kidney, adrenal gland, and bone.

Although this discussion is confined to squamous cell carcinoma, other malignant tumors of the esophagus should be mentioned. The rare lesions include leiomyosarcoma, rhabdomyosarcoma, carcinosarcoma, pseudosarcoma, and melanoma. Adenocarcinomas may be mucoepidermoid or adenocystic in type. Of particular interest are those adenocarcinomas arising from Barrett's esophagus. The latter have been recognized more frequently in recent years.

Finally, multiple malignancies, either synchronous or metachronous, are reported in from 0.6% to 8.0% of various series. Associated head and neck malignancy is the most frequent type.

Symptoms

Dysphagia is the first symptom in about 90% of these patients. This usually causes the patient to seek medical help relatively early, but unfortunately by then the carcinoma is already pathologically far advanced all too often. A number of reasons have been suggested for the late onset of dysphagia, but most likely the cause is that one-half to two-thirds of the circumference of the esophagus may be involved before dysphagia develops. Once experienced, the dysphagia is rapidly progressive, so that in just a few weeks the patient may not even be able to swallow water.

Rarely, acute obstruction is the first symptom. The patient may be able to indicate the level of the lesion fairly accurately. Regurgitation is, of course, frequent.

Pain develops in about 20% of these cases, and although variable in character, severity, location, and precipitating factors, the pain is usually associated with swallowing. Continuous pain, especially with radiation to the back, is an ominous sign as this usually indicates spread of tumor outside the esophagus. Respiratory symptoms may be due to aspiration or to direct extension into the respiratory passages.

Weight loss is almost uniformly present and may be severe in a very short period of time. Weakness develops as starvation and dehydration progress.

Bleeding, either as hematemesis or hemoptysis, occurs in only a small number of patients. Other symptoms, such as hoarseness, may indicate the spread of carcinoma.

Diagnosis

Physical examination usually provides no objective findings, but may detect metastases, show complications or concomitant disease, and aid in the evaluation of the patient as an operative risk. Laboratory determinations are also not specific, but provide evaluation of nutrition and hydration, hematologic status, and cardiac, pulmonary, liver, and renal function. Hypercalcemia may be found in as many as 15% of the patients and usually indicates advanced disease.

The important diagnostic examinations are radiologic and endoscopic. The characteristic roentgenographic finding with barium swallow is narrowing of the lumen with irregularity and rigidity of the wall. Shelving may be seen. The lumen may be angulated and eccentric; Akiyama et al. (28) emphasized the axis deviation as a factor in determining resectability. Occasionally the lesion may be polypoid; infrequently the lumen is not decreased appreciably. A lower-third carcinoma may resemble a benign stricture, but some asymmetry will be present. Plain films will, of course, be necessary in excluding metastases.

Computed tomography is useful in showing extraesophageal extension. Thompson et al. (30) summarized the experience with this study at the Duke-VA Medical Center. Demonstration of mediastinal invasion had a sensitivity of 93%, specificity of 83%, and accuracy of 90%. For enlarged celiac nodes, all three were 78%.

Esophagoscopy is necessary in any patient suspected of having carcinoma, regardless of the radiologic findings. Cellular material must be obtained for histologic study (cytology, biopsy). The upper extent of the lesion is determined, and some idea of tumor fixation to the surrounding structures can be formed. The typical lesion is ulcerated, irregular, granular, and red, gray, or white in color. The edges are usually elevated. The lesion is friable and bleeds easily. Occasionally, submucosal invasion and edema proximal to the carcinoma may make visualization of the actual ulceration difficult. In the small lesion, staining with Lugol's solution may be of value. Usually the normal mucosa stains and the tumor does not.

Bronchoscopy is an equally important procedure in any carcinoma of the esophagus because of the frequency of invasion of the trachea or a bronchus, usually left main.

Operability and Resectability

"Operable" is defined as those patients in whom the operation is started with a reasonable chance for complete removal of the tumor. "Resectability" defines those patients whose carcinoma actually can be removed. This resection may be palliative when the tumor is known not to have been entirely removed. A curative resection is defined as one in which the carcinoma has been completely resected as far as can be determined. Most authors state only the total number of resections, rather than divisions into palliative and possibly curative procedures.

The author has collected reports since 1940 totaling 22,514 patients; 10,861 or 48.24% were operable, and 6959 were resectable (5). The resectable cases represent 30.86% of all patients and 63.98% of the operable group. In the past decade, resectability has increased to 38.76% of all cases. Reports from China show much higher resectability rates.

The causes of inoperability may be illustrated by the Duke VA series in which 539 (54.8%) of the 983 patients were found to be inoperable after the initial examination. In the cervical and thoracic inlet group of 126 patients, tracheal invasion was present in 25, a large tumor in 18, cord paralysis in 17, neck node metastases in 18, and a fixed neck mass in 11. For upper thoracic lesions in 304 patients, tracheal or bronchial invasion was present in 89 as were metastases to neck nodes in 39, to lungs in 12, to liver in 13, and to bone in 13. Of 109 with lower-third lesions, metastases to the liver were found in 16 and to neck nodes in 10. A variety of other reasons for no operation were found in the other patients. For the entire group, 14 were determined to be senile, 27 were nutritionally depleted and had other disease, 21 were terminal, and 25 had severe cardiac or pulmonary disease.

Resection was abandoned after abdominal exploration in 27 patients of the Duke VA series, usually because of a large mass of fixed celiac nodes. Exploratory thoracotomy in 88 patients resulted in no resection because of invasion of trachea or bronchus in 26, posterior fixation in 36, and fixation to the pulmonary hilum in 27 and into the aorta in 24 (more than one cause was found in several patients).

Limited information is available on resectability of cancer of the esophagus in the elderly. Berman et al. (31) in a collective review found that 5% to 18% of patients with carcinoma of the esophagus were over 75 years of age. In their own series of 10 patients over 75 years, 9 were resected with only one postoperative death. They encourage aggressiveness in this older age group. Sugimachi et al. (32) reported 231 patients divided into three age groups; of the 80 patients in Group I who were aged 36 to 59, 44 were resected (55%), with 33 being considered curative. Sixty-two of 100 patients in Group II aged 60 to 69 years had resection (42 curative); in Group III, resection was possible in 30 of 51 patients (59%) aged 70 to 81 years with 25 classified as curative. There is no significant difference in the resection rate for the three groups. Williamson (33) utilized abdominocervical (transhiatal) esophagectomy in five patients aged 75 to 88 years with no deaths or serious complications. He states that the elderly can tolerate this operation well and satisfactory results can be obtained.

Selection of Treatment

Currently only surgical removal or irradiation treatment offers any hope of cure for esophageal cancer. Adjunctive measures may be of value, and additional methods are applicable for palliation. Whatever the treatment selected, these objectives should be observed: (1) to eradicate all carcinoma when possible, (2) to prolong an acceptably comfortable life, (3) to restore swallowing, (4) to prevent complications, such as pulmonary aspiration, and (5) to relieve pain.

A number of factors should be considered in the selection of treatment. Obviously, if invasion or metastases are demonstrated, only palliation will be possible. Assuming the tumor appears localized, evaluation of the patient's physiologic age, nutritional status, and concomitant diseases will influence the decision. As indicated above, chronologic age is less important than physiologic age; the senile patient can be expected to have an increased operative risk. The cachectic patient will not tolerate well any definitive treatment. Although such measures as total parenteral nutrition are of definite help, the tumor continues to grow, invade, or metastasize when the effort to restore weight and good nutritional status is prolonged. Pulmonary disease, cardiac lesions, hepatic damage, and impaired renal function alter operative risk and require proper evaluation.

If the patient is a candidate for definitive treatment, choices include attempted surgical excision of the carcinoma, preoperative irradiation with or without chemotherapy, or irradiation alone or combined with chemotherapy. Resectability is highest for lower-third lesions, and the consensus is reasonably uniform that operation for these lesions is indicated. In the cervical region, irradiation had been the primary treatment in the past because reconstruction after resection was unsatisfactory, but restoration methods have greatly improved and now resection is commonly employed. In the absence of definite contraindications, the author believes carcinoma of the middle third should be explored and resected when possible.

The role of preoperative irradiation has not been established; most reported series utilize historical controls, which makes interpretation difficult, although favorable results are usually reported. Gignoux et al. (34) randomized preoperative irradiation in 192 patients and found no effect on postoperative mortality and no apparent effect on survival. Launois et al. (35) also randomized 124 patients, giving 4000 rads to those who had irradiation. They found no difference in resectability, postoperative mortality, or 5-year survival.

Two groups in this country, Steiger et al. (36) and Kelsen et al. (37), have combined chemotherapy and irradiation in non-randomized series. Steiger (36) administers 5-fluorouracil and cisplatin plus 3000 rads with a 3- to 4-week delay before operation. Of 48 carcinomas resected, 15 had no residual tumor in the specimen. Kelsen (37) before operation gives cisplatin, vindestine, and bleomycin and, after resection, 5500 rads. Both groups report encouraging results, but final evaluation of long-term survival has not been made.

An extensive review of irradiation therapy alone, describing 8489 patients, was published by Earlam and Cunha-Melo (38). Definitive radiotherapy was given to 49% of the patients with a 5-year survival of 6%. They note that a controlled trial had not been reported. Pearson (39) reported a 5-year survival of 19% of 169 patients; later from the same clinic, Newaishy et al. (40) found a 9% 5-year survival of 444 additional patients. As far as can be determined, no one has been able to reproduce the excellent results reported by Pearson (39).

Response to chemotherapy alone has been variable; Kelsen (37) has published an excellent current review.

The need for controlled studies is evident from the above discussion.

Resection of Esophageal Carcinoma

Detailed descriptions of operative technique are readily available and need not be repeated; a brief outline of operations follow. A one-stage operation is much preferred over multiple-stage procedures.

Carcinoma in the cervical region is rarely small and localized enough to permit limited resection. Usually removal will be combined with laryngectomy and partial pharyngectomy. The otolaryngologist may participate in the excision, with the thoracic surgeon performing the reconstruction. Colon interposition offers an alternative to the restoration of continuity, but more often the stomach is used. Cervical resection may be combined with blunt thoracic esophagectomy, a maneuver recommended to ensure clear margins and to remove the occasional multicentric carcinoma. A free jejunal transplant into the neck has gained popularity, in part because of good functional outcome, but it has the problem of delicate microvascular anastomoses.

A carcinoma that crosses the thoracic inlet is difficult to resect because of the periesophageal extension. Ong et al. (41) have reported some success. Resectability is determined through a neck incision. If resectable, the sternum is split, or alternatively, a right thoracotomy is performed.

Carcinoma of the middle third is usually removed by the Ivor Lewis (42) operation, modified to one stage. Laparotomy is first performed to mobilize the stomach and to exclude metastases. The abdomen is then closed and the patient repositioned for right thoracotomy. The tumor is resected and the stomach brought into the chest for anastomosis. The esophagus should be divided high in the thorax, but if a safe margin cannot be obtained, the division and anastomosis can be made in the neck, as recommended by McKeown (43).

The surgical approach for lower-third lesions depends on the judgement of the surgeon regarding the safe level for resection and anastomosis, i.e., above or below the aortic arch. A right thoracotomy may be necessary, but a left thoracotomy may suffice. Occasionally a thoracoabdominal incision is most satisfactory as this will allow better lymph node removal.

Two additional operations should be noted. Skinner (44) has described an en bloc resection with removal of the tumor with a wide margin, along with all the tissues adjacent to the esophagus within the anatomic constraints of the mediastinum. Early results are encouraging and may provide improved survival. Mainly through the work of Orringer (45), esophagectomy without thoracotomy has gained increasing acceptance. Briefly, through neck and abdominal incisions, the esophagus is dissected from its bed, partly by blind blunt dissection. The stomach is elevated into the neck for anastomosis. For 116 intrathoracic carcinomas, postoperative mortality was

5.2% A number of surgeons have been concerned about the use of this operation in middle-third carcinoma because of the limited exposure and the possible danger of damage to adjacent structures.

Postoperative Morbidity and Mortality

Esophagectomy patients are subject to all the complications that may follow any major operation that includes thoracotomy. Two should be noted: pulmonary complications and anastomotic leak. In the lungs, tracheobronchitis, atelectasis, pneumonitis, and respiratory failure are all due to excessive mucus secretion, limited expansion, incomplete bronchial clearing, arteriovenous shunting, and poor gaseous exchange. Pulmonary problems account for the most frequent complications and are the most frequent causes of death.

An anastomotic leak in the past has been reported in approximately 10% of patients. A minor leak that closes promptly may occur. Large anastomotic defects including complete separation of the anastomosis are the serious problem. More recent reports, particularly where the end-to-end stapler has been used, indicate a decreasing frequency of these complications. An anastomotic leak can lead to fatal sepsis and in some series was the most frequent cause of death.

A survey of reports shows a decreasing operative mortality rate, from nearly 40% in the early days of esophageal resection to about 17% recently. Reports published in the past 5 years record a postoperative mortality of 0.8% to 37.5%, the lowest being reported by Akiyama et al. (46) who had only one death after 132 resections.

Mohansingh (47) reported 241 esophageal operations in patients less than 70 years old with a mortality of 4.2%; for 68 operations in patients over 70 years, mortality was 5.9%. Fifty-five resections for carcinoma in the younger group had a 9% mortality; in the older group, 15 resections resulted in a 20% mortality. He states that the elderly are more susceptible to general complications, such as myocardial infarction (but not anastomotic leak), and the approach for carcinoma should be radical with age being no barrier. Sugimachi et al. (48) in the report referred to above of 231 resections found pulmonary complications to be significantly more frequent in the 70-to 81-year age group. Anastomotic leak was not more frequent, however. Postoperative mortality, however, was significantly higher as age increased: age 36 to 59, 3.7%; age 60 to 69, 6.0%; age 70 to 81, 13.7%.

Palliative Treatment

The patient who requires palliation has advanced carcinoma, and the choice of treatment may be limited. The primary objective is, of course, to restore swallowing and the following methods have been utilized:

1. Dilatation and intubation
2. Irradiation
3. Chemotherapy
4. Laser
5. Surgical: resection, bypass, or gastrostomy

Endoesophageal tubes have been used for many years. The largest current experiences are from South Africa. Procter (49) used the Procter-Livingstone tube in 2000 patients, many of whom were terminal. Hospital death occurred in 720. Although the mean duration of life was 11 weeks, relief of dysphagia was obtained in over 90%. This tube is passed under endoscopic control. The second most frequently used tube, the Celestin, requires laparotomy and gastrostomy for fixation. Problems with these tubes include obstruction, migration, bleeding, and perforation.

Irradiation treatment has long been the major method of palliation, with the possibility of occasional cure. If the patient can tolerate a full course of radiation treatment, improved swallowing can be expected in over two-thirds of the patients. The duration of the improvement, however, is extremely variable.

Chemotherapy has been reviewed by Kelsen et al. (50) Various investigators have utilized bleomycin, cisplatin, 5 flurouracil, adriamycin, and methotrexate. Response is not consistent, and further study is indicated. The same is true of laser resection. Early reports have been encouraging, however.

Palliative resection will prolong life only moderately, but does consistently improve swallowing and prevent aspiration. Bypass operations may utilize jejunum, colon, stomach, or a greater curvature gastric tube placed in the chest, substernally or subcutaneously. The postoperative mortality rate is high, but the one situation in which this is acceptable is for malignant tracheoesophageal fistula. Patients with these fistulae face a miserable terminal course because of the aspiration. The author's preference is that of substernal placement of the stomach or the use of a greater curvature gastric tube.

Gastrostomy alone is rarely indicated, but may be the only means of allowing some patients to return home.

Results of Resection

The most extensive review, totalling 83,783 patients, was published by Earlam and Cunha-Melo. (51) They found 5-year survival to be 4% of the total group, 9% for those who had operation, 12% for those resected, and 18% for those surviving resection. The author's survey of reports published in the past 10 years, referring only to resection, showed 5-year survival ranged from 3.0% to 34.7%. (5) Most of the results were in the 10% to 25% range. A reasonable approximation of reported results would agree with the 18% 5-year survival found by Earlam and Cunha-Melo (51), although reports from China exceed this rate.

An interesting addendum to this discussion was the evaluation of 64 patients who had survived at least a year after resection of thoracic esophageal carcinoma published by Sugimachi et al. (48). Thirty-two were 60 to 69 years of age, and 21 were over 70 years. As judged by appetite, swallowing, and general activity, they conclude that the quality of life at that age is not diminished, and they continue to recommend operation.

MISCELLANEOUS LESIONS

Brief note should be made of several other esophageal lesions, even though they are not predominantly seen in the elderly.

A number of patients over 60 years of age have been reported with an apparently congenital H-type tracheoesophageal fistula. Approximately 20% of cysts of the esophagus are found in patients over 50 years old. The congenital form of Barrett's esophagus is compatible with normal function and may be discovered in the elderly

when ulcer, stricture, or adenocarcinoma develops. The Mallory-Weiss syndrome may, of course, occur at any age.

Reynolds et al. (52) note that the elderly are particularly prone to develop candidal and herpetic esophagitis.

REFERENCES

1. Pelemans W. Vantrappen G: Oesophageal disease in the elderly. *Clin Gastroenterol* 14:635–656, 1985.
2. Khan TA, Shragge BW, Crispin JS, Lind JF: Esophageal motility in the elderly. *Dig Dis* 22:1049–1054, 1977.
3. Hollis JG, Castell DO: Esophageal function in elderly men, a new look at "presbyesophagus." *Ann Intern Med* 80:371–374, 1974.
4. McGiffin D, Lomas C, Gardner M, McKeering L, Robinson D: Long oesophageal myotomy for diffuse spasm of the oesophagus. *Aust NZ J Surg* 52:193–197, 1982.
5. Postlethwait RW: *Surgery of the Esophagus.* East Norwalk, CT, Appleton-Century-Crofts, 1986.
6. Lock JR, Ellis H: Achalasia of the cardia in elderly patients. *Postgrad Med J* 54:538–540, 1978.
7. Templeton FE: Movements of the esophagus in the presence of cardiospasm and other esophageal disease. *Gastroenterology* 10:96-, 1948.
8. Kramer P, Ingelfinger FJ: Cardiospasm, a generalized disorder of esophageal motility. *Am J Med* 7:174–179, 1949.
9. Heiss FW, Tarshis A, Ellis FH Jr: Carcinoma associated with achalasia, occurrence 23 years after esophagomyotomy. *Dig Dis* 29:1066–1069, 1984.
10. Bortolotti M, Labo G: Clinical and manometric effects of nifedipine in patients with esophageal achalasia. *Gastroenterology* 80:39–44, 1981.
11. Vantrappen G, Janssens J: To dilate or to operate? That is the question. *Gut* 24:1013-1019, 1983.
12. Orringer MB: The treatment of achalasia: controversey resolved? *Ann Thorac Surg* 28:100–102 1979.
13. Ochsner A, DeBakey M: Surgical considerations of achalasia: review of the literature and report of three cases. *Arch Surg* 41:1146–1183, 1940.
14. Steichen FM, Heller E, Ravitch MM: Achalasia of the esophagus. *Surgery* 47:846–876, 1960.
15. Ellis FH Jr, Olsen AM: Achalasia of the esophagus. *Maj Prob Clin Surg* 9:1–221, 1969.
16. Heller E: Extramucous cardioplasty in chronic cardiospasm with dilatation of the esophagus. *Mitt Grenzgeb Med Chir* 27:141–149, 1913-1914.
17. Zaaijer HJ: Cardiospasm in the aged. *Ann Surg* 77:615–617, 1923.
18. Murray GF, Battaglini JW, Keagy BA, Starek PJ, Wilcox BR: Selective application of fundoplication in achalasia. *Ann Thorac Surg* 37:185–188, 1984.
19. Zenker FA, von Ziemssen H: Diseases of the oesophagus. In *Cyclopedia of the Practice of Medicine*, vol 8. New York, William Wood, 1878, p 1–214.

20. Katz D: Morbidity and mortality in standard and flexible gastrointestinal endoscopy. *Gastrointest Endos* 14:134–141, 1967.

21. Silvis SE, Nebel O, Rogers G, Sugawa C, Mandelstam P: Endoscopic complications, results of the 1974 American Society for Gastrointestinal Endoscopy Survey. *JAMA* 235:928–930, 1976.

22. Ancona E, Semonzato M, Peracchia A: Iatrogenic perforation of the esophagus. *Acta Chir Belg* 76:211–218, 1977.

23. Blichert-Toft M: Spontaneous esophageal rupture, an evaluation of the results of treatment of 1944–1969. *Scand J Thorac Cardiovasc Surg* 5:111–115, 1971.

24. Grillo HC, Wilkins EW Jr: Esophageal repair following late diagnosis of intrathoracic perforation. *Ann Thorac Surg* 20:387–399, 1975.

25. London RL, Trotman BW, DiMarino AJ, Oleaga JA, Freiman DB, Ring EJ, Rosato EF: Dilatation of severe esophageal stricture by an inflatable balloon catheter. *Gastroenterology* 80:173–175, 1981.

26. Taub S, Rodan BA, Bean WJ, Koerner RS, Mullin DM, Feng TS: Balloon dilatation of esophageal structure. *Am J Gastroenterol* 81:14–18, 1986.

27. Mercer CD, Hill LD: Surgical management of peptic esophageal stricture. *J Thorac Cardiovasc Surg* 91:371–378, 1986.

28. Stout AP, Lattes R: Tumors of the esophagus. In *Atlas of Tumor Pathology* Sect 5, Part 20, Washington DC, Armed Forces Institute of Pathology, 1957.

29. Akiyama H, Koguri T, Itai Y: The esophageal axis and its relationship to the resectability of carcinoma of the esophgus. Ann Surg 179:30–36, 1972.

30. Thompson WM, Halvorsen RA, Foster WL, Roberts L, Korobkin M: Computed tomography for staging esophageal and gastroesophageal cancer-a re-evaluation. *AJR* 141:951–958, 1983.

31. Berman JK, LaLonde AH, Fisher C: Esophageal carcinoma treatment in patients of 75 to 85 years of age. *Arch Surg* 82:353–359, 1961.

32. Sugimachi K, Matsuzaki K, Matsuura H, Kuwano H, Ueo H, Hnokuchi K: Evaluation of surgical treatment of carcinoma of the oesophagus in the elderly—20 years experience. *Br J Surg* 72:28–30, 1985.

33. Williamson RLN: Abdominocervical oseophagectomy in the elderly. *Ann Roy Coll Surg Engl* 67:344–348, 1985.

34. Gignoux W, Buyse M, Segol P, Roussel A, Paillot B, Kunlin A, Duez N: Multicenter randomized study comparing preoperative radiotherapy with surgery only in cases of resectable oesophageal cancer. *Acta Chir Belg* 4:373–379, 1982.

35. Launois B, Delarue G, Campion JR, Kerbaol M: Preoperative radiotherapy for carcinoma of the esophagus. *Surg Gynecol Obstet* 143:690–692, 1981.

36. Steiger Z, Franklin R, Wilson RF, Leichman L, Asfaw I, Vaishanpayan G, Rosenberg JC, Loh JJ, Dindogru A, Seydel H, Hoschner J, Miller P, Knechtges T, Vaitkevicious V: Eradication and palliation of squamous cell carcinoma of the esophagus with chemotherapy. *J Thorac Cardiovasc Surg* 82:713–719, 1981.

37. Kelsen DP, Bains M, Hilaris B, Martini N: Combined modality therapy of esophageal cancer. *Semin Oncol* 11:169–177, 1984.

38. Earlam R, Cunha-Melo JR: Oesophageal squamous cell carcinoma II, a critical review of radiotherapy. *Br J Surg* 67:457–461, 1980.

39. Pearson JG: The value of radiotherapy in the management of squamous oesophageal cancer. *Br J Surg* 58:794–798, 1971.

40. Newaishy GA, Read GA, Duncan W, Derr GR: Results of radical radiotherapy of squamous cell carcinoma of the oesophagus. *Clin Radiol* 33:347–352, 1982.

41. Ong GB, Tam KH, Lam THM, Wong J: Resection for carcinoma of the superior mediastinal segment of the esophagus. *World J Surg* 2:497–504, 1978.

42. Lewis I: The surgical treatment of carcinoma of the esophagus with special reference to a new operation for growths of the middle third. *Br J Surg* 34:18–31, 1946.

43. McKeown KC: Resection of mid-esophageal carcinoma with esophagogastric anastomosis. *World J. Surg* 5:517–525, 1981.

44. Skinner DB: En bloc resection for neoplasms of the esophagus and cardia. *J Thorac Cardiovasc Surg* 85:59–71, 1983.

45. Orringer MB: Transhiatal esophagectomy without thoracotomy for carcinoma of the thoracic esophagus. *Ann Surg* 200:282–288, 1984.

46. Akiyama J, Tsurumaru M, Watanabe G, Ono Y, Udagawa H, Suzuki M: Development of surgery for carcinoma of the esophagus. *Am J Surg* 147:9–16, 1984.

47. Mohansingh MP: Mortality of oesophageal surgery in the elderly. *Br J Surg* 63:579–580, 1976.

48. Sugimachi K, Maekawa S, Koga Y, Ueo H, Inokuchi K: The quality of life is sustained after operation for carcinoma of the esophagus. *Surg Gynecol Obstet* 162:544–546, 1986.

49. Procter DSC: Esophageal intubation for carcinoma of the esophagus. *World J Surg* 4:451–461, 1980.

50. Kelsen DP, Heelan R, Coonley C, Bains M, Martini N, Hilaris B, Golbey RB: Clinical and pathological evaluation of response to chemotherapy in patients with esophageal carcinoma. *Am J Clin Oncol* 6:539–546, 1983.

51. Earlam R, Cunha-Melo JR: Oesophageal squamous cell carcinoma I, a critial review of surgery. *Br J Surg* 67:381–390, 1980.

52. Reynolds JC, Ouyang A, Cohen S: Recent advances in dx and rx of esophageal disease. *Geriatrics* 37:91–104, 1982.

Chapter 18

Hiatal Herniae and Diaphragmatic Disorders in the Elderly

Mark K. Ferguson, M.D., David B. Skinner, M.D., F.A.C.S.

As the percentage of the elderly in the United States population rises with each census, disorders associated with advanced age are becoming more common. Gastrointestinal problems worsen and increase in the elderly because of the continuing changes and alterations of physiology and anatomy associated with aging. Polypharmacy contributes to the frequency and severity of many gastrointestinal disorders in the geriatric population. Although most symptoms are secondary to functional disorders, many have an organic basis and should not be dismissed as a normal part of aging. The evaluation of upper gastrointestinal symptoms is usually straightforward, consisting of plain chest and abdominal radiographs, barium esophogram and upper gastrointestinal contrast studies, and endoscopy.

The results of such evaluation show that the prevalence of hiatal herniae increases with age, largely as a result of loss of connective tissue integrity. These are anatomic defects that result from aging and that are associated with physiologic disorders, such as gastroesophageal acid reflux. These disorders are sometimes accompanied by serious complications, including hemorrhage, obstruction, incarceration, and strangulation. The increase in the incidence of these and other disorders of the diaphragm makes their proper management of vital importance in the elderly, a problem that is profoundly influenced and often complicated by the aging process.

A number of factors may affect the decision to offer the elderly patient the aggressive medical and surgical treatment approach that is generally indicated for these disorders. Advanced age alone is not normally a contraindication to standard therapy. However, advanced age is often accompanied by multisystem problems that can adversely affect the outcome of aggressive treatment. Pharmacologic therapy of reflux, for example, may be accompanied by profound mental status changes when H2 receptor blockers are used. Changes in colonic function are apt to accompany the persistent use of antacids. Although the likelihood of controlling reflux symptoms surgically is similar when middle-aged patients are compared to elderly patients, the latter group experiences a higher risk of operative morbidity, particularly when such procedures are performed on an emergency basis.

Physicians must judge, together with the patients and their supporting families, the overall risks of surgical intervention and balance this risk estimate with the potential benefit of the procedure to the patient. It is always advisable and often beneficial to question patients about their personal expectations. Some doctors and families assume that the elderly patient is always interested in achieving the optimal health status and level of comfort. Some elderly patients, however, are not willing to take even a small risk to gain potentially great benefits from surgical treatment. This is true particularly when the older person has learned to coexist for many years with problems that some people would consider incapacitating. Other elderly patients will expect and demand the same treatment that would have been offered to them at a younger age. Whatever the case, the patient's wishes must be respected.

ANATOMY

Diaphragm

The diaphragm is a fibromuscular structure separating the thoracic and abdominal cavities. Its peripheral portion consists of muscular fibers originating from three areas: the back of the xiphoid anteriorly, the lower six ribs postero-laterally, and the lumbar vertebrae posteriorly. The muscular portions converge into a central tendon at the apex of this dome-shaped structure. There are three openings in the diaphragm that allow passage of structures between the thoracic and abdominal cavities: the aortic hiatus contains the aorta, azygos vein, and thoracic duct; the esophagus and accompanying vagus nerves pass through the esophageal hiatus; and the vena cava passes through the caval hiatus. Motor innervation is supplied by the phrenic nerves.

Esophageal Hiatus

Understanding the anatomy of the esophageal hiatus is fundamental for recognizing the differences among and the implications of the various types of hiatal herniae. The diaphragmatic muscle arising posteriorly forms two bundles, the right and left crura, which surround the esophagus on their passage to the central tendon. Most of the margins of the actual opening of the hiatus appear to arise from the right crus. The esophageal hiatus is composed of several additional layers separating the thoracic and abdominal cavities. The phrenoesophageal membrane, an extension of the endoabdominal fascia, is joined by the endothoracic fascia to form fibrous attachments to the esophageal muscle and submucosa 3 to 4 cm above the esophagogastric junction. The esophagus below this point is subject to intra-abdominal, rather than intrathoracic, pressure. At the distal end of the tubular esophagus lies the lower esophageal high pressure zone, or distal esophageal sphincter (DES). This has important functional characteristics and serves as the main barrier to gastroesophageal reflux.

HIATAL HERNIAE

Hiatal herniae occur through the esophageal hiatus. They are generally divided into three types, the Type I or sliding hernia, the Type II

or paraesophageal (rolling) hernia, and the combined form or Type III hernia. The Type I hernia is common and is without clinical significance in most cases. It occurs when there is dilatation of the esophageal hiatus and attenuation of the phrenoesophageal membrane. This allows a portion of the gastric fundus to slide above the diaphragm. (Figure 18.1) The Type II hernia is less common, but is clinically more significant. In this type of hernia, a defect in the phrenoesophageal membrane allows a protrusion of the peritoneum into the thoracic cavity, creating a true hernia sac. The relatively greater intra-abdominal pressure eventually tends to force abdominal contents through the defect and into the sac. Because there is a defect in only a portion of the phrenoesophageal membrane, the esophagogastric junction often remains in its usual position below the diaphragm. As the Type II hernia enlarges and the membrane becomes further attenuated, a combined (Type III) hernia may develop with elements of both the sliding and paraesophageal components present.

Type I Herniae and Gastroesophageal Reflux

Etiology

The Type I (sliding) hiatal hernia is found in about 10% of patients who are submitted to barium swallow. Etiologic factors associated with the development of a Type I hernia include age, obesity, and the habitual wearing of tight, restrictive clothing. Obesity and tight clothing appear to promote the stretching of the phrenoesophageal membrane by increasing intra-abdominal pressure.

Diagnosis

Radiographic demonstration of a Type I hernia (Figure 18.2) is enhanced by placing the patient in a recumbent position and applying abdominal pressure by hand or with an inflatable corset. Variations in technique and effort account for a large discrepancy in the frequency of these herniae that are reported (1–7). (See Table 18.1) A consistent finding, however, is the fact that the prevalence of Type I hiatal herniae increases with age (Figure 18.3) and that they are found in over two-thirds of patients aged 60 years and above. They occur twice as often in

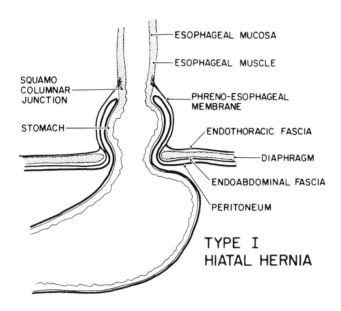

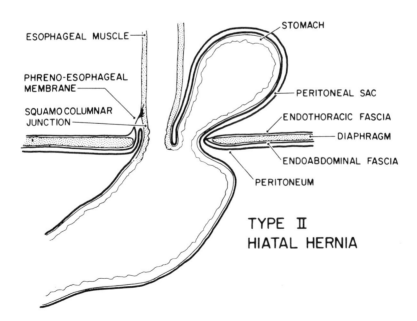

Figure 18.1. Diagrammatic illustration of Type I and Type II hiatal herniae. The Type I hernia has an attenuated but intact phrenoesophageal membrane with no true hernia sac. In the Type II hernia a defect in the phrenoesophageal membrane is associated with a true intrathoracic hernia sac. (Reproduced by permission from Skinner DB: Hiatal hernia and gastroesophageal reflux. In Sabiston DC Jr. (ed): *Textbook of Surgery,* ed 12. Philadelphia, WB Saunders, 1981, pp 821–833.)

Figure 18.2. A Type I hiatal hernia in which the esophagogastric junction and gastric fundus are found sliding above the esophageal hiatus.

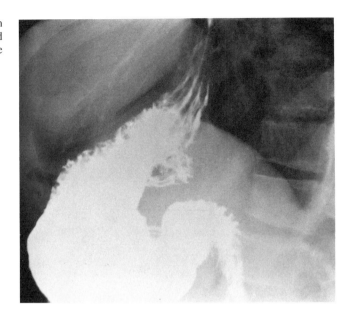

women as in men in the elderly population (8).

Symptoms

There are no specific symptoms associated with a Type I hernia. When symptoms are present, they are usually characteristic of those associated with gastroesophageal reflux. These include heartburn that tends to occur postprandially. Symptoms are worse while bending over or when lying down. Regurgitation and, less commonly, respiratory symptoms of coughing, shortness of breath, or pneumonia secondary to aspiration also occur as the effects of reflux and scarring progress. Other symptoms may not be at all characteristic for reflux esophagitis and may mimic angina or other serious cardiac disorders.

Gastroesophageal Reflux

The sliding hiatal hernia as an isolated entity does not normally give rise to gastroesophageal reflux in the absence of other contributing factors. Although up to 80% of patients with symptomatic reflux have a Type I hernia, only 1 in 20 of those people with a Type I hernia has pathologic reflux (9). The etiology of gastroesophageal reflux in these patients is not clearly understood. A variety of factors contribute to its severity. These factors may be separated into those affecting esophageal body

function, those affecting sphincter function, and those affecting gastric function.

The predominant factor in controlling gastroesophageal acid reflux (GER) is the anatomic and physiologic integrity of the distal esophageal sphincter (10). The importance of the Type I hernia in gastroesophageal reflux lies in its relationship to the anatomy and function of the distal esophageal sphincter. The three characteristics of the distal esophageal segment that are important in preventing gastroesophageal acid reflux are the overall length of the DES, the intrinsic pressure of the DES, and the overall length of the esophagus lying below the insertion of the phrenoesophageal ligament and exposed to intra-abdominal pressure. The presence of a sliding hernia should not normally affect the pressure or length of the DES (2, 11). However, such a hernia may be associated with a lower effective insertion of the phrenoesophageal membrane due to inflammatory adhesions or congenital variations, thus reducing the length of esophagus exposed to intra-abdominal pressure. Patients with larger hiatal herniae do have a higher incidence of reflux, which is associated with a shorter length of intra-abdominal esophagus (12).

Other substances that adversely influence the function of the DES include nicotine, fats, chocolate, alcohol, and peppermint. Pharmacologic agents with a negative influence include theophylline, anticholinergics, beta-adrenergic

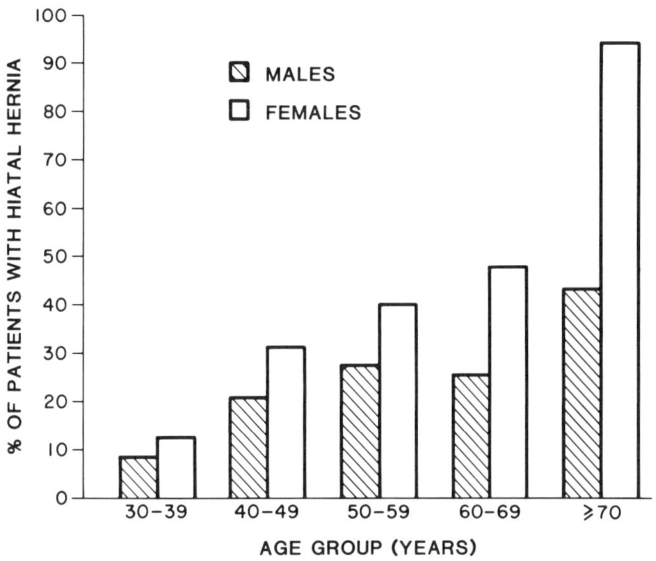

Figure 18.3. The prevalence of hiatal herniae found on barium swallow in relation to age. (Adapted from Pridie RB: Incidence and coincidence of hiatus hernia. *Gut* 7:188–189, 1966.)

agonists, alpha-adrenergic antagonists, diazepam, calcium channel blocking agents, and natural and synthetic opiates.

When acid reflux does occur, the rate of acid clearance from the distal esophagus is an important determinant of whether other complications from reflux will occur. Esophageal acid clearance may be impaired in the elderly by esophageal motor disorders, including presbyesophagus and other nonspecific motor disorders. (See Chapter 17) Factors included in the gastric phase of digestion that influence acid reflux consist of those that elevate intragastric pressure and those that increase gastric acid. Those factors that affect pressure include obesity and the wearing of tight, restrictive clothing, whereas factors that affect gastric acid content consist of ingestion of acidic foods (including citrus juices, tomato

products, coffee) and eating shortly before sleeping. Gastric motility disturbances increase in frequency and severity with advanced age, making gastric emptying slower than normal and predisposing to acid reflux.

Evaluation and Treatment

When symptoms of reflux are atypical or severe, a complete evaluation of esophageal function should be performed. We find that pathologic gastroesophageal reflux cannot be demonstrated in 25% of patients with typical symptoms of reflux. Evaluation of esophageal function involves a few minimally invasive tests that are well tolerated by most patients, including the elderly. These tests often provide very specific diagnoses from which appropriate therapeutic decisions can be made in most cases. The tests include extended esophageal pH monitoring, which is designed to quantitate the number and duration of acid reflux episodes, allowing the physician to correlate these objective data with the patient's symptoms. Due to recent improvements in ambulatory monitoring, this test may be performed on an outpatient basis. Esophagoscopy is strongly recommended to determine the degree of esophagitis, to evaluate the existence and extent of Barrett's esophagus, and to look for any other associated problems in the upper gastrointestinal tract. It may be done safely and on a routine basis, even in the elderly, (13)

Table 18.1 Radiographic Evidence of Sliding Hiatal Hernia in Patients with Gastroesophageal Reflux

Source	Year	Patients	Patients with Hernia	Percentage
Kramer[1]	1969	413	188	45.5
Cohen[2]	1971	25	12	48.0
Bucher[3]	1978	30	14	46.7
Wara[4]	1979	45	23	51.1
Jonsell[5]	1983	44	24	54.5
Berstad[6]	1986	101	64	63.4
Kaul[7]	1986	101	22	21.8
	Total	759	347	45.7

and should always be performed in anyone with symptoms related to the esophagus that are severe enough to initiate a visit to a physician.

When pathologic GER is diagnosed, a trial of medical therapy is usually indicated. Initial medical therapy consists of elevation of the head of the bed 6 inches, refraining from eating several hours before bedtime, elimination of foods and drugs that affect the distal esophageal sphincter pressure, and the use of antacids when symptoms become bothersome. More intensive medical management includes administration of an H2 receptor blocker, such as cimetidine or ranitidine. Drugs that improve esophageal motility and lower esophageal sphincter function and promote gastric emptying include bethanachol or metoclopramide. These drugs may be used to reduce symptoms of reflux esophagitis when inadequate improvement results from the usual modalities listed above.

The vast majority of patients with reflux experience significant symptomatic improvement using these medical measures. When symptoms become severe or fail to respond to adequate medical management, surgical correction is often indicated. An operation is also indicated to control reflux when complications from GER occur, including ulcerative esophagitis and stricture, severe bleeding, Barrett's esophagus, or aspiration with pneumonia or chronic pulmonary fibrosis.

Paraesophageal Hiatal Herniae

Paraesophageal hiatal herniae comprise less than 5% of all hiatal herniae. As with the sliding type of herniae, they are more common in women than in men, and their prevalence increases with age. The Type II hernia is much more likely to produce symptoms than is a sliding hernia, and thus they comprise 15% of all symptomatic herniae (14–19). (see Table 18.2) Symptoms include pain, which is present in 70% of these patients; it is characterized by a full feeling in the epigastrium or substernally and is frequently associated with postprandial cramping. Vomiting or dysphagia occurs in about 20% of patients. Although heartburn is not usually a prominent symptom, 20%–25% of patients are found to be anemic, which is presumably due to chronic blood loss from gastric or esophageal irritation or ulceration.

Table 18.2 Symptomatic Hiatal Hernia: Relative Frequency of Sliding and Paraesophageal Types

Source	Year	Sliding Hernia	Paraesophageal or Mixed Hernia
Johns[15]	1961	81	24
Krupp[16]	1966	388	85
Skinner[17]	1967	829	82
Windsor[18]	1967	326	74
Ellis[19]	1986	166	51
Totals		1790 (85%)	316 (15%)

Physiology

The Type II hernia is typically described as one in which the distal esophageal sphincter is tethered in its usual position below the diaphragm, providing a normal barrier to reflux. However, recent evidence shows that over half of those patients with a Type II hernia do have pathologic gastroesophageal acid reflux on extended esophageal pH monitoring (20). The finding of abnormal reflux is unrelated to the presence or absence of typical reflux symptoms, including heartburn and regurgitation. Individuals with a paraesophageal hernia and reflux typically have a very short distal esophageal sphincter length, a normal sphincter tone, and a short length of esophagus exposed to abdominal pressure. In contrast, patients with a Type I or sliding hernia have a DES of normal length but with low pressure. Acid clearance from the distal esophagus is similar in both groups.

Diagnosis

The diagnosis of a paraesophageal hernia can often be made on plain chest radiograph. (Figure 18.4) A large retrocardiac shadow containing an air-fluid level distinguishes this abnormality from the Type I hernia. An upper gastrointestinal examination usually reveals that more than half of the gastric mass is above the level of the diaphragm. (Figure 18.5) Occasionally the entire stomach migrates into the hernia sac, which then predisposes it to volvulus. A variety of other organs can migrate into the sac, the most common being the colon, but others include the spleen, small bowel, and the left lobe of the liver.

Complications

In spite of the frequency with which pathologic

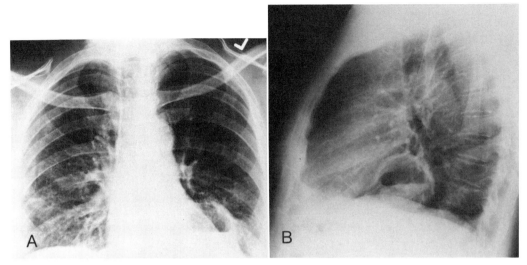

Figure 18.4. A paraesophageal or Type II hernia is often evident on a chest radiograph. It is characterized by a gastric bubble containing an air-fluid level located lateral (**A**) and posterior (**B**) to the cardiac shadow.

GER can be documented, endoscopic examination in patients with a Type II hernia rarely reveals direct evidence of esophagitis (20). Linear gastric erosions or frank gastric ulcerations are frequently found, and these defects usually correspond to the site upon the gastric wall that is immediately adjacent to the rim of diaphragm making up the hernia ring (21). It is believed that the constricting nature of the hernia ring and movement of the stomach across this defect result in a mechanical, rather than acid-peptic, injury.

Major complications occur with a paraesophageal hiatal hernia with much greater frequency than with a Type I hernia. They include gastrointestinal hemorrhage, gastric volvulus, ulceration with perforation, obstruction, and strangulation. The absence of symptoms associated with a Type II hernia should not prevent consideration of aggressive therapy for these patients when the diagnosis of such a hernia is made. As early as 1955, fatal complications secondary to intestinal obstruction in a diaphragmatic hernia were well known, (22) and many subsequent reports have confirmed the serious nature of this problem (23–28). Skinner and Belsey reported a group of 21 patients with a Type II hernia treated medically because of minimal symptoms and found that 6 (28.5%) died directly from complications resulting from the unrepaired hernia (17). As a result of these and other experiences, a general recommendation has evolved that a

Type II or combined (Type III) hernia should be electively repaired at the time of or soon after the diagnosis is made.

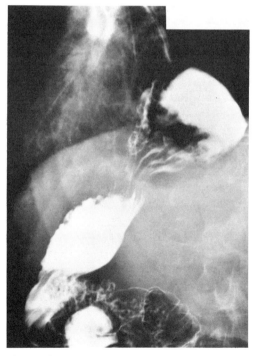

Figure 18.5. A paraesophageal (Type II) hernia in this 84-year-old woman caused obstructive symptoms and profound anemia.

Operative Techniques

In a general discussion of operative procedures designed to correct hiatal hernia, it must be emphasized that the indications and goals of these operations vary considerably when comparing the Type I to the Type II or Type III herniae. The indication for surgical intervention in a Type I hernia is almost exclusively failure of a trial of medical management or the development of complications not amenable to medical therapy. The objective of such a procedure is the prevention of continued reflux, and the elimination of the hernia is merely a side benefit of the operation. In some cases, in fact, an antireflux operation may be successfully performed without reduction of the hernia. In contrast to this, the indication for surgical intervention for a Type II or Type III hernia is the mere existence of such a hernia, regardless of whether or not symptoms are present. The goal of the surgical procedure here is not the elimination of complications, but it is the prevention of complications.

Once the indications for operation are met and the patient is medically prepared for the procedure, the next important consideration is the operative approach. Antireflux operations and hernia repairs may be performed either through an abdominal or a thoracic incision. Most antireflux operations are performed transabdominally. This approach is selected when there are other intra-abdominal conditions that require examination or intervention, such as peptic ulcer disease or gallbladder disease. The transabdominal approach eliminates the need for a chest drainage catheter and may be associated with less postoperative pain. Although an abdominal incision is smaller than a thoracotomy, it carries a 10% risk of developing a ventral hernia and has a higher risk of wound infection.

A transthoracic approach is indicated in obese patients and in those with a very large hiatal hernia. This technique allows complete mobilization of the esophagus and permits division of adhesions involving abdominal organs within the hernia sac under direct vision. It should be used routinely in reoperative cases involving the esophagus and gastroesophageal junction or in the presence of intrathroacic pathology requiring evaluation. The primary contraindication to a transthoracic approach is poor pulmonary function.

Successful operations to prevent reflux are designed to restore normal function, as opposed to normal anatomy, of the cardia. Most operations that successfully control reflux create an intra-abdominal segment of eosphagus during the repair. The length of intra-abdominal esophagus appears to correlate inversely with the degree of pathologic reflux in anatomic studies (11). This finding is supported by clinical studies from our laboratory (29). Wrapping the distal esophagus with a portion of the gastric fundus maintains an abrupt change in diameter from the esophagus to the stomach, bringing the Law of LaPlace into play (10) and resulting in a flap valve mechanism that has antireflux properties. The wrap also alters the angle of the esophagogastric junction, another element that may reduce pathologic reflux.

The three standard antireflux operations currently in use in the United States all satisfy these criteria. The selection from among these operative procedures will depend upon whether a transabdominal or transthoracic approach is desired. The selection is also influenced to some extent by each surgeon's training and experience. The Nissen fundoplicaton is the most frequently performed antireflux operation, and it may be done through either incision. It produces a higher incidence of gas bloat and results in the greatest increase in DES pressure, frequently causing dysphagia in the early postoperative period. In the elderly patients, who frequently have abnormalities in the esophageal body peristaltic function, a fundoplication of less than 360 degrees, such as the Belsy Mark IV procedure, should always be considered. This operation may be performed only through a transthoracic approach. We find that the Hill operation is particularly useful in patients who have had prior gastric resection and in those in whom a total fundoplication would unnecessarily limit gastric capacity.

In most instances it is important to mobilize the esophagus sufficiently to allow the fundoplication wrap to rest without tension beneath the diaphram. The total fundoplication operation requires that several of the proximal short gastric vessels be divided so that one has adequately freed the fundus and cardia for the wrap. The distal esophagus should also be completely mobilized, with careful preservation of the vagus nerves, including the hepatic branch, which is frequently injured at its takeoff just below the hiatus. The fat pad should be dissected off of the the anterior aspect of the gastroesophageal junction to allow the gastric serosa to heal to the esophageal muscle, preventing slippage and breakdown of the repair. The final preparatory step is the placement of crural stitches to close the enlarged hiatal hernia opening. These sutures should be of heavy nonabsorbable material and should be placed 1 cm apart, beginning posteriorly. These posterior buttress sutures should be left untied in most instances until completion of the fundoplication, at which time the size of the hiatus may be properly calibrated by approximating the crura to allow a single finger alongside the esophagus.

A total fundoplication, or Nissen fundoplication, is performed by wrapping the fundus posteriorly around the esophagus just above the gastroesophageal junction and suturing it to the remaining fundus anteromedially. We normally use 2–0 or 3–0 nonabsorbable sutures spaced 1 cm apart and incorporate a generous bite of esophagus between the fundic bites to prevent slippage. Marking the gastroesophageal junction with a hemoclip is helpful when the sutures are being spaced; this is useful when identifying the junction on the plain chest radiographs postoperatively. Placing three to four sutures will create a wrap of 2–3 cm in length. It is useful to perform the wrap over a 60 Fr. Maloney dilator to ensure the maintenance of an adequate caliber of the esophageal lumen. The crural stitches are then tied.

The Belsey Mark IV antireflux operation, or partial fundoplication, must be performed transthoracically. Two rows of mattress sutures, with three stitches in each row, are placed to create a 270 degree anterolateral wrap. The first-row sutures enter the gastric seromuscular layer 2 cm below the gastroesophageal junction and are then passed through the two muscle layers of the esophagus 2 cm above the junction. A mattress effect is created by reversing the direction of the sutures, passing them through the esophagus and stomach. Following completion of the first row of sutures, they are gently tied down to avoid tearing the delicate esophageal muscle. The second-row sutures are placed in a similar fashion, but pass first through the diaphragm at the junction of the central tendon and the mus-

cular ring of the hiatus. The sutures are placed in the stomach 4 cm below the gastroesophageal junction and in the esophagus 4 cm above the junction. A similar mattress effect is created, and the suture is finally brought through the diaphragm again. The second-row sutures are not tied until the stomach and gastroesophageal junction are manually reduced below the diaphragm. The posterior buttress sutures are then tied to approximate the crura.

The Hill repair is performed transabdominally. The fibrofatty tissue is dissected from the celiac axis, and the median arcuate ligament is elevated from the aorta and the axis, developing the plane between the preaortic fascia and aorta. The crural sutures are tied down. Beginning at the level of the gastroesophageal junction, nonabsorbable sutures are placed through the anterior and posterior bundles of phrenoesophageal fascia and through the median arcuate ligament. A series of four or five additional sutures are placed in a similar fashion extending caudally along the lesser curve. It is customary to perform intraoperative manometry to calibrate the suture tension, with the goal of obtaining a sphincter pressure between 35 and 55 mm Hg greater than the gastric pressure.

The management of a Type II or combined-type hernia (Figure 18.6) differs from that of a Type I hernia to some extent. There is no consensus as to whether an abdominal or a thoracic approach is best. We have had good results with both, but tend to favor the transthoracic approach. This is particularly useful when a large hernia is present or when other abdominal organs have migrated into the hernia sac. The transthoracic approach facilitates dissection of adhesions that often occur in the true hernia sacs. In contrast to the operative management of the Type I hiatal hernia, it is important to excise the peritoneal hernia sac in the Type II hernia to allow healing of the diaphragmatic hiatal defect, reducing the potential for recurrence. Closing the hiatal defect is more difficult than in the usual Type I hernia, and mobilization of the diaphragm from the pericardium, facilitated by the thoracic approach, may reduce tension on the repair.

There is no consensus whether an antireflux operation should be performed routinely in patients with a pure Type II hiatal hernia who have no clinical evidence of gastroesophageal reflux.

It is useful in such patients to evaluate the distal esophageal sphincter characteristics preoperatively and in some cases to perform extended esophageal pH monitoring, but this is not always feasible. The presence of a paraesophageal component to the hernia may alter the manometric characteristics of the sphincter such that prediction of the likelihood of reflux occurring postoperatively is impossible. It is our feeling that antireflux procedures should be performed routinely on these patients, as the normal anatomic relationships in the esophageal hiatus are usually destroyed both by the development of the hernia and by intraoperative dissection. A partial or total fundoplication also tends to anchor the gastroesophageal junction below the diaphragm and blocks herniation of the stomach or other abdominal organs through any remaining potential defect. Those who do not routinely perform a fundoplication usually advocate the addition of a gastrostomy, which functions in a fashion similar to an anterior gastropexy.

OTHER DIAPHRAGMATIC DISORDERS

Herniae

Although they are relatively rare in the elderly, a variety of diaphragmatic herniae may occur through defects other than the esophageal hiatus. Congenital defects may exist posterolaterally (Bochdalek) or anteriorly (Morgagni or retrosternal). The posterolateral diaphragmatic hernia is congenital in origin and is almost always diagnosed in the newborn period or during childhood. In contrast, a retrosternal (or Morgagni) hernia may be asymptomatic in childhood, only to produce symptoms during middle age or later following increases in intraabdominal pressure due to obesity (30, 31). Such a hernia normally contains transverse colon, and symptoms are due to partial or total colonic obstruction. This hernia does not ordinarily require surgical intervention unless it is symptomatic. Repair is most easily performed through a laparotomy with reduction of the hernia contents, excision of the hernia sac, and direct suture of the defect.

A traumatic hernia may occur following either blunt or penetrating trauma. Blunt injury to the

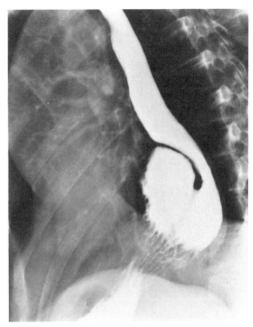

Figure 18.6. This barium study in a patient with a Type III hernia reveals the esophagogastric junction to be above the esophageal hiatus and clearly demonstrates the paraesophageal component.

abdomen can result in a bursting force that ruptures the weakest portion of the diaphragm, the central tendon. This normally occurs on the left side, as the right hemidiaphragm is somewhat protected by the liver. Penetrating diaphragmatic injuries do not usually result in immediate herniation of abdominal viscera and are initially asymptomatic. When herniation does not occur initially, most patients who are eventually affected present within the first few years following injury, having passed through an asymptomatic "interval phase."

When herniation does occur through a traumatic defect, symptoms normally consist of respiratory distress and cyanosis or bowel obstruction. There may be mediastinal displacement accompanied by hypotension. Bowel sounds may be present in the affected chest, and the diagnosis can often be made on plain chest film. Repair should be performed at the time of diagnosis, keeping in mind the association of acute traumatic diaphragmatic herniae with associated intra-abdominal injuries and fluid and electrolyte disorders. Direct closure is usually performed, although in some cases a prosthetic patch of Marlex® or Gortex® may be necessary.

Eventration

Eventration of the diaphragm occurs as a result of paralysis, aplasia, or atrophy of the diaphragmatic muscle fibers. Acquired eventration is said to occur nine times more often on the left side than on the right and is found twice as often in men as in women. Recent information shows that right sided eventration occurs more often than was heretofore thought (32). There is an age-related increase in the incidence of right-sided diaphragmatic eventration, reaching over 5% in those over 70 years of age. In contrast to left-sided eventration, right-sided eventration is much more common in females than in males. In the vast majority of patients, this disorder is very well tolerated, causing no symptoms. The diagnosis is usually made when a chest radiograph is obtained for other reasons. However, eventration may be symptomatic, causing respiratory embarrassment and can be mistaken for an intrathoracic mass. Diaphragmatic plication is indicated when respiratory symptoms accompany an acquired eventration. However, symptomatic and radiographic results may be disappointing, and the operative risk for the elderly patient should be considered.

Tumors

Primary tumors of the diaphragm are quite rare, consisting of cysts and benign or malignant neoplasms. Two-thirds of these tumors are benign, and the malignant tumors are usually sarcomas, particularly fibrosarcoma (33, 34). Symptoms of diaphragmatic tumors are not specific, and the diagnosis is frequently not suspected. A resection is indicated in most cases for both diagnosis and treatment. It is best to repair any defects primarily, although the addition of a prosthetic patch of Marlex® or Gortex® is frequently necessary to achieve adequate closure.

REFERENCES

1. Kramer P: Does a sliding hiatal hernia constitute a clinical entity? *Gastroenterology* 57:422–448, 1968.
2. Cohen S, Harris LD: Does hiatus hernia affect competence of the gastroesophageal sphincter? *N Engl J Med* 284:1053–1056, 1971.
3. Bucher P, Lepsien G, Sonnenberg A, Blum AL: Verlauf und Prognose der Refluxkrankheit bei konservativer und chirurguischer Behandlung. *Schweiz Med Wochenschr* 108:2072–2078, 1978.
4. Wara P, Oster MJ, Funch-Jensen P, Andresen J, Ottosen P: A long term followup of patients resected for benign esophageal stricture using the inkwell esophagogastrostomy. *Ann Surg* 190:214–217, 1979.
5. Jonsell G: The incidence of sliding hiatal hernias in patients with gastroesophageal reflux requiring operation. *Acta Chir Scand* 149:63- 67, 1983.
6. Berstad A, Weberg R, Larsen IF, Hoel B, Hauer-Jensen M: Relationship of hiatus hernia to reflux oesophagitis. *Scand J Gastroenterol* 21:55–58, 1986.
7. Kaul B, Petersen H, Myrvold HE, Grette K, Roysland P, Halvorsen T: Hiatus hernia in gastroesophageal reflux disease. *Scand J Gastroenterol* 21:31–34, 1986.
8. Pridie RB: Incidence and coincidence of hiatus hernia. *Gut* 7:188–189, 1966.
9. Ellis FH: Esophageal hiatal hernia. *N Engl J Med* 287:646–649, 1972.
10. Skinner DB: Pathophysiology of gastroesophageal reflux. *Ann Surg* 202:546–556, 1985.
11. Pettersson GB, Bombeck CT, Nyhus LM: Influence of hiatal hernia on lower esophageal sphincter function. *Ann Surg* 193:214–220, 1981.
12. DeMeester TR, Lafontaine E, Joelsson BE, Skinner DB, Ryan JW, O'Sullivan GC, Brunsden BS, Johnson LF: Relationship of a hiatal hernia to the function of the body of the esophagus and the gastroesophageal junction. *J Thorac Cardiovasc Surg* 82:547–558, 1981.
13. Stanley TV, Cocking JB: Upper gastro-intestinal endoscopy and radiology in the elderly. *Postgrad Med J* 54:257–260, 1978.
14. Ozdemir IA, Burke WA, Ikins PM: Paraesophageal hernia. *Ann Thorac Surg* 16:547–553, 1973.
15. Johns TNP, Clements EL: The relief of anemia by repair of hiatus hernia. *J Thorac Cardiovasc Surg* 41:737–747, 1961.
16. Krupp S, Rossetti M: Surgical treatment of hiatal hernias by fundoplication and gastropexy (Nissen repair). *Ann Surg* 164:927–934, 1966.
17. Skinner DB, Belsey RHR: Surgical management of esophageal reflux and hiatus hernia. *J Thorac Cardiovasc Surg* 53:33–54, 1967.
18. Windsor CWO, Collis JL: Anaemia and hiatus hernia: experience in 450 patients. *Thorax* 22:73–78, 1967.
19. Ellis FH, Crozier RE, Shea JA: Paraesophageal hiatus hernia. *Arch Surg* 121:416–420, 1986.
20. Walther B, DeMeester TR, Lafontaine E, Courtney JV, Little AG, Skinner DB: Effect of paraesophageal hernia on sphincter function and its implication on surgical therapy. *Am J Surg* 147:111–116, 1984.
21. Cameron AJ, Higgins JA: Linear gastric erosion. *Gastroenterology* 91:338–342, 1986.
22. Sellors TH, Papp C: Strangulated diaphragmatic hernia with torsion of the stomach. *Br J Surg* 43:289–292, 1955.
23. Hill LD: Incarcerated paraesophageal hernia. *Am J Surg* 126:286- 291, 1973.
24. Beardsley JM, Thompson WR: Acutely obstructed hia-

tal hernia. *Ann Surg* 159:49–62, 1964.

25. Hoffman E: Strangulated diaphragmatic hernia. *Thorax* 23:541–549, 1968.

26. McDonald CF, Walbaum PR, Sircus W, Grant IWB: Intrapleural perforation of peptic ulcer in association with diaphragmatic hernia. *Br J Dis Chest* 79: 196–199, 1985.

27. Pearson FG, Cooper JD, Ilves R, Todd TRJ, Jamieson WRE: Massive hiatal hernia with incarceration: a report of 53 cases. *Ann Thorac Surg* 35:45–51, 1983.

28. Wichterman K, Geha AS, Cahow CE, Baue AE: Giant paraesophageal hiatus hernia with intrathoracic stomach and colon: the case for early repair. *Surgery* 86:497–506, 1979.

29. O'Sullivan GC, DeMeester TR, Joelsson BE, Smith RB, Blough RR, Johnson LF, Skinner DB: Interaction of lower esophageal sphincter pressure and length of sphinc-ter in the abdomen as determinants of gastroesophageal competence. *Am J Surg* 143:40–47, 1982.

30. Comer TP, Clagget OT: Surgical treatment of hernia of the foramen of Morgagni. *J Thorac Cardiovasc Surg* 52:461–468, 1966.

31. Dawson RE, Jansing CW: Foramen of Morgagni hernias. *J Ky Med Assoc* 75:325–327, 1977.

32. Okuda K, Nomura F, Kawai M, Arimizu N, Okuda H: Age related gross changes of the liver and right diaphragm with special reference to partial eventration. *Br J Radiol* 52:870–875, 1979.

33. Wiener MF, Chou WH: Primary tumors of the diaphragm. *Arch Surg* 90:143–152, 1965.

34. Olafsson G, Rausing A, Holen O: Primary tumors of the diaphragm. *Chest* 59:568–570, 1971.

Chapter 19

Endoscopy in the Elderly

George R. Avant, M.D., R. Benton Adkins, Jr., M.D., F.A.C.S.

Endoscopic examinations performed in the elderly may be diagnostic and lead to elective, corrective action before an emergency situation develops, may provide treatment that will obviate the need for a larger procedure, and may in general be beneficial in the patient's care. The techniques of examination are the same as those performed in younger patients; nonetheless, more attention should be directed toward avoiding complications that might arise from the patient's fragile condition or coexisting diseases. In general the amount of sedation required for endoscopic procedures in the elderly is considerably less than the dosages required for younger patients. In many cases, only pharyngeal anesthesia will be required; in other cases only small amounts of narcotics and benzodiazepines will be needed. The exact dose of medication is difficult to determine in any individual, and the dose should be titrated to minimize adverse affect. Adjustments will be required for patients with coexisting cardiac, pulmonary, or hepatic diseases. We have tended to monitor elderly patients very closely during these procedures, and when risk factors are great, the anesthesiology service may manage both medication and monitoring throughout the procedure.

UPPER GASTROINTESTINAL ENDOSCOPY

Upper gastrointestinal (GI) endoscopy is perhaps the easiest of the endoscopic procedures in the elderly. This procedure can be very productive and in many cases is simpler and may be more helpful in making the diagnosis than an upper GI series. Certainly, the results of directly visualizing the mucosa of the upper GI tract are more efficacious than a barium meal.

Many elderly patients will complain of dysphagia. This may be a reflection of an esophageal motility disorder or a structural abnormality of the esophagus. Carcinoma of the esophagus can be easily diagnosed by endoscopy with direct biopsies or cytologic brushings of the lesion. Cancer of the esophagus in a markedly debilitated patient where there is little hope of cure may occasionally be treated with various types of palliation as mentioned in Chapter 17. Another option for palliation is to use the laser to do photodestruction of bleeding and obstructing tumors as described by Nath and coworkers in 1973 and modified and improved especially since 1983 (1–3). We would recommend these procedures as a palliative effort for elderly debilitated patients whenever other types of treatment are unsafe.

Lower esophageal strictures can be easily diagnosed and dilated under direct vision with the endoscope. Dilatation is frequently successful in offering significant relief of symptoms of dysphagia. Some elderly patients will develop dysphagia related either to a distal esophageal ring or to minimal esophageal strictures because of the presence of poorly masticated food that is usually secondary to ill-fitting or absent dentures. The acute food impaction that occurs in this setting can easily be relieved by endoscopic treatment. If flexible endoscopy is unsuccessful, the rigid esophagoscope is easily used.

Gastric lesions can be directly visualized and biopsied. Gastric ulcerations can be better characterized as either benign or malignant by visualization and biopsy. In the elderly patient, there is the special tendency to develop proximally located gastric ulcers, giant gastric ulcers, lymphomas, sarcomas, and various types of gastritis. Repeated endoscopy and biopsy of all suspicious, unhealed, hypertrophic, ulcerated, nodular, or otherwise unusual areas will be especially productive in surgically treatable pathologic conditions in the elderly patient. The unusual delay in diagnosis of many of these upper GI tract problems in the elderly can be significantly reduced and avoided if an aggressive approach toward repeated endoscopy, visualization, and biopsy of all possibly abnormal areas is vigorously pursued. (See Chapters 17 and 20)

Many elderly patients are now receiving nonsteroidal anti-inflammatory drugs that cause symptoms of dyspepsia and in fact can lead to both gastric and duodenal ulceration. These lesions can best be defined by endoscopic examination.

Upper GI bleeding in the elderly patient can be an event associated with major mortality. The mortality depends on repetitive and uncontrolled blood loss, as well as on the presence of underlying pulmonary and cardiac disease. Endoscopic evaluation early in the acute upper GI tract bleeding episode will help differentiate between bleeding esophageal varices and mucosal lesions, such as Mallory-Weiss tears, gastric or duodenal ulcerations, or vascular lesions. We try to proceed with endoscopy after 500–1000 cc of bleeding in the elderly patient. Sclerotherapy of esophageal varices performed by flexible instruments has been shown to be moderately effective in acute bleeding, as well as for temporary obliteration of the esophageal varices. This may be followed by repetitive sclerotherapy in the elderly cirrhotic patient. Visualization of a bleeding site in the stomach or duodenum has some predictive value: Lesions with a visible vessel suggest that the patient will continue to bleed or have a recurrent bleed.

It is our policy to be very aggressive with elderly patients with upper GI bleeding, especially in those with cardiac or pulmonary disease. If there is any evidence of unrelenting or of recurrent bleeding or if the patient exhibits any cardiovascular instability, an operative procedure is felt to be necessary for the early control of the bleeding site before the situation becomes irreversible. The indications for surgical control of upper GI bleeding from stomach and duodenum are outlined in Chapter 20 where the volume of bleeding per given episode is shown to be related to the prognosis in the elderly patient.

ENDOSCOPIC RETROGRADE CHOLANGIOPANCREATOGRAPHY

Diseases of both the biliary tree and the pancreas occur more frequently in the elderly. Endoscopic examination of the second portion of the duodenum with contrast injection into the biliary system and the pancreatic ductal system is a relatively non-invasive method of x-ray diagnosis. Certainly, endoscopic retrograde pancreatography is the only convenient method of outlining the pancreatic duct. Endoscopic pancreatography may be useful in the patient in whom carcinoma of the pancreas is suspected. If this suspicion is based on clinical evidence and imaging modalities, the diagnosis may be confirmed by finding such characteristic changes as abrupt ductal obstruction and/or irregularity of the pancreatic duct. Pancreatography is helpful also in defining the exact location of a malignancy in the pancreatic gland itself. In the elderly patient with known chronic pancreatitis, the pancreatogram gives information regarding dilatation of the pancreatic duct, thereby allowing critical decisions to be made regarding operability.

Evaluation of jaundice and cholestasis in the elderly is first achieved by non-invasive measures, such as ultrasound and CT scanning. Depending on the results of these imaging modalities in conjunction with the remainder of the evaluation, direct visualization of the papilla and endoscopic cholangiography may be most helpful. Carcinoma of the ampulla of Vater can be easily diagnosed by endoscopic visualization of the area with appropriate biopsies. Because carcinoma of the papilla is a malignant tumor that can be cured by resection if diagnosed early, it is important to take special measures to rule out this disease.

Diagnostic cholangiography can be most productive. A normal cholangiogram in the jaundiced patient would suggest intrahepatic cholestasis possibly due to a drug. In this case no operative intervention would be required. An abnormal cholangiogram is helpful in planning an operative procedure should one be required. Some biliary tract diseases can be treated with therapeutic endoscopy. The elderly patient who is found to have common bile duct stones, whether or not a previous cholecystectomy has been performed, can have endoscopic sphincterotomy with common duct stone extraction. This technique has low morbidity and mortality and affords relief of obstruction and potential sepsis. Some strictures of the bile duct can be successfully dilated with hydrostatic balloons. Patency of obstructing malignant lesions of the biliary tract can be guaranteed by insertion of stents.

LOWER GI ENDOSCOPY

Flexible sigmoidoscopy and colonoscopy have added to our ability to visualize the anus, rectum, and colon in a way that has been previously unavailable with the rigid anoscopes and sigmoidoscopes. However, the anoscope and rigid sigmoidoscope may still be used to great advantage in certain situations and can probably better complement the findings of digital examination than a flexible instrument. These rigid instruments allow visualization of the area of the anus, lower rectum, and anal canal in a way that can never be achieved with flexible instruments because of the direct view that is afforded the examiner of the area of fissures, fistulae, hemorrhoids, and condyloma. Many of these conditions, which are common in the elderly, can be treated in a definitive manner using the rigid endoscopes.

The flexible fiberoptic sigmoidoscope is more expensive, causes less discomfort, allows the examiner to see well beyond the area of the rigid sigmoidoscope, and should be clearly indicated for use in the diagnosis, surveillance, and treatment of problems above the level of the rigid sigmoidoscope. We agree, however, with Marks (4) that never should the need for total colonoscopy be pre-empted by the exclusive use of flexible fiberoptic sigmoidoscopy. The complete examination of the entire colon and rectum can be done only by the use of the full length colonoscope.

Lesions within reach of the flexible fiberoptic sigmoidoscope and those above that area within reach of the flexible colonoscope include polyps, carcinoma, inflammatory lesions, intussusception, volvulus, diverticula, and other conditions that can be diagnosed and sometimes treated in a definitive manner by the use of these fiberoptic instruments. In the aging individual in whom the avoidance of extensive anesthetic and surgical intervention may be very desirable, these instruments have indeed been found to be of great value.

The diagnosis of lower GI tract bleeding, the removal of benign and malignant growths, the diagnosis of inflammatory and neoplastic conditions, the relief of areas of obstruction and pseudo-obstruction, and the surveillance for residual or recurrent disease make these instruments a necessary part of the armamentarium of all surgeons and gastroenterologists involved with the care of elderly individuals.

Special Considerations in the Elderly

We have tended to perform upper and lower GI endoscopy in the high-risk elderly individual under conditions that are carefully monitored and in some instances attended by nurse anesthetists or anesthesiologists. Occasionally this has been helpful and perhaps life saving. When arrhythmias, respiratory changes, unusual complaints, and the rare incidence of perforation were encountered, careful monitoring has been especially valuable. In the elderly individual who may be on chronic steroid therapy for pulmonary or musculoskeletal disorders, a special word of caution should be given. In our experience, endoscopic polypectomy with the use of the cautery has occasionally been associated with delayed perforation at the site of the polypectomy. These problem are recognized immediately and solved expeditiously and without mortality. When monitoring of this magnitude is not available for the elderly patient undergoing prolonged and significant endoscopy, it is advised that close attention be paid to any signs of distress that might occur during the procedure at which time the procedure should be aborted prematurely, rather than too late. Most well-equipped endoscopy laboratories have sufficient modern monitoring devices to satisfy these requirements for most elderly patients.

BRONCHOSCOPY

The rigid bronchoscope is used primarily by

thoracic surgeons to diagnose pulmonary and bronchial disorders. The fiberoptic bronchoscope has a wide variety of uses, and flexible bronchoscopy is now used by many other medical specialists.

In the postoperative patient, flexible bronchoscopy is useful in cases of respiratory failure to clear secretions from the airway or to treat atelectasis. Frequent bronchoscopy in burn patients or in those who have smoke inhalation is an effective means of irrigation, suction, and removal of desquamated epithelium.

Aspiration of gastric contents is not uncommon in the elderly patient. Flexible bronchoscopy should always be employed immediately to clear the bronchi of these aspirated contents; in some situations, rigid bronchoscopy may be necessary for a more thorough washing and cleansing of the tracheobronchial tree.

As with other types of endoscopic procedures, careful monitoring of the high-risk elderly patient is essential during the procedure. Cardiac arrhythmias may occur as a result of hypoxia or vagal stimulation. For this reason, many surgeons have chosen to perform most of the diagnostic endoscopies on the surgical service in the operating room under local anesthesia with full monitoring and attendance by the anesthesiologists. Therapeutic endoscopy can be done easily in the intensive care suite with full monitoring as required.

As with obstructing lesions of the esophagus, the occasion will arise when it is appropriate to use the laser, multiple biopsies, the cautery, and other instruments for the dilatation and clearing of the airway in the elderly individual who has obstructing strictures and tumors of the bronchi and trachea. With a cooperative effort between the endoscopists and the anesthesiologists, major airway-obstructing tumors can also be handled in elderly individuals using the YAG laser technique (5, 6).

CHOLEDOCHOSCOPY

The incidence of retained stones in the elderly patient following cholecystecomy and exploration of the common bile duct is at least as high as the usual reported incidences of this occurrence in the general population, and it is our impression that it may be higher. Reports of 5% to 10% are usually given, but the true incidence obviously is never known because some retained stones never have clinical manifestations. When instances of retained stones in elderly individuals arise and a second laparotomy is necessary, most surgeons prefer the rigid endoscope with a right angle viewing arm that is very similar to the nephroscope employed for kidney stones. An excellent description of the use of this instrument including its indications can be found in *Common Bile Duct Exploration* (7) and subsequently discussed by Berci in *Surgical Endoscopy* (8). We prefer the flexible fiberoptic choledochoscope, which can be used both intraoperatively and postoperatively through a well-established T-tube drainage tract. Our experience with the use of this instrument both during the initial duct exploration and also in the postoperative patient has been most gratifying. This is especially true in cases of elderly individuals in whom a formal second surgical procedure can be successfully avoided.

SUMMARY

Perhaps more than in any age group, the technique of endoscopy can be used in the elderly patients to the greatest benefit. Both the diagnostic and therapeutic uses of these instruments are especially suited to the elderly patient who needs especially careful surveillance and ultra-safe nonoperative therapy whenever possible. These techniques should not, however, take the place of more definitive procedures when they are indicated for the appropriate treatment of our elderly patients.

REFERENCES

1. Nath G, Gorisch W, Kreitmair A, Kiefhaber P: Transmission of a powerful argon laser beam through a fiberoptic flexible gastroscope for operative gastroscopy. *Endoscopy* 5:213–215, 1973.
2. Fleischer D, Kessler F: Endoscopic Nd:YAG laser therapy for carcinoma of the esophagus: a new form of palliative treatment. *Gastroenterology* 85:600–603, 1983.
3. Fleischer D: Palliative therapy of esophageal carcinoma. In Fleischer D, Jensen D, Bright-Asare P (eds): *Therapeutic Laser Endoscopy in Gastrointestinal Disease.* Boston, Martinus Nijhoff, 1983, pp 117–129.
4. Marks G: Guidelines for the use of flexible fiberoptic colonoscopy in the management of patients with colorectal neoplasia. *Dis Colon Rectum* 22:302–305, 1979.

5. Warner M, Warner M, Leonard PF: Anesthesia for neodymium-YAG (Nd-YAG) laser resection of major airway obstructing tumors. *Anesthesiology* 60:232–235, 1984.

6. Rontal M, Rontal E: Laser treatment of tracheal and endobronchial lesions. In Dent TL, Strodel WE, Turcotte JG (eds): *Surgical Endoscopy.* Chicago, Year Book, 1985, pp 391–406.

7. Cuschieri A: Exploration of the common bile duct. In Cuschieri A, Berci G (eds): *Common Bile Duct Exploration.* Boston, Martinus Nijhoff, 1984, pp 81–84.

8. Berci G: Choledochoscopy. In Dent TL, Strodel WE, Turcotte JG (eds): *Surgical Endoscopy.* Chicago, Year Book, 1985, pp 349–361.

Chapter 20

Diseases of the Stomach and Duodenum in the Elderly

R. Benton Adkins, Jr., M.D., F.A.C.S., H. William Scott, Jr., M.D., F.A.C.S.

Many gastrointestinal symptoms appear as we grow older, and other symptoms that are already present tend to worsen with aging. The symptoms imposed upon the elderly patient by the changes of aging are often considered to be purely functional in nature, but they tend to become increasingly bothersome with time and may cause the older patient much anxiety. When the seemingly functional symptoms of dyspepsia, "gas," flatulence, fullness, epigastric discomfort, and frank pain persist in the elderly they should always be investigated (1).

Most studies have shown that the gastrointestinal tract complaints of the elderly are 60% functional, 10% malignant disease, 8% biliary tract, 7% duodenal ulcer, 3% gastric ulcer, 3% diverticulitis, and 9% all other causes (2).

Dyspeptic symptoms and epigastric distress, so common in the elderly, may be caused by ulcer disease, gastritis, or malignant disease, or they may be purely functional (3). Cancer of the stomach may cause such unexpected symptoms as left upper quadrant pain and diarrhea in the elderly. These symptoms should always prompt immediate investigation. Exact localization of pain from benign or malignant ulcerations of the stomach is difficult enough for any patient, but is notoriously imprecise in the elderly (3).

ANATOMY AND PHYSIOLOGY

The changes of aging that are seen throughout the gastrointestinal tract are most easily studied in the stomach. Endoscopes, suction tubes, biopsy forceps, and sensors of pressure, pH, and motility find easy access to the esophagus, stomach, and duodenum. With aging, there

is variable but definite evidence for a decrease in the quality and quantity of the secretions of digestive enzymes and acid in the stomach.

The anatomic and physiologic changes that are associated with many senile stomachs include mucosal atrophy, decreased blood supply, decreased motility, diminished absorption, and a degree of hypochlorhydria (4). Gastric emptying times for elderly individuals are not that different from younger controls when no gastric lesions are present (5). A few studies show that there is slightly delayed gastric emptying after age 70 (6).

After age 50, the level of acid and pepsin secretion begins to decline, and this reduction continues until it reaches one-third of the levels of normal young adults by age 70–80. There is thinning of the gastric mucosa that parallels the decrease in mucosal secretions; there is also an increase in submucosal fibrosis, a drop in mucin secretion, a fall in the number of parietal cells, and metaplasia of the fundic glands (2).

These changes leave the aged stomach vulnerable to gastric ulcer, gastric polyps, and atrophic gastritis. All of these are of significance, but especially alarming is the latter, which is associated with a 20-fold increased risk of gastric cancer. The ratio of prevalence of duodenal to gastric ulcer changes from 10 to 1 in the young to 2 to 1 in the aged.

More fat is found in the elderly stomach wall as the muscle layers thin out and become slightly atrophic and as the submucosa becomes infiltrated with leukocytes, monocytes, and poorly formed elastic fibers. There is a progressive and definite proximal migration of the line of junction between fundic and antral mucosa with aging (7). This migration may account for the onset of hypochlorhydria and atrophic gastritis and for the more proximal location of gastric ulcers and gastric cancers in the aged stomach.

STUDIES AND INVESTIGATIONS

Investigation of the gastrointestinal symptoms of the elderly should be done in a careful and thorough manner to identify organic problems. When the studies are done well, they will be helpful and in themselves therapeutic for the worried elderly patient. If done routinely for complaints expressed by elderly patients, the usual long delay in the diagnosis of serious upper gastrointestinal tract diseases in the elderly can be avoided. Unfortunately, the early symptoms of the elderly are frequently ignored. A delay in investigative efforts and in diagnosis has become the hallmark of upper gastrointestinal problems of the aged. The usual clinical picture of advanced cancer and complicated, urgent peptic ulcer disease is the typical introduction of the elderly patient to the surgeon.

PATHOLOGY

Chronic Gastritis

In 1980, Correa (8) presented a synopsis of his epidemiologic, etiologic, and pathogenetic studies of chronic gastritis in which he modified the concepts of Strickland and McKay (9) and earlier students of this subject. His new classification was established in an effort to classify the major forms of chronic gastritis into groups that reflect the best theory of etiopathogenic factors based on currently available information. Correa's synthesis of the principal causes of chronic gastritis on a worldwide basis, the morphologic substratum of which is a chronic inflammation of the gastric mucosa, includes three types of gastritis.

1. Type of chronic gastritis that accompanies the pernicious anemia (PA) syndrome: Because this syndrome is related to autoimmune mechanisms, he labels this type *autoimmune chronic gastritis* or *ACG*.
2. Type of gastritis seen in patients with duodenal ulcer disease whose excessive gastric acid peptic secretion is thought to be of psychosomatic or neurogenic origin: Correa labels this group *hypersecretory chronic gastritis* or *HCG*.
3. Type of gastritis most common in populations with a high frequency of gastric cancer: Because this type of gastritis is probably related to diet, an important component of the environment, he labels it *environmental chronic gastritis* or *ECG*.

Figure 20.1 shows topographic diagrams of the three types of chronic gastritis that Correa has described (8).

Autoimmune chronic gastritis is the type classified in the past by Strickland and McKay and others as Type A gastritis (9). For many years, complete atrophy of the parietal cell mass has been recognized as an important component of the pernicious anemia syndrome. This occurs in less than half of patients; chronic atrophic gastritis and intestinal metaplasia are found on gastric biopsy in the majority of patients with involvement of the corpus and fundus, leaving the antrum undisturbed as shown in the Figure 20.1. The pathogenesis of the gastric lesion is injury by autoantibodies against parietal cells and intrinsic factor. The intestinal metaplasia that accompanies ACG has a high risk of undergoing dysplastic changes with the development of gastric cancer with advancing age. The tumors that result are characteristically located in the corpus and fundus of the stomach.

Correa has pointed out that there are at least two etiologic entities that can produce peptic ulcer: hypersecretory chronic gastritis (HCG), which can also be called psychosomatic or neurogenic gastritis, and environmental gastritis (ECG). For all practical purposes, duodenal ulcers constitute a part of the HCG syndrome, whereas gastric ulcers may form a part of either the HCG or ECG complexes. As indicated in Figure 20.1 the topographic localization of gastritis in patients with duodenal ulcer is confined to the antrum while the corpus and fundus are normal or show minimal focal, acute, superficial gastritis. On the contrary, when the ulcer that accompanies the HCG complex is located in the stomach, the gastritis is present in the antrum, but according to Correa may also extend to the body of the stomach.

HCG is characterized histologically by

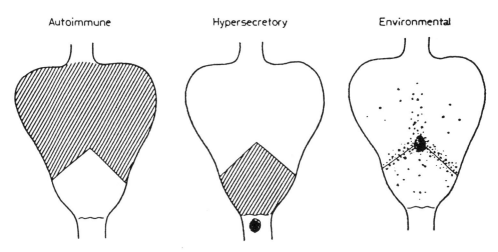

Figure 20.1. Topographic diagrams of the three types of chronic gastritis described by Correa. (Reprinted with permission from Correa P: The epidemiology and pathogenesis of chronic gastritis: three etiologic entities. *Frontiers in Gastrointestinal Research,* Basel, Karger, 1980, pp 98–108.)

mucosal distortion caused by regenerative hyperplasia of epithelial cells and lymphocytic infiltration of the lamina propria, often with large lymphoid follicles and germinal centers. Correa believes that antral gastritis precedes duodenal ulcers. He further indicates that, when HCG results in gastric ulcers, they are most frequently pyloric in location. Hypersecretory chronic gastritis is associated with excessive secretion of acid and pepsin. Surgeons have learned empirically to treat prepyloric ulcers because of these associations, as they treat duodenal ulcers.

Environmental chronic gastritis is Correa's third categorization of chronic gastritis and includes the so-called intestinal or epidemic type that is frequent in populations with a high risk of gastric cancer. He has indicated that epidemiologists have gradually realized that both this form of chronic gastritis (Figure 20.1) and gastric carcinoma quite likely share the same etiology. Multiple studies of populations that are at high risk for gastric carcinoma in various parts of the world have identified chronic gastritis as a cancer precursor. In the early stages, there are few symptoms, but as gastritis progresses in severity, postprandial epigastric discomfort, heartburn, and development of gastric ulcer may occur, requiring medical and, less frequently, surgical treatment. The distribution of the lesions of ECG in the mucosa of the stomach is multifocal and involves both antrum and body, as seen in Figure 20.1.

The early histologic lesions of ECG are those of acute superficial gastritis. As it progresses, a dense lymphocytic inflammatory infiltrate develops, and the stomach slowly enters into a condition of gastric atrophy with hypochlorhydria and ultimately achlorhydria. With loss of the gastric glandular epithelium, regeneration takes place and is usually faulty, and the gastric cells gradually are replaced by cells normally found in intestinal mucosa. This is intestinal metaplasia of the gastric mucosa, a common result of the atrophic changes of ACG and ECG types of gastritis; it rarely occurs with HCG.

In Correa's opinion, most patients with ECG live a normal life without further complications from the gastritis. However, a small group of them have atypical changes in their intestinalized gastric mucosa and develop gastric dysplasia. These alterations are progressive and can lead to invasive adenocarcinoma. The type of carcinoma that develops under these conditions is the so-called epidemic or intestinal type. Correa indicates that a quite different type of gastric carcinoma known as the diffuse variety is not associated with ECG, intestinal metaplasia, or dysplasia and is called endemic because it does not have the geographic clustering of the epidemic type.

Hyperplastic Gastropathy

Hyperplastic gastropathy is a term introduced by Ming in 1973 to designate a group of uncommon conditions that are characterized by gross and sometimes gigantic enlargement of the rugal folds of the gastric mucosa (10). Ming's term replaced the older term "hypertropic gastritis," which is considered a misnomer because rugal enlargement is caused neither by inflammatory gastritis nor hypertrophy, but by hyperplasia of the mucosal epithelial cells.

Fieber and Rickert (11) have strongly endorsed the pathologic classification of hyperplastic gastropathy suggested by Ming in 1973, in which three types are defined:

1. Mucous cell type: Hyperplasia involves the mucous surface and the foveolar cells. The glands are normal or atrophic. Systemic dilatation of glands can frequently be observed, and occasionally intestinal metaplasia is found.
2. Glandular cell type: Hyperplasia involves the gastric glands with an increase in the numbers of parietal and chief cells. Often the foveolae are shortened, and the number of mucous cells may be reduced.
3. Mixed mucous-glandular type: According to Ming, hyperplasia involves both the mucous and the specialized cells.

In 50 cases selected from the literature by Fieber and Rickert (11), the incidence by Ming's pathologic type was (1) mucous cell hyperplasia, 33 cases; (2) glandular cell hyperplasia, 11 cases; and (3) mixed mucous-glandular cell hyperplasia, 6 cases.

The 33 cases of mucous cell hyperplasia seem to be cases of Menetrier's disease both with and without protein losses (11). In our opinion, the Zollinger-Ellison syndrome represents the most frequently encountered clinical manifestation of Ming's glandular cell hyperplasia, and gastrinomas of pancreas or duodenum are the specific cause (10).

Menetrier's disease may occur in the very young and also in the elderly. Its etiology is no better known today than when described by Menetrier in 1888 (12). On pathologic examination, the enlarged rugal folds of Menetrier's disease are caused by enormous hyperplasia of the mucous cells of the gastric epithelium. There is a concomitant atrophy with disappearance of the parietal and chief cells of the gastric mucosa. In Fieber and Rickert's collected series, the average age was 40 years, with a range from 5 to 87 years. The ratio of males to females was 39:11. X-rays studies show the enlarged rugal folds in the upper part of the stomach with sparing of the antrum, which may be quite small. Gastroscopy shows massive enlargement of rugal folds, and gross examination cannot determine differences between mucous-glandular forms of hyperplasia. Menetrier's disease must be differentiated from the mucosal hyperplasia of the Zollinger-Ellison syndrome and from the forms of hyperplastic gastropathy to which Schindler gave the name hypertrophic glandular gastritis and which Stempien classified as hypertrophic hypersecretory gastritis. These conditions are all known to be possibilities in the elderly patient. A carefully done endoscopy with multiple biopsies is mandatory when any of these abnormalities are discovered on x-ray studies of elderly patients.

Peptic Ulcer Disease

Unlike neoplasia, the incidence of peptic ulcer does not appear to increase with age. The type and location of ulcers seen in the elderly population change from an almost exclusively duodenal prevalence in the young (10:1) to a prevalence of only 2:1 of duodenal ulcer over gastric ulcer as age progresses (13). The decreased quality of mucus and possibly some impaired circulation to the gastric mucosa contribute to these increases of gastric ulcers in the elderly. Middle-aged men are 10 to 11 times as apt to have a duodenal ulcer as middle-aged women. In old age, this ratio drops to 5:1. Old men and old women have gastric ulcers at the same rate. The peak incidence for both gastric and duodenal ulcers is in the fourth and fifth decade (14).

Symptoms of duodenal ulcers in the elderly are usually not severe, are frequently ignored, may be called functional, and are notoriously atypical. These features account for many of the serious and often complicated problems of advanced peptic ulcer disease that present so often in the elderly. Even when advanced to the point of bleeding, penetration, and/or perforation, duodenal ulcers may present in a very undramatic way and be difficult to diagnose in an aged patient (15).

Gastric ulcers also may be very atypical in the aged and may cause the elderly patient to complain of vague upper abdominal pain, left upper quadrant fullness, weight loss, anorexia, nausea, and vomiting. Fever, leukocytosis, and abdominal signs may be minimal or entirely absent even with perforation (2). Older people often gradually adjust to the onset of pyloric obstruction when it occurs secondary to chronic peptic ulcer disease, and it may be very far advanced before complaints are elicited. It should be stressed again that none of the vague complaints that could be from peptic ulcer disease, but that are often thought to be functional, should be dismissed in the elderly patient. Although such symptoms can be functional, they can also stem from duodenal or gastric ulcer, chronic gastritis, or worse, from carcinoma of the stomach!

It is of interest to note here that the symptoms of cancer of the stomach and of gastric ulcer in the elderly may include diarrhea and other changes in bowel habits that are not usually associated with diseases of the stomach.

Perforation, gastric outlet obstruction, and bleeding are the complications of peptic ulcer that will lead to emergency or urgent surgical attention. It must be remembered that over 50% of the patients over age 60 with peptic ulcer who present with these serious complications will present as *new* cases. Such patients will usually have no previous history of ulcer, and it will often be the first time for that patient to complain of these symptoms (13, 16, 17). Fewer than 40% will recall any previous symptoms that could be those of peptic ulcer disease, and the symptoms that they do recall tend to be atypical. Approximately 80% of all deaths from peptic ulcers occur in the elderly age group, and bleeding is the most common complication in this group and the leading cause of death (18).

There is also general agreement that among all elderly patients with peptic ulcer disease who are symptomatic and who are followed long enough, more than half will eventually have a serious, complicated course and only one-fourth will ever become permanently asymptomatic (19).

An even poorer prognosis can be expected if bleeding is the first symptom to occur in an elderly patient with peptic ulcer disease (20). If bleeding is the reason for hospitalization, 20%–40% of gastric and 40%–50% of duodenal ulcer patients who present with this problem will need immediate surgical treatment at that time (21).

There is another subset of problems to be seen in the group of elderly patients who have had previous symptoms of peptic ulcer disease. Many older persons with established peptic ulcer disease who have been under treatment for 10, 15, or even 20 years will eventually reach 65 years of age. At that time and at that age, they are entering into the period of maximal susceptibility for the major complications that have just been mentioned as occurring in the group of elderly patients with no previous symptoms. Martin and Lewis predicted many years ago that approximately 50% of those patients who bleed massively would be in the category of patients in whom peptic ulcer disease had been present for over 10 years (22).

Bleeding Ulcers in the Elderly

The most common complication of a peptic ulcer in an elderly patient is massive arterial bleeding (See Table 20.1). Bleeding accounts for one half to two thirds of fatal cases (16). One-half of the bleeding cases occur in the absence of previous symptoms (23). A patient over age 50 with a peptic ulcer is twice as likely to bleed as a patient less than 50 (24).

In an excellent report from England by Watson, Hooper, and Ingram, half of their patients

Table 20.1 Complications in 100 Consecutive Patients Over Age 70 Admitted with Peptic Ulcer.

Complication	Gastric Ulcer	Duodenal Ulcer	Combined Gastric Ulcer and Duodenal Ulcer	Total
Bleeding	40	41	2	83
Perforation	5	3		8
Severe abdominal pain	1	5	1	7
Obstruction		2		2
	46	51	3	100

(Reprinted with permission from Narayanan M, Steinheber FU: The changing face of peptic ulcer in the elderly. *Med Clin N Am* 60:1159–1172, 1976)

over 65 with duodenal ulcers presented with bleeding (25). Half of the bleeders required surgical treatment, and half of the deaths in their patients were from bleeding. Ten percent of their surgically treated bleeders died after the operation, and 20% of the non-surgically treated patients died from bleeding. These figures agree with those of Antler who also noted that the operative mortality rate for patients who were operated upon for bleeding was similar in the very young and the elderly (26). Middle-aged patients who were operated on for bleeding fared better than either the old or very young in their experience.

Of patients over 65 years of age who require a surgical procedure for uncontrolled bleeding, there is a 10% to 20% mortality rate that varies directly with the duration of bleeding prior to operative intervention. Nonoperative mortality will usually be much greater because most elderly patients tolerate a surgical procedure far better than they do prolonged or recurrent bleeding (19, 25).

Perforation of Peptic Ulcer

Perforation of duodenal ulcer and gastric ulcer ranks second to bleeding as a cause of death and accounts for about one-fourth of ulcer-related deaths in the elderly. Kane, Fried, and McSherry reported 17% mortality rate in those treated surgically within 12 hours of perforation in a group of patients aged 60 years or older (27). One hundred percent of those treated non-operatively died. Feliciano and his co-workers in Houston recently reported their experience with perforated peptic ulcers in the elderly and found that only about one-half of them had a previous history of peptic ulcer, that it was difficult to make the diagnosis at the time of admission, and that the time from perforation to operation ranged from 3–72 hours or an average of about 18 hours, despite the fact that 75% had intraperitoneal free air when radiographs were finally obtained (28). Approximately 70% of their cases of perforated peptic ulcers in the elderly were duodenal, and 30% were gastric. The operative mortality rate was 18% for patients with duodenal and 19% for those with gastric ulcer perforations (28).

Walt recently reported a significant rise in the frequency of perforated ulcer in elderly people from all over the United Kingdom. This has been most marked since 1977, with rates of perforation in older women increasing faster than those for elderly men. Smoking and the use of anti-inflammatory drugs were suggested as important etiologic factors (29).

Watson and his associates also noted a high proportion of their patients who perforated (30%) and an even higher percentage of those who bled to be on anti-inflammatory drugs, especially phenylbutazone (25). Pillay et al reported an overall operative mortality rate of 23.5% for emergency procedures for bleeding and perforation in patients aged 65 years and older; all of those who died were over age 75 (30).

Gastric Outlet Obstruction

If chronic peptic ulceration occurs at or near the pylorus, a gastric outlet obstruction may result. Bouts of inflammation, edema, and fibrosis will lead to obstruction that will cause vomiting, dehydration, and electrolyte disturbances. Birkett outlines a good treatment plan for the elderly patient with this complication (31). It consists of 7–10 days of nasogastric suction, rehydration, correction of hypochloremia, and careful correction of hypokalemia. If the obstruction is not resolved by 7–10 days the patient should be operated upon. The likelihood is good that the procedure can then be done safely as an elective operation upon an elderly patient who is in good condition.

Gastric Ulcers

Gastric ulcers in the elderly behave in a slightly different fashion than they do in younger patients. Even in the elderly, duodenal ulcers still account for more of the actual number of patients with peptic ulcers than do gastric ulcers, but gastric ulcers account for two of every three deaths from peptic ulcer disease in the elderly (32). Ulcers greater than 3 cm in diameter, also called giant gastric ulcers, tend to occur more often in the elderly than in the young (33). Gastric ulcers also tend to be more proximally located and are more apt to occur within the cardia or within a hiatal hernia in the elderly patient.

The symptoms of gastric ulcer in the elderly are vague, misleading, bizarre, or absent. A high percentage (50%) of the cases present with a serious complication and with no previous history of symptoms. As previously mentioned, many gastric ulcers will have caused bleeding, perforation, or gastric outlet obstruction at the time the elderly patient makes the first visit, which will be as an emergency because of the major complication.

When symptoms of gastric ulcer do exist they may include pain in the left upper quadrant or the left lower quadrant, pain radiating to the chest, pain worsened with eating, weight loss, loss of appetite, anemia and weakness, dysphagia, constipation, or angina. It is the wise doctor indeed who will first suspect gastric ulcer or cancer of the stomach in this confusing setting.

The giant gastric ulcer is particularly troublesome because it has a high complication rate and is difficult to differentiate from ulcerated cancer. Giant ulcers heal slowly or not at all, and they can be difficult to resect. Fifty percent will bleed, only one third will heal with medical treatment, and when they occur in the elderly, they have a predictable overall mortality rate of 20%. Repeated endoscopy is necessary to monitor healing and to rule out cancer in the course of treatment of patients with this troublesome problem (19).

Intractable Pain in Peptic Ulcer Disease

Young and middle-aged peptic ulcer patients often have intractable pain and related symptoms suggestive of deep penetration of the chronic ulcer. However, pain that is unresponsive to medical management is an unusual problem in the elderly patient with peptic ulcer disease, no matter how deeply penetrating the ulcer. This is reflected by the fact that operation for intractable pain accounts for less than 5% of operations done for ulcer disease in patients above age 70 (19).

If an elderly patient with known duodenal or gastric ulcer develops severe or intractable pain, it usually means that the ulcer has penetrated into an adjacent organ, such as pancreas or liver, or into the lesser sac, mesocolon, or biliary tract. A large (giant) duodenal bulbar ulcer may occupy the entire duodenal bulb and be difficult to identify accurately on upper gastrointestinal x-ray examination. This uncommon type of ulcer may be the cause of intractable pain even in the elderly.

Although intractable pain is an uncommon symptom, when it does exist or when it develops in the elderly patient with a known peptic ulcer, it is a symptom that usually indicates that the patient needs prompt surgical intervention.

Surgical Treatment of Peptic Ulcer Disease in the Elderly

In older patients with bleeding peptic ulcer disease, we have tended to follow a general policy of management that is a close modification of the recommendations of Kaplan in 1972 (21) and of Christianson of Denmark, who reported a review of gastric ulcer in old age in 1978 (34). These recommendations are as follows:

1. Elderly patients with upper gastrointestinal bleeding should have prompt endoscopy to determine the site of bleeding. This should be done after only 500–1500 cc of bleeding.
2. If *active* bleeding from an artery in a gastric or duodenal ulcer is seen and the patient is a reasonable risk, he or she is operated on promptly before 2000–2500 cc of blood replacement is needed.
3. If active bleeding stops after 500–1500 cc and no arterial bleeding is seen on endoscopy, elective medical treatment is given. If the bleeding stops after 2000+ cc, elective surgical treatment is employed later unless medical problems are too great.
4. If it is the second bleed or more within 2 years and the total bleeding has been 2500 cc or more, we would plan to operate electively if possible.
5. Elderly patients with serious medical problems who have stopped bleeding should be treated for the medical problems before operative intervention is considered.
6. All bleeding gastric ulcers, even those in patients with massive medical problems, should be considered for operative treatment, rather than permitting exsanguination to occur.
7. Hemorrhagic gastritis usually is treated by non-operative means.

It has been fairly well shown by Kaplan et al. that the elderly patient with peptic ulcer disease tolerates bleeding very poorly (21). The report from Australia in 1981 agreed (30). Kaplan showed 7.5% mortality if bleeding was less than 3000 cc, 26% for 3000–5000 cc, and 35% for bleeding over 5000 cc (21). Their study and many other reports have shown that elderly patients tolerate exploratory laparotomy and suture of the bleeding site and even resection and vagotomy better than they tolerate prolonged bleeding (4, 19, 35).

We continue to do vagotomy, pyloroplasty, and suture of the bleeding *duodenal* ulcer in elderly patients (35). We recommend vagotomy and antrectomy to include the ulcer for *gastric* ulcer whenever possible in the elderly group (36).

Treatment of Perforation of Peptic Ulcer

Perforation is the second most common complication of peptic ulcer disease in the elderly population and accounts for about one-fourth of ulcer-related deaths. The risk of perforation doubles after age 50, and as mentioned before, the diagnosis may be delayed because of the lack of specific symptoms to suggest the diagnosis in the elderly patient. Only about one-half of the cases will be operated on in the first 12 hours of perforation. This delay affects the decision that the surgeon must make as to the proper type of surgical treatment. The best recent study on this subject is from the group at Baylor in Houston (28). They recommend a definitive resection of the ulcer if the patient's condition warrants it and primary closure of the perforation only if the condition of the patient is very poor. We agree with them that the operation done for elderly patients with perforated peptic ulcers should be selected in the same manner as for younger patients with the same findings. We recommend a gastrectomy to include the perforation site for perforated gastric ulcers when the patient's condition is good. If the patient is in poor condition, a vagotomy with pyloroplasty is done after the perforated gastric ulcer is excised. A generous biopsy should be done on all perforated gastric ulcers that are not resected or excised to exclude malignant disease if closure alone is used (36). In elderly patients with *duodenal* perforations, we do vagotomy with either an antrectomy or drainage procedure in patients with a long history of symptoms.

Gastric Polyps

Less than 5% of the elderly patients who have endoscopy or gastric resections for all reasons will be found to have gastric polyps. It has not been shown that this incidence increases with further advance of age. Hyperplastic epithelioid polyps, adenomatous polyps, and the hyperplasiogenous polyp are the types often seen (37, 38).

There is a definite relationship between polyps and cancer of the stomach, with foci of malignant areas often being seen within gastric polyps that are removed. The other frequently described relationship is that of one or more associated benign polyps being seen elsewhere in those stomachs that are resected for cancer (39). The adenomatous polyp is the type of polyp most often associated with atrophic gastritis and also the one with the greatest malignant potential. Most reports show that about 10% of patients with adenomatous gastric polyps developed cancer of the stomach if they were followed long enough (40). Any gastric polyp seen on x-ray or at endoscopy should be removed. It should always be studied by microscopy. The large ones and the ones that are not true polyps but are sessile adenomas are those most likely to be malignant (38).

Benign Gastric Neoplasms

The adenomatous polyp has already been discussed and is the most common benign gastric neoplasm. The leiomyoma of the stomach is the next most common benign lesion of the stomach, followed by lipoma (41).

Leiomyomas are submucosal or subserosal. They are usually asymptomatic and only produce symptoms if they become large, ulcerated, and bleed or cause pressure symptoms. They should be removed to rule out malignant change.

Lipomas are submucosal and tend to be sessile and may project into the lumen and become pedunculated. They have the same symptoms as leiomyomas, and the same treatment considerations should be given as for leiomyomata.

Neurilemmoma, fibroma, aberrant pancreas, and angiomas of various types appear in the stomach. They have all the same diagnostic and therapeutic implications as any mucosal or gastric wall lesion. In the elderly patient they should be removed and frozen section studies done to rule out cancer.

There is an association between atrophic gastritis and gastric carcinoids. Helling and Wood have reported 14 patients with atrophic gastritis, pernicious anemia, and gastric carcinoids, one of which was an 80-year-old woman (42). They point out that in this setting the carcinoid tumors may be multiple at the time of diagnosis; they recommend local excision for diagnosis and gastrectomy for multiple or diffuse involvement. We would agree and recommend that all carcinoid tumors larger than 2 cm be treated as malignant tumors (43).

Villous adenomata of the pylorus and duodenum are not common, but tend to occur in middle aged and older age groups. They should all be excised and treated with local excision if benign, more aggressively with *in situ* carcinoma, and as any cancer of the stomach or duodenum if invasion is present (44).

Cancer of the Stomach

Gastric cancer is more common in the later years of life, and most series of cases now report a peak age of 62–65, whereas some series show a peak age of 70 or above (45). Adenocarcinoma of the stomach may arise from or be found in a pre-existing adenoma, in the margin of a giant ulcer, in an area of chronic gastritis, or within sites of gastric mucosal atrophy. About half of the gastric cancers that occurred in this country in the first half of this century were located in the antrum or distal body of the stomach. Recently, however, most series are reporting a more proximal location of the primary site of the cancer, especially in men who are in the older age groups at the time of onset (46). These more proximally located tumors are rarely if ever of the signet ring cell type. The signet ring cell types still occur, but are now seen more often in women. In female patients most tumors still arise in the traditional, distally located antral sites (47).

Gastric Ulcer-Cancer Relationship

From 2%–6% of apparently benign gastric ulcers in every reported series are found to be cancerous on close examination at endoscopy and by careful biopsy or at the time of resection (36,

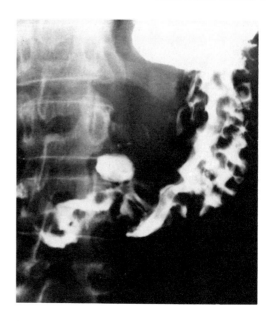

Figure 20.2. Upper gastrointestinal series shows a deep, lesser curvature gastric ulcer in the upper antral area. The presence of an associated duodenal ulcer characterizes this lesion as a Type II gastric ulcer. The radiologic, endoscopic, and gross pathologic appearance of the lesion were all typical for benign gastric ulcer. Final pathological report of the resected specimen was that of gastric adenocarcinoma. (Reprinted with permission from Adkins RB, et al: The management of gastric ulcers. *Ann Surg* 201:741–751, 1985)

48, 49). If there is an associated duodenal ulcer with the gastric ulcer, as shown in Figure 20.2, the likelihood that the latter will be malignant drops to 1%–2% (50). With good endoscopic techniques most malignant gastric ulcers should be detected (36, 51–53).

One problem that has developed in the past 8–10 years with the prolonged treatment of patients for "benign" gastric ulcer using H2 blockers, diet, and antacids is that some undiagnosed malignant ulcers placed on this regimen will heal (54–55).

The giant gastric ulcer larger than 3 cms is hard to distinguish from cancer, is more likely to have bleeding and perforation, and has a much greater likelihood of malignancy as it increases in size (50, 56).

As is true of benign gastric ulcers, it has recently been observed that gastric cancers have migrated more and more proximally in the stomach with advancing age (4). Steinheber also has pointed out that two paradoxes exist: First, when we assume that more gastric cancers occur in the elderly and we know there are many more elderly people now available to develop gastric cancer, we would expect to see more gastric cancers (4). Yet, there has been a dramatic decline in the incidence of gastric cancer in the United States in the last 30 years. This decline in incidence has not occurred in Japan and China. In the United States, a much lower percentage of a much larger group of elderly people have developed gastric cancer. A new observation also has been that even more of those cancers of the common adenocarcinoma cell type are being seen in a more proximal location.

The second paradox with cancer of the stomach is that, in spite of improved x-ray technique, better endoscopy, earlier detection by history, and improved surgical techniques, we are doing no better with cure. Hoerr in 1973 (57) and Diehl in 1983 (58) reported the results from Cleveland Clinic. Comparable patients from both decades had the same results: One-fourth were resected for cure, and a 5-year cure rate of 40% was observed in those few who were resected for cure. Diehl noticed that the number of early cancers that they detected actually declined over the last decade at their institution (58). In Japan, the incidence of gastric cancer has continued to rise over the past 30 years in all age groups, and the incidence of "early cancer" has increased.

"Early" Gastric Cancer

We have found very few early gastric cancers in our hospitals (51). In contrast, in Japan where there is the highest rate of occurrence of cancer of the stomach in the world, there are reports of increased rates of "early" cases of up to to 30% of all cases, and the reported 5-year cure rate has increased to 95% for that special group (59, 60). The reports from the United States and Europe reveal a few series of 10%–13% early cancer of the stomach (61). We observed only 7 early cases in a series of 213 patients with gastric carcinoma reported in 1985. Similar experience is reflected in most American reports (4, 51, 61).

We believe that any complaint in an elderly patient that may possibly be from gastric ulcer or gastric cancer should be investigated. Further, we agree with Steinheber that upper gastrointestinal contrast radiography and endoscopy with biopsy should be done on all elderly patients with such complaints with the hope of identifying *early* gastric cancer in the age group in which most cases of cancer of the stomach occur in this country (4).

Lymphoma and Sarcoma of the Stomach

As the incidence of carcinoma of the stomach has declined over the past 20–30 years, lymphoma and sarcoma have gradually increased in the percentage of the overall number of malignant tumors of the stomach. In cases of disseminated lymphoma, 10%–20% will involve the gastrointestinal tract. Primary lymphoma of the gastrointestinal tract accounts for about 20% of all gastric cancers (62), and sarcomas account for about 3% of all gastric malignancies (63). We found that these tumors occur most often in the 60- to 80-year-olds and that survival with "aggressive search and destroy" attitudes is good. The 5-year cure rates for patients with these tumors is better than for adenocarcinoma of the stomach (64). This general subject of lymphoma and sarcoma of the stomach has been covered recently in the book by Scott and Sawyers. (43).

Surgical Management of Cancer of the Stomach

We have followed an aggressive approach in the surgical treatment of cancer of the stomach for some years now and in resections for cure have combined gastric resection with node dissection of the hepatic pedicle and celiac axis as suggested by Arhelger, Lober, and Wangensteen in 1955 (65). The last 23 years of our experience has reflected no change in this attitude (51). Resection for cure has been done whenever possible. Radical subtotal gastrectomy with node dissection for antral carcinomas and total gastrectomy and extended total gastrectomy with node dissection for more extensive and all more proximal lesions have been the operations of choice. Palliative resections and bypass procedures have been offered to those patients in whom no chance of cure is seen. (Fig. 20.3)

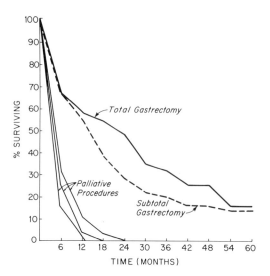

Figure 20.3. Life table survival curves in "curative" resections and in palliative procedures used in surgical treatment of gastric carcinoma. (Reprinted with permission from Scott HW, et al: Results of an aggressive surgical approach to gastric carcinoma during a twenty-three year period. *Surgery* 97:55–59, 1985.)

We have held the same aggressive philosophy for patients of all ages with gastric lymphoma and sarcoma (64). This approach is shared by many, and the best recent report of an especially aggressive surgical approach to gastric cancer of all types in the elderly is from Bittner et al. from West Germany (66). He reported upon the results of total gastrectomy in 186 patients of whom 74 were older than 70. An operative mortality rate of only 4.4% occurred in those patients who were above 70 years of age operated upon during the 1979–1984 time period as compared to a 3.67% operative mortality in those less than 70 operated upon during those 5 years. A much higher operative mortality was sustained by these authors in the years before 1978. They have, as have we, liberalized the indications for total gastrectomy in the older age group. We and others have noticed a significant increase with age in the number of gastric cancer patients and have seen a more proximal location in a few of them. Meyers, Postlethwait et al. recently reported their experience at Duke with carcinoma of the stomach and they too have noticed a recent, startling tendency for a more proximal location of malignant tumors (46). They as we have continued to aim for curative resection,

regardless of age. They acknowledge the poor prognosis and the singular lack of improved success in recent years, but continue to recommend an aggressive surgical approach and a much more aggressive diagnostic attitude in hopes of finding the tumors early.

Effects of Gastric Resection upon the Elderly

We have been impressed with the ability of members of the elderly population of modern-day America to tolerate surgical procedures of all magnitudes. In a report of our experience over a recent 5-year period with operations of all types in 75 patients, all over age 90, there was an operative mortality rate of 2.3% for 42 elective cases, 10% for 32 urgent cases, and 45% for 11 emergency cases (67). The relationship of operative risk for the elderly patient with upper gastrointestinal problems and the urgency with which the procedure is done is the most important factor and outweighs the factor of associated medical problems in every instance. Following vagotomy, pyloroplasty, antrectomy, subtotal gastrectomy, and total gastrectomy, elderly patients do very well. A recent report from Sweden outlined the follow-up results of 449 postgastrectomy men who were 70 years old in 1971–1972 (68). Three hundred and thirty one of these men were 75 years old in 1976 and 1977. Some had had partial gastrectomy as long as 20–30 years ago. The authors compared these elderly gastrectomy patients with controls of the same age and concluded that there was some slight increased risk of iron deficiency, B12 deficiency, osteopenia, and weight reduction. Post-resection patients and controls both considered themselves to be in equally good health. We have had the same experience and continue to offer the elderly patient the same operative procedure for problems of the stomach and duodenum that we would offer a younger patient with the same condition.

REFERENCES

1. Sklar M: Functioning gastrointestinal disease in the aged. *Am J Gastroenterol* 53:570–575, 1970.
2. Schuster MM: Disorders of the aging GI system. *Hosp Pract* 11:95–103, 1976.
3. Altman DF: Gastrointestinal diseases in the elderly. *Med Clin N Am* 67:433–444, 1983.
4. Steinheber FU: Aging and the stomach. *Clin Gastroenterol* 14:657–688, 1985.

5. Kupfer RM, Heppell M, Haggith JW, Bateman DN: Gastric emptying and small-bowel transit rate in the elderly. *J Am Geriatr Soc* 33:340- 343, 1985.

6. James OFW: Gastrointestinal and liver function in old age. *Clin Gastroenterol* 12:671–691, 1983.

7. Kimura K: Chronological transition of the fundic-pyloric border determined by stepwise biopsy of the lesser and greater curvatures of the stomach. *Gastroenterology* 63:584–592, 1972.

8. Correa P: The epidemiology and pathogenesis of chronic gastritis: three etiologic entities. *Frontiers in Gastrointestinal Research* Basel, Karger, 1980, pp 98–108.

9. Strickland RG, Mackay IR: A reappraisal of the nature and significance of chronic atrophic gastritis. *Dig Dis Sci* 18:426–440, 1973.

10. Ming SC: *Tumors of the Esophagus and Stomach.* Washington, DC, Armed Forces Institute of Pathology, 1973.

11. Fieber SS, Rickert RR: Hyperplastic gastropathy: analysis of 50 selected cases 1955–1980. *Am J Gastroenterol* 76:321–329, 1981.

12. Menetrier P: Des Polyadenomes gastriques et de leurs rapports avec le cancer de l'estomac. *Arch Physiol Norm Pathol* S4, 1:32–55; 236, 1888.

13. Levrat M, Pasquier J, Lambet R, Tissot A: Peptic ulcer in patients over 60. Experience in 287 cases. *Am J Dig Dis* 11:279–285, 1966.

14. Colin-Jones DG: Problems of peptic ulceration in the elderly. *Postgrad Med J* 51(suppl 5):41–45, 1975.

15. Cohen N: Gastroenterology in the aged. *Mt Sinai J Med* 47:142–149, 1980.

16. Schanke K: Gastroduodenal ulceration in old age. *Acta Chir Scand* 104:227–235, 1952.

17. Stafford CE, Jorgenson EJ, Murray GC: Complications of peptic ulcer in the aged. *Calif Med* 84:92, 1956.

18. Tsai N, Weiser MM: Gastrointestinal problems in the elderly. *Prim Care* 9:33–44, 1982.

19. Narayanan M, Steinheber FU: The changing face of peptic ulcer in the elderly. *Med Clin N Am* 60:1159–1172, 1976.

20. Fry J: Peptic ulcer: a profile. *Br Med J* 2:809–812, 1964.

21. Kaplan MS, List JW, Stemmer EA, Connolly JE: Surgical management of peptic ulcer disease in the aged patient. *Arch Surg* 104:667–671, 1972.

22. Martin L, Lewis N: Peptic ulcer cases reviewed after ten years. *Lancet* 2:1115–1120, 1949.

23. Weinckert A, Borg I, Lindblom P: Review of medically treated bleeding gastric or duodenal ulcers. *Acta Chir Scand* 120:66–78, 1960.

24. Pulvertaft CN: Comments on the incidence and natural history of gastric and duodenal ulcer. *Postgrad Med J* 44:597–602, 1968.

25. Watson RJ, Hooper TL, Ingram G: Duodenal ulcer disease in the elderly: a retrospective study. *Age Aging* 14:225–229, 1985.

26. Antler AS, Pitchumoni CS, Thomas E, Orangio G, Scanlan BC: Gastrointestinal bleeding in the elderly: morbidity, mortality, and cause. *Am J Surg* 142:271–273, 1981.

27. Kane E, Fried G, McSherry CK: Perforated peptic ulcer in the elderly. *J Am Geriatr Soc* 29:224–227, 1981.

28. Feliciano DV, Bitondo CG, Burch JM, Mattox KL, Jordan GL, DeBakey ME: Emergency management of perforated peptic ulcers in the elderly patient. *Am J Surg* 148:764–767, 1984.

29. Walt R, Logan R, Katschinski B, Ashley J, Langman M: Rising frequency of ulcer perforation in elderly people in the United Kingdom. *Lancet* 1:489–492, 1986.

30. Pillay SP, Hardie IR, Burnett W: Emergency surgery for the complications of peptic ulcer in the elderly. *Aust NZ J Surg* 51:590- 594, 1981.

31. Birkett DH: When do you recommend surgery for peptic ulcer? *Geratrics* 36:83–88, 1981.

32. Sterup K, Mosbeck J: Trends in the mortality from peptic ulcer in Denmark. *Scand J Gastroenterol* 8:49–53, 1973.

33. Strange SL: Giant innocent gastric ulcer in the elderly. *Gerontol Clin* 5:171–189, 1963.

34. Christiansen P, Jensen HE, Amdrup E, Fenger C, Lindskov J, Nielsen J, Nielsen SAD: Gastric ulcer in old age. *Acta Chir Scand* 144:491–494, 1978.

35. Herrington JL, Scott HW, Sawyers JL: Experience with vagotomy- antrectomy and Roux-en-Y gastrojejunostomy in surgical treatment of duodenal, gastric, and stomal ulcers. *Ann Surg* 199:590–597, 1984.

36. Adkins RB, DeLozier JB, Scott HW, Sawyers JL: The management of gastric ulcers. *Ann Surg* 201:741–751, 1985.

37. Koch H: Endoscopic therapy of premalignant and malignant changes in the stomach. *Endoscopy* 13:148–151, 1981.

38. ReMine SG, Hughes RW, Weiland LH: Endoscopic gastric polypectomies. *Mayo Clin Proc* 56:371–375, 1981.

39. Tomasulo J: Gastric polyps: histologic types and their relationships to gastric carcinoma. *Cancer* 27:1346–1355, 1971.

40. Kamiya T, Morishita T, Asakura H, Miura S, Munakata Y, Tsuchita M: Long term followup study on gastric adenoma and its relation to gastric protruded carcinoma. *Cancer* 50:2496–2503, 1982.

41. Fernandez MJ, Davis RP, Nora PF: Gastrointestinal lipomas. *Arch Surg* 118:1081–1083, 1983.

42. Helling TS, Wood WG: Gastric carcinoids and atrophic gastritis. *Arch Surg* 118:765-n-768, 1983.

43. Adkins RB, Gray GF: Gastric lymphomas, sarcomas, and carcinoids. In Scott HW, Sawyers JL (eds): *Surgery of the Stomach, Duodenum, and Small Intestine.* Boston, Blackwell Scientific Publications, 1987, pp 463–479.

44. Geier GE, Gashti EN, Houin HP, Johnloz D, Madura JA: Villous adenoma of the duodenum, a clinicopathologic study of five cases. *Am Surg* 50:617–622, 1984.

45. Borch K, Hammarstrom LE, Liedberg G: Gastric cancer: diagnosis, treatment, and prognosis in clinical routine. *Acta Chir Scand* 148:517–523, 1982.

46. Meyers WC, Damiano RJ, Rotolo FS, Postlethwait RE: Adenocarcinoma of the stomach: changing patterns over the last four decades. *Ann Surg* 205:1–8, 1987.

47. Antonioli DA, Goldman H: Changes in the location and

type of gastric adenocarcinoma. *Cancer* 50:775–781, 1982.

48. Christiansen P, Amdrup E, Fenger C, et al: Gastric ulcer III: Non- surgical treatment. *Acta Chir Scand* 139:466–469, 1973.

49. Ihre BJE, Barr H, Havermark G: Ulcer-cancer of the stomach. *Gastroenterologia* 102:78–91, 1964.

50. Wenger J, Brandborg LL, Spellman FA: The Veterans Administration Cooperative Study on gastric ulcer. Cancer, Part I: Clinical aspects. *Gastroenterology* 61:598–621, 1971.

51. Scott HW, Adkins RB, Sawyers JL: Results of an aggressive surgical approach to gastric carcinoma during a twenty-three year period. *Surgery* 97:55–59, 1985.

52. Winawer SJ: Tissue diagnosis in upper gastrointestinal malignancy. *Gastroenterology* 82:379–382, 1982.

53. Goldstein F, Kline TS, Kline IK, Thornton JJ, Abramson J, Bell L: Early gastric cancer in a United States hospital. *Am J Gastroenterol* 78:715–719, 1983.

54. Sakita T, Oguro Y, Takasu S, Hisayuki F: Observations on the healing of ulcerations in early gastric cancer. The life cycle of the malignant ulcer. *Gastroenterology* 60:835–844, 1971.

55. Isenberg JI, Peterson WL, Elashoff JA, Sandersfeld MA, Reedy TJ, Ippoliti AF, VanDeventer GM, Franke H, Langstreth GF, Anderson DS: Healing of benign gastric ulcer with low-dose antacid or cimetidine. A double-blind, randomized placebo-controlled trial. *New Engl J Med* 308:1319–1324, 1983.

56. Cohen I, Sartin J: Giant gastric ulcer. *Ann Surg* 147:749–758, 1958.

57. Hoerr SO: Prognosis for carcinoma of the stomach. *Surg Gynecol Obstet* 137:205–209, 1973.

58. Diehl JT, Hermann DE, Cooperman AM, Hoerr SO: Gastric carcinoma: a ten-year review. *Ann Surg* 198:9–12, 1983.

59. Murakami T: Early cancer of the stomach. *World J Surg* 3.685–692, 1979.

60. Bralow SP: Diagnosis and staging of esophageal and gastric cancer. *Cancer* 50:2566–2570, 1982.

61. O'Brien M, Burakoff R, Robbins EA, Golding RM, Zamcheck N, Gottlieb LS: Early gastric cancer. *Am J Med* 78:195–202, 1985.

62. Craig O, Gregson R: Primary lymphoma of the gastrointestinal tract. *Clin Radiol* 32:63–71, 1981.

63. Bedikian AY, Khankhanian N, Valdivieso M, Heilbrun LK, Benjamin RS, Yap BS, Nelson RS, Bodey GP: Sarcoma of the stomach: clinicopathologic study of 43 cases. *J Surg Oncol* 13:121–127, 1980.

64. Adkins RB, Scott HW, Sawyers JL: Gastrointestinal lymphoma and sarcoma: a case for aggressive search and destroy. *Ann Surg,* 205:625–633, 1987.

65. Arhelger SW, Lober PH, Wangensteen OH: Dissection of the hepatic pedicle and the retropancreatic-duodenal areas for cancer of the stomach. *Surgery* 38:675, 1955.

66. Bittner R, Schirrow H, Butters M, Roscher R, Krautzberger W, Oettinger W, Beger HG: Total gastrectomy. A 15-year experience with particular reference to the patient over 70 years of age. *Arch Surg* 120:1120–1125, 1985.

67. Adkins RB, Scott HW: Surgical procedures in patients aged 90 years and older. *South Med J* 77:1357–1364, 1984.

68. Mellstrom D, Rundgren A: Long-term effects after partial gastrectomy in elderly men. *Scand J Gastroenterol* 17:433–439, 1982.

Chapter 21

Diseases of the Liver, Gallbladder, and Biliary Tract in the Elderly

Joel J. Roslyn, M.D., F.A.C.S., Ronald K. Tompkins, M.D., F.A.C.S.

The number of elderly patients undergoing major abdominal surgical procedures has increased significantly over the past 20 years (1). This finding, coupled with the observation that hepatobiliary procedures account for over one-third of all abdominal operations performed in this age group (2), underscores the importance of a clear understanding of diseases affecting the liver, gallbladder, and bile ducts as they occur in the geriatric population. Although the pathogenesis and pathology of these disorders are similar in young and old alike, the clinical manifestations and sequelae vary appreciably in the different age groups, thereby necessitating different treatment strategies.

There are numerous factors (aside from a mere increase in population) that may account for the increasing frequency of hepatobiliary procedures in the elderly. In recent years there has been a revolution in technological advances that has facilitated both the diagnosis and management of individuals with either benign or malignant diseases of the liver and extrahepatic biliary tract. The emergence of skilled interventional endoscopists and radiologists has promoted and fostered original areas of investigation, which in turn have provided the clinician with new information and insight, and, perhaps more importantly, innovative options for patient care. Moreover, our understanding of the effects of jaundice and hepatic dysfunction on other organ systems, and our ability to care for patients with these problems, has been greatly expanded in recent years. The net effect is that elderly patients with complicated hepatobiliary disorders can now be managed either non-operatively or surgically in a safe and effective manner.

Consideration of issues unique to geriatric surgery is essential prior to and during the formulation of management strategy for the elderly patient with hepatobiliary disease. Many of these patients have associated medical disorders that should be carefully evaluated, with the goal being stabilization and optimization of medical condition prior to operation. A delay in operation for several hours in order to permit a more definitive diagnosis, restoration of normal hemodynamics, and detailed discussion with the patient and family is often appropriate in the elderly patient with acute disorders of the biliary tract. In the case of a patient with a hepatobiliary malignancy, it is incumbent upon the surgeon to measure carefully the potential merits of radical resection as opposed to biliary diversion without resection. Often, excellent palliation can be provided for the patient with a bile duct tumor without subjecting the individual to a higher risk from a more radical procedure that might offer the only, albeit minimal, chance for cure. These decisions are often quite difficult to make under any circumstances, but particularly so when dealing with the geriatric population. In addition to the obvious medical issues, careful consideration must be given to such social issues as quality of life, the patient's ability to recognize and to deal emotionally with the prognosis of the underlying malady, who will provide long-term care and in what setting, and what is the patient's rehabilitative potential. An ongoing dialogue with the patient and his or her family, as well as with a social worker, can often provide insight into the family's expectations and may prove quite helpful in the resolution of what is typically a challenging and often frustrating decision-making process.

The purpose of this chapter is to review the

surgical management of disorders affecting the liver, gallbladder, and biliary tract as they occur in the elderly patient. Prior to discussing specific diseases, the effects of aging on the hepatobiliary tract will be considered.

PHYSIOLOGIC CHANGES OF AGING

Liver

Morphologic changes occur in the liver with advancing age. The liver gradually becomes smaller in both absolute size and relative to body weight, so that by age 90 it accounts for only 1.6% of total body weight, as compared to 2.5% in patients prior to age 50 (3). In addition, there is frequently molding of the liver to conform with other organs, which becomes more pronounced with increasing age (4). Although the factors that regulate hepatic blood flow are not well defined, it has been previously shown that a diminution in hepatic blood flow (0.3% to 1.5% per year) occurs such that total liver blood flow is 40% less in patients 60 years and older than in those individuals less than 25 years of age (5). The decrease in liver size would appear to be due to an actual reduction in the number of hepatocytes, even though individual liver cells increase in mean volume (6). In addition to the documented change in hepatocytes, there is also evidence of bile duct proliferation with increasing age (7). The effects of these macro- and microscopic changes on hepatic function, however, would appear to be minimal. Recent reports have confirmed that standard liver function tests—total bilirubin, alkaline phosphatase, and serum glutamic oxalacetic transaminase (SGOT)—are unaltered despite increasing age (8). Moreover, biliary excretion as determined by retention of sodium sulfobromophthalein (BSP) and rose bengal scan remains normal in elderly patients (9). Although it has been thought that the pharmacokinetics of drug metabolism are abnormal in elderly patients, recent evidence would support a contrary view. Several studies have shown that liver metabolism of most drugs proceeds normally in elderly patients and that any isolated drug reactions that occur in this group are the result of multiple factors, rather than aging alone (10).

It is well known that the incidence of cholesterol gallstones increases with age. It is generally felt that a major factor responsible for this trend is the alteration in biliary metabolism that occurs with aging. Studies in Chilean women indicate that the proportion of biliary cholesterol and the cholesterol saturation index are significantly increased in elderly females as compared to younger subjects (11). The increased incidence of gallstones observed in elderly men has been linked to changing ratios of androgen to estrogen and this effect on biliary lipid metabolism. These data support the hypothesis that the increased incidence of gallstones observed in the elderly is due in part to an age induced increase in canalicular secretion of biliary lipids.

Gallbladder

The effects of aging on gallbladder motor activity have not been well defined. Recent ultrasonographic studies suggest that gallbladder sensitivity to cholecystokinin (CCK) decreases with aging, although this is balanced by increased fasting and fat-stimulated levels of CCK (12). Serum levels of a second gut peptide, pancreatic polypeptide, a substance released postprandially by the pancreas, increase with aging (13). The recent observation that pancreatic polypeptide enhances postcontractile gallbladder filling (14) suggests that another possible mechanism responsible for the increased incidence of gallstone formation in the elderly may be related to alterations in gallbladder motility. Further studies are needed to clarify the effects of these peptides and others on gallbladder contractility in the geriatric population.

LIVER DISEASE

Malignant Tumors

Metastatic Cancer

Malignant tumors of the liver are considerably more frequent in elderly patients than are benign lesions. Therefore, the finding of a filling defect on ultrasonography or liver scan is reason for grave concern. Metastatic cancer is 20 times more common than primary tumors in the liver. It has been estimated that approximately one-half of all patients dying with cancer will have liver metastases. Although carcinomas of the breast, lung, kidney, and ovary can metastasize to the liver, the overwhelming majority of metastatic lesions in the liver arise from a gastrointestinal primary site. The correlation between incidence of gastrointestinal malignancy and increasing age underscores the importance of metastatic neoplasms of the liver in the geriatric population.

Elderly patients with hepatic metastases may have vague symptoms or no symptoms whatsoever referrable to the liver lesions. Usually, however, these patients will have constitutional symptoms of weight loss, anorexia, and easy fatigability. Right upper quadrant pain, jaundice, and ascites are generally associated with advanced disease in which much of the liver substance has been replaced by tumor. Abnormal liver tests (bilirubin, alkaline phosphatase, SGOT) may be the only indicator of liver involvement in an otherwise asymptomatic patient. These findings should prompt further evaluation, particularly in the elderly patient. Although there are currently no data that define the frequency with which this occurs, it has been our experience that it is not at all unusual for elderly patients with an occult primary to have their initial manifestation of malignancy as metastases to the liver.

The treatment of liver metastases has been the subject of numerous studies and innovative interventions during the last several years. Liver resection, intra-arterial catheters, and implantable pumps and reservoirs have all been used to treat patients with metastatic disease. Most of these patients have had colorectal carcinomas. The role of these modalities in the elderly patient has not been well defined in the literature. It is essential that the clinician carefully weigh and measure the potential risk versus benefit before electing to proceed with a particular treatment option in an elderly patient with metastatic tumor involving the liver. Such factors as the relationship between the presentation of the metastases and the primary (precocious, synchronous, or metachronous) lesion, the size and location of the hepatic lesions, and the patients' associated medical problems should all be considered prior to final decision. Age itself is not as important to this decision-making process as

is the patients' overall medical and mental state, the rehabilitative potential, and other social issues. Obstruction of the major bile ducts can occur in the presence of metastatic cancer and may be due to tumor debris (15) or extrinsic compression. Intubation of the biliary tract usually provides good palliation for these patients and can generally be achieved without significant morbidity or mortality.

Primary Liver Cancer

The recent identification of specific etiologic factors in the development of hepatoma, coupled with the worldwide frequency with which this tumor occurs, has been responsible for intense investigative and clinical interest in this, the most common of all primary liver tumors. The prevalence of hepatoma varies widely around the world and even within countries. Hepatoma is the most common cancer observed in Taiwan, the third most common in China, but ranks 22nd among cancers seen in the United States (16). Hepatocellular carcinoma is more frequent in males than females, and its incidence increases with increasing age. There does appear to be, however, a leveling off of this progressive rise in the elderly population. Recent reports, however, indicate that the incidence of hepatoma over the last 8 years is actually increasing (17). This finding, coupled with the increasing age of our population, suggests that hepatocellular carcinoma may become a problem of greater magnitude in the elderly population in the future.

The insidious presentation of hepatoma in the vast majority of patients reduces the likelihood of early diagnosis, especially in the elderly patient. Symptoms of pain, hepatomegaly, sudden deterioration in a previously stable cirrhotic patient, and/or acute illness with fever and abdominal pain are late manifestations and are suggestive of rapid progression of a hepatic neoplasm.

Most hepatomas can be demonstrated using computed tomography (CT) or ultrasonography. In addition, CT-guided or ultrasound-guided biopsies can generally be performed percutaneously, facilitating tissue diagnosis. However, recent experience with seeding of tumor into the chest wall following percutaneous biopsy of liver tumors makes us hesitant to do this procedure in patients who are candidates for operation. If resection is contemplated or if further delineation of tumor involvement is required, then arteriography can be quite beneficial. Once a tissue diagnosis has been established, we generally reserve arteriography only for those patients in whom resection is contemplated. Increasing experience with major liver resections and improved parasurgical care have expanded the indications for liver resection. Nonetheless, recent studies suggest that the duration of operation in a major university medical center is still in excess of 4 1/2 hours and that the estimated blood loss is in excess of 3,000 ccs (18). These facts, coupled with the significant morbidity that may follow these procedures, should temper enthusiasm for major hepatic resection in the very elderly with advanced primary hepatocellular carcinoma. Certainly, the presence of jaundice is a contraindication to resection in most patients.

It is important to distinguish between a limited wedge resection and an anatomic formal lobectomy. The potential complications from each are considerably different. Wedge resections can be performed safely in most instances and are generally well tolerated in elderly patients. The decision to proceed or not with a limited or anatomic resection should be made by a surgeon experienced in hepatic surgical procedures.

Cholangiocarcinomas account for approximately 15% of all primary hepatic tumors. They usually spread diffusely throughout the liver, and extrahepatic metastases occur with great frequency. The symptoms and signs associated with this type of liver tumor may be quite similar to that of hepatoma. The chance for resection, however, is even less with this type of lesion than with the more common hepatocellular carcinoma. Because most elderly patients with primary cancer of the liver (either hepatoma or cholangiocarcinoma) are unsuitable for resection, great interest has been generated in other forms of therapy. These other modalities have included ligation of the hepatic artery, intra-arterial chemotherapy, and hyperthermia. To date there is only anecdotal evidence that one or more of these modalities will increase patient survival.

Benign Tumors and Cysts

Benign tumors and noninfectious cysts of the liver are unusual in elderly patients. Hepatic adenomas and focal nodular hyperplasia are generally found in female patients during the childbearing years. Asymptomatic lesions that are, however, discovered in elderly patients, such as cavernous hemangiomas, should be observed unless their size is of such concern as to warrant resection or the patient has symptoms related to the mass. Cystic disease of the liver, either solitary unilocular or polycystic liver disease, should be treated symptomatically. When these lesions are managed surgically, biopsies should always be performed to rule out cystadenoma or cystadenocarcinoma. It has been our practice to unroof simple cysts containing water-clear fluid. Drainage of cysts into a Roux-en-Y limb of jejunum is indicated if there is evidence of communication with the bile ducts.

Hepatic Abscess

The epidemiology of abscesses involving the liver has changed appreciably during recent years. Most cases of hepatic abscesses seen in the 1980s are due to cholecystitis and/or suppurative cholangitis. It is unusual that either appendicitis or diverticulitis is complicated by the formation of hepatic abscesses by spread through the portal vein, although these possible sites of infection should certainly be considered. In approximately 10% to 50% of the patients, no antecedent infection can be identified; these have been termed cryptogenic abscesses. Although hepatic abscesses may be parasitic, fungal, or bacterial, the majority of such lesions in the United States are pyogenic. The clinical course may be indolent, with the only symptoms being a low-grade fever and generalized malaise, or it may be fulminant with significant toxicity, high fever, jaundice, and right upper quadrant pain. Often the liver is enlarged, and the pain may actually be severe. Jaundice is unusual in the absence of significant biliary obstruction, multiple abscesses, or rapid deterioration.

There may be many clues to the diagnosis of liver abscess in the elderly patient. In addition to the clinical setting, one often sees either a basilar atelectasis or pleural effusion on chest x-ray. When the process involves the right lobe of the liver, it is not unusual to see an elevated right hemidiaphragm. Ultrasound and CT scans are the most useful diagnostic tests and will often allow definitive diagnosis. We have had reasona-

Table 21.1 Gallbladder Disease Prevalence by Age Group[a]

Age	Percentage with stones	
	Female	Male
10–39	5.0	1.5
40–49	12.0	4.4
50–59	15.8	6.2
60–69	25.4	9.9
70–79	28.9	15.2
80–89	30.9	17.9
90+	35.4	24.4

[a]Reproduced with permission from Bateson MC: Gallbladder disease and cholecystectomy rates are independently variable. *Lancet* 2:621–624, 1984.

ble success using percutaneous drainage of solitary liver abscess. Unfortunately, however, in our patient population, single lesions are the exception, rather than the rule (19). Most often, these patients will have multiple liver abscesses secondary to biliary obstruction from either benign or malignant causes. Therapy should be aimed at treating the underlying cause if possible, relieving the obstruction, and drainage of the infection.

GALLBLADDER DISEASE

Cholelithiasis

Incidence

It has previously been stated that biliary tract disease in the elderly is almost exclusively associated with gallstones or cancer. Numerous studies (20–22) have in fact demonstrated an almost linear increase in the prevalence of gallstones with advancing age. (See Table 21.1) The actual frequency with which gallstones are found in any given ethnic group or country varies considerably and is dependent on multiple factors. Nonetheless, there appears to be a direct correlation between gallstone prevalence and increasing age, regardless of the locale. In the United States, the incidence of gallstones in Caucasian women increases from 5% at age 20 to 10% at age 40 and up to 25% by age 60 (23). In Scandinavia, the incidence of stones is higher, with nearly 60% of women between the ages of 60 and 69 having stones (24). Perhaps most impressive is the 20% incidence of gallstones among Pima (American Indian) women aged 15 to 24,

which rises to over 60% by 35 years of age (25). Similar trends exist for males, although the absolute prevalence remains less than in women for any given age. Over 50 years ago, an autopsy study indicated that gallstones were present in more than 50% of the patients over the age of 70 (26). More recent autopsy studies confirm these earlier observations (27).

Natural History

The basis for decision making in the elderly patient with gallstones is a clear understanding of the natural history of this disease. Unfortunately, there are little prospective data that address this issue. Considerable evidence suggests, however, that gallstone disease in the elderly may be more virulent than in a younger population. This is based on clinical observations of an increased percentage of elderly patients who develop choledocholithiasis (28, 29), emphysematous cholecystitis (30), perforation of the gallbladder (31), and septic complications of cholecystitis (32, 33). Whether these increased complications represent actual differences in the evolution of the disease process or merely the byproduct of delayed diagnosis and treatment remains unclear. We suspect that the increased risk of biliary complications in elderly patients can be attributed to a reluctance on the part of many surgeons to recommend early elective surgery in the elderly patient with cholelithiasis. In actuality, recent studies suggest that elective cholecystectomy can be safely performed in elderly patients with minimal morbidity and mortality (29, 34). In contrast, the mortality rate increases by at least five-fold when emergency cholecystectomy is performed in this same population. Although it is becoming increasingly clear that a more aggressive attitude is warranted in the elderly patient with symptomatic gallstone disease, a critical question remains unanswered: What are the chances that a patient over age 65 with asymptomatic gallstones will develop symptoms in the future and require cholecystectomy?

Treatment of Asymptomatic Stones in the Elderly

Despite renewed interest in the prevention and the dissolution of gallstones, cholecystectomy remains the gold standard of treatment for patients with cholelithiasis. Nonetheless, the selection of elderly patients for operative intervention and the timing of the procedure itself continue to be issues that are controversial. Should elderly patients with asymptomatic gallstones undergo cholecystectomy, or should a period of watchful waiting be instituted? Reliable, definitive data to answer this question are not currently available. Those recommending watchful waiting point to the frequency with which gallstones are found at autopsy, suggesting that many patients live with silent gallstones. Recent epidemiologic studies suggest that, in non-elderly patients with asymptomatic gallstones, the likelihood of developing any complication of gallstone disease requiring cholecystectomy is 7% (35). These authors conclude that routine prophylactic cholecystectomy for asymptomatic gallstone disease is unnecessary.

Can these data, derived from a university faculty, be extrapolated to the geriatric population? Although this is clearly an unanswerable question at this time, we strongly feel that the complex situation that is usually present in elderly patients necessitates an individual and rational approach. When one hears that gallstones were discovered accidently in a patient who is "asymptomatic," one must consider why that study was being done and, therefore, whether that patient is truly asymptomatic. Traditionally, we think of biliary colic as being the only manifestation of gallstone disease. It is clear that a significant number of patients do not have postprandial pain, but instead have dyspepsia, vague epigastric discomfort, or perhaps even mild increased flatulence as the primary manifestation of biliary lithiasis. In an elderly patient who may have a variety of non-specific functional (or physiologic) complaints, it may be quite difficult for the clinician to define an exact cause-and-effect relationship. Often, the physician is asked to decide what therapy to recommend in an elderly patient with documented cholelithiasis who has atypical symptoms of biliary tract disease. As previously stated, it is difficult to predict what the natural history of this patient's gallstone disease will be, and the ultimate decision to proceed or not with cholecystectomy is generally based on the physician's intuitive feeling and the patient's overall medical condition.

The operative mortality for elective cholecystectomy in patients under 50 years of age is 0.3% and rises to 5% in those individuals over 65 years of age (36). However, when cholecystectomy is performed on an emergency basis in the elderly, the mortality from operation actually increases five-fold. It would therefore appear prudent to avoid the need for emergency operation in an elderly patient with gallstone disease. Although we do not routinely advocate prophylactic cholecystectomy in an elderly patient with truly asymptomatic gallstones, we do consider removal of the gallbladder in an elderly patient to be appropriate in certain settings.

Postoperative cholecystitis has the potential to be a particularly lethal condition, and for this reason in part, we recommend removal of the gallbladder in an elderly patient who is undergoing laparotomy for other reasons if it is technically easy to do. The classical example of this situation is the individual undergoing aortic aneurysmectomy who in addition has cholelithiasis. Our experience supports that of the literature (37, 38), which indicates that incidental cholecystectomy can be safely performed in combination with major intra-abdominal surgical procedures. (See Table 21.2) For patients with abdominal aortic aneurysms, our approach is to conclude aortic revascularization, close the retroperitoneum, and isolate this field from the right upper quadrant. We then proceed with routine cholecystectomy. This approach prevents the potential evolution of gallstone disease, as well as the sequelae of postoperative cholecystitis.

Table 21.2 Indications for Primary Abdominal Procedure[a]

Condition	Number of Cases
Carcinoma of colon	12
Diverticular disease of colon	2
Sigmoid volvulus	2
Peptic ulcer disease	10
Carcinoma of stomach	3
Aortic aneurysm	3
Small bowel obstruction	2
Carcinoma of pancreas	1
Hiatus hernia	3
Trauma	1
Other	5
Total	44

[a]Reproduced with permission from Schreiber H, et al: Incidental cholecystectomy during major abdominal surgery in the elderly. *Am J Surg* 135:196–198, 1978.

Acute Cholecystitis

Clinical Presentation

With the increase in longevity of our population, the incidence of cholecystitis among the elderly has become increasingly frequent. The textbook description of cholecystitis, including persistent right upper quadrant pain, fever, and leukocytosis, which is so typical in the young patient, may be partially present or absent completely in the elderly patient. It is therefore of paramount importance that the clinician consider this diagnosis in an elderly patient with gallstone disease who presents with abdominal pain. In addition, nausea and vomiting are frequent complaints (39) and may be the only sign of an intra-abdominal process. Although the mechanism by which it occurs is not clear, alterations in mental status have been reported to occur in elderly patients with cholecystitis (40). Deterioration in intellectual function may be the primary manifestation of hepatobiliary disease in an elderly patient and may occur in the absence of any clinical signs usually associated with acute cholecystitis.

Diagnosis

It has been our practice to consider the diagnosis of acute cholecystitis in elderly patients with gallstone disease who have right upper quadrant pain lasting for more than 12 hours, whether or not they have a febrile course or an elevated white blood cell count. Furthermore, the diagnosis of acute cholecystitis should be pursued in the elderly patient who presents with sepsis of undetermined etiology (41). This aggressive approach facilitates early diagnosis and implementation of management that is aimed at correction of altered fluid and electrolyte status and restoration of normal hemodynamics. It is essential that the diagnosis of acute cholecystitis be confirmed in an expeditious manner.

Since its introduction by Graham and Cole (42) over 50 years ago, the oral cholecystogram has been the gold standard for the diagnostic evaluation of patients with cholelithiasis. When used in appropriate clinical situations, the reported accuracy for oral cholecystography is 90% to 95% (43). There are, however, several specific limitations that apply to this test, especially in elderly

patients: (1) This modality is not appropriate in the acutely ill patient; (2) there is a significant false-negative rate associated with oral cholecystography; and (3) patients who are noncompliant or who have emesis, malabsorption, diarrhea, jaundice, or any significant hepatic dysfunction may have a false-negative study. Because of these limitations and the advances in ultrasonography and biliary scintigraphy, the oral cholecystogram is not recommended in the elderly patient and certainly not in an individual who is acutely ill.

During the past several years, abdominal ultrasonography has become a mainstay in the evaluation of patients with suspected gallstone disease or cholecystitis. This technique has significant advantages over oral cholecystography: (1) There is no radiation exposure for the patient, (2) the test is not dependent on patient compliance, and (3) normal intestinal absorption, hepatic secretion, and gallbladder concentration of a dye are not required for this procedure to be accurate. An additional advantage, especially in the elderly patient, is the information provided about the anatomy of the bile ducts and pancreas. Often in the elderly patient, it is not clear whether the primary pathologic problem is an inflammatory process or a neoplasm. Cholecystosonography is most accurate in diagnosing cholelithiasis. Chronic and acute cholecystitis and choledocholithiasis may be diagnosed as well, but with less accuracy. The use of ultrasonography in the diagnosis of patients with calculous disease of the biliary tract has been well described, and certainly it is a safe and effective diagnostic tool in the elderly patient.

Biliary scintigraphy is emerging as an important diagnostic test in the elderly patient with suspected acute cholecystitis. Its reported accuracy and specificity approaches 98% (44). One of the primary advantages of radionuclide imaging is its ability to demonstrate cystic duct obstruction despite serum bilirubin levels in excess of 15 mg%. Significant information regarding focal hepatic masses, parenchymal function, and gallbladder motor activity can be obtained using imaging techniques. In most patients with biliary disease, the intrahepatic bile ducts, gallbladder, common bile duct, and duodenum can all be visualized within 30–60 minutes. It should be emphasized that radionuclide imaging is not a suitable diagnostic test for cholelithiasis. However, these scans are the most accurate tool for diagnosing cystic duct obstruction, which is the "sine qua non" for acute cholecystitis. False positives have been reported in patients on prolonged fasting as well as those being given morphine analgesics. The importance of biliary scintigraphy in the evaluation and management of elderly patients with acute cholecystitis is underscored by a recent report of 74 elderly patients in whom scans confirmed the clinical impression of acute cholecystitis (45). In this group, cholecystectomy was performed in a timely manner, and the operative mortality was zero (45).

The choice of whether to obtain an abdominal ultrasound or a hepatobiliary scan in a patient with right upper quadrant symptoms continues to be debated. It is important to emphasize that, although abdominal ultrasonography is a reasonable means of diagnosing cholelithiasis, its ability to diagnose acute cholecystitis accurately is limited. In contrast, radionuclide imaging, as currently employed, is a very accurate test for acute cholecystitis, but in turn does not detect gallstones per se. In many clinical situations, however, knowledge of the presence of gallstones is all that is needed. We feel that there are advantages to both ultrasonography and biliary scintigraphy and that the decision to proceed with one or the other should be based on the individual clinical situation. It should be recognized that prior scintigraphy may delay the ability to obtain an ultrasound of the gallbladder due to possible radiation exposure to ultrasound technicians.

Management

Acute cholecystitis in patients 65 years of age and older continues to be a serious problem that is best treated surgically. The initial goals of management should include restoration of homeostasis; treatment of any underlying medical problems, such as diabetes, ischemic heart disease, or pulmonary dysfunction; correction of any associated coagulopathy due to warfarin, aspirin, or persantin; institution of broad spectrum antibiotic therapy; verification of diagnosis; and preparation for operation. Many of these patients will not have a prior history of biliary tract disease, and it is crucial that therapy be initiated while the diagnosis is being pursued.

Natural History

It is generally accepted that early cholecystectomy is preferable to delayed operation in patients with acute cholecystitis (46, 47). The reluctance of physicians to adhere to this principle in the treatment of elderly patients may, in part, be responsible for the increased morbidity and mortality that have been previously reported for this age group. Glenn (48) reported that patients 65 years of age and older accounted for 70% of all deaths at the New York Hospital resulting from acute cholecystitis. In that study, the two most common causes of death were sepsis and cardiovascular disease. Similarly, the overall mortality rate in a recent series of 88 elderly patients undergoing cholecystectomy was 7% (49), nearly ten times the rate for younger patients. The importance of timing of treatment in the elderly patient with acute cholecystitis is underscored by a more careful analysis of these data. Medical therapy consisting of intravenous fluids and antibiotics was attempted in 44% of these 88 patients with cholecystitis. Emergency cholecystectomy became necessary in 97% of this subgroup because of failure to respond to conservative, supportive treatment. The morbidity and mortality rates were 44% and 10%, respectively, in patients who required emergency cholecystectomy. In contrast, the morbidity and mortality rates were only 22% and 2% in the group of patients who underwent semi-urgent operation. In our experience, elderly patients with acute cholecystitis are best managed by timely diagnosis, early stabilization, and semi-urgent cholecystectomy.

Operative Strategy

For over 100 years, cholecystectomy has been the treatment of choice for patients with acute choleycstitis. The procedure remains the primary and only curative treatment for cholelithiasis and acute cholecystitis (50). Under certain circumstances, however, we do not hesitate to perform other procedures. Sub-total cholecystectomy with cauterization of the posterior wall adherent to the hepatic bed may be life saving in the elderly cirrhotic patient with portal hypertension and acute cholecystitis. Amputation of the gallbladder with intubation of the infundibulum may be appropriate in the critically ill patient with significant inflammation and/or perforation.

Although cholecystostomy was first performed in 1867 (51), this procedure has been relegated to second-class status and is viewed by some as a procedure of compromise. Nonetheless, cholecystostomy may convert a potentially grave medical situation to one that is manageable. Cholecystostomy may be performed at the time of laparotomy (under general anesthesia) when a particularly difficult situation is encountered.

The usual indication for cholecystostomy is the critically ill individual with serious hepatic, cardiovascular, or pulmonary problems who in addition has developed acute cholecystitis. In this setting, cholecystostomy may be performed safely at the bedside using local anesthesia. This temporizing maneuver may allow for the performance of a safe cholecystectomy at a later date. When performing a cholecystostomy, it is essential to document radiographically the patency of the common bile duct. The overall operative mortality from cholecystostomy varies from 15%–40% (52–54). However, this high mortality probably reflects the severe medical diseases of the elderly patient, rather than the selection of the operation itself. In addition to dealing with an acute and immediate problem, cholecystostomy provides subsequent access to the biliary tract. In those patients with retained common bile duct stones, radiologic and endoscopic techniques can be employed to remove these calculi (55). The significantly increased incidence of choledocholithiasis in elderly patients mandates an intraoperative cholangiogram in all geriatric patients undergoing cholecystectomy. When this is not feasible in the usual manner, it can generally be performed by placement of a "butterfly" needle directly into the choledochus.

Cholecystitis and Diabetes

A significant percentage of elderly patients have diabetes mellitus. In addition, it has long been suggested that there is an increased incidence of cholesterol gallstone disease among diabetics (21) and that these patients are more likely to develop acute cholecystitis and its associated complications (56). However, in a recent prospective review of 175 diabetic and non-diabetic patients undergoing cholecystectomy, the incidence of gallbladder perforation,

wound infection, and overall morbidity and mortality was not significantly different between the two groups (57). The conclusion that diabetes itself is not a significant risk factor for severe biliary tract disease should be tempered because the study cited was not controlled for timing of operation. Nonetheless, we continue to recommend aggressive preoperative evaluation and treatment with early operation in the elderly diabetic patient with presumed acute cholecystitis.

Complications of Gallstone Disease

Choledocholithiasis

In addition to acute cholecystitis, there is an increased incidence of complications associated with gallstone disease in the elderly. For reasons that remain obscure, choledocholithiasis has been reported to be present in 20%–54% of elderly patients undergoing cholecystectomy (29, 49). It is generally accepted that this is a byproduct of the surgeon's reluctance to perform elective procedures in the elderly patient. The natural corollary is that the incidence of common duct stones could be significantly reduced by a more aggressive surgical approach to cholelithiasis when these patients are younger. The clinical impact of the increased incidence of choledocholithiasis in the elderly is underscored by the mortality rates for common bile duct exploration, which increase with age. The mortality rate associated with choledochotomy is 0.9% in patients less than age 50 (58) and rises to 7.6%–29% in patients older than 70 (59).

Some authors have recommended a protective or prophylactic choledochoduodenostomy in the elderly patient with multiple common bile duct stones (60). The rationale for this is the difficulty in extraction of retained stones from patients, coupled with the low morbidity and mortality associated with this type of biliary enteric bypass. It has generally been our policy not to perform a bypass prophylactically, but to do so only if there is a clear-cut indication, regardless of the patient's age. The ability of our radiologic colleagues to basket the stones, as well as that of the endoscopist to perform sphincterotomy, has encouraged us to do only what is necessary at the time of laparotomy. In general, the acutely ill elderly patient should have a meticulous and expeditious operation.

Gallblabber Perforation

The incidence of gallbladder perforation is between 3% and 10% of all patients with acute cholecystitis. Gallbladder perforation can be classified into three types: acute free perforation with bile-stained peritoneal fluid, subacute perforation with pericholecystic or right upper quadrant abscess, and chronic perforation with formation of either cholecystocutaneous or cholecystoenteric fistula. It has long been recognized that gallbladder perforation occurs more frequently in the aged population. Although the explanation for this observation is not evident, the presumption is that circulatory changes in the elderly are an important etiologic factor (61). Cholecystoenteric fistulae are found in the majority of patients with perforation of the gallbladder and are particularly important in the elderly (31, 62, 63). Most often, the fistulous communication is between the gallbladder and duodenum, although other areas of involvement have been reported (62). Depending on the size of the fistulous communication, gallstones may pass through this tract and ultimately cause bowel obstruction.

Gallstone ileus is a relatively rare condition and accounts for less than 5% of all causes of intestinal obstruction. However, in the elderly population, gallstone ileus accounts for 20%–25% of all cases of small bowel obstruction (64). As one would anticipate, this condition is more typically seen in women and represents one of the more common causes of small bowel obstruction in this subset of patients. Frequently the stone becomes impacted in the terminal ileum, and the presentation is typical of a distal small bowel obstruction. Occasionally, the diagnosis is suspected preoperatively based on the finding of intrahepatic biliary air noted on abdominal radiography (65). In most cases the diagnosis is made at the time of laparotomy when a gallstone is palpated at the site of obstruction. The primary therapeutic goals at laparotomy in a patient with gallstone ileus are correction of the obstruction and removal of the offending stone. Because most of these elderly patients are quite ill, cholecystectomy and takedown of the biliary-enteric fistula probably should not be performed at that time. Although early reports indicated that the mortality associated with this condition approached 40%, more recent studies suggest a mortality rate of 5%–15% (64, 66, 67). Our current practice is to correct the bowel obstruction by removing the impacted stone by enterotomy proximal to the impaction site and retrograde extraction of the stone. Cholecystectomy is not done unless there is evidence of acute biliary tract disease or the cholecystectomy could be quite easily performed and safe for the patient. Our experience supports the recent literature (67) and suggests that most of these patients will not require subsequent cholecystectomy for recurrent symptoms.

Emphysematous Cholecystitis

Acute emphysematous cholecystitis is an unusual clinical entity that is characterized by the radiographic demonstration of gas either within the gallbladder lumen or wall (68). This entity is more common in elderly men and diabetics and is associated with gangrene and perforation of the gallbladder. Clostridial organisms are present in most patients with emphysematous cholecystitis, although other gas-forming organisms may also be found. The pathogenesis of this disorder is not clear, although up to 50% of patients may not have associated gallstones. Ischemia has been implicated as a potential etiologic factor in this process. The associated mortality is high, and prompt cholecystectomy is indicated.

Biliary Sepsis

Much has been written in recent years about biliary sepsis in the aged population, particulary in regard to gallstone disease. Elderly patients, presumed to be asymptomatic, may have septic shock as their initial manifestation of cholelithiasis (69). Prospective studies have demonstrated that the incidence of positive bile cultures in patients with acute cholecystitis increases linearly with age. The reported incidence of positive bile cultures in patients under 50 years of age is 30% and increases to over 50% in patients 70 years or older (70). Most bacteria are of enteric origin, with *E. coli* being the most common. *Bacteroides fragilis* has been recovered from 28% of elderly patients undergoing biliary tract procedures (71). In their now classic article, Chetlin and Elliott (72) identified high risk-factors for the development of septic complications following cholecystectomy. Among other factors was age over 70 years.

The importance of this observation has been

clarified by studies that have looked at the role of prophylactic antibiotic therapy (73, 74). Antibiotic prophylaxis is now an accepted feature of gallstone surgery in the elderly. We administer a broad spectrum antibiotic (a second-generation cephalosporin) 1 hour preoperatively to all elderly patients undergoing elective cholecystectomy. An intraoperative gram stain is generally performed only to identify those patients who may have an anaerobic infection. We generally give one or two doses of antibiotics postoperatively unless there are clinical indications to extend treatment. We tend to be more aggressive in the elderly patient with acute cholecystitis and will frequently employ a therapeutic regimen with good anaerobic coverage and coverage for *Enterococcus*. In general, septic complications in the elderly can be minimized by the judicious use of appropriate antibiotics.

Gallstone Dissolution in the Elderly

The medical dissolution and prevention of gallstones have been goals of clinicians dating back to ancient times. Two agents, chenodeoxycholic acid (CDCA) and ursodeoxycholic acid (URSO), have been shown to be effective in the dissolution of cholesterol gallstones in a limited number of carefully selected patients. These two bile salts dissolve cholesterol stones by decreasing hepatic cholesterol synthesis and expanding the bile acid pool, thereby reducing the degree of cholesterol saturation of bile. In the most complete and comprehensive study of stone dissolution, performed under the supervision of The National Cooperative Gallstone Study, the rate of complete stone disappearance was only 13.5% and partial response was an additional 28% (75). In addition to this disappointingly low success rate, other problems with the use of these agents, especially in the elderly, include (1) the need for lifetime therapy to prevent the recurrence of stones (50% of patients), (2) the need for strict compliance, (3) the long period of time required to achieve a response, and (4) the potential toxic side effects. Although intuitively the ideal candidate for dissolution therapy would be the elderly, infirm patient with symptomatic gallstones, this is the very individual who can be predicted to have the least chance of responding to this type of therapy. Currently, we do not feel that dissolution therapy has a role in the management of elderly patients with gallstone disease. Recently, the concept of local dissolution of gallbladder stones by percutaneous instillation of specific agents (methyl tert-butyl ether) directly into the gallbladder has been introduced (76). The efficacy of this procedure and its potential role in the management of elderly patients with asymptomatic or symptomatic gallstone disease remain to be defined.

Colon Carcinoma and Cholecystectomy

Recent preliminary clinical studies have suggested that there may be an increased risk of colorectal carcinoma following cholecystectomy. The implication of this finding in the elderly patient, if it were true, is obvious. The theoretical basis for this proposal is the alteration in the relative concentrations of primary and secondary bile acids that occurs in the bowel following cholecystectomy and the observation that the relative concentrations of secondary bile acids (deoxycholic and lithocholic acid) seem to be increased among patients with colorectal cancer (77). The evidence to support this hypothesis is based on retrospective and circumstantial studies (78, 79). A more recent prospective study of over 16,000 patients undergoing cholecystectomy suggests that there is no etiologic association whatsoever between cholecystectomy and the subsequent development of a colorectal carcinoma (80). Therefore, we feel that the decision to proceed or not to proceed with cholecystectomy in an elderly patient with symptomatic biliary tract disease should be based on the biliary tract disease process, and the issue of whether or not he or she will be at increased risk for colon carcinoma should not be weighed heavily.

Gallbladder Carcinoma

Carcinoma of the gallbladder is an uncommon though not rare malignancy that occurs more frequently in male patients whose median age is 65 years (81–83). The association between cholelithiasis and cancer of the gallbladder has long been recognized. Recent studies have shown that calcium carbonate stones are associated with a much higher risk than cholesterol stones and

Table 21.3 Optimum Treatment for Carcinoma of Gallbladder[a]

Stage I (Nevin): Intramucosal
　Cholecystectomy alone: probably adequate in most cases
　Consider hepatic radiation (gallbladder bed)

Stage II (submucosa), III (serosal), IV (cystic node metastasis)
　Surgery: resection of gallbladder and its fossa (wedge resection of liver with portahepatic node dissection) (common and hepatic ducts and periduodenal); mark with clips
　Adjuvant: consider radiation; chemotherapy (?)

Stage V: Protocol study/palliative radiation, chemotherapy(?)

[a]Reproduced with permission from Wanebo HJ (ed): *Hepatic and Biliary Cancer.* New York, Marcel Dekker, 1987, p 441.

that patients with gallbladder stones over 2.5 cm in diameter are at much higher risk than patients with smaller stones. However, it is important to re-emphasize that the incidence of carcinoma in the gallbladder is sufficiently low so that, by itself, it should not be an indication for cholecystectomy. The clinical presentation of this disease is similar to that seen in patients with symptomatic cholelithiasis. Most often, the diagnosis is made at the time of laparotomy, and it is rare that the diagnosis is actually made preoperatively. Occasionally, carcinoma in situ will exist, and cholecystectomy performed for biliary calculous disease may be curative. Unfortunately, this is the exception, and most often the disease is advanced and unresectable at the time of diagnosis. The overall prognosis is poor, and the 5-year survival rate is generally reported to be less than 5% (84). Several strategies have been developed for the optimal treatment for carcinoma of the gallbladder (See Table 21.3). In our experience, rather aggressive treatment, including local hepatic resection and lymphadenectomy, is generally not indicated nor is it technically feasible in most elderly patients with carcinoma of the gallbladder. Most of these patients go on to develop local recurrence with jaundice arising from tumor involvement in the porta hepatis. These patients may often receive excellent palliation with the intubation of the biliary tract (either endoscopically or percutaneously) by the placement of transhepatic tubes.

The role of radiotherapy or chemotherapy in the management of patients with gallbladder carcinoma has not been well defined. Insofar as local spread of this disease occurs through the lymphatics and venous drainage of the gallbladder, radiotherapy has been advocated as an effective means of controlling local disease. In patients with more advanced disease, combination therapy with concomitant radiotherapy and chemotherapy may offer some advantage. The clinician caring for the elderly patient with carcinoma of the gallbladder must weigh the potential advantages and benefits of this type of aggressive adjuvant therapy against the impact that it will have on the patient's lifestyle and quality of his or her remaining life.

MANAGEMENT OF THE JAUNDICED PATIENT

Overview

The elderly patient with jaundice often presents considerable diagnostic and therapeutic challenges for even the experienced clinician and surgeon. The differentiation among jaundice secondary to hepatocellular disease, drug-induced cholestasis, or extrahepatic obstruction may be quite difficult in the geriatric population, especially in those individuals with multiple associated medical problems. The presence of jaundice is associated with increased operative morbidity and mortality, and it is therefore essential that the diagnosis be precise and that nonoperative interventions be considered prior to development of a surgical therapeutic plan. Studies from the mid-1970s suggested that the mortality for jaundiced patients over the age of 70 years who undergo operations for gallstone disease was in excess of 30%. Although biliary sepsis was a contributing factor, the predominant cause for this high mortality appeared to be renal failure. Currently, with our increased awareness of nephrotoxic agents and improved parasurgical techniques, the mortality is appreciably less. Nonetheless, the widespread use of non-operative means, such as endoscopic sphincterotomy, has led to a critical re-evaluation of the need for operative intervention in the jaundiced elderly patient.

Diagnostic Evaluation

The basic question to be answered when confronted with an elderly patient with jaundice is to decide whether this individual has a medical cause or a surgical cause (extrahepatic obstruction) for the jaundice. Although biochemical tests may provide a clue, further evidence to substantiate a clinical impression is often mandated. The typical profile of a patient with extrahepatic biliary obstruction includes elevated levels of total bilirubin and alkaline phosphatase with normal or minimally elevated transaminases. The pattern for a patient with hepatocellular disease or drug-induced cholestasis frequently consists of elevated serum transaminases and only mild increases in the alkaline phosphatase levels. Ultimately, the key to differentiating medical versus surgical jaundice lies in diagnostic imaging of the intra- and extrahepatic bile ducts. Ultrasonography has been shown to be a simple, safe, and accurate tool for the identification of the dilated intra- or extrahepatic ducts, which may be due either to gallstones or tumor. Once biliary ductal dilatation has been identified, it is essential to define the anatomy and if possible establish a definitive diagnosis prior to consideration of laparotomy. This may be greatly facilitated by a CT scan that may show a mass in the head of the pancreas or some other lesion to explain the biliary obstruction. If the diagnosis is still in doubt and/or if anatomic delineation of the biliary tract is deemed essential, then one should proceed with either percutaneous transhepatic cholangiography (PTC) or endoscopic retrograde cholangiopancreatography (ERCP), depending on local expertise. In patients with a lesion suspected in the distal common bile duct, an ERCP provides certain advantages over a transhepatic cholangiogram, including the ability to visualize and do a biopsy of the ampulla of Vater. However, for those lesions believed to be in the mid-or proximal bile duct, the transhepatic cholangiogram is much more helpful in delineating the intrahepatic anatomy, which will aid in the preoperative decision making.

Management of Obstructive Jaundice

The realization that most causes of extrahepatic jaundice in the elderly patient can be treated without surgical intervention has led to a re-evaluation of therapeutic guidelines in this patient population. Studies from the 1970s suggested that the operative mortality for elderly patients with jaundice who undergo cholecystectomy is considerable (85). The widespread use of endoscopic sphincterotomy has provided a reasonable alternative for the management of elderly patients with biliary obstruction secondary to calculous disease. The reported mortality rate in elderly patients who undergo endoscopic sphincterotomy and gallstone removal approaches 2% (86). In addition, the procedure generally requires minimal hospitalization, and the recovery period is usually shorter than that of laparotomy. Certainly, cholecystectomy, operative cholangiography, and common bile duct exploration (when indicated) remain the gold standard of treatment. Endoscopic sphincterotomy should be weighed in view of available expertise and the patient's overall condition.

Unfortunately, most studies would suggest that malignant tumors are the cause of twice as many cases of jaundice in the elderly as benign gallstone disease (87, 88). Although the most common malignant lesion causing jaundice in the elderly patient is carcinoma of the head of the pancreas, the lesions most amenable to surgical treatment are ampullary tumors. These lesions are associated with a 5-year survival rate of 25%–30% (89). Based on these data, we feel that age alone should not preclude aggressive surgical management in a patient with a potentially resectable tumor. In contrast, tumors that involve the more proximal bile duct and the gallbladder are associated with shorter survival rates, and in these situations, good palliation should be the goal.

Currently, there are several different methods available for treatment of obstructive jaundice due to a malignancy. These include surgical resection, biliary enteric bypass, insertion of an endoprosthesis either via the percutaneous or endoscopic route, and endoscopic sphincterotomy. In a recent report of 180 patients (90), many of whom were elderly, there was no difference in overall survival between the patients who were treated by biliary enteric bypass and those treated by the placement of biliary stents. Experience with the non-operative modalities for the management of obstructive jaundice is increasing worldwide. At our own institution, the interventional radiologists have gained considerable experience with the placement of transhepatic tubes for the purpose of internal drainage of an obstructed biliary system. The placement of these tubes often obviates the need for an operation and generally provides excellent palliation. There are, however, certain problems that arise with the use of these tubes. If the tumor is high in the biliary tree, a definitive tissue diagnosis may not be feasible unless a laparotomy is performed; cytologic analysis of biliary drainage is generally not conclusive in establishing a diagnosis of malignancy. Furthermore, these tubes frequently become occluded with debris leading to sepsis and in our experience generally require changing every 2 to 4 months. Endoscopically placed prostheses are being used with increasing frequency and can generally be placed through a malignant stricture without difficulty. When palliation is contemplated for the jaundiced patient with underlying malignancy, the goal should be internal drainage, rather than the creation of an external biliary fistula. The symptoms associated with jaundice, which include anorexia and pruritus, can be greatly ameliorated by the percutaneous or endoscopic placement of internal biliary stents. As stated previously, the most common tumor causing extrahepatic obstruction is carcinoma involving the head of the pancreas. This is discussed in detail in Chapter 22.

Despite the increasing use of non-operative means for the treatment of the elderly jaundiced patient, laparotomy and biliary exploration continue to be done in most centers. The elderly patient with gallstone disease undergoing operation should be treated in a manner similar to the younger patient. Although several authors have advocated either sphincteroplasty and/or choledochoduodenostomy for the elderly patient with common duct stones, we have elected to apply the same principles to the elderly patient that would govern our operative strategy for the younger patient. In the elderly patient with multiple common duct stones, our goal is to remove each and every gallstone. If this is feasible and there does not appear to be any distal biliary obstruction, we would then insert a T-tube and would not perform either a sphincteroplasty or a biliary enteric bypass. If on the other hand, we are unable to extract all the stones or find that there is an abnormality of the distal duct, then we would perform a biliary enteric bypass. In summary, it is important to recognize that, although our ability to treat biliary obstruction non-operatively has been vastly improved in recent years, operative management remains the mainstay in most situations.

THE FUTURE OF BILIARY TRACT SURGERY IN THE ELDERLY

The recent radiologic and technical advances, which have already been discussed, have had a profound effect on the management of diseases of the liver, gallbladder, and biliary tract as they occur in the geriatric population. The indications and applications of this technology will continue to influence the care that these patients receive in the future. Endoscopic manipulation of the biliary tract, for either benign or malignant disease, has revolutionized our thinking about disease processes in these patients. In addition to these technical advances, our ability to perform radical surgical procedures safely has been greatly facilitated in recent years. Age by itself, therefore, should never preclude the aggressive treatment of a biliary disorder in an elderly patient, either by non-operative or operative means. The value of our gained knowledge and capabilities is only as great as our rational ability to apply these principles to individual patients. The problems associated with the elderly patient in particular mandate an overall understanding of the surgical principles as outlined in this and other chapters.

REFERENCES

1. Reiss R: Moral and ethical issues in geriatric surgery. *J Med Ethics* 6:71–77, 1980.
2. Reiss R, Deutsch AA: Emergency abdominal procedures in patients above 70. *J Gerontol* 40:154–158, 1985.
3. James OFW: Gastrointestinal and liver function in old age. *Clin Gastroenterol* 12:671–691, 1983.
4. Okuda K, Nomura F, Okuda H, Shimokaha Y: Ageing and gross anatomical alterations of the liver. In Kitan K (ed): *Liver and Ageing*. Amsterdam, North Holland, Elsevier, 1978, pp 159–176.
5. Mooney H, Roberts R, Cooksley WGE, Halliday JW, Powell LW: Alterations in the liver with ageing. *Clin*

Gastroenterol 14:757–771, 1985.

6. Watanabe T, Tanaka Y: Age-related alterations in the size of human hepatocytes. *Virchows Arch* 39:9–20, 1982.

7. Schaffner F, Popper H: Nonspecific reactive hepatitis in aged and infirm people. *Am J Dig Dis* 4:389–399, 1959.

8. Kampmann JP, Sinding J, Moller-Jorgensen I: Effect of age on liver function. *Geriatrics* 30:91–95, 1975.

9. Koff RRS, Garvey AJ, Burney SW: Absence of an age effect on sulfobromophthalein retention in healthy men. *Gastroenterology* 65:300–302, 1973.

10. Woodhouse KW: Drugs and the ageing gut, liver, and pancreas. *Clin Gastroenterol* 14:863–880, 1985.

11. Valdivieso V, Palma R, Wunkhaus R, Antezana C, Severin C, Contreras A: Effect of aging on biliary lipid composition and bile acid metabolism in normal Chilean women. *Gastroenterology* 74:871–874, 1978.

12. Khalil T, Walker JP, Wiener I, Fagan CJ, Townsend CM Jr, Greeley CH Jr, Thompson JC: Effect of aging on gallbladder contraction and release of cholycystokinin-33 in humans. *Surgery* 98:423–429, 1985.

13. Floyd JC, Fajans SS, Pek S, Chance RE: A newly recognized pancreatic polypeptide: Plasma levels in health and disease. *Recent Prog Horm Res* 33:519–570, 1977.

14. Conter RL, Roslyn JJ, DenBesten L, Taylor I: Pancreatic polypeptide enhances post-contractile gallbladder filling. *Gastroenterology* 92:771–776, 1987.

15. Roslyn JJ, Kuchenbecker S, Longmire WP Jr, Tompkins R: Floating tumor debris: a cause of intermittent biliary obstruction. *Arch Surg* 119:1312–1315, 1984.

16. Linsell A: Primary liver cancer: Epidemiology and etiology. In Wanebo HJ (ed): *Hepatic and Biliary Cancer*. New York, Marcel Dekker, 1987, p. 4.

17. Saracci R, Repetto F: Time trends of liver cancer. *JNCI* 65:241–247, 1980.

18. Fortner JG, MacLean BJ, Kim DK, Howland WS, Turnbull AD, Goldiner P, Carlon G, Beattie EJ Jr: The seventies evolution in liver surgery for cancer. *Cancer* 47:2162–2166, 1981.

19. Conter RL, Pitt HA, Tompkins RK, Longmire WP Jr: Differentiation of pyogenic from amebic hepatic abscesses. *Surg Gynecol Obstet* 162:114–120, 1986.

20. Heaton KW: The epidemiology of gallstones and suggested etiology. *Clin Gastroenterol* 2:67–83, 1973.

21. Lieber MM: The incidence of gallstones and their correlation with other disease. *Ann Surg* 135:394–405, 1952.

22. Friedman GD, Kannel WB, Dawber TR: The epidemiology of gallbladder disease: Observations in the Framingham study. *J Chronic Dis* 19:273–292, 1966.

23. Bateson MC: Gallbladder disease and cholecystectomy rates are independently variable. *Lancet* 2:621–624, 1984.

24. Lindstrom C, Wenchkert A: Paper given to meeting of the Gallstone Study Group, UMGE, Copenhagen, 1970.

25. Sampliner RE, Bennett PH, Comess LJ, Rose FA, Burch TA: Gallbladder disease in Pima Indians. Demonstra-

tions of high prevalence and early onset by cholecystography. *N Engl J Med* 283:1358–1364, 1970.

26. Crump C: The incidence of gallstones and gallbladder disease. *Surg Gynecol Obstet* 53:447–455, 1931.

27. Newman HF, Northup JD: The autopsy incidence of gallstones. *Int Abstr Surg* 109:1–13, 1959.

28. Ibach JR Jr, Hume HA, Erb WH: Cholecystectomy in the aged. *Surg Gynecol Obstet* 126:523–528, 1968.

29. Krarup T, Sonderstrup J, Kruse-Blinkenberg HO, Schmidt A: Surgery for gallstones in old age: do we operate too late? *Acta Chir Scand* 148:263–266, 1982.

30. Mentzer RM, Golden CT, Chandler JG, Horsley JS III: A comparative appraisal of emphysematous cholecystitis. *Am J Surg* 129:10–15, 1975.

31. Roslyn J, Busuttil R: Gallbladder perforation: pitfalls in management. *Am J Surg* 137:307–312, 1979.

32. Fry DE, Cox RA, Harbrecht JP: Gangrene of the gallbladder. *South Med J* 74:666–668, 1981.

33. Norman DC, Yoshikawa TT: Intraabdominal infections in the elderly. *J Am Geriatr Soc* 31:677–684, 1983.

34. Sullivan DM, Hood TR, Griffen WO Jr: Biliary tract surgery in the elderly. *Am J Surg* 143:218–220, 1982.

35. Gracie WA, Ransohoff DF: The natural history of silent gallstones. The innocent gallstone is not a myth. *N Engl J Med* 307:798–800, 1982.

36. Glenn F: Silent gallstones. *Ann Surg* 193:251–252, 1981.

37. Schreiber H, Macon WL IV, Pories WJ: Incidental cholecystectomy during major abdominal surgery in the elderly. *Am J Surg* 135:196–198, 1978.

38. Quriel K, Ricotta JJ, Adams JT, DeWeese JA: Management of cholelithiasis in patients with abdominal aortic aneurysm. *Ann Surg* 198:717–719, 1983.

39. Huber DF, Martin EW Jr, Cooperman M: Cholecystectomy in elderly patients. *Am J Surg* 146:719–722, 1983.

40. Cobden I, Venables CW, Lendrum R, James OFW: Gallstones presenting as mental and physical debility in the elderly. *Lancet* 1:1062–1064, 1984.

41. Madden JW, Croker JR, Beynon GPJ: Septicaemia in the elderly. *Postgrad Med J* 57:502–506, 1981.

42. Graham EA, Cole WH: Roentgenologic examination of the gallbladder: preliminary report of a new method utilizing the intravenous injection of tetrabromophenolphthalein. *JAMA* 82:613–614, 1924.

43. Baker HL, Hodgson JR: Further studies on the accuracy of oral cholecystography. *Radiology* 74:239–245, 1960.

44. Suarez CA, Block F, Bernstein D, Serafini A, Rodman G Jr, Zeppa R: The role of HIDA/PIPIDA scanning in diagnosing cystic duct obstruction. *Ann Surg* 191:391–396, 1980.

45. Van Rensburg LCJ: The management of acute cholecystitis in the elderly. *Br J Surg* 71:692–693, 1984.

46. Van der Linden W, Sunzel H: Early versus delayed operation for acute cholecystitis. A controlled clinical trial. *Am J Surg* 120:7–13, 1970.

47. Lahtinen J, Alhava EM, Aukee S: Acute cholecystitis treated by early and delayed surgery. A controlled clinical trial. *Scan J Gastroenterol* 13:673–678, 1978.

48. Glenn F: Trends in surgical treatment of calculous dis-

ease of the biliary tract. *Surg Gynecol Obstet* 140:877–884, 1975.

49. Glenn F: Surgical management of acute cholecystitis in patients 65 years of age and older. *Ann Surg* 193:56–59, 1981.

50. Morrow DJ, Thompson J, Wilson SE: Acute cholecystitis in the elderly. A surgical emergency. *Arch Surg* 113:1149–1152, 1978.

51. Thorbjarnarson B: History of biliary tract surgery. In Thorbjarnarson B (ed): *Surgery of the Biliary Tract.* Philadelphia, WB Saunders, 1982, pp 1–2.

52. Welch JP, Malt RA: Outcome of cholecystostomy. *Surg Gynecol Obstet* 135:717–720, 1972.

53. Costello C: Cholecystostomy in modern surgery. *Am Surg* 22:1079–1094, 1956.

54. Skillings JC, Kumal C, Hinshaw JR: Cholecystostomy: a place in modern biliary surgery? *Am J Surg* 139:865–869, 1980.

55. Patterson HC, Bream CA: Cholecystostomy—an old dog with new tricks. *South Med J* 70:187–188, 1977.

56. Turrill FL, McCarron UM, Mikkelsen WP: Gallstones and diabetics: an ominous association. *Am J Surg* 102:184–190, 1961.

57. Walsh DB, Eckhauser FE, Ramsburg SF, Burney RB: Risk associated with diabetes mellitus in patients undergoing gallbladder surgery. *Surgery* 91:254–257, 1982.

58. Haff FC, Butcher HR, Ballinger WF: Biliary tract operations: a review of 1000 patients. *Arch Surg* 98:428–434, 1969.

59. Lygidakis NJ: Operative risk factors of cholecystectomy—choledochotomy in the elderly. *Surg Gynecol Obstet* 157:15–19, 1983.

60. Moesgaard F, Nielsen ML, Pedersen T, Hansen JB: Protective choledochoduodenostomy in multiple common duct stones in the aged. *Surg Gynecol Obstet* 154:232–234, 1982.

61. Glenn F, Moore SE: Gangrene and perforation of the wall of the gallbladder. A sequela of acute cholecystitis. *Arch Surg* 44:677–686, 1942.

62. Ramanujam P, Shabeeb N, Silver JM: Unusual manifestations of gallstone migration into the gastrointestinal tract. *South Med J* 76:30–32, 1983.

63. Williams NF, Scobie TK: Perforation of the gallbladder: analysis of 19 cases. *Can Med Assoc J* 115:1223–1225, 1976.

64. Cooperman AM, Dickson ER, ReMine WH: Changing concepts in the surgical treatment of gallstone ileus. *Ann Surg* 167:377–383, 1968.

65. Rigler LG, Borman CM, Nobel JF: Gallstone obstruction: pathogenesis and roentgen manifestation. *JAMA* 117:1753–1759, 1941.

66. Kurtz RJ, Hermann TM, Kurtz AB: Gallstone ileus: a diagnostic problem. *Am J Surg* 146:314–317, 1983.

67. Heuman R, Sjodahl R, Wetterfors J: Gallstone ileus: an analysis of 20 patients. *World J Surg* 4:595–600, 1980.

68. Hegner CG: Gaseous pericholecystitis with cholecystitis and cholelithiasis. *Arch Surg* 22:993–1000, 1931.

69. Faber RC, Ibrahim SZ, Thomas DM, Beynon GPJ, Le-

Quesne LP: Gallstone disease presenting as septicaemic shock. *Br J Surg* 65:101–105, 1978.

70. Reiss R, Eliashiv A, Deutsch AA: Septic complications and bile cultures in 800 consecutive cholecystectomies. *World J Surg* 6:195–199, 1982.

71. Shimada K, Inamatsu T, Yamashiro M: Anaerobic bacteria in biliary disease in elderly patients. *J Clin Infect Dis* 135:850–854, 1977.

72. Chetlin SH, Elliott DW: Biliary bacteremia. *Arch Surg* 102:303–307, 1971.

73. Chetlin SH, Elliott DW: Preoperative antibiotics in biliary surgery. *Arch Surg* 107:319–323, 1973.

74. Keighley MRB, Baddeley RM, Burdon DW, Edwards JAC, Quoraishi AH, Oates GD, Watts GT, Alexander-Williams J: A controlled trial of parenteral prophylactic gentamicin therapy in biliary surgery. *Br J Surg* 62:275–279, 1975.

75. Schoenfield LJ, Lachlin JM: Chenodiaol (chenodeoxycholic acid) for dissolution of gallstones: the National Cooperative Gallstone Study. A controlled trial of efficacy and safety. *Ann Intern Med* 95:257–282, 1981.

76. Allen MJ, Borody TJ, Bugliosi TF, May GR, LaRusso NF, Thistle JS: Rapid dissolution of gallstones by methyl tert-butyl ether. Preliminary Observations. *N Engl J Med* 312:217–220, 1985.

77. Hill MJ, Draser BS, Williams REO: Faecal bile acids and clostridia in patients with cancer of the large bowel. *Lancet* 1:535–538, 1975.

78. Turunen MJ, Kivilaakso EO: Increased risk of colorectal cancer after cholecystectomy. *Ann Surg* 194:639–641, 1981.

79. Turnbull PRG, Smith AH, Isbister WH: Cholecystectomy and cancer of the large bowel. *Br J Surg* 68:551–553, 1981.

80. Lowenfels AB, Domellof L, Lindstrom CG: Cholelithiasis, cholecystectomy, and cancer: a case-control study in Sweden. *Gastroenterology* 83:672–676, 1982.

81. Richard PF, Cantin J: Primary carcinoma of the gallbladder: study of 108 cases. *Can J Surg* 19:27–32, 1976.

82. Blalock JB Jr: An analysis of 15 cases of gallbladder carcinoma. *Am Surg* 44:286–289, 1978.

83. Piehler JM, Crichlow RW: Primary carcinoma of the gallbladder. *Surg Gynecol Obstet* 147:929–942, 1978.

84. Wanebo JH, Castle WN, Fechner RE: Is carcinoma of the gallbladder a curable lesion? *Ann Surg* 195:624–634, 1982.

85. Lee E: Obstructive jaundice. In Truelove SC, Trowell J (eds): *Topics in Gastroenterology* 2nd ed. Oxford, Blackwell, 1974, pp 255–270.

86. Mee AS, Vallon AG, Croker JR, Cotton PB: Nonoperative removal of bile duct stones by duodenoscopic sphincterotomy in the elderly. *Br Med J* 283:521–523, 1981.

87. O'Brien GF, Tan CV: Jaundice in the geriatric patient. *Geriatrics* 25:114–127, 1970.

88. Eastwood HD: Causes of jaundice in the elderly: a survey of diagnosis and investigations. *Gerontol Clin* 13:69–81 1971.

89. Longmire WP Jr, McArthur MS, Bastounis EA, Hiatt J: Carcinoma of the extrahepatic biliary tract. *Ann Surg* 178:333–345, 1973.

90. Leung JWC, Emery R, Cotton PB, Russell RCG, Vallon AG, Moson RR: Management of malignant obstructive jaundice at The Middlesex Hospital. *Br J Surg* 70:584–586, 1983.

Chapter 22

Surgical Management of Pancreatic Disease in the Elderly

Keith D. Lillemoe, M.D., John L. Cameron, M.D., F.A.C.S.

Pancreatic disease is a significant health care problem in the elderly. Although the entire spectrum of benign and malignant disease of the pancreas can occur in all age groups, many conditions are quite common in older patients. Acute pancreatitis primarily of biliary origin and pancreatic carcinoma are by far the most common disorders seen in the elderly. As the population ages, these pancreatic diseases are likely to become more common. This trend is already apparent as the incidence of pancreatic cancer is clearly rising with more older patients presenting with this condition. Gallstone disease also is much more common in older patients. Many older patients can be expected to present with gallstone pancreatitis as a complication of biliary stone disease.

The management of diseases of the pancreas is no different in older patients. Both acute pancreatitis and pancreatic cancer are associated with significant increases in morbidity and mortality in older patients. However, with early efforts at diagnosis, good supportive care, and aggressive surgical management, elderly patients can be managed successfully with these disorders. An aggressive attitude toward the diagnosis and management is important for avoiding complications. The surgical management of patients in the older age group will always be associated with significant risks, but with proper management many of these patients can be restored to a healthy and active state.

CHANGES IN THE PANCREAS WITH AGING

Anatomic Changes

Changes in the anatomy of the pancreas in the

elderly have been well described. An understanding of these changes is necessary for the accurate interpretation of radiographic studies of the pancreas in older patients. First, the duodenal C loop and the pancreas may be displaced inferiorly in older patients. The head of the pancreas is often located as low as the body of the second sacral vertebra (1). This "low-lying" pancreas may lead to difficulty in visualization of the pancreas by imaging techniques if they are not projected low enough.

Changes in the pancreatic ductal anatomy have also been described. Kreel and Sandin performed retrograde pancreatography at necropsy in 120 cases (1). Of the 120 cases, 107 were at least 60 years of age, and 84 were 70 years or older. Pancreatic duct width was noted to increase with age at the rate of 8% per decade. This increase occurs throughout the whole pancreas—head, body, and tail—at proportionally the same rate. The dilated duct in the elderly retains its uniform tapered appearance with smooth margins, with only scattered and intermittent branch dilatation. Peripheral single or conglomerate tiny cysts were also noted frequently. Cyst formation is more common in association with greater duct width, and there was a significant correlation of the presence of cysts with increasing age.

Pathologic Changes

Pathologic changes in the pancreas of the elderly are seen in almost all patients. In 1921, Rossle showed that the weight of the pancreas decreased after the age of 70 from a normal mean weight of $60 +/- 20$ g to 40 g or less at the age of 85 (2). Histologic changes affect both glandular tissue, as well as pancreatic ducts. The glandular changes involve most frequently fatty infiltration and fibrosis. The fatty infiltration appears to be a replacement phenomenon, with small remnants of lobules completely surrounded with adipose tissue. The fibrosis noticed was fine and patchy and unassociated with destruction of exocrine parenchyma as seen in chronic pancreatitis.

Ductal changes consisting of proliferation and metaplasia of ductal epithelial cells also are noted (3). This proliferation often led to the formation of a solid cord of cells, which was followed by lumen formation, expansion, and cavitation. Cavity formation was a consistent finding in older patients. Metaplasia of the pancreatic duct occurred to the extent that ductal epithelium eventually became a stratified squamous epithelium in the interlobular ducts. These findings provide the pathologic support for the radiographic changes noted above by Kreel and Sandin (1). Histologic examination following pancreatography showed that the dilatation was present in both the interlobular and intralobular ducts, giving additional explanation for the diminished pancreatic endocrine and exocrine function noted in aging.

Functional Changes

Pancreatic exocrine function in the elderly patient may also be altered. Early reports showed reduced levels of pancreatic exocrine enzymes in duodenal aspirates of elderly subjects. Later work using secretin stimulation has failed to demonstrate changes in volume and output of bicarbonate and amylase in elderly patients (4, 5). However, with repeated secretin stimulation, the pancreas of older subjects appears to show fatigue and diminished function when compared to younger individuals (5). Analysis of specimens of pure pancreatic juice collected endoscopically has also demonstrated that pancreatic function does diminish with age. Significant decreases in volume of pancreatic secretion in response to secretin stimulation and pancreatic protein and lipase concentration in response to cholecystokinin stimulation have been observed in subjects over 65 years of age (6). Thus, some physiologic decline in exocrine pancreatic function does indeed occur, but because only 10%–15% of pancreatic secretion is needed for normal digestion,

it is unlikely that these changes are of any clinical significance.

There is experimental information suggesting a diminished endocrine cell function with aging. However, beta-cell function in the human has been demonstrated to be normal, elevated, or decreased in various studies. A recent report by Chen and colleagues has demonstrated both a significant B-cell defect in insulin secretion and diminshed peripheral response to insulin in the elderly (7). It may be that pancreatic endocrine changes contribute to the pathogenesis of age-related glucose intolerance.

INFLAMMATORY DISEASES OF THE PANCREAS

Acute Pancreatitis

Acute pancreatitis has an incidence of 0.5% in the general population. Aging itself is not associated with an increased risk of acute pancreatitis. It is an important cause of abdominal pain in the elderly, and when it occurs, it is associated with increased morbidity and mortality.

In large series of patients with acute pancreatitis, the proportion of elderly patients varies considerably. In series in which alcohol is the leading cause of pancreatitis, elderly patients make up a very small percentage of the patients. However, in series in which gallstones are the leading cause of pancreatitis, elderly patients make up a much greater proportion. In one such series, 45% of patients were in their seventh, eighth, or ninth decades. Similarly, the sex distribution of elderly patients with acute pancreatitis reflects the biliary tract etiology, with elderly females affected more often than males.

Etiology

As in younger patients, there are a multitude of causes of acute pancreatitis in the elderly (Table 22.1). Although gallstones and alcohol are etiologic factors in up to 90% of cases of all age groups, gallstones are by far the most common cause of acute pancreatitis in the elderly, and alcohol is an infrequent factor. In the elderly patient, external trauma is an uncommon cause of pancreatitis. However, the elderly patient who is undergoing operation for unassociated condi-

Table 22.1. Causes of Acute Pancreatitis in the Elderly

Biliary tract disease—gallstones
Alcohol consumption
Trauma
  External
  Operative
  Retrograde pancreatography
Ischemia
Drugs
Metabolic and endocrine
  Hypercalcemia
  Hyperlipidemia
Pancreatic duct obstruction
  Tumor
  Duodenal diverticula
  Pancreas divisum
  Papillary stenosis
Idiopathic

tions appears to be susceptible to postoperative pancreatitis, which presumably is at least in part secondary to pancreatic trauma. In the recent report by Park, the second leading cause of pancreatitis in the elderly was operative trauma (12.5%) (8). Injury to the pancreas can occur during almost any upper abdominal or retroperitoneal operation, but is frequently observed following biliary or gastric operations, splenectomy, or aortic reconstruction. Endoscopic retrograde cholangiopancreatography (ERCP) performed to evaluate the pancreaticobiliary tree is often associated with a transient elevation of serum amylase. However, less than 5% of patients actually develop clinical pancreatitis. Acute pancreatitis has also been noted following translumbar aortography.

Ischemia has been recognized recently as an initiating factor in some patients with acute pancreatitis. This etiology would appear to play an important role in the elderly. Acute pancreatitis has been noted in up to 50% of patients with oligemic shock following repair of a ruptured abdominal aortic aneurysm (9). Similarly, 20% of patients who died following cardiac operations had pathologic evidence of acute pancreatitis (10). These findings are felt to be secondary to ischemic injury incurred during the low flow state of hypovolemic shock or cardiopulmonary bypass.

A multitude of drugs have been suspected of initiating acute pancreatitis (11). For most of those suspected, the incidence is extremely low, and the pathogenic mechanisms are entirely

unknown. A list of drugs in which evidence exists to suggest causation of acute pancreatitis is provided in Table 22.2. In the elderly population, the most important drugs of this group are probably the diuretics.

Endocrine and metabolic abnormalities, such as hypercalcemia and hyperlipidemia, have also been associated with acute pancreatitis. Hypercalcemia may be masked by a low serum calcium at the time of presentation due to pancreatic inflammation. Hypercalcemia should always be considered in the elderly patient with recurrent pancreatitis without evidence of gallstones. Acute pancreatitis has also been well documented to occur in hyperlipoproteinemia, types I and V. Finally, diabetes mellitus and uremia have recently been suggested as etiologic factors. However, the evidence in support of these latter conditions is weak, and the diagnosis of pancreatitis may be falsely based on elevation of serum amylase unassociated with pancreatic disease.

Obstruction of the pancreatic duct may cause acute pancreatitis. Pancreaticobiliary abnormalities, such as periampullary duodenal diverticula, papillary stenosis, and pancreatic divisum, are rare causes of acute pancreatitis. The most important cause of pancreatic duct obstruction resulting in acute pancreatitis in elderly patients is pancreatic cancer. In a large series of patients with pancreatic cancer, clinical pancreatitis occurred in 3% of cases (12) and frequently led to delay in diagnosis and an unfavorable outcome. Although only approximately 1% of cases of acute pancreatitis will be secondary to pancreatic cancer, this relationship should not be overlooked especially in the elderly, a group at high risk for pancreatic cancer.

Finally, in any large series of patients with acute pancreatitis, the etiology in a proportion of patients will remain unknown or idiopathic. In the recent series of elderly patients reported by Park, 30% of the cases remained idiopathic

Table 22.2. Drugs Implicated in the Etiology of Pancreatitis

Azathioprine	L-asparaginase
Thiazides	Steroids
Furosemide	Ethacrynic acid
Estrogens	Methyldopa
Sulfonamides	Phenformin
Tetracyclines	Procainamide
	Clonidine

(8). In that series, however, ERCP was not routinely performed, and thus, anatomic abnormalities of the pancreatic or biliary ductal system may have remained undetected. Such abnormalities have been shown to account for 45% of cases previously thought to be idiopathic (13). It is our feeling that regardless of a patient's age, a thorough evaluation for the etiology of acute pancreatitis should be completed, including ERCP.

Clinical Presentation of Acute Pancreatitis

The presentation of acute pancreatitis in the elderly is similar to that in younger patients, except that the findings may be more subtle than expected in the presence of severe disease. The most common symptom is pain, which is characteristically located in the epigastrium, radiates to the back, and is occasionally referred to the left shoulder. In the elderly population, in which gallstones may be the cause of pancreatitis, the pain may be sensed in the right upper quadrant. The onset of pain is usually gradual, but occasionally may be sudden, mimicking that of a perforated duodenal ulcer. The pain is often steady and severe. Patients with pancreatitis typically seek relief from their pain by leaning forward. Constant agitation and movement are typical as opposed to the patient with peritonitis who will often lie as motionless as possible. Nausea and vomiting almost invariably are present and are often a prominent early feature. The vomiting may be repeated, is usually not copious, and contains gastric and duodenal contents.

The physical findings can vary widely. The patient may be restless with a rapid pulse and respiratory rate. The temperature is usually elevated in the range of 38 °C, but elevations up to 40° may be seen. The abdomen is usually moderately distended, and bowel sounds are diminished. Diffuse tenderness with guarding and rebound is usually most marked over the epigastrium, upper abdomen, and sometimes the left flank. True rigidity of the abdomen, however, is uncommon. It is not unusual, especially in elderly patients, for the clinical presentation to be out of proportion with physical findings. Rarely with necrotizing or hemorrhagic pancreatitis a bluish discoloration may appear in the flank (Grey-Turner's sign) or periumbilical

Table 22.3. Causes of Hyperamylasemia in the Elderly

Intra-Abdominal Disorders	Extra-Abdominal Disorders
Pancreatic disorders	Salivary gland disorders
Acute pancreatitis	Parotitis
Chronic pancreatitis	Trauma
Trauma	Surgery
Pseudocyst	
Pancreatic ascites	Impaired amylase ex-
Carcinoma	cretion
	Renal failure
	Macroamylasemia
Nonpancreatic disorders	Miscellaneous
Biliary tract disease	Cerebral trauma
Peptic ulcer with	Severe burns
perforation or	Diabetic ketoacidosis
penetration	Pneumonia
Intestinal obstruction	Prostate surgery
Mesenteric infarction	
Acute appendicitis	
Ruptured aortic aneurysm	
Peritonitis	

area (Cullen's sign). Jaundice may be noted especially in cases of gallstone pancreatitis. However, it is more usual for the patient to be anicteric at presentation. Frequently in severe pancreatitis patients will present with respiratory distress. Findings of respiratory difficulty, as well as peripheral signs of hypoxemia, may be obvious, especially in the elderly patient.

Diagnosis

The diagnosis of acute pancreatitis is made on the basis of the clinical presentation, with laboratory determinations serving to confirm the diagnosis. Serum amylase elevations can occur from a multitude of causes (Table 22.3), many of which may mimic acute pancreatitis clinically. In a recent report, only 68% of patients with hyperamylasemia and abdominal pain had acute pancreatitis (14). The acute extrapancreatic abdominal conditions that are commonly associated with serum amylase elevations include perforated peptic ulcer, mesenteric infarction, small bowel obstruction, and acute biliary tract disease. Many of these conditions require urgent operation, and thus, it is of the utmost importance to differentiate these conditions from acute pancreatitis. It does not appear that amylase elevation is a less sensitive indicator of pancreatitis in the elderly. However, elderly patients may be particularly susceptible to other serious conditions causing hyperamylasemia.

The level of hyperamylasemia is not a reliable indicator of the severity of pancreatic inflammation, but is often valuable in establishing the etiology of pancreatitis. Biliary pancreatitis is frequently associated with marked elevation in serum amylase, often to a five- to ten-fold increase, whereas alcoholics with pancreatitis often have a relatively low degree of hyperamylasemia. Patients with postoperative pancreatitis, an important cause in the elderly, frequently present with only minimal or no elevation of serum amylase.

Urinary amylase or amylase-creatinine ratio determinations have been employed in attempts to increase the specificity of amylase determinations. Similarly, serum lipase levels may be useful because elevations may persist longer than elevated serum amylase levels. Unfortunately, none of these methods has been found to be extremely useful in elderly patients. Other abnormal laboratory measurements in patients with acute pancreatitis include a leukocytosis of 10,000 to 15,000 cells/mm³, elevation of the hematocrit secondary to extracellular fluid sequestration, or a low hematocrit due to retroperitoneal bleeding. Hyperglycemia and hypocalcemia may be observed in severe acute pancreatitis and are uncommon with other acute abdominal conditions.

The radiologic findings associated with acute pancreatitis include a small left pleural effusion, segmental small bowel ileus (sentinel loop), dilatation of the transverse colon with absence of air in the left colon, the so called cut-off sign, and duodenal ileus. In patients with acute relapsing pancreatitis, calcifications in the region of the pancreas may also be noted. An upper gastrointestinal series with water-soluble contrast medium can be exceedingly valuable in ruling out perforation of the stomach or duodenum or by demonstrating bowel obstruction. Ultrasonography is especially useful in the diagnosis of elderly patients with acute pancreatitis because of the high incidence of gallstones causing pancreatitis in this age group. Although somewhat difficult because of gaseous distention of the bowel, imaging of the pancreas may show generalized enlargement, localized swelling, or cyst formation. However, in a high percentage of patients, ultrasonography of the pancreas is normal.

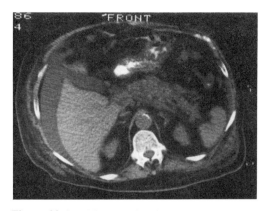

Figure 22.1. CT scan of a 68-year-old male with acute pancreatitis. The scan demonstrates inflammation and edema of the body of the pancreas and the surrounding small bowel mesentery. The presence of pancreatic ascites is also noted.

More recently, computed tomography has been used in the evaluation of patients with acute pancreatitis. The CT scan provides a quick, noninvasive, generally accurate assessment of the pancreas and peripancreatic retroperitoneum. Abnormal CT findings are present in up to 90% of cases (15–16) (Figure 22.1), and they include diffuse pancreatic enlargement, obliteration of peripancreatic fat planes, and inflammation of the anterior perirenal space. Peripancreatic fluid collections can also be visualized (17). There appears to be a direct correlation between the degree of CT abnormalities and the severity of acute pancreatitis (15). In addition, Ranson and his colleagues have used CT scanning to define and identify groups of patients with increased risk of pancreatic abscess (16). We thus believe that CT scanning should be included in both the diagnosis and hospital management of all elderly patients with acute pancreatitis. After the diagnosis of acute pancreatitis is confirmed, we often perform serial CT scans in the severely ill patient in hopes of demonstrating complications of pancreatitis at an early stage.

Attempts to visualize the biliary tree radiographically using oral or intravenous contrast agents are rarely successful in the patient with acute pancreatitis. Endoscopic retrograde cholangiopancreatography (ERCP) is an invasive technique that can provide excellent visualization of the biliary tree. Although ERCP can be performed safely in most patients with acute pancreatitis, its use is not indicated routinely in the early assessment of acute pancreatitis because of potential exacerbation of the inflammation. In those patients with gallstone pancreatitis, preoperative ERCP is useful in demonstrating bile duct anatomy and/or stones. This procedure should not be performed until after the resolution of inflammation except in the severely ill elderly patient in whom it is felt that a stone may be present and obstructing the common bile duct and pancreatic duct. In this setting, endoscopic sphincterotomy and stone extraction may be useful as an alternative to surgical intervention (18). Percutaneous transheptic cholangiography can also provide visualization of the biliary tree without the potential for adversely affecting the pancreas by manipulation of the sphincter. This technique also allows percutaneous drainage of the biliary tree should evidence of obstruction be present on cholangiography.

Historically, diagnostic exploratory laparotomy played an important role in the diagnosis of acute pancreatitis. At the present time, the diagnosis of acute pancreatitis can be made based on a careful, non-operative evaluation in most patients. By the aggressive use of CT scanning, the need for diagnostic laparotomy has been almost completely eliminated in the diagnosis of acute pancreatitis. It must be remembered, however, that the presence of acute pancreatitis does not rule out the possibility of coexisting intra-abdominal pathology in elderly patients. Older patients have a much higher probability of other intra-abdominal catastrophies, such as mesenteric ischemia, gangrenous cholecystitis, or perforated viscus. Diagnostic laparotomy should still be employed to avoid the disastrous complications of non-operative management of these disorders. It is clear from recent studies that simple diagnostic laparotomy does not significantly increase morbidity and mortality of acute pancreatitis, and certainly the risk is justified should the potential for other intra-abdominal pathology exist.

Clinical Course

Because of improvements in supportive care, the overall mortality has decreased in recent years to a level of approximately 5%. Moreover, in many series of patients with mild to moderate pancreatitis, no hospital mortalities are noted.

The clinical course of all patients with acute pancreatitis is highly dependent on the severity of disease. Most patients (approximately 75%) have relatively mild edematous pancreatitis with improvement noted within 48 to 72 hours of hospitalization. Most of the morbidity and mortality that does occur is in that small group of patients with severe and/or hemorrhagic pancreatitis.

Elderly patients represent the extreme in the spectrum of patients with acute pancreatitis. Most authors consider age over 55 years as a significant risk factor for death associated with acute pancreatitis (19–22). In a recent large review by Cornfield and colleagues, the mortality for patients aged 60 or greater was 28% versus 9% for patients below that age ($p < .001$) (22). In a review of pancreatitis in patients 70 years of age or older, a mortality rate of 20% was noted, with an average hospital stay in excess of 3 weeks (8). This is significantly higher than the mortality in the general population, but represents an improvement over the mortality rate of 40% observed by Pollock in his report of pancreatitis in the elderly published in 1959 (23). Thus, it must be concluded that elderly patients are at significant risk for death from acute pancreatitis, and supportive care and intensive care monitoring should be instituted early to avoid a disastrous outcome.

During early clinical assessment, those patients with a high risk of complications can be predicted. Perhaps the most important tool in assessing the severity of acute pancreatitis early in its course has been described by Ranson and his colleagues (19). They were able to identify 11 early prognostic signs (including age over 55) that strongly correlated with subsequent occurrence of serious prolonged illness or death. (Table 22.4) In a retrospective study (19), and subsequently in a prospective study (24), they have found excellent correlation between the number of grave prognostic signs and the subsequent clinical course. In almost 80% of patients, fewer than three positive signs were present, and there was an overall mortality of 0.9%. In those patients with three to four positive signs, the mortality rose to 16%; in those with five to six positive signs it was 40%, and for those with seven or more signs, the mortality was 100%. The number of grave prognostic signs also corre-

Table 22.4. Ranson's Early Prognostic Signs of Acute Pancreatitis

AT ADMISSION
Age greater than 55 years
WBC count greater than 16,000/cu mm
Blood glucose level greater than 200 mg/dl
Serum lactic dehydrogenase greater than 350 IU/liter
SGOT greater than 250 units/dl

DURING INITIAL 48 HOURS
Hematocrit fall greater than 10%
BUN elevation greater than 5 mg/dl
Serum calcium fall to less than 8 mg/dl
Arterial PO_2 less than 60 mm Hg
Base deficit greater than 4 mEq/liter
Estimated fluid sequestration greater than 6 liters

lates well with the days of intensive care required. These grave signs were initially described in patients with pancreatitis secondary to alcohol abuse, and their value in elderly patients with gallstone pancreatitis has been questioned. Subsequently, however, they have been shown to achieve good prognostic separation in patients with biliary, postoperative, and other forms of acute pancreatitis (25).

The value of these signs is that they may identify, by early assessment, those patients (approximately 25%) who are at risk for serious, prolonged, and complicated hospitalizations that may result in death. They can be immediately admitted to the intensive care unit and monitored carefully with appropriate supportive care. It is for this group of patients that non-operative measures, such as peritoneal lavage, broad spectrum antibiotic coverage, and stress ulcer prophylaxis, should be considered. In addition, frequent CT scans should be obtained for early identification of peripancreatic fluid collections and/or pancreatic abscess so that early aggressive operative management can be instituted.

Treatment

The initial management after the diagnosis of acute pancreatitis consists of resuscitation and correction of deficits of fluids and electrolytes. There is little difference in this initial management in patients of any age. Meticulous replacement of fluid and electrolyte losses with adequate maintenance therapy is of utmost importance. Constant attention to the urinary output, central venous pressure, and, in those elderly patients with evidence of heart failure, pulmonary capil-

lary wedge pressure is mandatory. A urinary catheter and central venous line should be utilized in all elderly patients with pancreatitis. Replacement of extracellular fluid loss is accomplished by administration of a crystalloid solution. In patients with severe hemorrhagic pancreatitis, blood transfusion may be required. In those patients with evidence of glucose intolerance, control must be obtained with administration of insulin. Hypocalcemia should be corrected by intravenous administration of calcium gluconate.

Several other steps have been advocated through the years in the specific treatment of acute pancreatitis. (Table 22.5) These modalities are designed to decrease the severity of pancreatic inflammation by inhibition of pancreatic secretion and enzyme activity. They will interrupt the development of complications, support the patient, and treat the complications. Of all these modalities, only the institution of ''nothing by mouth'' (NPO) and intravenous (IV) fluids are universally accepted management techniques of patients with acute pancreatitis. Resumption of oral feedings prior to resolution of pancreatic inflammation is associated with reactiviation of the pancreatitis. Thus, the patient should remain NPO until the complete resolution of abdominal pain, tenderness, fever, and leukocytosis.

In addition to nothing by mouth, IV fluids, and pain control, elderly patients with gallstone pancreatitis or severe pancreatitis should also receive broad spectrum antibiotic coverage. Nasogastric suction is also recommended for patients with persistent vomiting or evidence of ileus. H_2 blockers or antacids should be used in patients at risk for stress ulceration and gastrointestinal hemorrhage. Parenteral nutrition can also pro-

Table 22.5. Proposed Nonoperative Measures for the Treatment of Acute Pancreatitis

Measures to Suppress Pancreatic Secretion or Enzyme Activity	Supportive Measures
Nothing by mouth	Intravenous fluid replacement
Nasogastric suction	Electrolyte replacement
Anticholinergics	Analgesics
Glucagon	Nutritional support
Histamine antagonists	Respiratory support
Aprotinin (Trasylol)	Peritoneal dialysis
	Antibiotics

vide a means of nutritional support in select patients requiring prolonged periods of fasting for pancreatic inflammation.

Finally, peritoneal dialysis may be effective in removing potentially toxic compounds from the peritoneal cavity. Two prospective randomized trials of early institution of peritoneal dialysis, within 24 to 48 hours of hospitalization, appear to show a favorable influence on the early clinical course of acute pancreatitis (24, 26) by reducing the duration of hyperamylasemia, leukocytosis, and hypocalcemia. Peritoneal dialysis does not, however, reduce the incidence of subsequent pancreatic abscess formation, and thus, overall mortality does not appear to be improved with dialysis. Despite this, we continue to advocate early peritoneal lavage in those elderly patients with severe acute pancreatitis. If rapid improvement is not noted or late deterioration is observed, one should consider the presence of associated biliary or pancreatic sepsis. Close monitoring of the patient's metabolic and respiratory status in the intensive care unit is required during peritoneal dialysis. Lavage should be continued for at least 48 hours or longer depending on the status of the patient.

Operative Management

The operative management of acute pancreatitis can be divided into three categories: (1) laparotomy for diagnosis purposes; (2) operation for drainage, debridement, or resection; and (3) operation for biliary tract disease causing pancreatitis.

In the small group of patients in whom diagnosis cannot be made non-operatively, diagnostic laparotomy may be necessary to avoid acute intra-abdominal catastrophes. In addition, even strong non-operative evidence of acute pancreatitis does not exclude the presence of coexistent conditions, such as gangrenous cholecystitis, mesenteric infarction, or other conditions that would require laparotomy. Such coexistent conditions may be a significant problem in elderly patients who may frequently suffer from many abdominal conditions. We feel that early diagnostic laparotomy should not be withheld if the diagnosis remains uncertain. If only mild pancreatitis is found at exploration, there is little evidence that any procedure will ameliorate the patient's course. If gallstones are present in such

cases, definitive biliary tract procedures may be performed. The placement of drains in the pancreatic bed should be avoided because this may lead to an increase in late peripancreatic sepsis. If more severe pancreatitis exists, there seems to be no clear benefit in performing extensive resection or drainage in the absence of necrotic tissue or secondary infection, and thus, with the exception of placement of a peritoneal lavage catheter, no further operative procedures would appear to be indicated.

Operative intervention to drain aggressively or resect pancreatic tissue in patients with severe necrotizing acute pancreatitis has been advocated in those patients with clinical deterioration despite optimal conservative management. Despite this, operative management has been studied in only one randomized controlled trial (19). Ranson and others reported a small controlled trial of early wide sump drainage plus cholecystostomy, gastrostomy, and jejunostomy in patients with "severe" acute pancreatitis. Although no deaths occurred, patients undergoing operative management had a dramatically increased frequency of intra-abdominal sepsis, more severe respiratory complications, and longer ICU stays than patients managed by non-operative means. Moreover, Ranson and Spencer reported in 1978 on five patients who had undergone pancreatic resection for acute pancreatitis, all of whom died (27). In addition, early operation of any type was associated with a 67% hospital mortality compared to 16% in patients managed non-operatively. Thus, it is our conclusion that early operation for drainage, debridement, or resection of pancreatic tissue is not advocated routinely in any group of patients with acute pancreatitis, no matter the extent or severity. Such procedures, however, are indicated in the face of pancreatic sepsis. In these cases, the use of CT scanning provides a valuable technique to determine the extent of pancreatic inflammation, pancreatic phlegmon, or abscess formation.

The management of gallstone pancreatitis is also somewhat controversial. The vast majority of patients with gallstone pancreatitis do well with conservative treatment. When it is assumed that the stone has passed, there is no need for early operation. Acosta and associates challenged this premise by performing a definitive biliary tract procedure within the first 2 days after presentation (28). In this group, a gallstone was found to be impacted in the ampulla of Vater in 70% of the cases. By utilizing this approach, they decreased their hospital mortality from 16% to 2%. Hospital stay was also decreased from 25 days to 13 days. Stone and others have also performed early definitive operation in gallstone-associated pancreatitis (29). In a controlled trial, there was one death in the operated group and no deaths in the non-operative group. The length of initial hospital stay was similar. However, two deaths occurred in 29 patients who underwent subsequent elective biliary tract operations, and an additional 12 days of hospital stay were required. Because of this unexplained high mortality rate for elective biliary procedures, the authors advocate early biliary tract operations. Ranson reviewed the results of early operative treatment of biliary tract disease within 7 days of admission with pancreatitis (30). There were five deaths in 22 patients undergoing operation, but no deaths in 58 patients managed non-operatively. Biliary tract surgical procedures were undertaken later during the same admission in 37 patients with no deaths. Although there is some controversy, the majority of clinicians feel that in patients with gallstone pancreatitis, operative treatment should not be performed until resolution of pancreatic inflammation.

In the past, 4 to 6 weeks of convalescence has been recommended before an elective biliary tract operation is performed. However, it is now clear that cholecystectomy can be performed safely during the initial hospitalization. This eliminates the risk of recurrent pancreatitis during the interval and reduces the overall length of hospital stay. We strongly advocate a definite biliary tract procedure in all elderly patients with gallstone pancreatitis, because the risk of elective cholecystectomy in the elderly is minimal compared to the risk of recurrent pancreatitis.

In elderly patients with severe gallstone pancreatitis, endoscopic sphincterotomy for removal of the impacted stone has become an alternative for management. This is a Sinak procedure. Safrany and Cotton have employed this technique in 11 patients, 5 of whom were 75 years of age or older (18). Successful stone removal was done in all patients, with marked improvement in the clinical course in 10 patients with only one death. The patients who survived all underwent the procedure early in their course. It would appear then that this procedure can be a safe, non-operative means of managing the patient with severe gallstone pancreatitis who has not responded rapidly during the course of acute pancreatitis. We would feel that this provides a valuable alternative to an early biliary tract operation in the elderly patient with gallstone pancreatitis.

Complications of Acute Pancreatitis

Despite optimal management of both simple edematous pancreatitis and hemorrhagic pancreatitis, complications can occur. Elderly patients are not only susceptible to an increased risk of complications, but have a worse prognosis when such complications develop. The older patient, often with a number of pre-existing medical conditions, poorly tolerates the significant hemodynamic, respiratory, or septic complications occurring with severe acute pancreatitis. The lack of essential organ reserve often leads to multisystem failure and death. The initial therapeutic efforts in the management of acute pancreatitis are designed to resuscitate the patient and prevent the catastrophic outcome related to shock. Elderly patients are very sensitive to hypovolemic shock resulting from extensive fluid sequestration and/or pancreatic hemorrhage. Progressive fluid resuscitation and blood transfusion are required at the time of presentation and during the initial few hours. In addition, significant early complications related to metabolic abnormalities can occur. Hyperglycemia should be treated aggressively with insulin administration. Significant hypocalcemia may also occur, and administration of calcium gluconate intravenously may be required to correct this abnormality. Acidosis may occur and should be corrected with bicarbonate administration to avoid cardiovascular dysfunction.

The most serious complications noted in elderly patients with severe pancreatitis are respiratory. Respiratory complications, which occur in 20% to 60% of all patients, occur much more frequently in older patients. Ranson noted such complications in two-thirds of his patients over 55 years of age as opposed to only 20% of younger patients (31). These respiratory complications include left-sided pleural effusions, characterized by an elevated amylase content, due to seepage of pancreatic inflammatory fluid through the diaphragm into the thoracic cavity. Atelectasis and pneumonia may be due to elevation of the diaphragm secondary to abdominal distension, splinting because of abdominal pain, or compression of parenchyma by pleural effusions.

The most serious respiratory complication that occurs is respiratory failure with resulting hypoxemia. In a series of 116 patients, Ranson was able to associate the development of severe respiratory insufficiency with a number of factors, including PaO_2 of less than 66 mm Hg at presentation, age greater than 55 years, amylase of greater than 1000 Somogyi units/100 ml, serum calcium less than 8.5 mg/dl, fluid sequestration of greater than 4.5 liters during the first 48 hours, and early laparotomy (31). Despite the liberal use of intubation and respiratory support, a 25% mortality was noted in this group of patients. The development of pulmonary edema in acute pancreatitis was reviewed by Warshaw, who noted the occurrence of pulmonary edema in the absence of heart failure or fluid overload in 8% of patients (32). The pathogenesis of this severe pulmonary dysfunction is unclear, but most hypotheses suggest that a circulating factor possibly released from the pancreas during the acute attack may play a role.

The management of respiratory complications of early pancreatitis includes recognition and intensive respiratory support. Patients with massive fluid requirements, underlying cardiorespiratory disease, or clinical evidence of early respiratory insufficiency require monitoring of arterial blood gases and pulmonary artery pressures with a Swan-Ganz catheter. Aggressiveness in the monitoring of elderly patients is necessary because of the likelihood of underlying cardiorespiratory diseases. Hypoxemia improves as pancreatitis resolves. If there is progressive respiratory insufficiency or a recent laparotomy has been done, full respiratory support is indicated. Albumin and diuretic therapy have been recommended with monitoring of pulmonary arterial pressure. Using these modalities, Ranson was able to demonstrate diminished need for ventilatory support and hospital mortality (31). The administration of intravenous steroids is not felt to be of any value in preventing pulmonary complications of pancreatitis.

Pancreatic Phlegmon and Abscess

Other life-threatening complications facing patients with acute pancreatitis are development of pancreatic phlegmon and abscess. A phlegmon is pancreatic swelling due to inflammation and edema with localized areas of pancreatic infarction and occurs in up to 30% of cases. A mass may be palpable in 15% to 20% of the patients, but the CT scan is the most sensitive method for detection of a pancreatic phlegmon. The patient may be asymptomatic, but the most likely course is continued pain, low-grade fever, and hyperamylasemia with a mass effect of the pancreatic phlegmon that may cause biliary, gastroduodenal, or colon obstruction. In addition, localized ileus due to inflammation or irritation of adjacent bowel segments is also common. The preferred treatment of a pancreatic phlegmon is the conservative non-operative approach. Liquefaction and possible abscess formation should be monitored by CT scan. Seldom is surgical intervention necessary for obstruction of the biliary tree, duodenum, or colon, because most of these obstructions will resolve as pancreatic inflammation subsides. Parenteral hyperalimentation should be instituted, as the duration of symptoms can often be prolonged to 4 to 6 weeks.

Extensive necrosis of the pancreas and surrounding retroperitoneal fat may occur. This tissue provides an excellent culture medium for invading bacteria and pancreatic abscess formation. Abscess occurs in up to 10% of these patients, and it is influenced by both the etiology and severity of the pancreatitis (33). It is more common in patients with postoperative pancreatitis than in those with alcoholic, biliary, or miscellaneous causes. Pancreatic abscesses develop in 2.7% of patients with fewer than three early prognostic signs, 32% of patients with three to five signs, and 50% in those with more than five prognostic signs. Because age over 55 is included in these prognostic signs, advancing age can be expected to be associated with an increased risk of pancreatic abscess. In addition, because postoperative pancreatitis is a relatively more important cause of pancreatitis in the elderly, the aged are at significant risk for this disastrous complication.

The diagnosis is made by clinical suspicion and is confirmed by CT scanning. Between the first and fourth week following a severe bout of acute

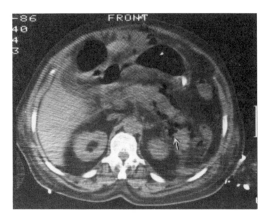

Figure 22.2. CT scan of an 80-year-old man with a pancreatic abscess. The presence of air bubbles *(arrow)* in the inflammatory pancreatic phlegmon is pathognomonic of pancreatic abscess.

pancreatitis, fever, abdominal pain and tenderness, and ileus may develop. On CT scan are seen a fluid collection and the demonstration of gas bubbles in the pancreatic and peripancreatic tissue (Figure 22.2).

Once the diagnosis of pancreatic abscess is made, prompt surgical drainage is necessary, no matter how old the patient because mortality of undrained abscesses is 100%. Broad spectrum antibiotics, including an aminoglycoside, a penicillin-like drug, and anaerobic coverage, should be instituted. There is no role for antibiotics alone. Laparotomy should be performed through a midline or transverse abdominal incision. The lesser sac should be entered, and all necrotic pancreatic and peripancreatic tissue should be debrided by blunt dissection as sharp dissection may lead to debridement of viable tissue and significant hemorrhage. Extensive drainage with Penrose and sump drains is necessary. Recurrent abscess requiring reoperation occurs in approximately 30% of cases. The reported mortality of pancreatic abscess following drainage ranges from 20% to 50%.

Because of this high mortality, some authors have advocated more aggressive debridement and open packing of the lesser sac with multiple antibiotic-soaked gauze pads with the abdomen being left open or else closed loosely. At 24 to 48 hours, the packs are removed, and further blunt dissection is performed, removing all necrotic tissue. The pads tamponade any hemorrhage and debride any necrotic tissue when they are removed. At reexploration, the tissues are more delineated, and further debridement can be performed. Eventually debridement can be done in the intensive care unit with simple analgesia. This technique was developed for both control of hemorrhage that frequently accompanies debridement of pancreatic abscesses, as well as for preventing the complication of recurrent abscess formation. Two recent series using this technique have reported reduced mortality in the range of 9%–15% (34, 35). This technique requires multiple general anesthetics in the elderly and may seem to be extremely risky, but in these reports of several elderly patients, including one who was 91 years old, they have been managed very successfully.

Pancreatic abscesses and phlegmon can lead to significant necrosis of surrounding tissue. Major visceral vessel erosion of the splenic, gastroduodenal, or colic branches of the superior mesenteric artery can occur, resulting in massive hemorrhage into the retroperitoneal space or the GI tract. The management of such bleeding usually requires the identification of the vessel by angiography and embolization for control of hemorrhage. This allows time for operation and further control of bleeding and debridement of necrotic and infected tissues. Thrombosis of a major arterial blood supply to the small intestine or colon in the abscess area may result in bowel necrosis. Bowel necrosis and intestinal fistulization can occur with perforations of the colon, duodenum, stomach, or small intestine. Patients usually present with an enterocutaneous fistula through the wound or from a drain site. Maintaining the patient NPO on parenteral nutrition may allow closure of some fistulas, but reoperation with resection of the damaged bowel will usually be necessary.

Complications of pancreatic abscess remain a significant cause of mortality, and most series continue to report mortality for this complication in the 30% to 50% range. Newer techniques of reoperation and/or open packing, earlier detection using CT scanning, and early aggressive surgical drainage and debridement should improve survival.

PANCREATIC PSEUDOCYSTS

A pancreatic pseudocyst develops when a pancreatic duct disruption occurs and pancreatic secretions leak into and are walled off by the inflammatory adherence of the adjacent structures that contain the pancreatic fluid and the surrounding tissue planes, usually in the lesser sac. The pancreatic pseudocyst will persist and enlarge until the pancreatic ductal disruption seals. The pancreatic secretions will then resorb, and the pseudocyst will collapse and disappear. Peripancratic fluid collections occur acutely in approximately 50% of patients with acute pancreatitis (17). The majority of these probably are not associated with duct disruption, resolve spontaneously, and are not of clinical concern. Pseudocysts occur in only 5%–10% of cases of acute pancreatitis. Most are alcoholic and thus are uncommon in the elderly.

Pseudocysts may be asymptomatic and shown by routine examination of patients with pancreatitis, or they may be detected because of symptoms of persistent pain or amylase elevation after an episode of acute pancreatitis. A palpable abdominal mass, or symptoms from extrinsic compression by the enlarging pancreatic mass may also suggest a pseudocyst. Sonogram and CT scan will demonstrate the cystic nature of the mass, distinguishing it from a pancreatic phlegmon or abscess (Figure 22.3). Contrast studies of the stomach or colon may also demonstrate the presence of a pseudocyst by extrinsic compression of these organs.

If the patient has persistent pain and symptoms, he or she should be maintained on nothing by mouth and parenteral nutrition. The size of the pseudocyst is not a factor and if the patient is pain free, attempts at oral intake may be made.

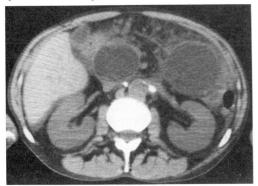

Figure 22.3. CT scan showing two large pancreatic pseudocysts located in the head and body of the pancreas in a 65-year-old man.

If no pain recurs, the patient can be advanced to a regular diet. We recommend a conservative approach unless complications develop. If resolution has not occurred in 2–3 months, surgical drainage is advised. The chance of resolution is small after this time, and the risk of complications is increased. Complications include gastric outlet obstruction, colon obstruction, obstructive jaundice, hemorrhagic complications from erosion into surrounding visceral vessels, or free rupture of the pseudocyst into the peritoneal cavity resulting in pancreatic ascites (36). Pseudocysts may also become secondarily infected, requiring urgent drainage as in a pancreatic abscess.

The surgical management of pancreatic pseudocysts consists of drainage. Young pseudocysts are friable and hold sutures poorly, and a significant risk of anastomotic disruption and subsequent complications exists. After 6 to 8 weeks of observation, the pseudocyst wall is usually mature and fibrous in nature and is optimal for the preferred treatment of internal drainage. Most pancreatic pseudocysts requiring operation at less than 6 weeks duration will require external drainage. The specific form of drainage advised depends upon the location of the pseudocyst with respect to adjacent structures. We prefer internal drainage of most pseudocysts by cystojejunostomy to a Roux-en-Y loop. This allows drainage of the pancreatic fluid into a defunctionalized limb and minimizes the reflux of intestinal contents into the pseuodcyst cavity. Cystogastrostomy should be performed in all situations where the pseudocyst is tightly adherent to the posterior gastric wall. This is carried out by performing an anterior gastrostomy and creating a cystogastrostomy through the posterior gastric wall. Hemostasis must be ensured by continuous hemostatic suture at the anastomosis. Cystoduodenostomy is a tempting route of drainage but should be avoided if at all possible because of the potential development of disastrous complications associated with anastomatic leak. A small pseudocyst located at the tail of the gland can be treated sucessfully by a distal pancreatectomy.

The radiologic drainage of pancreatic pseudocyst using ultrasound or CT guidance has been advocated by some. Our experience with this technique is limited, but it appears that such drainage is associated with a very high rate of early recurrence. In the elderly, however, percutaneous drainage may in some instances be the treatment of choice.

Reported mortality from drainage of pancreatic pseudocysts ranges from 3 to 11%. The incidence of recurrent pseudocysts ranges from 5% to 23% and is usually related to the operative technique employed. Internal drainage is associated with a much lower recurrence rate than is external drainage.

PANCREATIC ASCITES AND PLEURAL EFFUSIONS

Pancreatic ascites and pancreatic pleural effusions are forms of internal pancreatic fistulae representing a communication from the pancreatic duct to the peritoneal or pleural cavity. Both entities involve disruption of the main pancreatic duct with free leakage of pancreatic juice. The surrounding inflammation usually walls off the leak and forms a pseudocyst. In pancreatic ascites or pleural effusions this inflammation does not occur, and the duct communicates with the entire peritoneal or pleural cavity. When the duct disrupts anteriorly, pancreatic ascites may occur. A posterior pancreatic duct disruption allows pancreatic secretions to enter the retroperitoneal space where they most commonly follow the path of the aorta or esophagus into the mediastinum. Here they may again wall off and form a mediastinal pseudocyst. If the mediastinal pleura is penetrated and the secretions enter one or both pleural cavities, the result is an internal pancreatic fistula between the pancreatic duct and the pleural cavity and formation of a pancreatic pleural effusion. These effusions are not to be confused with small self-limiting left-sided pleural effusions that may accompany acute pancreatitis. Such effusions require no therapy.

Pancreatic ascites or pleural effusions occur most commonly in the absence of any clinical history of acute pancreatitis. As with pseudocysts, these disorders occur mainly in young alcoholics and are thus uncommon in the older age groups. Ductal disruption may also follow abdominal or surgical trauma.

Most patients with pancreatic ascites present with few symptoms other than discomfort from abdominal distension. Many are totally asymptomatic. The fluid must be documented as being pancreatic in origin. Thoracentesis or paracentesis will yield fluid with amylase levels in the thousands and albumin elevations in the range of 3 g/dl. The serum amylase is also usually elevated, from reabsorption of amylase from the ascitic fluid into the blood.

The initial treatment is conservative and should consist of efforts to decrease pancreatic secretion, including nothing by mouth, parenteral nutrition, and multiple paracentesis or thoracentesis to decrease the volume of fluid. This regimen should continue for a 2- to 3- week period. In a series reported from the Johns Hopkins Hospital, 17 patients with pancreatic ascites were treated initially by non-operative methods (37). In eight the ascites cleared and the patients were discharged from the hospital. Of seven patients with pancreatic pleural effusions, five were cured by the non-operative regimen. When non-operative therapy is not effective operative management should be carried out, and attempts to visualize the pancreatic duct disruption should be made. Endoscopic retrograde pancreatography (ERCP) should be done to define the area of leak (38). This procedure should be performed within 24 to 36 hours of operation to avoid infection of the ascitic fluid. The use of ERCP to define the area of ductal disruption will eliminate the need for duodenotomy and operative pancreatography. (Figure 22.4) If ERCP is unsuccessful, however, operative pancreatography should be performed. The area of ductal disruption should be drained by a Roux-en-Y jejunal loop.

CHRONIC PANCREATITIS

Acute pancreatitis has been recognized since antiquity, but chronic pancreatitis was not described until the middle of this century. For the purpose of this chapter, we will consider chronic pancreatitis to be a chronic inflammatory disease with some degree of endocrine and exocrine dysfunction and with either chronic unrelenting abdominal pain or recurrent attacks of abdominal pain. Perhaps 5% of all patients with chronic pancreatitis are asymptomatic with the diagnosis made by seeing pancreatic calcifications on x-ray or at laparotomy.

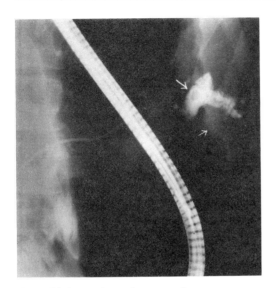

Figure 22.4. Endoscopic retrograde pancreatogram demonstrating a normal proximal duct, a distal duct pseudocyst *(large arrow)*, and extravasation into the free peritoneal cavity *(small arrow)*. (Reprinted from Cameron JL, et al.: Internal pancreatic fistulas: pancreatic ascites and pleural effusions. *Ann Surg* 184:587–593, 1976.)

Incidence and Etiology

Biliary tract disease, which is the commonest etiology for acute pancreatitis in the elderly, rarely progresses to chronic pancreatitis because in most cases, the biliary tract disease is recognized after one or two episodes of acute pancreatitis and proper surgical management can be obtained. Because alcoholism is by far the most common cause of chronic pancreatitis it is often seen in younger patients. Chronic pancreatitis in the alcoholic involves recurrent episodes of acute pancreatitis in which the gland becomes more involved with of inflammatory disease, atrophy, and fibrosis with each subsequent attack. The ductal system will develop segmental areas of fibrosis and stricture. At this point, even if abstinence from alcohol can be obtained, the disease often is progressive. Elderly patients occasionally have a chronic pancreatitis that is idiopathic and may manifest primarily as pancreatic insufficiency and no pain. Changes brought on by aging may account for the symptoms (39, 40).

Presentation and Course

Approximately 5% of patients may be asymp-

tomatic, but the majority of patients with chronic pancreatitis have chronic abdominal or back pain. The elderly patient, however, with idiopathic chronic pancreatitis may have little or no pain. Pain is usually located in the epigastric area with radiation into the back. It may come and go, but it is usually constant. The pain may be aggravated by eating. Some patients have recurring episodes of severe pain that may be associated with fever, nausea, and vomiting. The amylase and leukocyte count may be elevated. This scenario with chronic recurring attacks is most often seen in nonalcoholics whereas the chronic unrelenting pain is frequently seen in alcoholics. Addiction to narcotics frequently develops in the latter group.

Symptoms of exocrine and endocrine insufficiency may be the major component of chronic pancreatitis in the elderly. The diabetes of pancreatitis is very similar to that of adult onset diabetes; however, these patients frequently have a very unusual sensitivity to insulin. Fifteen percent of these patients will become insulin dependent, but the diabetes can usually be controlled easily with small insulin requirements.

Repetitive inflammatory response eventually results in acinar cell atrophy and fibrosis and significant reduction and secretion of amylase, lipase, and preotolytic enzymes in approximately 50% of patients with chronic pancreatitis. Steatorrhea, malabsorption, and weight loss occur in over three-quarters of the patients. These conditions are especially disabling in the elderly, with pancreatic exocrine insufficiency being the second most common cause of steatorrhea in patients over 65.

Diagnosis

Chronic pancreatitis is diagnosed by a history of frequent hospitalizations for alcoholic pancreatitis with the subsequent development of chronic pain. Amylase levels are infrequently elevated or normal. Pancreatic calcification is pathognomonic of chronic pancreatitis. (Figure 22.5) Endocrine insufficiency may be demonstrated. Exocrine insufficiency can be determined by measurement of bicarbonate and enzyme concentrations. A decrease in bicarbonate output in the duodenal aspirate is the most characteristic finding in chronic pancreatitis. Pancreatic insuffi-

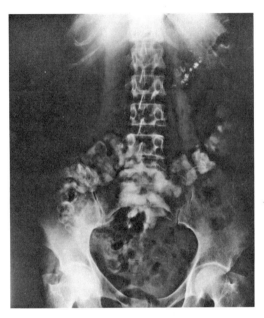

Figure 22.5. Plain abdominal radiograph demonstrating extensive pancreatic calcification in a patient with chronic pancreatitis.

ciency may also be documented by fecal fat collections.

CT scanning and sonograms are useful in the identification of the dilated ducts of the biliary tract and pancreas. Endoscopic retrograde cholangiopancreatography (ERCP) is the most valuable tool for demonstration of pancreatic ductal abnormalities. Dilated ducts, strictures, or the presence of strictures and dilatations (chain of lakes) in the pancreatic ductal system may be seen. (Figure 22.6) ERCP is mandatory for the determination of patients who might benefit from surgical procedures for chronic pancreatitis.

A major point for differentiation in the elderly is between chronic pancreatitis and pancreatic cancer. (Table 22.6) A number of characteristics, such as weight loss, chronic abdominal and back pain, and even jaundice, are shared by both diseases. Radiographic studies showing the presence or absence of calcification, ERCP appearance of the pancreatic and biliary ductal system, arteriography, or CT scan may differentiate a chronic inflamed gland from a mass in the head of the pancreas (41). Pancreatic secretory differences may also be useful (42). Percutaneous needle aspiration for cytology is helpful, but only if carcinoma is seen on cytology. In many cases the diagnosis cannot be made preoperatively, and even at laparotomy, there may be difficulty in distinguishing chronic pancreatitis from pancreatic cancer. An occasional pancreaticoduodenectomy is done for benign disease, or a ductal drainage procedure is done for presumed chronic pancreatitis only to have the patient subsequently develop evidence of metastases.

Management

The medical treatment for chronic pancreati-

Figure 22.6. Endoscopic retrograde cholangiopancreaticogram in patient with chronic pancreatitis demonstrating dilatation of the pancreatic and common bile ducts.

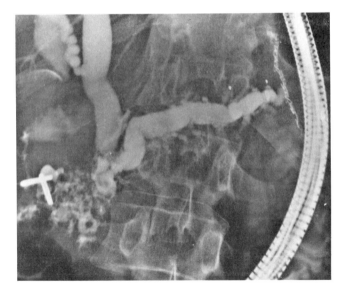

Table 22.6. Differential Diagnosis of Pancreatic Cancer and Chronic Pancreatitis

Assessment Measure	Pancreatic Cancer	Chronic Pancreatitis
History and physical examination	Jaundice, weight loss, older patients, cigarette smoker, palpable gallbladder (Courvoisier's sign), evidence of metastasis	Alcohol abuse, younger patients, frequent attacks of pancreatitis, steatorrhea
Laboratory data	Elevated bilirubin, liver enzymes, decreased serum albumin	Elevated bilirubin, alkaline phosphatase
Plain radiographs	Normal	Pancreatic calcification
ERCP	Ductal cut-off	"Chain of lakes" appearance, secondary and tertiary ducts, calculi, pseudocysts
CT scan/sonogram	Mass in pancreas, biliary ducts, metastasis	Diffuse enlargement, dilated pancreatic duct, pseudocyst
Angiography	Vessel encasement	Normal
Secretory tests	Decreased volume	Decreased volume, bicarbonate, enzymes
Cytology	Malignant cells	Inflammatory cells

tis is directed at the precipitating factors, such as alcohol or drugs, and its complications of pain, diabetes, steatorrhea, and weight loss. Surgical therapy is reserved for persistent jaundice or unrelenting pain. For recurrent pancreatitis, each attack is managed in a similar fashion to acute pancreatitis. In most cases, the episodes are mild, and the patients' hospitalization is only for a short period. Pancreatic diabetes frequently involves only dietary manipulation or possibly use of oral hypoglycemic agents. Insulin is necessary in only a minority of patients and should be avoided in almost all cases where alcohol continues to be a problem. Pancreatic insufficiency and weight loss can usually be well managed with the adminstration of exogenous enzymes (43). Supplements, such as viokase or pancrease, before each meal will decrease steatorrhea and prevent weight loss as the nutritional status improves. Cimetidine has also been used to increase gastric pH and thus increase the delivery of effective enzymes into the duodenum.

The most difficult problem is pain control and is the primary indication for operative management of chronic pancreatitis. If medical therapy can be maintained long enough, the disease will eventually "burn out" and subsequently require no therapy. Operative management of chronic pancreatitis in the elderly is uncommon and does not improve pancreatic insufficiency.

Biliary diversion, ductal decompression, and pancreatic ablation all have a role in managing patients with chronic pancreatitis. Either choledochoduodenostomy or choledochojejunostomy will bypass the obstructed biliary tree and restore bile flow, but play no role in the control of the pain of chronic pancreatitis. Sphincteroplasty may be useful in patients with chronic pancreatitis, but only in those with ampullary stenosis or a proximal single pancreatic ductal stricture.

The treatment for chronic pancreatitis is ductal decompression. ERCP is helpful in determining the form of ductal decompression to be performed. With a dilated ductal system and a single proximal stricture, retrograde drainage with a pancreatectomy and end-to-end pancreaticojejunostomy (Duvall procedure) will provide ductal decompression. If extensive areas of stricturing and dilatations are present throughout the entire gland, the side-to-side pancreaticojejunostomy (Puestow procedure) is indicated (44, 45).

In those patients with a clear ductal abnormality, ductal decompression by either the Duvall or Puestow procedure can provide successful relief of pain in up to 80% of cases (44, 45). Operative mortality is usually less than 2%, and although postoperative complications are frequent, most are well tolerated. The major factor in the failure to achieve pain relief and in latent mortality is continued alcoholism.

Pancreatic ablation may also be used for chronic pancreatitis. In disease involving the distal gland, resection of anywhere from 70% to 95% of the pancreas can be performed. Distal pancreatectomy may be successful in relief of pain in 70% to 90% of cases with an operative mortality of less than 5% (45–47). Such operations, however, are extensive and are mainly indicated for younger patients with disabling pain from pancreatitis. We would recommend only a ductal drainage procedure or distal pancreatectomy (less than 70%) in those rare elderly patients with significant pain from chronic pancreatitis who require operation.

NEOPLASMS OF THE PANCREAS

Cancer of the pancreas is now the fourth leading cause of cancer death in the United States, with almost 25,000 new cases diagnosed each year. It is an extremely lethal disease with an estimated cure rate of less than 1%, it now represents 2% to 3% of all cancers, and it causes 5.5% of cancer deaths.

Age is one of the principal risk factors for pancreatic cancer. The annual incidence in the age of 40 to 44 years is about 2 per 100,000, increasing thereafter to 100 per 100,000 in the age range of 80 to 84 years, an increase of 50-fold (48). Nearly three-fourths of patients with pancreatic cancer are 60 years of age or older. A male-to-female sex ratio of 1.7 to 1 is noted in the overall number, but older patients have a nearly equal sex ratio. Blacks have a higher risk of pancreatic cancer than non-blacks, and it is more common in smokers, diabetics, and in alcoholics. No evidence supports the role of pancreatitis, either

acute or chronic, in predisposing to carcinoma of the pancreas.

Exocrine Pancreatic and Periampullary Carcinoma

Periampullary tumors include tumors of the pancreas, ampulla of Vater, distal bile duct, and duodenum. Carcinoma of the pancreas is by far the most common periampullary tumor; however, there is often difficulty distinguishing many of these forms of tumors even at laparotomy, and most large series group all such tumors together. (See Chapter 21)

Pathology

Adenocarcinoma of the pancreas arises from pancreatic glandular or ductal tissue. The most common location for the tumor is the head, with 65% to 70% of cases located there. (Table 22.7) Tumors in the head of the pancreas average 5 cm in diameter, whereas tumors in the body and the tail average 12 cm. In a large review of over 500 cases from Memorial Hospital in New York, only 14% were limited to the pancreas, with 21% having involvement of regional lymph nodes. Sixty-five percent had advanced local disease with or without dissemination (49). These statistics reflect the late presentation seen in the vast majority of patients with pancreatic cancer. Adenocarcinomas originating from the distal bile duct, ampulla of Vater, or duodenum usually present with obstructive jaundice early in their course, resulting in more localized disease and thus a better chance for cure.

Clinical Presentation

Carcinoma of the pancreas often presents late and in a very insidious manner because of the lack of early diagnosis techniques. Screening techniques are not available, and the symptoms

Table 22.7. Relative Frequency of Periampullary Neoplasms

Location	Percentage
Pancreas	83
Head	70
Body and tail	30
Ampulla of Vater	10
Duodenum	4
Common bile duct	3

of pancreatic cancer are often vague, non-specific, and similar to functional gastrointestinal disorders. For tumors arising in the pancreatic head, jaundice frequently leads to the diagnosis. Lesions in the tail of the pancreas have a more insidious presentation with pain, weight loss, and early satiety or nausea; by the time these symptoms have occurred, the disease is almost always locally invasive and metastatic. The duration of symptoms typically proceeds diagnosis by 3 to 6 months, and survival from the time of diagnosis to the time of death is usually less than 6 months.

Abdominal pain occurs in 89% of patients and is the first symptom in 64%. The pain is most frequently located in the mid epigastrium. Back pain can be the initial symptom in up to 30% of patients. Typically, the pain is a dull, boring ache that becomes progressively worse. The pain may be aggravated by food if associated with some degree of biliary obstruction. Weight loss and anorexia occur in almost all patients.

Seventy-five percent of patients with carcinoma of the head of the pancreas will develop jaundice that is usually progressive, unremitting, and associated with abdominal pain. The popular concept of painless jaundice that is classically ascribed to victims of pancreatic cancer is atypical. In a report of 80 elderly jaundiced patients with a mean age of 75.7 years, malignant obstruction was the most common cause, with pancreatic cancer being the most common neoplasm (50).

Other symptoms, such as a change in bowel habits with either constipation or diarrhea, abdominal bloating, and distension, will add little to the diagnosis and may actually hinder focusing in on the pancreatic cancer as the etiology. Early satiety progressing to gastric outlet obstruction may occur from duodenal involvement by the tumor.

Uncommon presentations may include psychological changes, thromboembolic phenomenon, and the development of new onset diabetes or worsening of pre-existing diabetes. Patients may demonstrate more prominent psychiatric symptoms than with other malignancies. In a preoperative prospective study, psychiatric interviews and psychometric testing in 46 patients with carcinoma of the pancreas were evaluated and compared to a control group of 93 patients with other

GI malignancies (51). Seventy-six percent of the patients with pancreatic cancer had psychiatric symptoms as opposed to only 17% of patients with colonic malignancies. In almost half the patients, the psychiatric symptoms were reported to precede physical symptoms by 1 to 43 months, with a median interval of 6 months.

The association of carcinoma of visceral organs with thrombophlebitis (Trousseau's syndrome) has been recognized for centuries. Pancreatic cancer is one of the most prevalent tumors associated with this phenomenon, but it is also seen with lung, stomach, ovary, uterus and colon cancer. Trousseau's syndrome is a very late manifestation of the disease, but recognition of it is important for suggesting the diagnosis and appropriate treatment.

There appears to be a high proportion of patients who develop clinical diabetes or whose previously well-controlled diabetes changes with pancreatic cancer. There is an increased risk of pancreatic cancer in long-term diabetic patients. Patients with pancreatic cancer may have early diabetes mellitus for a duration of 1 year or less. This new-onset diabetes is likely due to pancreatitis and fibrosis that occur in association with the pancreatic cancer.

The physical findings of pancreatic cancer are jaundice (the most frequent physical finding), weight loss, malnutrition, and hepatomegaly. Palpable gallbladder (Courvoisier's sign) can be found in up to 30% of jaundiced patients with pancreatic cancer. Signs of advanced or metastatic disease are supraclavicular lymphadenopathy (Virchow's node), palpable abdominal mass, and peritoneal seedings in the cul de sac of Douglas (Blumer's shelf).

Diagnosis

There is no screening test available at this time for pancreatic cancer, and often there is usually significant delay in diagnosis. To make the early diagnosis of pancreatic cancer, the physician must have a very high index of suspicion. In a review of 200 patients with established pancreatic cancer, 70% had been investigated in a hospital during the year before the diagnosis was made. Even jaundice was associated with a mean duration of symptoms of 5 weeks prior to diagnosis.

An elevation of serum bilirubin, alkaline phosphatase, and liver enzymes does not distinguish

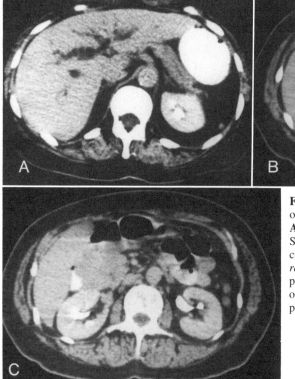
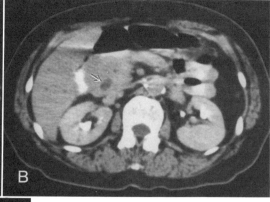

Figure 22.7. CT scan of 73-year-old female with obstructive jaundice due to pancreatic carcinoma. **A,** Scan shows dilated intrahepatic bile ducts. **B,** Scan demonstrates a mass in the head of the pancreas surrounding the dilated common bile duct *(arrow)*. **C,** Scan taken 1 cm inferiorly shows persistence of the pancreatic mass but the absence of the dilated common bile duct, representing complete obstruction of the duct by the tumor.

pancreatic cancer from other forms of obstructive jaundice. Serum albumin and transferrin may be diminished, and there may be other signs of malnutrition. The first investigative tests should be non-invasive imaging techniques of the pancreas and biliary tract. Computed tomography and ultrasonography of the pancreas are the most sensitive and specific for pancreatic disease. The two are complementary, with both tests showing dilatation of the biliary ductal system. Sonography is somewhat better for detection of gallstones, whereas CT scanning is better able to delineate pancreatic masses, pancreatic ductal enlargement, and liver metastases. (Figure 22.7)

If ductal obstruction is determined, more invasive techniques to image the biliary system are indicated. Endoscopic retrograde cholangiopancreatography (ERCP) provides an endoscopic view of the area of the ampulla, as well as visualization of the biliary and pancreatic system in a high percentage of patients. (Figure 22.8) Aspiration of pancreatic and biliary juice for cytologic examination and endoscopic biopsy of any masses present may also be performed.

An associated risk of 2% to 3% incidence of complications, including pancreatitis and cholangitis, are factors to consider.

The alternative to ERCP is percutaneous transhepatic cholangiography (PTC). The classic finding with a pancreatic neoplasm is a tumor meniscus with complete obstruction of the common bile duct at the knee of the biliary tree as it enters the glandular substance of the pancreas. (Figure 22.9) Bile can be aspirated for cytology, as well as brushings taken from the bile duct itself.

Angiography has been used as a tool for preoperative investigation in patients who are deemed to be candidates for major pancreatic resection. Major arterial (hepatic, splenic, superior mesenteric) or venous (portal, superior mesenteric, or splenic) encasement is virtually pathognomonic of unresectability. (Figure 22.10) Knowing the exact anatomy of important vascular structures is useful at the time of resection. Angiography is often a useful technique in avoiding exploration in high-risk patients. However, angiography can be associated with some risks

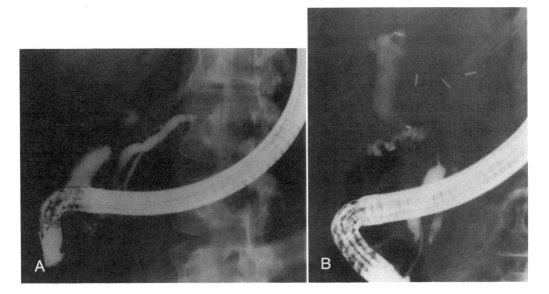

Figure 22.8. **A,** Endoscopic retrograde pancreatogram demonstrating an abrupt tapering of the pancreatic duct and pancreatic body due to pancreatic carcinoma in an 72-year-old female. **B,** ERCP of a 71-year-old female with obstructive jaundice due to pancreatic cancer. The cholangiogram demonstrates a long stricture of the common bile duct just distal to the cystic duct. Dilatation of the proximal bile duct is also seen.

related to catheter placement, with the possibility of vascular complications occurring in those patients with atherosclerotic disease. The contrast media administered during angiography provides an additional risk of renal failure, and intravenous hydration prior to angiography is important in jaundiced patients. It is not our policy to obtain visceral angiography in most patients prior to exploration for pancreatic resection.

Management

A number of important risk factors must be considered in the management of carcinoma of the pancreas. These risk factors include the age and life expectancy of the patient, associated medical condition, extent of the tumor, and the need for palliation of symptoms. Age cannot be an absolute contraindication for surgical management in any patient; yet, it is a factor in predicting surgical morbidity and mortality. For years the operative mortality for pancreaticoduodenectomy for periampullary cancer has been 15% to 25% in all patients. But this rate has fallen significantly in a number of recent series, with mortality rates of 5% or less (52–55). Advanced age, however, continues to be a factor associated with perioperative mortality. Herter et al., noting that

the major morbidity remained constant in all age groups, observed that the operative deaths rose from 7.7% in patients in the 41- to 50-year age group to 25% in patients 61 to 70 years of age (56). Lerut and others also noted a significant increase in mortality, (41% versus 5%, $p <$ .0001) and morbidity (58.8% versus 16.30% p < .001) in patients undergoing pancreaticoduodenal resection over the age of 65 (57). Obertop and others reported a 33% mortality following pancreaticoduodenectomy in patients over 70 compared to 4% in patients younger than 70. In those patients undergoing palliative bypass procedures, there were no deaths in 20 patients under 70 years of age. However, two of nine patients over 70 (22%) died postoperatively (58).

Our experience at the Johns Hopkins Hospital also reflects this trend (55). In the Hopkins series, seven deaths occurred in 29 patients who were 65 years of age or older compared to only three deaths in 59 patients under 65. Complications also occurred more frequently in the older patients, including delayed gastric emptying, abscess and sepsis, and upper GI bleeding.

The extent of operation necessary for resection or palliation of carcinoma of the pancreas often mitigates against surgical therapy in elderly

Figure 22.9. Percutaneous transhepatic cholangiogram demonstrating obstruction of the common bile duct due to pancreatic cancer in a 76-year-old woman. The area of obstruction is at the "knee" of the common bile duct where it enters the glandular substance of the pancreas.

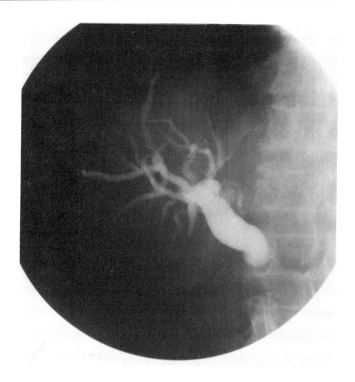

patients. The operation is frequently greater than 6 hours in length and is often associated with significant loss of extracellular fluid and blood. Postoperative respiratory support is frequently indicated. Metabolic derangements, GI bleeding, and infectious complications provide additional stress to patients undergoing either resection or palliative procedures. Patients with borderline cardiac, pulmonary, or renal function frequently do not tolerate such procedures and their associated complications. Alcoholism also appears to worsen the chances of survival following a

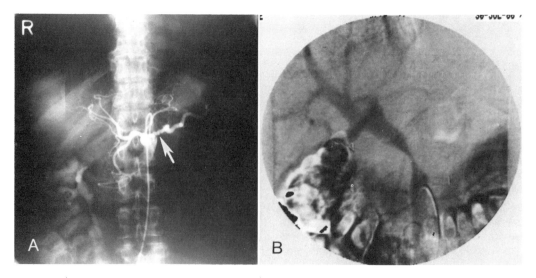

Figure 22.10. **A,** Selective arteriogram of celiac artery demonstrating encasement of splenic artery *(arrow)* in a 72-year-old female with pancreatic carcinoma. **B,** Venous phase of selective superior mesenteric arteriogram demonstrating encasement and narrowing of portal vein at the junction of the superior mesenteric vein.

pancreatic operation.

Preoperative findings can be valuable in determining resectability in these patients. The size of tumor on CT scan or ultrasound, local invasion into surrounding tissues, or lymph node involvement often predicts unresectability. Liver metastasis or ascites can also be detected using similar techniques. Visceral arteriography may be useful for determining whether invasion of major vascular structures has occurred. With these findings, the patients should be considered unresectable, and laparotomy should be avoided to decrease the patient's length of hospital stay and potential for morbidity and mortality.

Decompression of the biliary tree is important in palliative management of the jaundiced patient with pancreatic cancer. Pruritis, cholangitis, liver failure, and coagulopathy may be present. Decompression can be provided either by operative means or non-operatively. Surgical decompression of the biliary tree can be provided by a cholecystojejunostomy or hepaticojejunostomy. Using the gallbladder is the procedure of choice when the cystic duct is widely patent and enters the common bile duct a good distance away from the tumor mass. When the tumor is infringing on the cystic duct, its use may result in early recurrence of biliary obstruction. The common hepatic duct should then be used to form a hepaticojejunostomy. A loop of jejunum may be brought up in an antecolic fashion or as a Roux-en-Y jejunal limb. If a loop jejunostomy is used, an enteroenterostomy below the biliary-enteric anastomosis is useful in avoiding reflux of food into the biliary tree.

Palliative biliary procedures offer significant risks. In a collected review by Sarr and Cameron of over 8,000 cases from the English literature between 1965 and 1980, biliary bypass alone was associated with an operative mortality of 19% (59). No significant difference was noted between the common duct and the gallbladder when each was used for bypass. Mean survival in those patients undergoing biliary bypass was 5.4 months. Recurrent jaundice developed in 8% of patients who had a cholecystojejunostomy and in no patients undergoing hepaticojejunostomy. Great care must be taken in selecting those patients in whom the gallbladder will be used for bypass.

Because of this mortality risk, non-operative

drainage techniques have been advocated. These techniques can be successful in up to 95% of cases (60, 61). External drainage catheters have poor patient acceptance; however, newer endoprostheses that allow internal drainage are now available. Such prostheses can be placed either via the percutaneous route or endoscopically. They may become obstructed from sludge or further tumor growth and require periodic changing. They are advocated primarily for the elderly, poor-risk patients, or those with extensive tumor burdens.

Recently, Malangoni et al. compared the results of operative biliary decompression with percutaneous decompression for malignant biliary obstruction (62). Hospital mortality was 25% for those having percutaneous drainage and 17% for those drained operatively. Advanced age was associated with a significant increase in mortality following either procedure; it was 39% in all patients over 70. The long-term survival was 14 months following operation compared to 5 months after percutaneous drainage. Such comparisons may not be fair because of the more advanced state of disease in those patients managed non-operatively. It is clear that all palliative procedures can have significant morbidity and mortality, especially in the elderly.

Complete duodenal obstruction occurs in only 5% of cases, duodenal involvement can be demonstrated in 40% to 60% of patients, and obstructive symptoms (nausea, early satiety, and vomiting) can occur in up to 30% of patients. Mechanical obstruction or delayed gastric emptying can be relieved by gastrojejunostomy, which is suggested for all patients undergoing laparotomy with evidence of duodenal involvement. Sarr and Cameron found that 16% of patients who had biliary bypass without gastrojejunostomy later developed significant gastric outlet obstruction requiring reoperation prior to their death (63). Another 10% to 20% of patients had symptoms of gastric outlet obstruction, but were not reoperated on. Palliative gastrojejunostomy was not associated with any increase in operative mortality. Stomal ulceration occurred in only 3 of 100 patients in another review by Sarr (64). To protect against this complication a truncal vagotomy can be added in the good-risk patient. If not, H_2 blocking agents may be used for the remainder of his or her life. We recommend that a gastrojejunostomy be performed in all cases of unresectable pancreatic cancer. This is to prevent the occurrence of gastric outlet obstruction late in the course of the illness.

Pain is the last feature of pancreatic cancer that frequently requires palliation. Epigastric and back pain, which often are the most incapacitating and disabling symptoms, occur in up to 90% of patients some time during the course of their disease. Most of the pain is visceral pain due to tumor invasion of retroperitoneal autonomic nerves. Sphanchnicectomy by celiac axis injection with 50% alcohol or 6% phenol at the time of laparotomy for pancreatic cancer, as Flanigan and Kraft have demonstrated, is successful for pain relief in 88% of patients for a mean duration of 4.3 months (65). This technique is useful for palliation in patients undergoing laparotomy, but in those not undergoing laparotomy, similar short-term relief may be obtained via percutaneous injection of the celiac ganglia.

Preparation for Operation

To proceed with an operation for periampullary cancer requires proper preparation. The assessment of cardiopulmonary status, renal and hepatic function, and the state of hydration, nutrition, anemia, and coagulation abnormalities is necessary. Fluid administration is necessary to ensure adequate hydration when preoperative biliary decompression is used. Bile drainage needs to be replaced intravenously to correct potential fluid and electrolyte abnormalities. Hydration is especially important in the jaundiced patient who is at a significant risk for the development of renal failure. Adequate hydration is also very important to prevent renal injury during the use of intravenous contrast agents at the time of CT scanning or angiography. Some degree of malnutrition is present in almost all these patients, and parenteral hyperalimentation to correct these nutritional deficits is needed preoperatively. This is especially important in patients whose evaluation or bowel preparation has required significantly reduced oral intake in the days prior to operation.

Anemia should be corrected in anticipation of blood loss during pancreaticoduodenectomy. Carcinoma of the ampulla or duodenum is frequently associated with low grade GI bleeding and anemia. Prolongation of prothrombin time may occur in jaundiced patients with pancreatic cancer. Daily injection of vitamin K (IM) for several days prior to operation is indicated in all jaundiced patients whether the prothrombin time is abnormal or not. Fresh frozen plasma may also be necessary prior to such invasive procedures as PTC or ERCP to prevent hemorrhagic complications.

An issue of question today is the value of preoperative biliary decompression. Whipple, at the time of his initial pancreaticoduodenectomy for periampullary carcinoma, performed a staged procedure in which biliary drainage was initially performed via cholecystogastrostomy. He then returned the patient to the operating room several weeks later and performed the pancreatic resection. It was his opinion that biliary decompression allowed improvement in liver function and thus a safer operation. Percutaneous transhepatic drainage provides a non-operative method for biliary decompression. Initially, uncontrolled studies showed a benefit for such drainage in decreasing operative morbidity and mortality (66–68). Therefore, biliary decompression was once recommended for all jaundiced patients undergoing operation. Subsequently, prospective controlled studies have been carried out (69, 70). The largest of these studies in the United States came from Pitt and others at UCLA (71). No benefit was found in terms of morbidity and mortality from prolonged percutaneous biliary decompression in patients undergoing operation for obstructive jaundice. The length of hospital stay and hospital cost were significantly increased. In both benign and malignant obstruction, there was no difference in the results based on the nature of obstruction, advanced age, level of bilirubin, or other potential risk factors. Other prospective studies agree, and thus we can conclude that preoperative biliary decompression is not necessary in all patients undergoing operation for obstructive jaundice. We do advocate its use, however, in selected patients who are in need of prolonged parenteral hyperalimentation, have biliary sepsis, or require treatment of an intercurrent illness preoperatively.

Biliary sepsis is uncommon with malignant biliary obstruction. However, PTC and drainage invariably result in bacterial contamination and the risk of biliary sepsis. Antibiotic coverage is indicated prior to any biliary catheter manipulations, and we recommend broad spectrum antibiotic coverage prophylactically for all operations for pancreatic cancer. Finally, all of these patients should receive a mechanical as well as an oral antibiotic bowel preparation preoperatively.

Curative Resection of Pancreatic Cancer

Operative objectives for periampullary carcinoma include diagnosis and determination of resectability. Clinical diagnosis of periampullary carcinoma is based upon radiographic findings and the findings at operation. In a minority of cases, a histologic diagnosis based on cytology is available preoperatively. The surgeons's clinical judgement usually allows him or her to proceed without the necessity of a histologic diagnosis. In cases where histologic diagnosis is felt to be necessary, intraoperative biopsy with frozen section may be performed. The standard technique for intraoperative biopsy of a pancreatic mass employs a true-cut needle inserted through the intact duodenum into the suspicious area. In other cases, a direct biopsy through the pancreatic capsule is preferable.

In determining resectability of periampullary tumor, the surgeon will develop his or her own technique, which is thorough and meticulous yet not time consuming. Time can be wasted in determining resectability. In general, tumor involvement anywhere outside the area encompassed by en bloc resection of the pancreas precludes proceeding with resection. After inspecting for liver, peritoneal, and omental implants, a number of maneuvers are necessary to determine resectability. First, the duodenum and pancreas should be mobilized by a wide Kocher maneuver to determine if the mass is free of the inferior vena cava, aorta, and the superior mesenteric artery. Next, the superior mesenteric vein in the lesser sac should be found to be free of tumor. The hilum of the liver should be dissected to determine if an adequate margin can be obtained on the common bile duct and that the portal vein is free of tumor. Lymph nodes in the area of the liver hilum, as well as along the celiac axis, should be inspected and a biopsy performed if they are suspicious. Finally, the surgeon's finger should be passed along the superior mesenteric vein from below to the portal vein

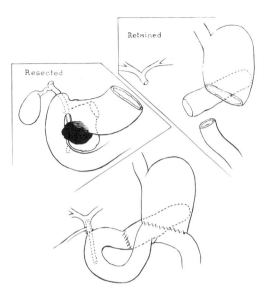

Figure 22.11. Standard pancreaticoduodenectomy. *Top left*, structures resected, including distal stomach, entire duodenum, head and neck of pancreas with tumor, gallbladder, and distal extrahepatic biliary tree. *Top right*, structures retained, including proximal stomach, body and tail of the pancreas, proximal biliary tree, and jejunum distal to the ligament of Trietz. *Bottom*, reconstruction: proximal pancreaticojejunostomy, hepaticojejunostomy over T-tube, and distal gastrojejunostomy.

above to determine that these vessels are not involved by tumor.

If no spread of the tumor is found, resection may be performed. The standard operation for periampullary carcinoma is a pancreaticoduodenectomy or the Whipple procedure (Figure 22.11), which entails resection of the duodenum, the head and neck of the pancreas, the distal common bile duct, gallbladder, and the distal 50% to 60% of the stomach. A modification of pancreaticoduodenectomy with pylorus preservation has been popularized by Traverso and Longmire (72) and Braasch and others (52). The entire stomach and pylorus and approximately 1 to 2 cm of duodenum are spared, avoiding gastric resection and postoperative problems, such as the dumping syndrome or stomal ulceration. This modification lessens the area of lymph node resection along the lesser curvature of the stomach. Many surgeons reserve this operation for tumors of ampullary, distal bile duct, or duodenal origin and for pancreatic resections for benign disease.

Following resection, the pancreatic remnant is usually anastomosed in an end-to-end fashion with the jejunum. The biliary anastomosis is performed end-to-side with the jejunum. This anastomosis may be stented with either the indwelling percutaneous biliary stent or a T-tube. The gastrojejunostomy (or duodenojejunostomy in a pylorus-preserving resection) is performed 18 inches distally. The editors recommend a truncal vagotomy (with Whipple procedure).

Postoperative Care and Complications

Adequate fluid and electrolyte maintenance, as well as glucose regulation, pulmonary care, nutritional support, and provision of antibiotics, is routine. We perform biliary tract contrast examination at about postoperative day 5 to demonstrate the biliary anastomosis. Gastrograffin upper GI series may follow, and if all studies are satisfactory, drains from the area of the biliary and pancreatic anastomosis may be removed and oral intake initiated slowly, watching for potential delays in gastric emptying. Antibiotics can be discontinued after cholangiography unless biliary tract infection exists.

Intra-abdominal hemorrhage is the most common early postoperative complication. Hemostasis should be meticulous during the entire operation. Adequate replacement of blood and coagulation factors during the procedure is essential. Reoperation is essential for ongoing postoperative bleeding or with indication that a collection of blood exists, as it may represent a potential site of sepsis.

Leakage at the pancreaticojejunostomy is a common complication that has been particularly disastrous in the past. Currently, however, with adequate drainage, antibiotics, and total parenteral nutrition, it is usually associated with a favorable outcome. Leakage is less likely to occur at either the biliary or gastric anastomosis. Sepsis, due to anastomotic leak or abscess, and postoperative pancreatitis are additional complications that may cause major postoperative problems. Other complications include upper GI hemorrhage from either stress ulceration or anastomotic ulceration, cholangitis, wound infection, delayed gastric emptying, or pneumonia.

In general, there have been improvements in the management of these complications, result-

Table 22.8. Operative Results and Long Term Survival Following Whipple Procedure

Series	Operative Mortality %	Operative Morbidity %	Actuarial 5-Year Survival %
Braasch[a] (52)	2	50	18
van Heerden (53)	4	33	4
Grace[a] (54)	4	32	3
Cameron (55)	2	36	18

[a]Operative morbidity and mortality represent operations for both benign and malignant disease.

ing in recent reports of reduced operative mortality. The elderly patient, however, frequently lacks the reserve to handle such complications, and failure to avoid these complications may be disastrous with ensuing multisystem organ failure and eventual death.

Results of Operation

For many years, operative mortality for pancreaticoduodenectomy from major centers has been 10% to 25%. Morbidity was often reported in the range of 50% to 60% of cases. Recent reports have shown significant improvement, with a number of reports showing mortality rates of less than 5% and morbidity of 20% to 30% (52–55). (Table 22.8) The reason for this improvement may be better patient selection, but probably represents the concentration of more patients in the hands of surgeons in major centers with extensive experience with the procedure.

The results of resection for pancreatic cancer remain dismal, with only 10% to 20% of patients in most series being resectable for cure and the percentage even lower nationwide. The resectability rate for ampullary, distal bile duct, and duodenal carcinoma is higher. The 5-year survival after resection for pancreatic cancer remains poor, with most series showing 5-year survival of less than 10% with a mean survival in the range of 12 months. Ampullary, distal bile duct, and duodenal carcinoma appear to be associated with a better 5-year survival, with reports of 5-year survivals of 40% to 60%. (See Chapter 21)

Cancer of the Body and Tail of the Pancreas

Survival for carcinoma of the body and tail of the pancreas is even more dismal than that for those of the pancreatic head. It is the silent, asymptomatic nature of tumors in this area that leads to their late presentation, usually long past consideration for resection. The diagnosis of such tumors can frequently be made by percutaneous techniques, thereby avoiding the need for operation. Although such masses on rare occasion may represent lymphomas or islet cell tumors with a somewhat better prognosis, the morbidity and operative mortality from simple exploratory laparotomy in the elderly patients with large pancreatic masses often preclude abdominal exploration. The occasional need for palliation in these cases usually involves the performance of gastrojejunostomy because of obstruction at the duodenal-jejunal junction.

Role of Chemotherapy in Radiation Therapy for Pancreatic Therapy

Because of the dismal results of resection in patients with pancreatic carcinoma, much attention has turned to chemotherapy or radiation therapy as both a primary treatment or in the treatment of recurrences. Unfortunately, the large tumor burden present at the time of diagnosis frequently hinders the response to chemotherapy. Single-agent chemotherapy has been studied extensively, with the best response rates noted with 5-flurouracil treatment in young patients, usually with lesions confined to the body of the pancreas. Current investigations are centering on the role of combination chemotherapy, and although various combination of agents have been employed, little enthusiasm can be gained from any of the results. This is especially true in elderly patients in whom performance status frequently will not allow vigorous chemotherapeutic regimens.

The effectiveness of radiation therapy for pancreatic carcinoma has been limited by the dose that can be tolerated by surrounding vulnerable structures, such as the kidneys, intestines, and spinal cord. Newer radiotherapeutic techniques have improved our ability to deliver radiation at more suitable doses with less morbidity. Median survivals, however, remain in the range of 10 to 12 months with significant morbidity associated with treatment. Intraoperative techniques of radiation therapy done at laparotomy, with adjacent tissues displaced and shielded from the radiation field so that the radiation can be directed directly at the tumor, are being evaluated. A similar form of local radiation involves the implantation of interstitial radioactive seeds. These techniques are frequently associated with a very high morbidity and mortality as laparotomy in this poor-risk group is still required. A combined approach using adjuvant chemotherapy or radiation after pancreaticoduodenectomy may prove useful in improving long-term survival in this group of patients.

Cystadenoma and Cystadenocarcinoma

Cystic lesions of the pancreas are a common finding with the increased use of computed tomography and ultrasonography. The majority of cysts are inflammatory pseudocysts. True cysts are classified as either congenital, retention, or proliferative. Cystadenoma (non-malignant) and cystadenocarcinoma (malignant) are examples of the proliferative form. Cystadenomas represent about 10% of non-malignant cystic lesions of the pancreas, and cystadenocarcinomas represent about 1% of the primary pancreatic malignant lesions. Cystadenoma appears primarily in middle-aged women. However reports of patients in their seventies and eighties have appeared. Cystadenocarcinoma occurs at about the same age as pancreatic exocrine malignancies, between 50 and 70 years of age. There is no sex predilection in this group.

The symptoms of cystadenoma and cystadenocarcinoma are virtually identical. Patients usually present with abdominal pain, weight loss, nausea, vomiting, anorexia, weakness, or an enlarging abdominal mass. Jaundice has been reported to occur in up to 28% of cystadenocarcinomas, but only 6% of cystadenomas (73, 74). Both can be found throughout the entire gland. However, cystadenomas are more frequent in the tail of the pancreas, whereas cystadenocarcinomas occur more frequently in the head.

The management of these lesions is surgical excision. Complete excision of the lesion for pathologic examination is important because needle biopsy is not suitable for detecting malignant potential. Cystadenocarcinomas occur half as frequently as do cystadenomas. The prognosis for cystadenomas is excellent. For cystadenocarcinoma, total excision is necessary to avoid recurrence and possible metastasis. In a series of 21 patients with cystadenocarcinoma from the Mayo Clinic, total excision was associated with a 68% 5-year survival versus only 14% for unresectable lesions (74).

Endocrine Tumors of the Pancreas

Tumors of the endocrine pancreatic islet cells are relatively rare, making up only 10% of pancreatic neoplasms (Table 22.9). They are of great interest, however, because of the unique clinical syndromes associated with the effects of the GI hormones that they produce. The pancreatic islet cells originate from the neural crest and share a common biochemical and ultrastructural feature related to polypeptide and amine synthesis. These features have lead to their classification as APUD cells (amine precursor uptake and decarboxylation). Similar cells have been identified in the pituitary, adrenal gland, and small intestine, which accounts for the association of islet cell tumors with tumors of other neural endocrine organs in the multiple endocrine neoplasia (MEN) syndromes. Although islet cell tumors are uncommon in older age groups, their occurrence has been reported and will thus be mentioned in this chapter.

Insulinomas

Insulinoma, a tumor of the pancreatic beta cells, was the first recognized and is the most common endocrine tumor of the pancreas. Insulinomas can occur in all age groups, but the age of presentation is usually in the range of 20 to 75 years, with a mean age in the mid-forties. In two large series, 25% to 33% of patients were over 60 years of age (75, 76). About 60% of cases are in females. These tumors produce insulin autonomously and thus produce symptomatic hypoglycemia with secondary symptoms related to a hypoglycemia-induced surge of catecholamines. These symptoms include tremor, restlessness, irritability, weakness, diaphoresis, and palpitations. Progressive and prolonged hypoglycemic attacks may lead to neu-

ropsychiatric symptoms that may be particularly confusing and hard to diagnose when seen in the elderly.

The diagnosis of insulinoma depends on documentation of fasting hypoglycemia and inappropriately elevated insulin levels. The classic triad of symptoms of insulinoma was described by Whipple in 1935. These include symptoms of hypoglycemia with fasting, blood sugar level of less than 50 mg/100 ml, and relief of symptoms with glucose administration. The addition of radioimmunoassay for insulin confirms the diagnosis by documenting an insulin level greater than 25 uu/ml. The measurement of concomitant serum levels of connecting peptide (C-peptide), which is released by the beta cell on a one-to-one basis with endogenous insulin, is valuable to rule out surreptitious insulin administration.

Preoperative localization of an insulinoma can now be done in the vast majority of cases. CT scan and ultrasonography frequently are not helpful because of the small size of the tumors, often less than 2 cm. Arteriography appears to be the most commonly available test for detection of insulinomas, identifying the tumor in between 80% to 90% of cases. (Figure 22.12) Selective pancreatic vein sampling for insulin can be successful in almost all patients when other techniques have failed.

Eighty percent of insulinomas are benign and single, with 10% benign and multiple. Ten percent of insulinomas are malignant. The presence of multiple insulinomas suggests a possible MEN syndrome. Ninety-eight percent of insulinomas are found in the pancreas, and the 2% ectopic insulinomas are located in a peripancreatic or periduodenal sites.

The treatment of insulinoma is surgical. At operation, if the tumor is identified and found to be located superficially, it can usually be enucleated without damage to the underlying duct. If the tumor is embedded in the tail or body, a distal pancreatectomy should be performed. In the rare case when the lesion is embedded in the head of the pancreas, pancreaticoduodenectomy may be indicated. It is extremely difficult on histologic examination to determine whether an insulinoma is malignant or benign, and thus, the diagnosis of malignancy usually depends on the

Table 22.9. Endocrine Tumors of the Pancreas

Tumor	Islet Cell Type	Major Hormone	Clinical Syndrome	Associated MEN Syndrome	Malignancy %
Insulinoma	Beta cell	Insulin	Hypoglycemia	MEN I—10	10
Gastrinoma	Non-beta cell	Gastrin	Peptic ulcer, diarrhea	MEN I—25	75
VIPoma	Non-beta cell	Vasoactive intestinal peptide	Watery diarrhea, hypokalemia, achlorhydria	MEN I—rare	50
Glucagonoma	Alpha-cell	Glucagon	Diabetes, skin manifestations	MEN I—rare	60
Somatostatinoma	Delta-cell	Somatostatin	Gallstones, diabetes	MEN I—rare	100

demonstration of metastasis. If metastasis is present, efforts should be made to debulk as much of the tumor as possible.

The results of surgical therapy for insulinoma are excellent, with complete cure after resection in 70% to 80% of cases. Ten percent of these patients will develop diabetes postresection no matter how much pancreas was removed. About 10% to 15% of patients have persistent or recurrent hypoglycemia. In those cases of malignant insulinoma, debulking procedures can provide significant palliation in 60% to 70% of cases. In a large series from the Mayo Clinic, operative mortality was reported as 0% for operations for insulinoma over the last 23 years (77).

In those patients with persistent hypoglycemia, drug therapy with diazoxide may be useful. Diazoxide suppresses insulin release and is successful in up to 60% of patients. Other suggested agents include phenytoin (Dilantin), calcium channel blockers, DL-propranolol, and, more recently, somatostatin analogues. Streptozotocin is a chemotherapeutic agent useful for malignant insulinomas that is used either alone or in combination with 5-fluorouracil with good response in up to 60% of patients.

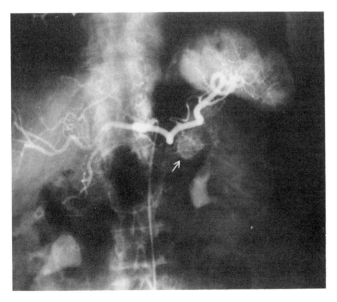

Figure 22.12. Selective arteriogram of the celiac artery in an 80-year-old female with an insulinoma. The *arrow* demonstrates the hypervascular well-circumscribed tumor in the inferior aspect of the pancreas.

Gastrinoma

The Zollinger-Ellison syndrome of gastric hypersecretion with virulent peptic ulcer disease and hypergastrinemia caused by non-B islet cell tumor has been recognized since the mid-1950s. As in other pancreatic endocrine tumors, the discovery of the causative peptide, gastrin, and the development of its radioimmunoassay have enabled us to improve our understanding of the disease and its diagnosis and management. Gastrinomas are now recognized to occur both in a sporadic form (75%) or as a component of MEN I syndrome. In contrast to insulinomas, the majority (60%) of gastrinomas are malignant with metastasis in up to 50% of these.

Gastrinomas account for only .1% of all peptic ulcer disease in the United States and for 2% of recurrent peptic ulcers following standard ulcer operations. Gastrinomas have been reported in all age groups, but as in other pancreatic endocrine tumors, the usual age of presentation is in the 40- to 50-year age group. Almost every series, however, includes patients over age 70. There is no sex or racial predilection.

The clinical presentation for most patients with Zollinger-Ellison syndrome (70% to 95%) is abdominal pain related to peptic ulcer disease. Approximately 20% of the patients have diarrhea as an initial symptom either with or without ulcer disease. Another 30% develop diarrhea later during their course. Because the incidence of severe peptic ulcer disease has decreased markedly in this country, consideration of gastrinoma should be given in all cases with severe complications or intractablity to the usual medical management.

The diagnosis of the Zollinger-Ellison syndrome is based on gastric analysis with a basal acid output of greater than 15 mEq per hour. Such levels of acid secretion would be uncommon in elderly patients. Because acid secretion is at a near maximally stimulated state, the pentagastrin-stimulated acid secretion is not much higher than the basal level. A ratio of basal to stimulated gastric acid secretion of 0.6 or greater suggests gastrionoma. The mainstay of the diagnosis of gastrinoma is the serum gastrin level. Most patients with gastrinoma have basal gastrin levels greater than 500 pg/ml with normals or those patients with peptic ulcer disease usually having levels less than 100 pg/ml. Intermediate levels may require stimulation testing with either secretin or calcium, which will show elevation in patients with gastrinoma but not in normal patients or those with peptic ulcer disease, antral hyperplasia, or retained antrum.

The initial management of patients with Zollinger-Ellison syndrome consists of control of acid secretion by histamine receptor antagonists. All patients should then undergo evaluation for localization of the gastrinoma using CT scan, selective arteriography, and selective venous sampling. In those good-risk patients, including the elderly with localized disease, surgical exploration and attempted resection are warranted. This is possible in 20% to 30% of patients, with most resectable lesions being in the duodenum or other sites, but not the pancreas. The management of those patients who preoperatively are found to have extensive disease or at operation are found to have unresectable tumors consists of control of acid secretion with H_2 receptor antagonists. This treatment is based on rigid control of acid secretion as determined by measurement of gastric acid output. It appears that nearly all patients can be controlled by this means, and failures are related to inadequate dosing. Surgical therapy for gastric hypersecretion should be left only for those patients with complications or who are failures of medical management. In those patients who are explored for gastrinoma and found to be unresectable, a parietal cell vagotomy should be performed to lessen the H_2 blocker requirements. At the present time, we do not advocate more radical resection of these tumors, nor would we recommend exploration for patients of significant operative risk because this tumor, although malignant, remains a slow-growing tumor with 5- and 10-year survivals of 42% and 30%, respectively, even without surgery. Failures of non-operative treatment remain candidates for total gastrectomy.

Other Pancreatic Endocrine Tumors

A number of other pancreatic endocrine tumors have been recognized. Such tumors are not only rare with less than 100 reported cases of each, but also reports of such tumors in elderly patients are quite uncommon. Most patients are in the 45- to 50-year age group. These tumors include (1) glucagonoma, known for its characteristic dermatologic manifestations and mild diabetes; (2) VIPoma, of the syndrome of watery diarrhea, hypokalemia, and achlorhydria (WDHA) described by Verner and Morrison; and (3) the rare somatostatinoma, which has been found in patients with gallstones and diabetes. In addition, nonfunctioning islet cell tumors occur. The majority of all of the tumors are malignant and frequently unresectable for cure. Aggressive surgical debulking is indicated in most cases, however, in hopes of decreasing the symptoms of the hormones produced by the tumors.

REFERENCES

1. Kreel L, Sandin B: Changes in pancreatic morphology associated with aging. *Gut* 14:962–970, 1973.
2. Rossle O: Beitrage zur Kentniss der gesunden und der kranken bauchspeicheldruse. *Beitraege zur pathologischen Anatomie und zur allgemeinen Pathologie* 163:69–79, 1921.
3. Andrew W: Senile changes in the pancreas of Wistar Institute rats and of man with special regard to the similarity of locule and cavity formation. *Am J Anat* 74:97–127, 1944.
4. Rosenberg IR, Friedland N, Janowitz HD, Dreiling DA: The effect of age and sex upon human pancreatic secretion of fluid and bicarbonate. *Gastroenterology* 50:191–194, 1966.
5. Bartos V, Groh J: The effect of repeated stimulation of the pancreas on the pancreatic secretion in young and aged man. *Geront Clin* 11:56–62, 1969.
6. Langier R, Sarles H: The pancreas. *Clin Gastroenterol* 14:749–756, 1985.
7. Chen M, Bergman RN, Pacini G, Porte D: Pathogenesis of age-related glucose intolerance in man: insulin resistance and decreased B-cell function. *J Clin Endocrinol Metab* 60:13–20, 1985.
8. Park J, Fromkes J, and Cooperman M: Acute pancreatitis in elderly patients. *Am J Surg* 152:638–642, 1986.
9. Warshaw AL, O'Hara PJ: Susceptibility of the pancreas to ischemic injury in shock. *Ann Surg* 188:197–201, 1978.
10. Feiner H: Pancreatitis after cardiac surgery. *Am J Surg* 131:684–688, 1976.
11. Mallory A, Kern F: Drug-induced pancreatitis: a critical review. *Gastroenterology* 78:813–820, 1980.
12. Gambill EE: Pancreatitis associated with pancreatic carcinoma: a study of 26 cases. *Mayo Clin Proc* 46:174–177, 1971.
13. Cooperman M, Ferrara JJ, Carey LC, Thomas FB, Martin EW, Fromkes JJ: Idiopathic acute pancreatitis: the

value of endoscopic retrograde cholangiopancreatography. *Surgery* 90:666–670, 1981.
14. Weaver DW, Bouwman DL, Walt AJ, Clink D, Resto A, Stephany J: A correlation between clinical pancreatitis and isoenzyme patterns of amylase. *Surgery* 92:576–580, 1982.
15. Hill MC, Barkin J, Isikoff MB, Silverstein W, Kalser M: Acute pancreatitis: clinical vs. CT findings. *AJR* 139:263–269, 1982.
16. Ranson JHC, Balthazar E, Cacarale R, Cooper M: Computerized tomography and prediction of pancreatic abscess in acute pancreatitis. *Ann Surg* 201:656–663, 1985.
17. Siegelman SS, Copeland BE, Sabe GP, Cameron JL, Sanders RC, Zerhouni EA: CT of fluid collections associated with pancreatitis. *AJR* 134:1121–1132, 1980.
18. Safrany L, Cotton PB: A preliminary report: urgent duodenoscopic sphincterotomy for acute gallstone pancreatitis. *Surgery* 89:424–428, 1981.
19. Ranson JHC, Rifkind KM, Roses DF, Fink SD, Eng K, Spencer FC: Prognostic signs and the role of operative management in acute pancreatitis. *Surg Gynecol Obstet* 139:69–81, 1974.
20. Imrie CW, Benjamin IS, Ferguson JC, McKay AJ, Mackenzie I, O'Neill J, Blumgart LH: A single-centre double-blind trial of Trasylol therapy in primary acute pancreatitis. *Br J Surg* 65:337–341, 1978.
21. Jacobs ML, Daggett WM, Civetta JM, Vasu MA, Lawson DW, Warshaw AL, Nardi GL, Barlett MK: Acute pancreatitis: analysis of factors influencing survival. *Ann Surg* 185:43–51, 1977.
22. Cornfield, AP, Cooper MJ, Williamson RCN: Acute pancreatitis: a lethal disease of increasing incidence. *Gut* 26:724–729, 1985.
23. Pollock AV: Acute pancreatitis. *Br Med J* 1:6, 1959.
24. Ranson JHC, Rifkind KM, Turner JW: Prognostic signs and nonoperative peritoneal lavage in acute pancreatitis. *Surg Gynecol Obstet* 143:209–219, 1976.
25. Ranson JHC: Etiologic and prognositc factors in human acute pancreatitis: a review. *Am J Gastroenterol* 77:633–638, 1982.
26. Stone HH, Fabian TC: Peritoneal dialysis in the treatment of acute alcoholic pancreatitis. *Surg Gynecol Obstet* 150:828–882, 1980.
27. Ranson JHC, Spencer FC: The role of peritoneal lavage in severe acute pancreatitis. *Ann Surg* 187:565–575, 1978.
28. Acosta JM, Rossi R, Galli OVR, Pellegrini CA, Skinner DB: Early surgery for gallstone pancreatitis: evaluation of a systematic approach. *Surgery* 83:367–370, 1978.
29. Stone HH, Fabian TC, Dunlop WE: Gallstone pancreatitis: biliary tract pathology in relation to time of operation. *Ann Surg* 194:305–312, 1981.
30. Ranson JHC: The timing of biliary surgery in acute pancreatitis. *Ann Surg* 189:654–663, 1979.
31. Ranson JHC, Turner JW, Roses DF, Rifkind KM, Spencer FC: Respiratory complication in acute pancreatitis. *Ann Surg* 179:557–566, 1974.

32. Warshaw AL, Lesser PB, Ric M, Cullen DJ: The pathogenesis of pulmonary edema in acute pancreatitis. *Ann Surg* 182:505–510, 1975.

33. Ranson JH, Spencer FC: Prevention, diagnosis, and treatment of pancreatic abscess. *Surgery* 82:99–106, 1977.

34. Bradley EL, Fulenwider JJ: Open treatment of pancreatic abscess. *Surg Gynecol Obstet* 159:509–513, 1984.

35. Stone HH, Strom PR, Mullins RJ: Pancreatic abscess management by subtotal resection and packing. *World J Surg* 8:340–345, 1984.

36. Bradley EL, Clements JL, Gonzalez AC: The natural history of pancreatic pseudocysts: a unified concept of management. *Am J Surg* 137:135–141, 1979.

37. Cameron JL, Keiffer RS, Anderson WJ, Zuidema GD: Internal pancreatic fistulas: pancreatic ascites and pleural effusions. *Ann Surg* 184:587–593, 1976.

38. Levine JB, Warshaw AL, Falchuk KR, Schapiro RH: The value of endoscopic retrograde pancreatography in the management of pancreatic ascites. *Surgery* 81:360–362, 1977.

39. Maimon S, Kirsner JB, Palmer WL: Chronic recurrent pancreatitis. *Arch Int Med* 81:56–72, 1948.

40. Bartholomew LG, Comfort MV: Chronic pancreatitis without pain. *Gastroenterology* 36:563–572, 1956.

41. Mackie CR, Cooper MJ, Lewis MH, Moossa AR: Nonoperative differentiation between pancreatic cancer and chronic pancreatitis. *Ann Surg* 189:480–487,1979.

42. Goodale RL, Condie RM, Gajl-Peczalska K, Taylor T, O'Leary J, Dressel T, Borner JW, Frick MP, Fryd DS: Clinical and secretory differences in pancreatic cancer and chronic pancreatitis. *Ann Surg* 194:193–198, 1981.

43. Dimagno EP: Medical treatment of pancreatic insufficiency. *Mayo Clin Proc* 54:435–442, 1979.

44. Prinz RA, Greenlee HB: Pancreatic duct drainage in 100 patients with chronic pancreatitis. *Ann Surg* 194:313–320, 1981.

45. Frey CF: Role of subtotal pancreatectomy and pancreaticojejunostomy in chronic pancreatitis. *J Surg Res* 31:361–370, 1981.

46. Frey CF, Child CG, Fry W: Pancreatectomy for chronic pancreatitis. *Ann Surg* 184:403–414, 1976.

47. Eckhauser FE, Strodel WE, Knol JA, Harper M, Turcotte JG: Near-total pancreatectomy for chronic pancreatitis. *Surgery* 96:599–607, 1984.

48. MacMahon B: Risk factors for cancer of the pancreas. *Cancer* 50:2676–2680, 1982.

49. Cubilla AL, Fitzgerald PJ: Surgical pathology of tumors of the exocrine pancreas. In Moossa AR (ed): *Tumors of the Pancreas,* Baltimore, Williams & Wilkins, 1980, pp 159–193.

50. Doll R, Muir M. Waterhouse J (eds): *Cancer Incidence in Five Continents,* Vol 2, *Internationalia Contre le Cancer,* Geneva, Switzerland, 1970.

51. Fras I, Lithin EM, Pearson JS: Comparison of psychiatric symptoms in carcinoma of the pancreas with those in some other intraabdominal neoplasms. *Am J Psychiatry* 123:1553–1562, 1967.

52. Braasch JW, Deziel DJ, Rossi RL, Watkins E, Winter PF: Pyloric and gastric preserving pancreatic resection: experience with 87 patients. *Ann Surg* 204:411–418, 1986.

53. van Heerden JA: Pancreatic resection for carcinoma of the pancreas: Whipple versus total pancreatectomy—an institutional perspective. *World J Surg* 8:800–888, 1984.

54. Grace PA, Pitt HA, Tompkins RK, DenBesten L, Longmire WP: Decreased morbidity and mortality after pancreatoduodenectomy. *Am J Surg* 151:141–149, 1986.

55. Cameron JL, Crist D: Improved hospital morbidity, mortality, and survival following the Whipple procedure. *Ann Surg* (In press)

56. Herter FP, Cooperman AM, Ahlborn TN, Antinori C: Surgical experience with pancreatic and periampullary cancer. *Ann Surg* 195:274–281, 1982.

57. Lerut JP, Fianello PR, Otte JB, Kestens PJ: Pancreaticoduodenal resection surgical experience and evaluation of risk factors in 103 patients. *Ann Surg* 199:432–437, 1984.

58. Obertop H, Bruining HA, Schattenkerk ME, Eggink WF, Jeekel J, Van Houten H: Operative approach to cancer of the head of the pancreas and the periampullary region. *Br J Surg* 69:573–576, 1982.

59. Sarr MG, Cameron JL: Surgical management of unresectable carcinoma of the pancreas. *Surgery* 91:123–133, 1982.

60. Dooley JS, Olney J, Dick R, Sherlock S: Non-surgical treatment of biliary obstruction. *Lancet* 2:1040–1044, 1979.

61. Mueller PR, van Sonnenberg E, Ferrucci JT: Percutaneous biliary drainage: technical and catheter-related problems in 200 procedures. *Am J Radiol* 138:17–23, 1982.

62. Malangoni MA, McCoy DM, Richardson JD, Flint LM: Effective palliation of malignant biliary duct obstruction. *Ann Surg* 201:554–559, 1985.

63. Sarr MG, Cameron JL: Surgical palliation of unresectable carcinoma of the pancreas *World J Surg* 8:906–918, 1984.

64. Sarr MG, Gladen HF, Beart RW Jr., vanHeerden JA: Role of gastroenterostomy in patients with unresectable pancreatic carcinoma. *Surg Gynecol Obstet* 152:597–600, 1981.

65. Flanigan DP, Kraft RO: Continuing experience with palliative chemical splanchnicectomy. *Arch Surg* 113:509–511, 1978.

66. Takada T, Hanyu F, Kobayashi S, Uchida Y: Percutaneous transhepatic cholangial drainage: direct approach under fluoroscopic control. *J Surg Oncol* 8:83–97, 1976.

67. Nakayama T, Ikeda A, Okunda K: Percutaneous transhepatic drainage of the biliary tract. *Gastroenterology* 74:554–559, 1978.

68. Gobian RP, Stanley JH, Soucek CD: Routine preoperative biliary drainage: effect on management of obstructive jaundice. *Radiology* 152:353–356. 1984.

69. Hatfield ARW, Tobas R, Terblanche J: Preoperative ex-

ternal biliary drainage in obstructive jaundice: a prospective controlled clinical trial. *Lancet* II:896–899, 1982.

70. McPherson GAD, Benjamin IS, Hodgson HJF: Preoperative percutaneous transhepatic biliary drainage: the results of a controlled trial. *Br J Surg* 71:371–375, 1984.

71. Pitt HA, Gomes AS, Lois JF, Mann LL, Deutsch LS, Longmire WP: Does preoperative percutaneous biliary drainage reduce operative risk or increase hospital cost? *Ann Surg* 201:545–553, 1985.

72. Traverso LW, Longmire WP Jr., Preservation of the pylorus during pancreatoduodenectomy. *Surg Gynecol Obstet* 146:959–962, 1978.

73. Hodgkinson DJ, ReMine WH, Weiland LH: Pancreatic cystadenoma—a clinicopathologic study of 45 cases. *Arch Surg* 113:512–519, 1978.

74. Hodgkinson DJ, ReMine WH, Weiland LH: A clinicopathologic study in 21 cases of pancreatic cystadenocarcinoma. *Ann Surg* 188:679–684, 1978.

75. Service FJ, Dale JD, Elveback LR, Jiang N: Insulinoma—Clinical diagnostic features or 60 consecutive cases. *Mayo Clin Proc* 51:417–429, 1976.

76. Glickman MH, Hart MJ, White TT. Insulinoma in Seattle: 39 cases in 30 years. *Am J Surg* 140:119–125, 1980.

77. van Heerden JA, Edis AJ, Service FJ: The surgical aspects of insulinomas. *Ann Surg* 189: 677–682, 1979.

Chapter 23

Diseases of the Small Bowel in the Elderly

R. Benton Adkins, Jr., M.D., F.A.C.S.

The normal physiologic and functional responses of the small bowel to the general process of aging are still not thoroughly understood. One might expect intestinal function to become sluggish with age, but actually, experimental and clinical evidence does not indicate any major functional abnormalities that occur in the aging intestine. Functional small bowel problems in the elderly are more often the result of systemic disorders and drug ingestion than any measurable effect of aging itself.

NORMAL EFFECTS OF AGING

The small intestine does decrease in weight after age 40. The mucosal parenchyma is reported to be replaced to some degree by fibrous tissue, and fewer healthy smooth muscle fibers are seen (1). However, anatomic and histologic changes in the aging intestine have been difficult to identify as a specific alteration due to the *normal* result of aging. In many of the earlier studies of the aging gut, neither the nutritional state nor the presence or absence of disease in the study group was addressed, although these conditions are known to have a considerable effect on mucosal structure and on protein and enzyme content of the small bowel. This fact should be kept in mind as the literature on the subject is reviewed.

In the mid- and late 1970s, several studies were published that reported abnormal small bowel histology in aged rats. The abnormalities included villus atrophy, decreased villus height, decreased length of the small bowel, disoriented microvilli, and increased collagen and amyloid within the mucosa. None of these reports, however, included mention of the overall health status of the older rats. In 1984, Holt et al. studied the effects of aging upon the small bowel in a large group of Fischer 344 rats (2). These animals were barrier-reared, checked regularly for infections, and were maintained since birth on the same diet. They found villus-crypt length and villus height in the duodenum and jejunum in the older rats to be identical to that in the young. Ileal villus height and crypt depth were actually greater in the older rats. Of course, normal histology does not artibrarily equate with normal function. Holt and his co-workers found that the functional expression of several enzymes in the epithelial cells of the intestinal villus was delayed in aged rats (2). This supports the paradoxical notion that the epithelial cells in the aged small bowel are more immature than those seen in the young.

Considerable experimental and clinical research has addressed the question of malabsorption in the elderly. Morphologic changes that might seem to lead to malabsorption in the aging bowel have not been absolutely proven to occur as a result of age. However, the general consensus of most researchers is that aging is accompanied by a slight degree of decreased absorptive capacity in the small bowel.

Carbohydrate absorption has been studied by many researchers (3–8). The results of their studies do not consistently provide evidence for, but are suggestive of proof for a reduction in carbohydrate absorption by the bowel that is age-related. Moreover, Fiebusch and Holt suggest that a further absorption impairment occurs in elderly subjects aged 75 and older (8). It has been suggested that this malabsorption in the "old" elderly is the result of some type of malfunction of the mucosal cells, specifically in the intestinal enzyme production.

Fewer studies have investigated xylose absorption in the elderly. The consensus is that xylose absorption may be decreased in the elderly, but mainly in those subjects over 80 years of age (3).

The investigations of fat absorption have been hampered by the problems involved with the use of institutionalized subjects. In these elderly individuals, systemic diseases and nutritional defects are likely to be present. However, most studies done with these subjects have suggested decreased absorption of fat with advanced age. Holt and Dominquez found that the intestinal absorption of triolein was reduced in the elderly apparently due to impaired luminal uptake and a delayed transintestinal transport (9).

Very little information is available about protein absorption in the elderly, and the studies that have been done have produced conflicting findings. There has been general agreement that overall protein absorption is not diminished by the aging process. There is disagreement, however, in the amount of protein normally required to maintain a positive nitrogen balance in the elderly. Gersovitz et al. have suggested that, in advanced age, the process of albumin synthesis responds less well to altered types and amounts of dietary protein (10).

There is some evidence that fat-soluble vitamins are absorbed as readily, if not more readily, in the elderly individual as in younger persons. Vitamin D may be an exception to this general hypothesis. Concentrations of plasma 25-hydroxycholecaliferol are also found to be lower in elderly subjects. Water-soluble vitamins do not appear to be poorly absorbed in the elderly (3).

For reasons as yet unexplained, calcium absorption has been shown to decrease with advancing age. The need for research in this area is very great because of the prevalence of osteoporosis and osteomalacia in the elderly. There is strong evidence to support the thesis that the major factor causing these conditions may be a defect in the absorption of Vitamin D as mentioned above, which may then prevent or alter normal calcium absorption as well (3).

Concentrations of serum iron and serum transferrin are generally expected to fall with advanced age, but the large number of studies reporting on this subject do not provide absolute proof of this decrease. A host of clinical conditions may also be responsible for the increased incidence of iron deficiency anemia in the elderly. Intestinal blood loss should be excluded first when iron deficiency or any type of anemia occurs in the elderly.

Intestinal Motility

Most studies have suggested that small intestinal function in normal elderly subjects is somewhat diminished compared to those of younger ages. This difference is not significant enough, however, to alter transit time from stomach to cecum. Small intestinal motility is most often hampered by systemic disease and/or medications.

INFLAMMATORY BOWEL DISEASE

Although inflammatory bowel diseases (IBD) are generally considered to be disorders of the young, they are not that uncommon in the elderly. In fact, in some series, a bimodal incidence curve is seen, with a secondary increase in the incidence of IBD in patients who are over age 60. It has been estimated that approximately 5%–10% of all patients with IBD are over age 60 (3).

Most reports indicate that recurrence of quiescent IBD is less likely in older patients than in younger age groups. This hypothesis is difficult to prove, however, based on the data available. In most series, those patients who develop IBD at age 60 or 65 are not separated from those who had the disease prior to that age (3).

In many series, distinction is not made between IBD of the small bowel and that of the colon. Shapiro describes the experience with IBD in 33 patients over age 60. Eighteen had disease confined to the small bowel, and four others had ileocolitis. The remaining eleven had colonic disease only (11).

The presenting symptoms of IBD in the elderly are much the same as those seen in younger patients. Diarrhea, weight loss, and abdominal cramps are the primary symptoms. In addition to the fact that Crohn's disease is not readily considered as a diagnosis in the elderly, making the diagnosis can be difficult because of the similarity of symptoms to ischemic bowel disease. Shapiro found this true in his series from Beth Israel Hospital (11).

Watts et al. have emphasized the severe morbidity and mortality associated with the initial onset of IBD in elderly patients, and therefore, they recommended early operative treatment (12). Others have pointed out that all inflammatory diseases are more poorly tolerated in older age groups and that postoperative mortality is greater in older patients. These authors call for a more conservative approach to the elderly with IBD (13). We would agree with Watts and his colleagues and suspect that Gupta's group could avoid the complications and postoperative deaths that they report if they would begin to treat their cases with early resection when indicated.

The medical treatment of Crohn's disease in the elderly is generally the same as with younger patients. One important difference, however, involves the use of corticosteroids. Steroids are more hazardous in older age groups because of the incidence of concomitant disease. Osteoporosis, atherosclerosis, diabetes, and hypertension may all be worsened by the use of steroids. Immunosuppressive agents should also be used judiciously in the elderly patients who may be more sensitive to these agents.

CIRCULATORY PROBLEMS

Intestinal problems resulting from circulatory disorders are seen almost exclusively in older age groups. In an early study, Brandfondbrener et al. showed that reduced mesenteric flow occurred in the elderly as a result of reduction in resting cardiac output (14). Another contributing factor may be a reduced responsiveness to physiologic need in the elderly. For example, the shift in blood volume occurring after a meal can produce hypotension in well, elderly subjects presumably because of age-associated blunting of sympathetic baroflex sensitivity. Concomitant diseases, such as congestive heart failure, may also result in poor intestinal perfusion.

Atherosclerotic vascular disease does not have the dramatic effect on the function of the small intestine that might be expected. Holt points out that complete proximal obstruction of the three major intestinal vessels can be accompanied at times by no symptoms and that a minimum of two vessels must be involved before signs of intestinal ischemia are seen (3).

Acute intestinal ischemia usually occurs abruptly with the onset of severe abdominal pain. It may be the result of a mesenteric artery embolus or thrombus or venous thrombosis. In these situations, immediate surgical intervention is the only hope for recovery and survival.

Gradual occlusion of abdominal vessels by progressive atherosclerosis produces pain that may be confused with peptic ulcer disease or cholelithiasis (15). Bouts of "abdominal angina" occur with meals. Ischemic ileitis usually occurs in patients older than 50 when inferior mesenteric artery disease is accompanied by congestive heart failure, hypertension, or other conditions that decrease blood flow to the abdominal vessels. Abdominal pain and bloody diarrhea are the most common symptoms, and they may occur in various degrees of severity. If not treated by revascularization, intestinal gangrene can occur that will require operative intervention and resection. Antibiotics and IV fluids are appropiate treatment for less serious cases.

Intestinal infarction in the absence of vascular occlusion is not uncommon. It usually occurs in the face of congestive heart failure, anoxia, or shock. In these situations, blood is shunted to the brain and other vital organs, and ischemic necrosis can therefore occur in the intestinal mucosa. Surgical resection is then necessary to prevent peritonitis.

DIVERTICULAR DISEASE

Uncommon in patients younger than age 40, diverticula occur with considerable frequency in older individuals. Approximately 20%–30% of patients over 60 and more than 40% of those over 70 have diverticular disease (16). Moreover, the number of diverticula usually found in a given individual is likely to increase in older persons.

Diverticula may occur singularly in the duodenum. Pearce has reported an incidence of duodenal diverticula of 20.1% in patients in a geriatric hospital (average age 80.1) compared to 6.5% in a general hospital (17). He found that these lesions are rarely responsible for nutritional deficiencies.

It has been reported that 60% of duodenal

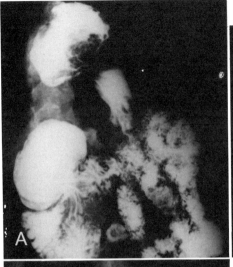

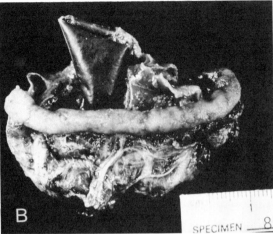

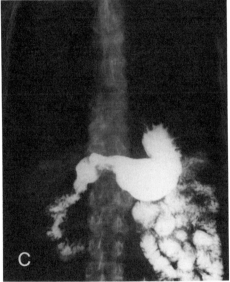

Figure 23.1. **A,** An upper gastrointestinal series done for chronic abdominal complaints and anemia in a 76-year-old female. It shows a moderate-sized hiatal hernia and an enormous juxtapapillary duodenal diverticulum. Notice the suggestion of foreign material inferiorly within diverticulum. **B,** Resected specimen showing duodenal diverticulum. The opening is 5 cm in diameter with receptacle-like appearance and contains debris, food particles, and fruit peelings. Notice the rim of ulcerated mucosa secondary to foreign body trauma. **C,** Postoperative film done 6 weeks after operation showing no evidence of hiatal hernia and absence of the large duodenal diverticulum. Patient remains symptom free with normal hematologic profile more than one year postoperatively at age 78.

diverticula are juxtapapillary (3). Duodenal diverticula have been associated with biliary calculi in some reports. It has been suggested that patients with juxtapapillary diverticula have an associated choledochoduodenal sphincter dysfunction (3). We would recommend a conservative surgical approach to duodenal diverticula in the elderly. We have tended to treat only those that bleed, perforate, or ulcerate. (Fig. 23.1 a–c)

Jejunal diverticula are seldom solitary lesions. Often occurring in the proximal jejunum, they can be asymptomatic for considerable periods of time. Perforation, hemorrhage, formation of enteroliths, and bezoars may result, however, in the more severe cases. The symptoms resulting from the consequential bacterial overgrowth are more insiduous. These may include abdominal cramps, distension, diarrhea, steatorrhea, and weight loss. These symptoms occasionally may be treated with antibiotics with success. Most often, however, surgical intervention and intestinal resection are necessary.

SMALL BOWEL OBSTRUCTION

Intestinal obstruction occurs frequently in older age groups. In one reported series, operations for intestinal obstruction were the second most common emergency surgical procedures in patients above age 70 (18). Characteristically, symptoms include abdominal pain, vomiting, abdominal distention, and obstipation. Elderly persons have a higher mortality rate from intestinal obstruction than found in younger patients, making prompt diagnosis and treatment imperative. In 1978, 70% of patient who died from small bowel obstruction were over 70 years of age (19). Usually, however, the mortality rate from intestinal obstruction resulting from nonmalignant conditions is much lower than in those instances of malignant obstruction (10% vs 41%). Reiss and Deutsch's work supports this notion; the mortality rate for their elderly patients with benign obstructive conditions was only 6% (18). Under elective conditions (i.e., in the absence of sepsis or gangrene), the mortality rate fell to 0. Obviously, early operative treatment of small bowel obstruction is important for a good result. Some authors have reported that elderly patients with intestinal strangulation do not always present with the classic signs of that disorder. Zadeh et al. found this to be true in 35% of the older patients they treated for small bowel obstruction (19). In one-half of these cases, operative treatment was delayed for some reason for more than 24 hours. In that group, the morbidity rate increased from 50% to 71%. They have concluded that in the absence of carcinomatosis, Crohn's disease, early postoperative obstruction, and partial small bowel obstruction, operative management of suspected small bowel obstruction should be done as expeditiously as possible.

SMALL BOWEL NEOPLASMS

Only 5% of all gastrointestinal tract neoplasms occur in the small bowel. This low incidence is surprising when one considers that the small bowel accounts for over 75% of the length and over 90% of the absorptive surface of the entire gastrointestinal tract (20, 21). Local factors in the small bowel, such as mild alkalinity or neutral pH and a rapid transit time, have been thought to help prevent the development of neoplasms. The incidence of benign and malignant small bowel tumors varies from author to author, but when taken in the aggregate, relatively equal incidence rates for benign and malignant small

bowel neoplasms are seen (22). The average age of patients who are diagnosed as having benign small bowel neoplasms is 62 years, whereas most patients with malignant tumors are slightly younger at diagnosis (57 years) (23). In some reports, as many as 62% of malignant tumors are seen in patients in their sixth and seventh decades of life (24). There is a higher incidence of small bowel neoplasms in cases of familial polyposis, Gardner's syndrome, Crohn's disease, and other inherited disorders of the gastrointestinal tract.

Benign Tumors

Almost 50% of all benign tumors of the small bowel are asymptomatic, and approximately one-third are found incidentally at the time of autopsy. When these tumors are symptomatic, pain is usually the presenting complaint. In more than 50% of these cases, the pain will be the result of partial or total obstruction. Intussusception, caused by the tumor, can also result in intestinal obstruction. Mild, chronic bleeding resulting from mucosal involvement with the tumor occurs in approximately one-quarter of patients who are symptomatic (25, 26). Benign tumors are usually not large enough to be palpable, but if so, they are generally freely movable. Rarely do benign tumors cause malabsorption, jaundice, or signs of an acute abdomen.

Approximately 35% of all benign small bowel tumors are adenomas (27, 28). These growths are the result of benign proliferation of epithelium from the mucosa or mucosal glands. Most of these lesions are polypoid, but villous adenomas and Brunner's gland adenomas also occur.

Adenomatous polyps occur in the duodenum more often than in other areas of the small intestine. Generally they are solitary, but multiple adenomatous polyps can occur. Although usually asymptomatic, these lesions can result in intussusception and obstruction or in chronic intestinal bleeding. If symptomatic or if found incidentally at laparotomy, surgical excision is indicated. When intussusception and/or obstruction has occurred, reduction of the twist and/or intussusception and segmental resection of the bowel will be necessary. As mentioned earlier, the risk incurred by emergency procedures in older patients is considerable, and the prognosis is improved significantly when elective procedures are possible (29).

Villous adenomas occur rarely in the small bowel and reportedly comprise less than 1% of all small bowel neoplasms (30). As are the adenomatous polyps, these lesions are usually asymptomatic unless they have grown to be quite large. Up to one-half of these lesions will become malignant if they are left untreated (31, 32). When they are symptomatic, crampy, intermittent pain and intestinal bleeding are usually present. Mucus diarrhea may rarely occur with large tumors. These lesions produce filling defects radiographically and are successfully diagnosed preoperatively in 75% of cases (33).

Surgical excision is the only treatment for villous adenomas. Large lesions may require segmental resection, and if there is evidence of malignancy, excision with wide margins (10 cm) and including all of the involved mesentery is necessary. For large duodenal lesions with malignant transformation, a pancreaticoduodenal resection should be done.

Adenomas of Brunner's glands occur rarely. When present, they may cause symptoms similar to those of peptic ulcer disease, i.e., duodenal obstruction and bleeding. Surgical excision is the treatment of choice.

Fibromas of the small intestine comprise approximately 8% of all benign small bowel tumors. Arising from the subserosa, these tumors usually extend intraluminally. Many of these tumors remain unknown because they do not typically produce symptoms. When they are symptomatic, intussusception and obstruction usually occur, and excision is necessary.

Malignant Tumors

Over 90% of patients with malignant tumors of the small bowel are symptomatic. Weight loss, pain, anemia, and nausea and/or vomiting account for the vast majority of symptoms (27). Sawyer and his co-workers described a symptom complex that they felt was a typical pattern for malignant tumors of the small intestine. The symptom complex consists of gurgling bowel sounds, a sense of abdominal fullness, cramps, nausea, and, finally, vomiting (28). This series of events occur intermittently at the same intervals of time following each of three daily meals. This complex of symptoms was more predictable with lesions of the proximal jejunum, but occurred with tumors at all small bowel sites.

When studied with upper gastrointestinal x-rays, 75%–80% of malignant tumors of the small bowel can be seen or their presence suspected (25). In those tumors of the duodenum, nearly 100% should be seen on upper gastrointestinal series (28). Those in the terminal ileum may be seen more easily with barium enema using reflux of the barium to the mid-ileum (24).

In Rochlin and Longmire's comprehensive review of small bowel tumors, the pertinent literature of the preceding 40 years was carefully reviewed, and the site of occurrence of 650 neoplasms of various types was documented (34). Carcinomas, sarcomas, carcinoids, and metastatic lesions were found to occur in the small bowel, with a general tendency of distribution of adenocarcinomas proximally and lymphosarcomas distally. (See Table 23.1) To the author's knowledge, a review of this magnitude has not since been reported. The current situation, however, continues to reflect this early report. In more recent series, adenocarcinoma occurs

Table 23.1 Review of the Literature, 1920 to 1960, on Malignant Tumors of the Small Intestine[a]

Location	Number
Total cases	
Duodenum	136
Jejunum	184
Ileum	308
Multiple	22
Total	650
Sarcomas	
Duodenum	12
Jejunum	61
Ileum	118
Multiple	17
Total	208
Carcinomas	
Duodenum	113
Jejunum	108
Ileum	98
Multiple	2
Total	321
Carcinoid Tumors	
Duodenum	11
Jejunum	15
Ileum	92
Multiple	3
Total	121

[a]Reproduced with permission from Rochlin DB, Longmire WP: Primary tumors of the small intestine. *Surgery* 50:586–592, 1961

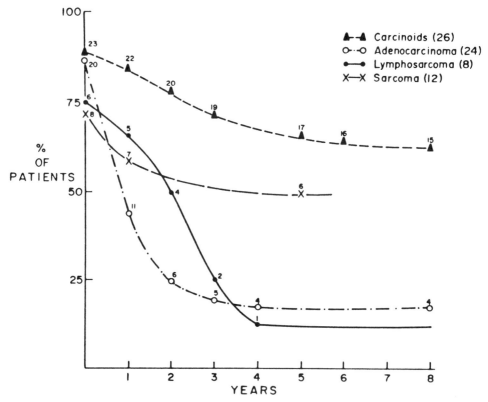

Figure 23.2. Survival of patients with malignant small intestinal tumors. The curve marked "sarcomas" includes nine leiomyosarcomas, two fibrosarcomas, and one hemangioendothelioma. (Reprinted with permission from Waterhouse G, et al: A clinical review of small bowel neoplasms. South Med J 74:1201–1203, 1981.)

primarily in the duodenum, then next most frequently in the jejunum. Carcinoids and lymphosarcoma occur mostly in the ileum, whereas the other types of sarcomas are usually evenly distributed in all parts (24, 25, 27, 28, 34, 35).

In an extensive review by Resnick and Cooper, 40% of the cancers of the duodenum are found to be suprapapillary, 40% are subpapillary, and only 20% are periampillary (36). Most of these tumors will require a major resection-usually a pancreaticoduodenectomy (Whipple procedure) (34).

Ileal and jejunal tumors will always require a wide segmental resection including the mesentery all the way to its base. We prefer a 10-cm margin proximally and 10 cm distally for all small bowel carcinomas or sarcomas (37–39).

Carcinoid tumors are the most common malignant small bowel tumors in most reported series (40, 35) and therefore deserve special mention. These are neuroendocrine tumors that occur in the ileum and appendix most often. When meta-static to the liver, they produce the "carcinoid syndrome." This syndrome is characterized by flushing, diarrhea, and cramps associated with an abdominal mass, an enlarged liver, and an elevated urinary 5-HIAA (41).

Resection of the primary carcinoid tumor and the metastatic lesions and the administration of drugs to block the neuroendocrine effects of the tumor are all indicated. All carcinoid tumors should be treated as malignant tumors whenever and wherever they are found.

The prognosis for patients with early detected and adequately resected malignant tumors of the small bowel is dependent upon many factors including the length of symptoms, extent of tumor, cell type of tumor, and its location within the small bowel. (Fig. 23.2)

We would continue to recommend the same vigorous, diagnostic search in the elderly patient with symptoms that could be from a small bowel neoplasm as we would for a younger patient with the same symptoms. The surgical and adjuvant treatment for these lesions must be tempered by the extent of the disease when discovered and by the overall physical condition of the patient. If discovered in a curable stage, the same surgical resection for a small bowel cancer that would be done in a middle-aged patient should be offered to the elderly patient with a similar tumor.

SUMMARY

The pathologic conditions that commonly lead to the surgical treatment for small bowel problems in the elderly tend to be dramatic. Vascular insufficiency, neoplasms (malignant and benign), inflammatory conditions, and various types of mechanical obstruction (see Chapter 24) attack the elderly population with alarming regularity. As with all surgical conditions in the elderly, if the problem is diagnosed early, the patient is prepared at leisure, the condition is treated with skill and care, and any complications are avoided, these problems can be solved for many of these patients who may seem beyond the hope of cure. It is the elderly patient in need of surgical treatment for one of these conditions, who is neglected until the situation is out of hand, who will have little hope of survival.

REFERENCES

1. Schuster MM: Disorders of the aging GI system. *Hosp Pract* 11:95–103, 1976.
2. Holt PR, Pascal RR, Kotler DP: Effects of aging upon small intestinal structure in the Fischer rat. *J Gerontol* 39:642–647, 1984.
3. Holt PR: The small intestine. *Clin Gastroenterol* 14:689–723, 1985.
4. Welch JD, Poley JR, Bhatia M, Stevenson DE: Intestinal disaccharidase activities in relation to age, race, and mucosal damage. *Gastroenterology* 80:94–98, 1978.
5. Vinardell P, Bolufer J: Age dependence changes on jejunal sugar absorption by rat in-vivo. *Exper Gerontol* 19:73–78, 1984.
6. Klimas JE: Intestinal glucose absorption during the life-span of a colony of rats. *J Gerontol* 23:529–532, 1968.
7. Calingaert A, Zorzoli A: The influence of age on 6-deoxy-D-glucose accumulation by mouse intestine. *J Gerontol* 20:211–214, 1965.
8. Feibusch J, Holt PR: Impaired absorptive capacity for carbohydrates in the elderly. *Am J Clin Nutr* 32:942, 1979.
9. Holt PR, Dominguez AA: Intestinal absorption of triglyceride and vitamin D3 in aged and young rats. *Dig Dis Sci* 26:1109–1115, 1981.
10. Gersovitz M, Munro HN, Udall J, Young VR: Albumin synthesis in young and elderly subjects using a new stable isotope methodology: response to level of protein intake. *Metabolism* 29:1075–1086, 1980.
11. Shapiro PA, Peppercorn MA, Antonioli DA, Joffe N, Goldman H: Crohn's disease in the elderly. *Am J Gastroenterol* 76:132–137, 1981.
12. Watts J McK, Dombal FT De, Watkinson G, Goligher JD: Early course of ulcerative colitis. *Gut* 7:16–31, 1966.
13. Gupta S, Saverymuttu SH, Keshavarzian A, Hodgson HJF: Is the pattern of inflammatory bowel disease different in the elderly? *Age Ageing* 14:366–370, 1985.
14. Brandfondbrener M, Londowne M, Shock NW: The relation of age to certain performance of the heart and the circulation. *Circulation* 12:567–576, 1955.
15. Cohen N: Gastroenterology in the aged. *Mt Sinai J Med* 47:142–149, 1980.
16. Bustin MP, Iber FL: Management of common non-malignant GI problems in the elderly. *Geriatrics* 38:69–76, 1983.
17. Pearce VR: The importance of duodenal diverticula in the elderly. *Postgrad Med J* 56:777–780, 1980.
18. Reiss R, Deutsch AA: Emergency abdominal procedures in patients above 70. *J Gerontol* 40:154–158, 1985.
19. Zadeh BJ, Davis JM, Canizaro PC: Small bowel obstruction in the elderly. *Am Surg* 51:470–473, 1985.
20. Braasch JW, Denbo HE: Tumors of the small intestine. *Surg Clin North Am* 44:791–809, 1964.
21. Schier J: Diagnostic and therapeutic aspects of tumors of the small bowel. *Int Surg* 57:789–792, 1972.
22. Sindelar WF: Cancer of the small intestine. In DeVita VT, Hellman S, Rosenberg (eds): *Cancer, Principles and Practice of Oncology.* Philadelphia, JB Lippincott, 1982, pp 616–642.
23. Botsford TW, Crowe P, Crocker DW: Tumors of the small intestine. A review of experience with 115 cases including a report of a rare case of malignant hemangio-endothelioma. *Am J Surg* 103:358–365, 1962.
24. Croom RD, Newsome JF: Tumors of the small intestine. *Am Surg* 41:160–167, 1975.
25. Ebert PA, Zuidema GD: Primary tumors of the small intestine. *Arch Surg* 91:452–455, 1965.
26. Schmutzer KJ, Holleran WM, Regan JF: Tumors of the small bowel. *Am J Surg* 108:270–276, 1964.
27. Silberman H, Crichlow RW, Caplan HS: Neoplasms of the small bowel. *Ann Surg* 180:157–161, 1974.
28. Sawyer RB, Sawyer KC Jr, Sawyer KC, Larsen RR: Benign and malignant tumors of the small intestine. *Am Surg* 29:268–272, 1963.
29. Adkins RB, Scott HW: Surgical procedures in patients aged 90 years and older. *South Med J* 77:1357–1364, 1984.
30. Kutin ND, Ransom JHC, Gouge TH, Localio SA: Villous tumors of the duodenum. *Ann Surg* 181:164–168, 1975.
31. Shulten MF, Dyasu R, Beal JM: Villous adenoma of the duodenum: a case report and review of the literature. *Am J Surg* 132:90–96, 1976.

32. Bremer EH, Battaile WB, Bulle PH: Villous tumors of the upper gastrointestinal tract. Clinical review and report of a case. *Am J Gastroenterol* 50:135–143, 1968.

33. Ring EJ, Ferrucci JT, Eaton SB, Clements JL: Villous adenomas of the duodenum. *Radiology* 104:45–48, 1972.

34. Rochlin DB, Longmire WP: Primary tumors of the small intestine. *Surgery* 50:586–592, 1961.

35. Miles RM, Crawford D, Duras S: The small bowel tumor problem. *Ann Surg* 189:732–740, 1979.

36. Resnick HLP, Cooper DR: Carcinoma of the duodenum; review of literature from 1948 to 1956. *Am J Surg* 95:946–952, 1958.

37. Waterhouse G, Skudlarick JL, Adkins RB: A clinical review of small bowel neoplasms. *South Med J* 74:1201–1203, 1981.

38. Kieffer RW, McSwain B, Adkins, RB: Sarcoma of the gastrointestinal tract: a review of 40 cases. *Am Surg* 48:167–169, 1982.

39. Adkins RB, Scott HW, Sawyers JL: Gastrointestinal lymphoma and sarcoma: a case for aggressive search and destroy. *Ann Surg* 205:625–633, 1987.

40. Rich JD: Malignant tumors of the intestine: a review of 37 cases. *Am Surg* 43:445–454, 1977.

41. Durning P, Galland RB, Nagorney DM, Welbourn RB: Neuroendocrine tumors of the gut. *World J Surg* 9:348–360, 1985.

Chapter 24

The Diagnosis and Management of Intestinal Obstruction and Herniae in the Elderly

Raymond Pollak, M.B., F.R.C.S. (Edin.), Lloyd M. Nyhus, M.D., F.A.C.S., F.R.C.S. (Eng)(Hon), F.R.C.S.I. (Hon)

The term "intestinal obstruction" connotes a clinical syndrome in which the contents of the intestine are unable to pass in the usual physiologic way, from proximal to distal, ultimately to reach the rectum. A hernia, on the other hand, may be defined as the protrusion of a viscus through a defect in the musculoaponeurotic structures that enclose that viscus. When this viscus is either the small or large intestine, it is apparent that a hernia may be a contributing cause to acute or chronic intestinal obstruction. As we will show, both intestinal obstruction and herniae of the abdominal wall are not uncommon in the population at large and as such also affect persons in our community who are considered elderly, i.e., those older than 65 years of age.

It is well to include a discussion of the principal factors that result in intestinal obstruction, including herniae of the abdominal wall, and the diagnosis, management, and the ultimate outcome of these conditions in the elderly population.

INCIDENCE

It is estimated that 10% of the population of the United States today are persons who are older than 65 years of age. By the year 2000 this number is predicted to approximate 30,000,000 persons (1, 2). As recently as 1985, it was estimated that 20% of surgical beds were occupied by elderly patients with serious and morbid surgical illnesses (3).

The incidence of intestinal obstructions rises progressively with age. There is a sharp increase in incidence after the age of 50 years and again after the age of 70 years (4). In a large series of 400 elderly Israeli patients admitted for emergency surgical therapy, 25% of patients had symptoms and signs of intestinal obstruction (5). An additional series, from the United Kingdom, described 375 patients, 218 of whom had symptoms and signs related to intestinal obstruction or incarcerated and strangulated abdominal wall herniae (6). There were 115 strangulated herniae (31% of all patients) and 103 episodes of intestinal obstruction (27.5% of all patients). These large series of patients serve to emphasize the fact that surgical intervention, especially emergency surgical intervention in the elderly, can be expected to increase dramatically in the future.

In the general population the incidence of hernia of the abdominal wall has been estimated to be approximately 15 per 1,000 (7). The incidence, however, for men in the sixth decade is 50 per 1000 and rises to 120 per 1000 for men over 75 years of age. Thus 3.75 million persons in the United States are estimated to suffer from some form of abdominal wall hernia or the complications thereof. Furthermore, approximately 550,000 persons, many of them elderly, undergo herniorrhaphy annually in the United States (8).

343

ETIOLOGY AND PATHOGENESIS

Traditionally causes of intestinal obstruction have been classified according to the nature of the obstructing process, i.e., where the process involves an intraluminal obstruction, where disease of the intestinal wall impinges on the lumen, or where a disease process from without compresses and obstructs intestinal transit. Most reviews of intestinal obstruction in elderly persons, however, divide the causes of obstruction into those that involve the large intestine, those that involve the small intestine, and herniae that result in intestinal obstruction themselves (3, 5, 6, 9). In the series described by Greene (9) in 1969, the large intestine, small intestine, and herniae each accounted for one-third of the number of patients who presented with symptoms and signs of intestinal obstruction. Colonic neoplasms, volvulus of the sigmoid, diverticulitis, fecal impaction, or volvulus of the cecum, in that order, were the major causes of large intestinal obstruction. The small intestine was obstructed for the most part by postoperative adhesions, gallstone ileus, metastatic tumors, mesenteric vascular accidents, regional enteritis, foreign bodies, and volvulus of the entire small intestine. In terms of the frequency of herniae encountered, inguinal herniae were the most common followed by femoral, umbilical, ventral, and internal herniae.

When the entire spectrum of emergency abdominal operations in elderly patients is examined in more detail, however, operations for intestinal obstruction usually account for about 25% of the operative procedures, closely following biliary tract operations (5). Again the obstructions are caused by incarcerated and strangulated herniae, as well as by mechanical obstruction resulting from adhesions, followed by mesenteric vascular accidents and malignant tumors. A similar series that examined emergency abdominal operations in elderly persons from the United Kingdom found operations for strangulated hernia and intestinal obstruction to be more common than all other forms of emergency abdominal procedures (6). In the latter series, strangulation was more common, with femoral herniae closely followed by inguinal, incisional, paraumbilical and obturator herniae. The causes of intestinal obstruction were also divided into those that affected the large and

those that affected the small intestine, with a similar spectrum of etiologic factors as previously mentioned. Conversely, when large series of elderly patients who are operated on for repair of abdominal wall herniae are examined, 16% of these patients present with incarceration, of whom 10% have strangulation (1). Only 3% of patients operated on electively for abdominal wall hernia have small intestinal obstruction as the presenting disease. In large series of elective repairs of groin herniae, about half are found to be indirect inguinal herniae, one-third to be direct inguinal herniae, 10% to be femoral herniae, and 8% to be pantaloon herniae. Men outnumber women by 6.5 to 1 in terms of the incidence of hernia, whereas the sex incidence is almost equal for patients who present with an acute abdominal surgical emergency or with acute intestinal obstruction (1, 3, 9).

Despite diverse causes, intraluminal obstructions, disease processes of the intestinal wall, and causes from without, such as postoperative adhesions, all produce a series of common pathologic events that eventually lead to compromise of intestinal viability and ultimate strangulation. These events are elegantly described by Stolar and Randolph in a rabbit model (10). When the obstructing mechanism causes an increase in the intramural tension of the intestinal wall, initially the low pressure venous and lymphatic flow within the wall becomes obstructed, resulting in engorgement and outpouring of extracellular fluid into the wall itself and into the lumen of the intestine. The proximal intestine makes spasmodic efforts to relieve the obstruction by active peristaltic movements, resulting in nonspecific symptoms of poorly localized abdominal pain, often accompanied by nausea and vomiting. Continued application of the obstructing mechanism results in a further outpouring of extracellular fluid into the intestinal lumen and a further increase in the intramural tension of the intestinal wall. As demonstrated by Stolar and Randolph, this process can continue unabated only for a few hours before a critical point is reached beyond which the intestine is unlikely to recover even though corrective measures are instituted. With increasing intraluminal and intramural tension, the arterial supply to the involved bowel part is jeopardized and strangulation ultimately occurs. Loss of the structural integrity of the intestinal mucosa, as well as stagnation, with absence of prograde intestinal movement, results in the overgrowth of a mixed flora of intestinal bacteria and migration of bacteria through the intestinal wall to involve the visceral peritoneum. Furthermore, the loss of the structural integrity of the intestinal wall, together with continuing intraluminal accumulation of fluid and bacteria and their products, eventually causes intestinal perforation and generalized peritonitis.

A clear understanding of the pathophysiology of intestinal obstruction and the resulting compromise of intestinal viability with strangulation should prompt timely and aggressive diagnostic and therapeutic measures to obviate progression to the state of generalized peritonitis, irreversible loss of portions of the intestine, and a possible threat to a patient's life.

CLINICAL SIGNS AND SYMPTOMS

A classic triad of crampy abdominal pain accompanied by nausea, vomiting, and absolute constipation may not always be present in the elderly patient with intestinal obstruction. In fact, delay in presentation is the factor most commonly seen in a large series of patients, and it is related to socio-economic factors, self-medication, and the minimizing of symptoms and signs by family, patient, and physician (9). Up to 4% of such patients in large series with late presentations died in the first few hours after their initial presentation without undergoing surgical treatment (9). A history of previous operations or history of treatment for intestinal obstruction may be elicited in up to 11% of patients. It is also important to establish a prior history of carcinoma, Crohn's disease, or the presence of a previously existing hernia. Many herniae in these elderly patients have been present for anywhere from 2 to 36 years (1).

The common presenting symptoms of herniae in a large elderly population are a mass in the groin or scrotum or localized inguinoscrotal pain. A prior history of hernia may be overlooked, however, in the setting of a seriously ill, toxic elderly patient who is in pain.

Concurrent co-morbid diseases, such as severe cardiovascular disease, obstructive chronic pulmonary disease and emphysema, chronic pyelonephritis, and senile dementia, may be present in more than 18% to 20% of persons (9). Diabetes mellitus may be present in about 6% of these patients (1).

Physical examination reveals a varying picture depending on the time of presentation and the progression of the disease process. Thus when the situation is of several hours duration, few physical signs are elicited other than that of vague abdominal tenderness. With more advanced disease, signs of extracellular fluid loss and dehydration are readily apparent. The mucous membranes are dry, oliguria is present, and the patient suffers from hypotension and tachycardia. The temperature may be normal or elevated. Hypothermia is an ominous sign and often denotes serious and far advanced disease, with an underlying septic process.

Examination of the chest, heart, and lungs may reveal the presence of co-morbid cardiovascular and respiratory disease.

Examination of the abdomen should be thorough and complete and should include an evaluation from "nipples to knees," with due respect being observed to patient modesty. Localized findings in the abdomen are infrequent apart from vague abdominal guarding and tenderness. Involuntary guarding and rebound tenderness can be expected to be found when the disease process has progressed to a state of generalized peritonitis. Even in elderly patients, however, these signs are often vague and ill defined. Auscultation of the abdomen for bowel sounds initially might reveal the presence of hyperactive rushes and "tinkles," but late in the course of the disease no bowel sounds may be heard. Examination of the inguinal region and hernial orifices and a rectal examination in men and a bimanual pelvic examination in women are all of the utmost importance. Occasionally the rare obturator hernia may be appreciated during the pelvic examination in women.

The presence of accompanying neurologic disorders, such as senile dementia and Parkinson's disease, should make one aware fairly soon that the elicitation of classic symptoms and signs may not be possible. Furthermore these disease processes, together with their attendant forms of therapy, may result in signs and symptoms that resemble those of intestinal obstruction, so-called pseudo-obstruction. The latter process, however, is a diagnosis of exclusion and should only be made when all chances of organic intestinal obstruction have been ruled out. Similarly the presence of surgical abdominal scars, atrial arrythmias, and jaundice might provide clues as to the nature of the obstruction. When a hernia in the groin is thought to be responsible for the problem, especially in obese persons, examination of the patient in the upright position to delineate more clearly the nature of any mass in the groin is important. The liberal use of proctoscopy, and flexible sigmoidoscopy and colonoscopy if indicated, complete the physical examination.

DIAGNOSTIC MEASURES

Initial x-ray studies of the abdomen and chest are likely to provide much useful information. We routinely recommend the so-called obstructive series, in which an upright chest x-ray, supine and upright films of the abdomen, and decubitus views of the abdomen are all obtained. Depending on the site of the obstructing process, a variety of x-ray findings might be seen. In large intestinal obstruction massively dilated loops of large and small intestine are visualized. When the ileocecal valve remains competent only the large intestine is distended with its typical haustral markings. Small intestinal obstruction is characterized by the presence of dilated loops of intestine with characteristic valvulae conniventes accompanied by numerous air fluid levels in a stepladder manner. Intestinal obstructions that are proximal and in the jejunum may demonstrate a nonspecific gas pattern and a distended stomach only. In situations of colonic pseudo-obstruction, or even with true obstruction of the large intestinal lumen, a low-pressure barium enema provides much diagnostic information. In the former situation the barium is seen to preceed proximally to the ileocecal valve without hindrance, whereas in obstruction of the lumen the barium does not pass by the obstructing process.

When air is noticed in the rectum on plain abdominal films, a situation of partial intestinal obstruction might be suspected. Under these circumstances and when there is no question of bowel viability a so-called enteroclysis may be performed. In this procedure thin barium is given orally, and its passage is followed through the intact intestinal tract to demonstrate the point of partial or complete obstruction in its lumen. Other features of note to be sought on x-rays include free air under the diaphragm, which is best seen on upright chest films. Fifty percent of patients with small intestinal obstruction due to gallstones, so-called gallstone ileus, might have air in the biliary tree, and 20% of patients may have the gallstones visualized in a supine view of the abdomen (11). Very few patients with gallstone ileus will have the classic triad of air in the biliary tree, ectopic stones, and small intestinal obstruction. Once again the use of thin barium may make the diagnosis in these patients by demonstrating barium in the biliary tree or in the fistulous tract between the biliary tree and the intestine. Oral and intravenous cholangiography rarely makes the diagnosis in the condition. Clues from the plain x-ray films allow us to make the diagnosis in one-third of patients, whereas contrast studies increase the rate to 80%–90% and are important studies to do when the patient is stable and the diagnosis of gallstone ileus is suspected (11).

Computed tomography, ultrasonography, and angiography are rarely required to make the diagnosis of bowel obstruction except under exceptional circumstances. When acute mesenteric ischemia is thought to be present, transfemoral abdominal aortography may be performed in the emergency setting. Similarly abdominal ultrasonography has been successfully used to diagnose occult herniae of the abdominal wall, such as Spigelian herniae and other such obscure herniae. Injection of contrast agents into the peritoneal cavity to demonstrate a hernial sac has also been used, especially when bilateral herniae are thought to be present.

For both elective hernia repairs and emergency procedures, important laboratory studies, such as a complete blood count, serum electrolyte values, and studies of the coagulation profile, are required before proceeding to the operating room. The results obtained may reflect the sequelae of some chronic co-morbid disease states, such as iron deficiency anemia that is characteristic of large intestinal cancer. Similarly the values vary with the current clinical disease state and may be grossly abnormal. Thus, with intestinal obstruction, the white cell count may be elevated, reflecting an ongoing inflammatory process. Electrolyte abnormalities are common as a result of the fluid shifts between the intracellular and vascular compartments and the extravascular compartmental space (the so-called third space). Although the combination of clinical features, such as an elevated temperature and laboratory values showing grossly elevated white cell counts, has been reported to be predictive of underlying intestinal ischemia and strangulation (12), well-designed prospective studies have failed to confirm these observations (13). Skillful interpretation, however, of the clinical, laboratory, and x-ray findings should provide accurate information and clues to the diagnosis in more than 80%–90% of patients (14).

Other invasive procedures, such as an abdominal tap and peritoneal lavage, occasionally reveal the presence of either purulent material, blood, or the "prune juice" fluid characteristic of mesenteric ischemia with infarction. Occasionally flexible sigmoidoscopy and colonoscopy reveal the absence of an organic obstructing lesion when the patient is suspected of having intestinal obstruction and is found to have pseuso-obstruction. The latter investigation might also reveal the cause of large intestinal obstruction and allow for biopsy, reduction of a volvulus, or the alteration of the approach to the planned therapy.

MANAGEMENT AND THERAPY

The Preoperative Phase

Rather than proceeding with an emergency surgical procedure, it is often prudent to delay the operation 4 to 6 hours to correct the fluid and electrolyte abnormalities and to allow for resuscitation of the elderly patient, especially when a number of co-morbid conditions exist. Thus admission to an acute care ward or to an intensive care unit is often required for these patients, many of whom have been ignored and who have become desperately ill. Immediate measures to relieve nausea and vomiting include the insertion of a nasogastric tube to aspirate air and intestinal contents. A Foley catheter is inserted into the bladder to monitor hourly urine output. Intravenous fluids in the form of dextrose-containing electrolyte solutions should be infused, preferably through catheters placed in large central veins to allow for accurate monitoring of filling pressures within the heart and of the extracellular intravascular compartmental space.

Assessment of Operative Risk

At this point in the resuscitation and management of these patients, an evaluation of operative risk is important to assess the need for the placement of invasive monitoring devices, such as Swan-Ganz catheters and arterial lines (15). A preoperative evaluation scale of the American Society of Anesthesiologists (grade 1–5) has been used to evaluate operative risk in 500 consecutive patients over 80 years of age (16). Mortality rose with increasing grade, and at class 5, (patients with severe life threatening disorders) 25% of patients died. The studies of DelGuercio and Cohn (17) employed an objective preoperative evaluation technique to assess cardiorespiratory risk factors in the elderly and allowed for a more scientific assessment of operative risk and the need for continued invasive monitoring. There are many age-related morphologic changes found in the heart, including conduction defects and valvular abnormalities, but the functional importance of these changes may vary considerably. Compounding these age-related changes are numerous pathologic conditions, the most serious and prevalent of which is atherosclerosis and its attendant sequelae of myocardial infarction and ventricular dysfunction. Similarly there is a normal decline in respiratory function that occurs with aging caused by changes in the chest wall, as well as in the lung. Chest wall compliance decreases, often because of increasing kyphosis, and perhaps is aggravated by vertebral collapse secondary to osteoporosis. Respiratory muscle weakness also is not uncommon and may result in a 50% decrease in maximum inspiratory and expiratory forces generated, with a resulting decrease in the strength of cough. Lung volume and function also change with age as the lung loses its reserve capacity, and many of these physiologic changes caused by increasing age are aggravated by disease processes active in elderly patients (15).

Evaluation and Management of Co-Morbid Conditions

Because more than 20% of elderly patients with emergency abdominal conditions have co-morbid conditions referable most often to cardiovascular or respiratory symptoms, evaluation and management of these disease processes before proceeding to the operating room might greatly influence the outcome. Thus treatment of arrhythmias, and when necessary insertion of a pacemaker, might be important to stabilize pulse and blood pressure. Similarly, uncontrolled hypertension may require the placement of an arterial line and the use of such potent agents as nitroprusside.

Because of the work of DelGuercio and others (17) the use of Swan-Ganz catheters preoperatively in elderly patients has now received wide acceptance, and for the most part the catheters should be used routinely in many emergency circumstances. The use of these catheters allows for both arterial and mixed venous blood gases to be obtained and for the determination of cardiac output. These data allow one to generate a ventricular functional curse, demonstrating left ventricular stroke work as a function of mean pulmonary capillary wedge pressure. On the basis on these data, inotropic agents to improve contractility and cardiac output can be administered, together with volume expansion or depletion to achieve optimal cardiac output. Similarly, patients who are at great risk for postoperative ventilatory failure can be identified early by the obtaining of a number of preoperative pulmonary function tests, of which the forced expiratory volume is the most valuable. When these pulmonary function tests are used with routine arterial blood gases, high-risk patients can be identified and treated appropriately (18).

In elective circumstances, such as routine hernia repairs, patients should be encouraged to cease from all smoking, and preoperative breathing exercises with emphasis on inspiratory efforts should be performed. Preoperative sputum cultures are often useful, as are the availability of humidification of inspired air and the use of nebulized bronchial dilators to keep secretions moist and to decrease bronchial spasm.

The appropriate use of modern monitoring equipment and devices should enable appropriate fluid and electrolyte replacement and maximize optimal renal function. Before going to the operating room an elderly patient needs to be in an ideal state of physiologic balance in order to tolerate the proposed operative procedure and a general anesthetic if such anesthesia is to be used.

Prophylactic Antibiotics

Another measure, perhaps equally important for ensuring a successful outcome, is the use of the appropriate combination of broad spectrum antibiotics. It is now well established that the intestinal microflora undergoes dramatic changes in the presence of intestinal obstruction, and this accounts for the so-called feculent vomitous of which patients with long standing intestinal obstructions often complain. Thus, appropriate broad spectrum antibiotics, to cover both aerobic and anaerobic intestinal flora, should be given intravenously. Single agents, such as second- and third-generation cephalosporins, appear to be adequate in most cases and are attractive choices in the elderly, especially because they provide a good range of broad spectrum coverage without the increase risk of nephrotoxicity. The use of prophylactic antibiotics for elective hernia repairs is rarely justified.

Prophylaxis of Deep Venous Thrombosis

On statistical grounds, all elderly patients, and especially those with an underlying carcinomatosis, are at risk to experience postoperative morbidity from deep venous thrombosis and possibly pulmonary embolism. In a study of hospitalized patients, it has been shown that those older than 60 years of age have a 25% incidence of pulmonary embolism as the primary cause of death, compared to a 3% incidence for those patients younger than 50 years of age (19). Because many of these venous thromboses occur during and after operations, it is prudent to provide some form of prophylaxis prior to, during, and after the operation. A wide variety of such prophylactic measures have been discussed and reported in the literature, with both mechanical external compression devices and the use of subcutaneous low-dose heparin being advocated by various proponents (20). For many elderly patients, early ambulation is the key to prevention once the operative procedure is completed.

Evaluation of Nutritional and Immune Status

Nutrition and immune function also have a bearing on the ability of elderly ill patients to withstand major operative morbidity. A number of physiologic, psychologic, and socio-economic factors influence the nutritional status of the elderly surgically ill population. Furthermore, it is often difficult to distinguish age-related changes in the immune system from altered immune functions caused by nutritional deficiencies. In otherwise healthy elderly patients undergoing elective hernia repairs preoperative immune deficiencies have been difficult to demonstrate by mitogen assay, mixed lymphocyte cultures, skin tests, or levels of immunoglobulins when compared to healthy younger control patients (21). Biochemical measurements of nutritional status do not vary significantly with age. Depressed levels of serum albumin, transferrin, and retinol-binding protein, however, are thought to be accurate indicators of nutritional status. Thus, malnutrition adds an additional burden to a potentially depressed immune system in elderly surgical patients, and it may very well lead to major problems with wound healing and ongoing sepsis in the postoperative period. When time allows and when such operations as elective herniorrhaphy can be deferred, it is of obvious benefit to improve the patient's nutritional status in some way. When nutritional support is thought to be necessary, the enteral route is to be preferred over the intravenous route whenever there is a choice (15). In emergency situations, however, little time is available to provide satisfactory alimentation to a patient who requires an immediate operation.

The Operative Procedure

Anesthesia

It is apparent from large series in which a mix of local, regional, and general anesthetic techniques were used that, for elective operations in the groin, the use of local anesthetic techniques is associated with the lowest incidence of postoperative complications and morbidity (1). However, skillfully applied general endotracheal anesthesia, using modern relaxation techniques, together with the infusion of potent narcotic agents, should allow for the successful recovery of even the most ill patient from a major abdominal exploration. As mentioned previously, the liberal use of invasive monitoring devices greatly aids the anesthesiologist today in intraoperative management so as to ensure that an elderly, seriously ill, surgical patient does survive the operation itself, all other factors being equal.

Abdominal Exploration

Exploratory procedures of the abdomen done on patients with intestinal obstruction due to postoperative adhesions or due to causes other than an incarcerated or strangulated inguinal hernia should be done through a generous midline or transverse incision. Our preference is to use a transverse supraumbilical incision whenever possible, especially when a previous midline incision has been made. The transverse incision allows for adequate exploration of the abdominal cavity and is associated with rapid healing and minimal compromise to respiratory function in the postoperative period. The editors prefer to use a midline incision in most instances.

Careful dissection in the abdominal cavity may be required regardless of the choice of the incision, especially when multiple adhesions are to be found. Proximal dilated loops of intestine should be sought and traced distally to the point of obstruction, where collapsed loops of small and large intestines are encountered. For the most part, gentle handling of the tissue is emphasized; unintentional or even deliberate enterotomies are associated with high postoperative morbidity.

When adhesions are thought to be the obstructing mechanism, simple incision of the adhesive band is usually all that is required. Extensive dissection of other adhesions, the use of techniques to layer the intestine in such a way as to prevent recurrent adhesive obstruction, and the use of long intestinal tubes have not been shown to be of great benefit (22). However, when proximal decompression of dilated fluid-filled loops of intestine is believed to aid the closure of the abdominal wound of entry, use of the Nelson-Nyhus long intestinal tube is preferable to making an enterotomy to facilitate this process (23). When prolonged postoperative intubation and nasogastric suction are anticipated, it might be prudent to perform a gastrostomy before closure of the abdomen to decompress the proximal intestine and to act later as a route for nutrition.

Numerous techniques have been proposed to evaluate the safety of leaving in situ loops of intestine of questionable viability. These methods include fluoroscein studies, Doppler ultrasonic examination, and the injection of radiolabeled microspheres into the mesenteric vasculature (24). None of these measures, however, has replaced experience and sound surgical judgement as to bowel viability. The presence of peristalsis and pulsatile vessels within the mesentery and the color and turgor of the intestinal wall are still the most reliable guides as to whether resection should be undertaken or not. The aphorism, ''when in doubt resect'', still holds should any doubt exist in the experienced surgeon's mind. These ill, frail patients only usually have one opportunity for survival, and a successful operation should be the goal. The opportunity for the surgeon to perform a second-look procedure often does not present itself because the elderly patient may die of ongoing sepsis and acidosis before it can be done.

If during the abdominal exploration, the entire small intestine is found to be dusky and ischemic, heroic measures at revascularization are required. These efforts can be greatly aided, as mentioned previously, by a preoperative aortogram and selective mesenteric arteriograms that might indicate a site of vascular occlusion at the celiac or superior mesenteric artery. Under these circumstances revascularization usually consists of a bypass procedure from the aorta to the artery that is predominantly involved, usually the superior mesenteric artery.

Unexpected internal herniae may be encountered at the time of laparotomy, and often only a minimal procedure is required to effect their cure. Most patients with this finding will have a satisfactory outcome. This subject has been dealt with extensively elsewhere (25).

Gallstone ileus as a cause of small intestinal obstruction is fairly common in elderly patients and should be suspected in most patients whose preoperative history, physical examination, and diagnostic studies have been appropriate. Incision of the intestine proximal to the obstructed stone should be made and the stone delivered proximally. As a rule, in poor risk elderly patients, no attempt should be made to correct the biliary-enteric fistula at the first operative procedure (11).

Hernia Repair

For all obstructing and incarcerated herniae of the groin, the preperitoneal technique is to be used routinely (26). Thus a transverse incision is made approximately 4 to 6 cm superior to the suprapubic ramus and is carried down through the abdominal wall musculature to the preperitoneal space. The hernial sac is seen to be incarcerated in any one of a number of hernial orifices (i.e., inguinal, femoral, or obturator), and skillful sharp dissection is required to reduce the sac and the entrapped viscera back into the abdominal cavity. The peritoneum can then be incised and the contained intestine examined critically for evidence of compromised viability. When the contained viscera do appear normal no further therapy is necessary, and the peritoneum can then be closed with absorbable suture material after excision of the redundant peritoneal sac. When compromise to intestinal viability is thought to be present, a small intestinal resection with an end-to-end anastomosis in a single layer usually suffices. After the return of the viscera to the abdominal cavity, attention can then be given to the herniorrhapy to effect a repair.

For nonrecurrent herniae of the inguinal region, approximation of the transversalis fascia to the ileopubic tract from the posterior approach using monofilament nonabsorbable suture material suffices. For femoral herniae closure of the femoral canal can be accomplished by sutures placed between the ileopubic tract and the tough Cooper's ligament inferiorly. For recurrent inguinal herniae, in addition to the aforementioned closure of the hernial defect, a reinforcing buttress of polypropylene mesh is now used routinely. No recurrences have been noted in long-term follow-up studies (27). For uncomplicated primary indirect and direct inguinal herniae of the groin, we still advocate the anterior approach of Condon to effect a sound repair (28). All primary uncomplicated femoral herniae, however, should be repaired by the posterior preperitoneal approach.

Epigastric, umbilical, incisional, and Spigelian herniae may also give rise to intestinal obstruction in the elderly patient, although they do so rarely. Detailed descriptions of the repair of these herniae have been provided elsewhere (29). In brief, the hernial sac and contained viscera are exposed by sharp dissection, and an attempt is made to define the margins of the fascial defect clearly. After inspection of the contents of the hernial sac and excision of redundant peritoneum, the fascial margins should be closed per primum whenever possible with monofilament nonabsorbable suture. Usually, simple mattress sutures suffice, and complex techniques (i.e., "vest over pants") and the use of a prosthesis (Polypropylene mesh or oxfascia) are rarely required.

Closure of Incision

At the conclusion of the operation, in situations in which the operative procedure has not involved spillage of intestinal contents, the wound may be closed in layers per primum. When there has been some contamination, when an enterotomy has been made, or when frank intestinal gangrene and peritonitis have been encountered, it is prudent to leave the skin and subcutaneous tissues open after the fascial closure. For the most part these patients should have the fascial closure performed with monofilament, long-lasting, absorbable suture material (polydioxane) or nonabsorbable monofilament suture material, such as stainless steel wire or polypropylene.

Treatment of Various Causes of Obstruction

Large intestinal obstructions are largely caused by inflammatory disorders, such as diverticulitis, or malignant disease in the distal colon. For the most part, when time allows, definitive therapy for these diseases should be undertaken because colostomies are associated with high morbidity and mortality in the elderly population (3). In the emergency setting, however, there is little choice other than to perform a resection of the diseased colon and create an end colostomy with a Hartmann procedure. This will effect an immediate relief of the problem at hand. A secondary operation to re-establish intestinal continuity is often not feasible in these elderly patients, especially when widespread carcinomatosis is present at the initial procedure. When the patient makes a satisfactory recovery, however, especially when complications from diverticular disease were the only findings at the initial operation, an attempt to restore intestinal continuity should be made at a later date. The use of the Prasad colostomy technique should greatly facilitate the latter goal (30).

Appendicitis and perforated appendicitis may present in the elderly as a small intestinal obstruction. It is interesting that 72% of elderly patients present with right lower quadrant pain and tenderness, but still have delayed diagnosis and appropriate therapy (31). The mechanism for the bowel obstruction is largely from the perforation of the appendix, with adherence of the small intestine to the periappendiceal phlegmon. A simple appendectomy with drainage of the right lower quadrant is usually all that is required in these circumstances.

Other rare causes of intestinal obstruction include paracolostomy herniae in the elderly. These herniae should always be repaired by relocation of the colostomy aperture within the rectus sheath itself and a repair or complete closure of the initial fascial defect (32).

Giant herniae of the abdominal wall even with incarceration of bowel rarely undergo strangulation. Liberal use of preoperative pneumoperitoneum allows for effective closure of these hernias. Optimal respiratory therapy pre- and postoperatively is very important if these repairs are to be successful (33, 34).

Postoperative Complications and Outcomes

The mortality for general surgical procedures in general increase linearly from the fifth to the tenth decade of life from 8.4% to a high of 22.1% overall. The mortality for elective operations only similarly shows a linear increase from a low of 1.3% for patients younger than 60 years of age to more than 11% for patients older than 89 years of age. The mortality for emergency operations, however, remains at a constant 25%–28% for all patients between 60 and 90 years of age. This mortality has not decreased significantly in 50 years, unlike the elective operative mortality (15).

More specifically, large series of patients who have emergency operations for intestinal obstructions do experience serious complications and a high mortality. Cardiovascular complications are the most frequent and are observed in 21% of patients. These complications include cardiac arrhythmias, digitalis toxicity, and cerebrovascular accidents. Pulmonary complications constitute 20% of the postoperative incidence of morbidity and include pneumonia, atelectasis, and the need for tracheostomy in some patients. Fever and sepsis are seen in 13.6% of patients, and half of the time these complications are caused by wound infections. Genitourinary disorders are not uncommon (8% of patients) and are largely related to episodes of urinary retention and acute renal failure. Patients unfortunate enough to experience acute renal failure also experience a high mortality—40% in some series (9).

In one large series of 300 elderly patients with intestinal obstruction, 84 (28%) of the patients died (9). Most of the patients who died were between 70 and 85 years of age. One-third of the deaths were caused by pneumonia alone; 27% of the deaths were the result of ongoing sepsis and 22% were the result of cardiovascular morbidity. Pulmonary embolism accounted for 6% of all deaths. Mortality and complications rates also are influenced significantly by the disease process present at the time of the operation. Thus, large intestinal obstructions caused by carcinoma carry a mortality of 40% to 50%, as seen on short-term follow-up studies (3, 14). When palliation or colostomy only is performed for intestinal carcinoma, the mortality may rise to 80% (3). Far fewer patients, about 30%, die of localized and resectable carcinomas of the large intestine. These mortality figures for carcinoma are increased significantly also by increasing age, especially for patients older than 70 years of age. No deaths were encountered in the absence of peritonitis or gangrenous intestine (3).

Wound infections are far more common when the skin is closed (21% vs 6%) than when the wound is left open. This is especially so in the presence of a contaminated field and when enterotomies have been made during the operative procedure.

The importance of elective repair of groin herniae in the elderly has been stressed previously. In a large series of 1500 elderly patients who underwent early elective hernia repairs, the complication rate was 2.6%; 14 of these patients died, for a total death rate of 1.3% (1.) Complications encountered included those referable to urinary retention, cardiorespiratory systems, and complications in the wound in 5%–10% of instances. When a hernia operation is undertaken for emergency indications or for small intestinal obstruction, 56% of patients experienced complications; 18 of these patients died, for a death rate of 7.5%. Both this large study and those of others emphasize that (1) elective repair of abdominal wall herniae is safe despite the usual co-morbid conditions in the elderly, (2) a higher morbidity and mortality can be expected with emergency repairs especially where the obstruction occurs in the femoral hernia position, and (3) the lowest complication rates are associated with the use of local anesthesia.

Attention to the appropriate preoperative preparation should obviate many of the cardiovascular and respiratory complications that have been reported in many historical series. Similarly, postoperative wound complications can be avoided by meticulous technique and the avoidance of accidental and even planned enterotomies (12, 14).

Postoperative chest physical therapy, optimization of cardiovascular function using the Swan-Ganz catheter as a guide, and early endotracheal extubation and ambulation are all features of postoperative care that will reduce the prohibitive morbidity and mortality that these elderly patients experience otherwise. Successful application of these newer techniques will reduce the mortality from the current 25% to more acceptable levels.

Less frequent and less severe complications can still be a source of some concern in the postoperative period. The most frequent of these troublesome problems is urinary retention, usually consequent upon occult urinary bladder outlet obstruction. The measurement of urinary flow rates (less than 10 ml per second) in men is a good diagnostic screening test for the presence of bladder outlet obstruction (35). Residual urine estimations are of little value. Thus, urinary retention can be expected to occur in approximately 7% of men undergoing elective hernial repairs. This number is often greatly increased by the use of spinal or regional anesthesia. Conversely, in a large series of men who experienced urinary obstruction due to prostatic hypertrophy (2810 patients) only 5.4% had associated groin herniae (36). Other annoying complications included uncontrolled hypertension, constipation, renal dysfunction, and deep venous thrombosis. An aggressive and dedicated nursing staff is often all that is required to obviate some of these postoperative conditions. (See Chapter 7)

CONCLUSIONS

Worldwide improvements in health care and living conditions have generated a great increase in the population older than 65 years of age. These people will become patients who will not only have elective and emergency clinical problems but also will have numerous degenerative and co-morbid conditions that adversely affect the outcome of any of our surgical endeavors. Sociocultural decisions and ethical and moral issues relating to the quality of life, dignity of death, and the expense to society for the care of these persons have not been addressed in this chapter. These are important issues, and although as physicians we may prefer to turn our attention away from them, society and elderly competent patients themselves are forcing these issues upon us. Especially troublesome are such cases where extensive carcinomatosis or other terminal diseases have already manifested themselves. As practicing physicians and surgeons, we can only advocate the earlier detection and surgical correction of any such disease states, including herniae of the abdominal wall and colonic neoplasms, that might result in intestinal obstruction. The application of these principles, together with the skills and use of modern preoperative, intraoperative, and postoperative therapeutic strategies, should result in a gratifying and successful outcome for most elderly patients with these problems.

Acknowledgements. We thank Ms. Catherine Judge for editorial assistance and Misses Suzanne M. Renfroe and Patricia Merced for the preparation of the manuscript.

REFERENCES

1. Nehme AE: Groin hernias in elderly patients. *Am J Surg* 146:257–260, 1983.
2. Tingwald GR, Cooperman M: Inguinal and femoral hernia repair in geriatric patients. *Surg Gynecol Obstet* 154:704–706, 1982.
3. Reiss R, Deutsch AA: Emergency abdominal procedures in patients above 70. *J Gerontol* 40:154–158, 1985.
4. Gleysteen JJ: Intestinal obstruction. In Condon RE, Nyhus LM (eds): *Manual of Surgical Therapeutics*, ed 2. Boston, Little, Brown and Co, 1985, pp 131–149.
5. Reiss R, Deutsch AA, Eliashiz A: Decision making process in abdominal surgery in the geriatric patient. *World J Surg* 7:522–526, 1983.
6. Blake R, Lynn J: Emergency abdominal surgery in the aged. *Br J Surg* 63:956–960, 1976.
7. Gentile A: The incidence of hernia in the United States. *Industr Med Surg* 31:19–21, 1962.
8. Pollak R, Nyhus LM: Complications of groin hernia repair. *Surg Clinic N Amer* 63:1363–1371, 1983.
9. Greene WW: Bowel obstruction in the aged patient. *Am J Surg* 118:541–545, 1969.
10. Stolar CJH, Randolph JG: Evaluation of ischemic bowel viability with a fluorescent technique. *J Pediatr Surg* 13:221–225, 1978.
11. Balthazar EJ, Schechter LS: Gallstone ileus. *Am J Roentgenol Radium Ther Nucl Med* 125:374–379, 1975.
12. Stewardson RH, Bombeck CT, Nyhus LM: Critical operative management of small bowel obstruction. *Ann Surg* 181:189–193, 1978.
13. Sarr MG, Buckley GB, Zuidema GD: Preoperative recognition of intestinal strangulation obstruction: prospective evaluation of diagnostic capability. *Am J Surg* 145:176–182, 1983.
14. Zadeh BJ, Davis JH, Canizaro PC: Small bowel obstruction in the elderly. *Am Surg* 51:470–473, 1985.
15. Rosenthal RA, Anderson DK: Surgery in the elderly. In Andres R, Bierman EL, Hazzard WR (eds): *Principles of Geriatric Medicine*. New York, McGraw Hill Book Company, 1985, pp 909–932.
16. Djokovic JL, Hedley-Whyte J: Prediction of outcome of surgery and anesthesia in patients over 80. *JAMA* 242:2301–2306, 1979.
17. DelGuercio LRM, Cohn JD: Monitoring operative risk in the elderly. *JAMA* 243:1350–1355, 1980.
18. Hodgkin JE, Dines DE, Didier EP: Pre-operative evaluation of patients with pulmonary disease. *Mayo Clin Proc* 48:114–118, 1975.
19. Morrell MT, Dunhill MS: The post mortem incidence of pulmonary embolism in a hospitalized population. *Br J Surg* 55:347–352, 968.
20. Lee BV, Thoden WR, Trainor FS, Kavner D: Noninvasive detection and prevention of deep vein thrombosis in geriatric patients. *J Am Geriatr Soc* 28:171–175, 1980.
21. Linn BS, Jensen J: Age and immune response to a surgical stress. *Arch Surg* 118:405–409, 1983.
22. Pollack R: Miscellaneous surgical techniques for the small intestine. In Nyhus LM, Baker RJ (eds): *Mastery of Surgery*. Boston, Little Brown and Co, 1984, pp 894–900.
23. Nelson RL, Nyhus LM: A new long intestinal tube. *Surg Gynecol Obstet* 149:581–582, 1979.
24. Pollak R: Strangulating external hernias. In Nyhus LM, Condon RE (eds): *Hernia*, ed 3. Philadelphia, JB Lippincott Co, 1987, (In press).
25. Pollak R, Nyhus LM: The unexpected internal hernia. *Prob Gen Surg* 1:226–237, 1984.
26. Nyhus LM: The preperitoneal approach and iliopubic tract repair of inguinal hernia. In Nyhus LM, Condon RE (eds): *Hernia,* ed 2. Philadelphia, JB Lippincott Co, 1978, pp 212–263.
27. Nyhus LM, Pollak R: Inguinal and femoral hernias. In Beahrs OH, Beart RW (eds): *General Surgery*

Therapy—Update Service. Media, PA, Harwal Publishing Co, 1986, pp 10-1 to 10-25.

28. Condon RE: Anterior iliopubic tract repair. In Nyhus LM, Condon RE (eds): *Hernia,* ed 2. Philadelphia, JB Lippincott Co, 1978, pp 195-211.

29. Pollak R, Nyhus LM: Hernias. In Schwartz SI, Ellis H (eds): *Maingot's Abdominal Operations,* ed 8. Norwalk, CT, Appleton-Century-Crofts, 1985, pp 297-350.

30. Prasad ML, Pearl RK, Abcarian H: End-loop colostomy. *Surg Gynecol Obstet* 158:380-382, 1984.

31. Smithy WB, Wexner SD, Dailey TH: The diagnosis and treatment of acute appendicitis in the aged. *Dis Colon Rect* 29:170-173, 1986.

32. Prian GW, Sawyer RB, Sawyer KC: Repair of peristomal colostomy hernias. *Am J Surg* 130:674-696, 1975.

33. Buddee FW, Coupland GAE, Reeve TS: Large abdominal wall herniae: an easy method of repair without prosthetic material, with the induction of pneumoperitoenum. *Aust NZ J Surg* 45:265-270, 1975.

34. Moreno IG: The rational treatment of hernias and voluminous chronic eventrations: preparation with progressive pneumoperitoneum. In Nyhus LM, Condon RE (eds): *Hernia,* ed 2. Philadelphia, JB Lippincott Co, 1978, pp 536-560.

35. Brugh R, Rous SN: Bladder outlet obstruction and inguinal hernia. *Urology* 19:550-552, 1977.

36. Riches E: Prostatic destruction: the treatment of associated conditions. *Proc Roy Soc Med* 55:744-746, 1962.

Chapter 25

Diseases of the Colon
and Rectum in the Elderly

John L. Sawyers, M.D., F.A.C.S., R. Benton Adkins, Jr., M.D., F.A.C.S.

The anatomic and pathologic changes seen in the aging bowel are similar to those that occur elsewhere in the gastrointestinal tract. In 1965, Yamagta described the anatomic changes of mucosal atrophy, increased connective tissue, and atrophy of the muscular layer in elderly subjects (1). In 1966, Pace reported that the thickness of the colon wall increased with aging and found the same to be true of the amount of elastin in the wall (2).

There is evidence that there is an overall weakness that is predominantly in the circular muscles and that most of the thickening is in the longitudinal layer of the teniae coli. The overall size of the colon increases both in diameter and in length as chronic constipation and "acquired megacolon" develop in those individuals who have poor bowel habits.

Several studies have addressed the question of whether bowel habits change as a person ages (3, 4). The major finding from these studies has been to show that a regular laxative-taking routine develops in the aged, and it is common among most older individuals, especially so among older women. However, constipation is not more common in the elderly patient than in the younger patient, but in immobile, elderly patients who are bedfast or confined to a chair, constipation can be a major problem. Milne and Williamson in a survey found that 70% of the elderly population had one bowel movement a day (4). Transit time through the colon is delayed in elderly people, particularly in those who are immobile. Immobile elderly people develop a condition described as the "terminal reservoir syndrome." The elderly patient lacks the stimulus of mobility to cause mass propulsion that is usually associated with a gastrocolic reflex combined with morning physical activity. Furthermore, the elderly person frequently depends on assistance to allow him or her to reach the toilet. If the call to stool is ignored, the rectal feces move back into the sigmoid colon, and the urge to defecate passes. Stool softeners and purgatives of the anthracene type are probably the most effective in relieving constipation in the elderly patient (5). The excessive use of laxatives may damage the myenteric neurons within the submucosa and intramural layers and result in functional disorders, such as constipation, acquired megacolon, and chronic colon ileus (6). Along with these changes, weakness of the muscularis propria develops at the intramural vascular passageway. These age-associated developments allow for the herniation of colonic mucosa and submucosa to form colonic diverticula alongside the neurovascular bundle. (Fig. 25.1) None of the changes seen in the aging colon seems to affect its absorptive ability.

LOWER GASTROINTESTINAL BLEEDING IN THE ELDERLY

Gastrointestinal bleeding is an important and common problem in elderly patients. In a study of 58 patients presenting with massive lower gastrointestinal bleeding, Cathcart et al. found an average age of 67.6 years (7). Many diseases associated with bleeding, such as diverticulosis, vascular ectasia, and cancer, increase in frequency in the elderly, and therefore the physician must consider a wide range of diseases when evaluating an elderly patient who has lower gastrointestinal bleeding.

Approximately 90% of acute episodes of gas-

355

trointestinal bleeding originate from sites proximal to the ligament of Treitz. Bright red bleeding from the rectum is usually indicative of a colonic or rectal bleeding site. A nasogastric tube should always be placed, however, to investigate the presence of upper gastrointestinal bleeding, although a negative aspirate does not completely rule out this possibility. Upper gastrointestinal endoscopy has been a rapid, accurate method of eliminating the esophagus, stomach, and duodenum as possible bleeding sites.

The evaluation of lower gastrointestinal bleeding should include a sigmoidoscopy and coagulation studies. Colonoscopy is performed if the rate of bleeding persists. In the face of active lower gastrointestinal bleeding an urgent angiographic study of the superior mesenteric, inferior mesenteric, and celiac arteries in this order is performed. Barium enema and small bowel series are deferred until after angiography (8). Infusion of technetium-tagged red cells is preferred by us as an initial evaluation in the slowly bleeding patient prior to the use of angiography.

The elderly patient does not tolerate episodes of bleeding as well as younger individuals. Therefore, stabilization and blood loss replacement are even more critical in the elderly patient. Immediate exploratory laparotomy is an avenue for diagnosis *and* treatment that may be necessary for patients in whom the bleeding continues and is not readily controlled.

If selective arteriography localizes the site of the bleeding, vasopressin can be infused at the time of arteriography into the vessels of the bleeding area. This technique is sometimes effective, but its benefit is often temporary. Matolo and Link have suggested the use of transcatheter embolization in selected patients in whom vasopressin infusion has failed and/or who are poor surgical risks (9). They have selectively embolized bleeding vessels using Gelfoam plugs or autologous clot. They further suggest that operative intervention can then be considered after the patient's bleeding is controlled and the operation can be done electively.

If the arteriogram demonstrates evidence of a vascular abnormality, such as an angiodysplastic lesion or ectasia, then this area may be removed electively. Such lesions are generally found in the right side of the colon, and right hemicolectomy is the preferred procedure. Even if the patient is not actively bleeding, an angiogram may identify a vascular ectatic lesion, which can be resected when the patient is brought to optimal condition for operation. It should be remembered that angiographic changes of the vessels within a cancer of the colon may mimic angiodysplasia. This makes elective resection an even more appropriate method of treatment.

When all studies including the angiogram are normal and the patient is still actively bleeding, urgent colectomy is performed with ileoproctostomy.

DIVERTICULOSIS

The incidence of diverticulosis steadily increases after age 40 and becomes more common in patients 60 and older (10). Approximately one-third of the population over age 45 has been estimated to have diverticular disease (11). Autopsies of patients 80 and older suggest an incidence of more than 50% in that age group (12).

The incidence of diverticulosis is significantly less in Africa and Asia than it is in the West. Apparently populations that have a diet high in vegetable fiber are protected from the development of diverticula (13). Persons on this diet do, however, develop colon volvulus at a very high rate!

In most cases (45%–65%) diverticular disease is confined to the sigmoid colon. Grossly, the colon involved with diverticulosis appears to be shortened and thickened. Upon examination, both the longitudinal and circular muscle show abnormally thickening, and the diameter of the lumen is decreased. The origin of the diverticula is found to be between the folds of the circular muscle fibers and adjacent to the teniae coli. If the bowel has been inflamed, fibrous tissue will also be evident (14).

Most individuals with diverticular disease never experience symptoms from the disorder. Only one of 70 will need hospital care for acute attacks of diverticulitis, and only one in 200 will require surgical treatment (15). Inflammation may spread along the serosa of the colon and eventually lead to the formation of adhesions in some cases. Other organs that might become adherent to the colon are therefore easily involved in the inflammatory process. Approximately 12%–25% of patients with inflammatory diverticular disease will develop a fistula, usually a vesicocolic fistula (14). If repeated episodes of diverticulitis are allowed to continue to recur, the colon will eventually obstruct due to increased fibrosis and stricture formation (16).

Bleeding is a very common consequence of diverticulosis, because of the proximity of the diverticulum to the blood vessels of the colon. (Fig. 25.1) It is likely that inflammation plays a part in this particular complication also. Usually the bleeding is substantial and always intraluminal (17).

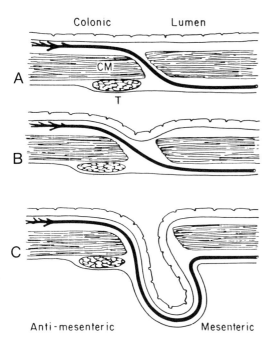

Figure 25.1. Structural dynamics of diverticular formation and vascular relationships. **A,** The long branch of the vas rectum penetrates the colonic wall through an obliquely oriented connective tissue gap in the circular muscle **(CM).** This occurs near the mesenteric side of a tenia **(T),** a longitudinal muscle band. **B,** Early mucosal protrusion widens the connective tissue cleft and begins to lift up the artery. **C,** With transmural extension of the diverticulum, the vas rectum is displaced over its fundus and penetrates to the submucosa on the antimesenteric side of its neck and orifice. (Reproduced with permission from Meyers MA, et al: Pathogenesis of bleeding colonic diverticulosis. *Gastroenterology* 71:577-583, 1976.)

Treatment of Diverticular Disease

The medical management of inflammatory diverticular disease with antibiotics and bowel rest is successful in most cases, but this inflammatory process, once it occurs, is almost always recurrent. Repeated acute episodes may result in extensive fibrosis and stenosis, leading eventually to colon obstruction. A high fiber diet aids in reducing the frequency of acute attacks of diverticulitis. Alexander and his colleagues at the University of Chicago reviewed 693 patients with diverticular disease and found that only 14% required surgical management (18). The most common indication for surgical intervention in their study was pericolic abscess. This was followed by bleeding, obstruction, and perforation as the causes for urgent or emergency surgical treatment. More than 50% of these operations were considered to be emergencies, and another 15% were urgent. We would agree with them, however, that older patients who have chronic, recurring episodes of bleeding and obstruction or in whom cancer cannot be ruled out should be managed with elective colon resection and primary anastomosis. In the absence of massive contamination and extensive inflammation, Alexander recommends a single-stage procedure (18). In their group of 44 patients managed by definitive resection and primary anastomosis, postoperative morbidity was low, no patient died, and the hospital stays were shorter.

Morgenstern and his colleagues have recognized an extremely severe form of diverticulitis that occurs primarily in the older age groups (19). They have called this variation "malignant" diverticulosis. It is characterized by (1) phlegmonous inflammation; (2) fistulazation to skin, bladder, or small bowel; (3) colonic obstruction; and (4) high postoperative morbidity and mortality. Clinically, it is very similar to granulomatous colitis. These authors suggest a conservative two- or three-stage surgical approach for these patients who have this severe form of diverticulitis as the safest plan of management.

Another complication that is rare but that also is seen largely in older patients is the formation of giant diverticula, usually on the antimesenteric border of the colon. The etiology of these large diverticula is unclear. Gallagher and Welch report that the symptoms of giant diverticula are similar to those of diverticulitis but that perforation is more likely to result in generalized peritonitis, rather than localized abscesses or inflammation (20). They recommend elective resection for all cases of giant diverticula in order to avoid an emergency operation.

COLONIC VOLVULUS

Of all patients in the United States and Western Europe who have intestinal obstruction, 3%–5% will have colonic volvulus as the etiologic factor. In Russia, India, and Eastern Europe, the incidence of colonic volvulus increases dramatically and results in 30%–50% of all cases of intestinal obstruction (6). This may be due in part to the bulky high fiber diet that is very common in that geographic region, which has been called by some the "volvulus belt."

Colonic volvulus is more common in older people than in younger individuals, and it usually affects the sigmoid colon in the elderly patient. Volvulus occurs at three major sites in the colon: about 75% in the sigmoid colon, 20% in the cecum, and 5% in the transverse colon (11). There are many factors that leave the elderly patient susceptible to the development of a colon volvulus. Enlargement of the colon, which can lead to volvulus, is not uncommon in the elderly and is the cause of most cases, especially in those patients who are physically inactive or institutionalized.

When managed nonoperatively, colon volvulus will likely recur. Arnold and Nance report a 55% recurrence rate of sigmoid volvulus in patients seen in the Charity Hospital in New Orleans (21). Elective resection is especially important in the elderly who are at a much higher operative risk with emergency procedures.

Diagnosis of Volvulus

Geriatric patients are susceptible to development of an asymptomatic "pseudo-megacolon" because of swallowing air, laxative abuse, and chronic constipation. The bowel becomes too long for its mesentery. The mesentery itself is then stretched and elongated, and this long, thinned pedicle has a disproportionate "short

base" upon which the sigmoid, cecum, or transverse colon can rotate. The pre-twisted or partially rotated condition of the bowel usually remains asymptomatic for years until volvulus occurs. The closed loop obstruction will lead to gangrene, perforation, and peritonitis if the volvulus is not promptly corrected.

Colonic volvulus is characterized by abdominal distention, tenderness, abdominal mass, and x-ray evidence of air in a distended loop of colon, which is described as the "bent inner tube" sign. Air fluid levels may be present in the distended small bowel. Barium enema contrast studies show a narrowing of the proximal rectum at the site of the obstruction, resulting in a "bird beak" deformity. Acute volvulus rapidly results in dehydration, fever, and electrolyte problems that progress to shock. The differential diagnosis includes toxic dilation of the colon, pseudo-obstruction (Ogilvie's syndrome), and distal colonic obstruction from tumor or anal stenosis.

Treatment

Once the diagnosis is suspected, measures to rehydrate, decompress the stomach and bowel, and correct the electrolyte imbalance should be begun. A sigmoid volvulus may be decompressed 70%–90% of the time by passing a rectal tube through the rigid sigmoidoscope. The rectal tube must be left in place for several days. A flexible colonoscope may be used, especially for volvulus of the transverse colon and cecum (22–25). If reduction of the volvulus is successful, there is a forceful evacuation of flatus and bowel contents. The operator is best advised to wear a protective gown and consider a face shield. Following successful reduction by endoscopy, the patient should be prepared for elective colon resection because of the high recurrence rate of colonic volvulus (60%–90%) (26). These nonoperative maneuvers should not be tried if there is questionable perforation, vascular compromise, suspected bowel necrosis, or peritonitis.

If nonoperative measures are unsuccessful emergency laparotomy, in spite of age, is indicated as soon as the situation will permit. If the bowel can be resected before gangrene, perforation, and peritonitis occur, the prognosis is usually good.

In 1985, Ballantyne and co-workers reported a series of patients with colon volvulus that covered the 20 years from 1960 to 1980 (25). Fifty percent were sigmoid, 40% cecal, and 3% were transverse colon or splenic flexure. Overall mortality was 14%, 17% for cecal, and 7% for sigmoid. These authors recommend elective laparotomy and resection of the involved segment of colon with primary anastomosis. If colon viability is in question, resection with colostomy, ileostomy, or appropriate other decompression is used, and re-anastomosis is planned for a later operation.

Cecal Volvulus

Although less common than sigmoid volvulus, cecal volvulus constitutes the surgical emergency situation because of the danger of cecal perforation. The "rule of nine" has been a standard, meaning that when the diameter of the cecum reaches 9 cm, the possibility of cecal perforation is greatly increased.

Cecal volvulus is generally thought to be due to incomplete fusion of the cecum to the parietal peritoneum. Torsion of the ileocecal intestinal segment usually occurs, with counter-clockwise rotation displacing the ileum and upward folding of the cecum in the so-called cecal bascule fashion. The diagnosis can usually be made with the presentation of a patient who has abdominal distention and the typical roentgenographic findings. On palpation of the abdomen, the right iliac fossa is generally found to be empty. Bowel sounds are typical of obstruction. A barium enema will help make the diagnosis.

Although attempts at reduction of cecal volvulus by colonoscopy have been reported, the preferred treatment is urgent laparotomy with detorsion of the cecal volvulus. If the bowel is viable, the colon may be fixed by cecopexy or a "blow-hole" cecostomy. Our preference is resection of the right colon with primary end-to-end anastomosis. The recurrence rate following cecopexy has been reported to be about 30%. Todd reports no recurrence rate in 31 patients managed by cecostomy. His overall mortality rate with cecal volvulus was 22.5%—14.5% if the bowel was viable and 41.2% mortality when the torsed cecum was gangrenous (27).

INFLAMMATORY BOWEL DISEASES

Crohn's Disease

Kyle has shown a small increase in the incidence of Crohn's disease in the sixth and seventh decades of life (28). Others have also noticed an increase in new cases in patients over age 60 (29). Most older patients are women and are likely to have involvement of the left colon (5).

Presenting symptoms are similar to those seen in patients who have diverticulitis and may include pain, diarrhea, and bleeding (30). Even the radiographic findings of Crohn's disease of the colon can be similar in appearance to those of diverticular disease.

Pathologic characteristics of Crohn's include inflammatory involvement of all layers of the bowel wall. Giant cell or epitheloid granulomas are usually present, and the formation of fissures or fistulae is not uncommon. Transmural fibrosis and inflammation are also major pathologic features.

Most patients, young and old, who have Crohn's disease are not seriously debilitated. Mayberry reported that 81% of patients in his study of Crohn's disease were employed full-time and that the amount of sick leave taken by this group was comparable to that of the total population (31).

Carr and Schofield reported that in their experience elderly patients with inflammatory bowel disease had an increased incidence of complications and an increased mortality when compared to younger patients (32). They stressed, therefore, the need for early, elective, surgical management. On the other hand, Gupta and colleagues determined that the majority of their 14 elderly patients with Crohn's disease were successfully managed medically (30). Surgical treatment in their study was reserved for complications of the disease. We would, like others (33), suggest that for older patients in whom medical management is not successful, surgical intervention should not be long withheld. If done under elective, controlled conditions, the elderly patient will tolerate bowel resection well and will then be able to avoid many of the serious complications of neglected Crohn's disease. In fact, it has been suggested that patients aged 60 or more who develop Crohn's disease are more likely to respond well to surgical treatment than are younger patients (34, 35).

Ulcerative Colitis

The occurrence of ulcerative colitis peaks between the ages of 20 and 40 and again between 60 and 65 years (11). This disease produces symptoms of severe, often bloody diarrhea and is associated with abdominal pain. Weight loss and anemia are not uncommon.

Pathologic involvement of the colon with ulcerative colitis usually begins at the rectum with diffuse mucosal ulceration. The ulcerative lesions bleed easily, and eventually all normal mucous membrane in the colon is replaced by the inflammatory process. The bowel wall becomes thickened and rigid as scar tissue develops. The granulomas associated with typical Crohn's disease are absent.

Medical therapy for ulcerative colitis includes dietary restrictions, steriods, and Azulfidine. When conservative management is unsuccessful, colon resection is indicated. When appropriately employed, surgical management generally results in alleviation of the symptoms associated with ulcerative colitis. If the rectum is disease free and can be safely spared, the elderly patient, like the younger one, should enjoy the benefit of an ileoproctostomy (36). The older, active individual would have the same difficult adjustment to a permanent colostomy that a younger individual experiences.

When surgical intervention is necessary as an emergency condition because of bleeding, perforation, or the development of toxic megacolon, the choice of procedure should be tailored to fit the patient's condition. A subtotal colectomy with end ileostomy and mucous fistula is usually indicated for situations of acute perforation. When there is massive bleeding, a total proctocolectomy is a definite consideration because of the probability that any remaining rectum will continue to bleed or will re-bleed. For toxic megacolon, a total proctocolectomy and ileostomy are the procedures of choice if perforation has not occurred. If there is free peritoneal perforation, subtotal colectomy, ileostomy, and sigmoid mucous fistula should be done. Ileo-anal pull through with ileal pouch has not been as successful in the older patient who has trouble adjusting to frequent stools. Proctocolectomy with a Brooke ileostomy is preferable in the elderly patient.

The complications of perforation and bleeding are poorly tolerated and can be devastating in all patients, especially the elderly (37, 38). Reiss and Deutsch found that the mortality rate for emergency procedures in which peritonitis was present was 32% compared to 8% in emergency cases in which peritonitis was not present (39). Therefore, in the older, otherwise healthy patient with ulcerative colitis, an early, aggressive, surgical approach may do much to preserve the well-being and lifestyle of the patient.

An equally important indication for early surgical treatment for patients with inflammatory bowel disease is the risk of colon cancer developing in the presence of ulcerative colitis and Crohn's disease (40, 41). Levinson and coworkers studied the risk of cancer developing in adults with ulcerative colitis (42). They found that in patients who had a 10-year history of the disease, the risk was 5%. This increased to 25% in 20 years and continues to rise as time goes on. Lightdale and Winawer estimate that the risk increases approximately 20% per decade (43). Although the symptoms of colonic carcinoma and inflammatory bowel disease are very similar, there are clinical features that might lead the physician to suspect a carcinoma. These include abrupt exacerbation of symptoms, new symptoms of bowel obstruction, abdominal pain not associated with defecation, unusual onset of constipation, palpable abdominal mass, and stricture formation (11).

Granular Proctitis

A form of granular proctitis occurring in older patients presents with an endoscopic appearance similar to ulcerative colitis (5). These patients have mild, intermittent symptoms characterized by moderate diarrhea and bleeding. The inflammatory process usually does not extend proximal to the distal sigmoid colon. Rectal biopsies of the diseased areas show a marked increase in cells containing IgE in the lamina propria (44). These patients usually respond favorably to medical management, such as steroid enemas.

VASCULAR DISORDERS OF THE COLON

Because atherosclerotic disease is a natural

process of aging, it is not surprising that ischemic disease of the colon occurs in the elderly. Both acute and chronic ischemic changes can affect the large bowel.

Mesenteric Vascular Occlusion

Acute Mesenteric Ischemia

Acute mesenteric vascular occlusion is usually secondary to an embolus. With the increased incidence of heart disease in elderly people, mural thrombi from the left ventricle following myocardial infarction or from a left atrium in fibrillation are the most frequent source of the emboli. Dissecting aortic aneurysms and arteriosclerotic occlusion of the superior or inferior mesenteric arteries may also be a precipitating factor of acute mesenteric occlusion. The patient is seized by sudden, severe abdominal pain usually associated with bloody diarrhea and the sudden onset of a shock-like state. A major embolus will rapidly result in infarction of the colon and requires emergency operation with surgical resection of the non-viable bowel. Proximal colostomy with later re-establishment of colonic continuity, if possible, is advised.

Acute superior mesenteric artery embolus is the etiologic factor in approximately 50% of the cases of acute intestinal ischemia (45). Almost half of these patients will admit to having had abdominal pain in the past weeks (46). These patients will then experience severe abdominal pain and rectal bleeding. A generalized abdominal pain then ensues; ileus and peritonitis follow. Death is certain in the absence of aggressive surgical intervention and is a real possibility in any instance (47).

Chronic Mesenteric Ischemia

Chronic mesenteric vascular ischemia occurs when atherosclerotic changes progress and occlusion results with obstruction of the major intestinal branches from the aorta. A characteristic syndrome known as abdominal angina may be seen. This is characterized by the presence of postprandial abdominal pain, usually occurring 20 to 30 minutes after eating and lasting for 2 to 3 hours. Patients dread eating and have weight loss and eventual malnutrition. Diarrhea, nausea/vomiting, and abdominal bloating are nonspecific symptoms. Physical findings are minimal, but occasionally an abdominal bruit may be heard on auscultation. The diagnosis may be confirmed by arteriogram that will show occlusion of at least two of the major visceral vessels. Surgical therapy is indicated to improve blood supply to the intestinal tract usually by a bypass procedure, but occasionally reimplantation of the artery or arterial endarterectomy may be performed.

Ileus is evident radiographically early in the disease. Barium enema shows spasm, irritability, thickening of the haustra, and submucosal hemorrhage. When necrosis of the mucosa occurs, ulceration then follows. As the disease progresses further, fibrosis and stricture will result.

Mild forms of this disorder may resolve spontaneously and result only in the fibrous stricture. Other cases will progress to fulminant gangrene that requires immediate, aggressive surgical intervention. Immediate resection of all affected areas of the colon is mandatory; primary anastomosis is usually not done under these circumstances (47).

A fair number of patients will present with pain and/or diarrhea without signs of perforation or clinical decline. In these situations, conservative management including IV fluids and intestinal decompression may be appropriate. Careful monitoring is extremely important in the elderly patient who might tolerate a complication and emergency operation poorly. If improvement is not evident within 48 hours, surgical management must be employed to avoid a lethal situation.

Non-occlusive vascular occlusion occurs from a low-flow state in patients with congestive cardiac failure, anoxia, and shock. Mesenteric blood flow is preferentially shunted to the brain and other vital organs, resulting in ischemic necrosis of the bowel. Angiography will show no occlusion of the vessels, but there may be spasm, narrowing, and irregularity of the vessels. Infusion of vasodilators and correction of the low-flow state are indicated. Surgical intervention is performed only if infarction of the intestine is strongly indicated, thereby requiring resection.

Ischemic Colitis

A clinical syndrome of abdominal pain and rectal bleeding associated with localized areas of colonic ischemia is known as ischemic colitis.

This is usually seen in elderly patients. The lesion usually involves the splenic flexure and descending colon. The disease is highly variable, depending upon the extent of disruption of blood supply to the colon. The onset may be acute with abdominal pain and bloody diarrhea, or a gradual onset of symptoms may be seen leading to a confusing diagnostic dilemma. The vascular lesion primarily involves the small arteries. Barium enema shows a characteristic appearance of intramural edema and hemorrhage. These lesions have been described as "thumbprinting." The disease is usually mild and subsides with non-operative treatment, which should be initially tried; it consists of stabilizing the patient and administering appropriate antibiotics. Occasionally a residual stricture results that will require surgical correction. Patients who develop acute fulminant stage of ischemic colitis may require emergency colectomy. The disease needs to be differentiated from inflammatory bowel disease. Ischemia may be the cause of an elderly patient's first episode of colitis. Angiography may be helpful, but frequently will not detect arterial occlusion that is localized to the small blood vessels. Barium enema is more often not helpful in this diagnosis.

Vascular Ectasias

Colonic angiodysplasias are reported with increasing frequency in the elderly. This lesion appears to be an ectasia of normal vasculature, rather than a malformation. Initially, the submucosal veins become dilated followed by dilation of the venules and capillaries (48). These ectasias are usually multiple, occurring in the right colon and cecum. Boley and associates believe that these degenerative lesions are produced by chronic, partial, intermittent, and low grade obstruction of the submucosal veins (48). This occurs repeatedly over many years during intestinal contraction and distention. As the capillary rings dilate, the competency of the precapillary sphincters is diminished, resulting in an arteriovenous communication. This final structural change results in the angiographic picture of "early filling veins." Whenever this condition is seen on arteriogram, it must always be remembered that some of these venous filling lesions will actually be vessels within cancer of the colon. In these instances, the vessels will be

tumor vessels, rather than vascular ectasias.

Vascular ectasias may sometimes be diagnosed at the time of colonoscopy, but in many cases, angiography is necessary for determining the presence of these lesions. Boley and co-workers have suggested that, when an elderly patient presents with active lower gastrointestinal bleeding and the site of the bleeding is not identifiable with NG suction or lower gastrointestinal hemorrhage, angiography should be done before barium enema or other studies (8). In cases in which the bleeding has stopped, the arteriogram may be deferred until after contrast intestinal x-ray studies are done. These authors recommend right hemicolectomy in all patients who have had an episode of bleeding and who have angiographic evidence of vascular ectasia.

Vasculitis of the Colon

Vasculitis with extensive necrosis of the small and large intestine can occur as a complication of rheumatoid disease, systemic lupus erythematosus, and polyarteritis nodosa. With vasculitis, patchy gangrene of the bowel occurs that is not reversible. Resection is necessary for survival, and even then the results can be dismal.

RECTAL PROLAPSE

Rectal prolapse occurs more frequently in elderly or debilitated patients. The basic problem is an unusually mobile rectum that moves freely into a vertical plane to form a straight tube in continuity with the rectosigmoid colon and anus. Increased intra-abdominal pressure with the rectum in this position results in an intussusception that protrudes through the anus as a prolapse of the rectum. Broden and Snellman agree with this concept of rectal prolapse resulting from an intussusception of the colon because of a laxity of the posterior attachments of the rectum (49).

Several procedures have been used to correct rectal prolapse. These include the Ripstein procedure (50), the Altemeier procedure (51), rectosacral suture fixation (52), and the modified Thiersch (53). In older patients who are unable to withstand a laparotomy, perineal resection procedures, such as the Altemeier operation, may be warranted. Whenever possible, however, we prefer the Ripstein procedure (transabdominal rectopexy) because of its definitive nature and the low recurrence rate (0%–10%) associated with it (54, 55). The Ripstein procedure secures the rectum into the hollow of the sacrum by a Teflon or marlex sling. This restores and maintains the normal posterior course of the rectum and prevents intussusception with subsequent prolapse.

ACUTE APPENDICITIS IN THE ELDERLY

As the proportion of elderly individuals in the general population has increased, so has the percentage of elderly patients who have acute appendicitis. Peltokallio and Tykka found the proportion of their patients aged 60 and older with appendicitis had risen from 4.6% to 8.8% in the years between 1975 and 1980 (56). Appendicitis in older individuals is more difficult to diagnose and is associated with a higher incidence of perforation than in younger patients. The incidence of perforation has also increased signficantly within the older age group. In Peltokallio's study, the incidence of perforation in older patients increased from 32.8% to 43.7%. In younger patients, they found that the incidence of perforation had increased also, but to a lesser degree than that seen in the older age group (56). Some authors have suggested that the symptoms of acute appendicitis are different in older patients from those seen in the young. Others have not found this to be true (56, 57). Peltokellio and Tykka also found the duration of the symptoms of acute appendicitis to be approximately the same in both age groups (56). The only significant difference in the symptoms of acute appendicits between young and older individuals is that there seems to be a faster progression of the disease in older patients. Peltokallio and Tykka suggest that this may be because of sclerotic arteries, atrophied mucous membranes, and scanty lymphatic tissue in the older appendix (56). These changes, coupled with the older person's tendency to delay seeking medical attention and perhaps a hesitancy by the physician to risk surgical intervention in an older patient, are all probably the combined reasons for the increased risk of perforation in these patients.

The mortality rate of elderly patients who have acute appendicitis is usually greater than 4% compared to less than 1% in the general population (56, 58). An aggressive diagnostic approach with early operation is the most effective method of managing appendicitis in the elderly.

COLON RESECTION IN THE ELDERLY

Most studies that have been done to evaluate intestinal operations in the elderly reflect a relatively higher postoperative mortality than seen in younger patients. This is especially true in emergency situations (59, 60). Greenburg and co-workers reviewed 464 patients, 163 of whom were 70 years of age or older (61). Emergency procedures were associated with an increased mortality; they suggest that the most effective way of avoiding the mortality associated with emergency procedures is to avoid emergency procedures. They promote an aggressive elective surgical approach. Of the patients who were 70 and older, those who died differed significantly from those who survived in the area of concomitant disease. Pre-existing renal and hepatic disease was much less common in the group of survivors than it was in the nonsurvivors. Likewise, Boyd and his associates found an 11-fold increase in postoperative mortality in patients over 70 year of age who had two or more diseased or abnormal physiologic systems (62).

Greenburg also examined the subgroup of patients who were 70 years of age or older who were without concomitant pulmonary, renal, hemopoeitic, and cardiac disease (61). The operative mortality in this group was 4%, which compared favorably to the mortality rate of 3.2% for patients younger than 70. They then concluded that age alone could be only a minor factor in operative risk in patients in whom the critical support systems are intact.

Blake and Lynn reviewed a series of 376 patients over 75 years of age undergoing emergency abdominal operations (63). The overall mortality of 31.7% was unrelated to age, but was related to the severity of the surgical condition and to cardiorespiratory complications.

Boyd and his associates reviewed operative risk factors in 357 patients over 50 years of age undergoing colon resection in West Virginia hospitals (62). Mortality rate (4.8%) correlated with the number of pre-existing conditions and not with age. There were no deaths in patients with no pre-existing conditions. The rate of infectious complications increased directly with the number of emergency operations. Morbidity and mortality rates in elderly patients undergoing colon resection may be lowered by careful preoperative assessment, correction of pre-existing pulmonary and nutritional deficiencies, and elective rather than emergency operations.

Cohen reported similar results in 101 patients aged 70 years or older undergoing colon resection (64). Complications occurred in 27.7%. The mortality rate was 4.95%, but no patient who underwent elective colon resection died. Elective colon resection can be performed safely in the elderly patient with careful preoperative evaluation and monitoring. Emergency operation has a higher mortality, especially from sepsis.

NEOPLASMS OF THE COLON AND RECTUM IN THE ELDERLY

Whenever the elderly patient has a complaint, history, signs, symptoms, or laboratory value, such as low hematocrit, that suggest a colon lesion, it should be investigated. Diarrhea, melena, anemia, frank rectal bleeding, abdominal pain, iron deficiency, guaiac positive stools, or change in bowel habits can all result from a benign or malignant colon tumor. The discovery of a benign neoplasm, or an atypical cell type adenoma, or a small Dukes' A cancer of the rectum or colon in an elderly patient is tantamount to saving him or her from a life-threatening series of events. Any of the previously mentioned symptoms in a younger person would most likely lead to a thorough, exhaustive search, but in individuals from the age group in which most of these lesions are found, there has been a tendency to procrastinate.

A stool exam that is positive for blood in an elderly patient on a meat-free diet for 5 days is due to neoplasm 50% of the time if an iron deficiency is also present. Rigid sigmoidoscopy will reveal a polyp in 5% to 10% of elderly adults. The flexible fiberoptic scope allows the surgeon to visualize the rectum and sigmoid colon with an even higher yield of discovering colorectal neoplasms.

The distribution of colon polyps is more widespread through the colon than previously suspected. This is true not only of polyps but is also true for cancer (65, 66). Bernstein and his colleagues in 1985 reported a study of polyp distribution in the elderly (67). They have shown a marked tendency for a change in distribution from rectosigmoid in the young patient to a right colon location for lesions in the elderly. (Figs. 25.2 and 25.3)

When a polyp, adenoma, area of ulceration, fungating lesion, or submucosal lesion is found, a biopsy or total removal should be done. If a rectal polyp or benign lesion is found in the rectum or sigmoid colon, there is a 30%–40% chance of another tumor being present elsewhere in the colon (68). An air contrast barium enema and/or colonoscopy should then be done to rule out other lesions.

Colonoscopy is useful to confirm positive barium enema findings, look for other lesions, do biopsies on lesions higher than the sigmoid, remove polyps, and to confirm negative findings of barium enema. Once a cancer or a benign polyp has been removed, colonoscopy or barium enema should be done yearly.

Benign Tumors

Polyps of the colon are the most common benign lesions. Ninety percent are hyperplastic and 10% neoplastic if all lesions less than 0.5 cm are examined. For lesions above 1 cm, 50% are neoplastic, and 1-cm polyps have a 10% chance of being malignant (69).

In elderly patients, the hyperplastic, inflammatory, and infectious polyps are the most frequently found benign lesions. An occasional lipoma, leiomyoma, and fibroma will be located (70, 71). The juvenile polyp is rare in adults, but occasionally a mixed juvenile-adenomatous polyp will be seen in the elderly. Berg and coworkers emphasize that the true identity of all "colon polyps" must be made by histologic examination and that only then can their behavior be predicted (72). This is an extremely important aspect of these lesions in the elderly in whom a large percentage of the "benign" tumors may have undergone malignant change. All polypoid, sessile, or ulcerated lesions of the colon should be removed or biopsied through the sigmoidoscope or colonoscope. All benign tumors that are

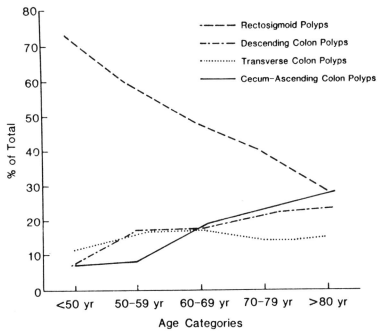

Figure 25.2. Percentage distribution of polyps by age, illustrating the decreasing incidence of rectosigmoid lesions and increase in lesions of the cecum and ascending colon. (Reproduced with permission from Bernstein MA, et al: Distribution of colonic polyps: increased incidence of proximal lesions in older patients. *Radiology* 155:35–38, 1985.)

symptomatic, enlarging, bleeding, or of uncertain etiology should be removed even if this requires a laparotomy with colon resection.

Malignant Tumors

The elderly patient is more apt to have a colon or rectal cancer than a younger person, with 25% of all cases of colon cancer occurring in patients over the age of 70 (73–75). Of those cases occurring in persons over 70 years of age, about 25% will be in patients above age 80. (Figs. 25.4 and 25.5) In high risk groups of elderly patients with anemia, melena, history of colon cancer, history of colon adenoma, ulcerative colitis, and Crohn's disease, patients should be studied every 6 months alternatively by barium enema and colonoscopy such that each of those are done each year until the patient no longer fits a high risk category. Once an adenoma is found, there is a 30%–50% chance that another will appear. If adenomas are allowed to grow to greater than 1 cm in size, the risk of cancer is increased. Adenomas that are 2 cm in diameter have a 35%–45% rate of malignancy. The incidence of cancer increases to 40%–60% in villous adeno-

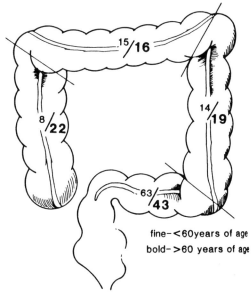

Figure 25.3. Percentage of lesions before and after the age of 60. The marked increase in right-sided lesions and decrease in rectosigmoid lesions are statistically significant. (Reproduced with permission from Bernstein MA, et al: Distribution of colonic polyps: increased incidence of proximal lesions in older patients. *Radiology* 155:35–38, 1985.

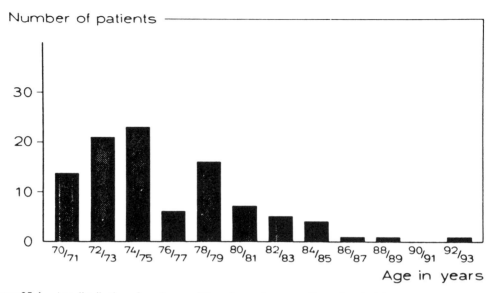

Figure 25.4. Age distribution of carcinoma of the colon and rectum. (Reproduced with permission from Wobbes TH: Carcinoma of colon and rectum in geriatric patients. *Age Aging* 14:321–326, 1985.)

mas (76). In patients who have had a previous cancer of the colon, 3%–5% will have another cancer. Patients who have had previous breast cancer are at increased risk for development of a colon cancer.

The distribution of cancer of the colon and rectum in the elderly is about the same as in the younger age group (Fig. 25.5), with some groups reporting a higher incidence of cancer in the right colon in the elderly (77).

Some observers report that cancer of the colon behaves less aggressively in the older patient (77,

78), but this is not the case (73). Because a 70-year-old person is expected to live another 10+ years and an 80-year-old person more than 6 years, it is our policy to do as aggressive or perhaps a little extra resection in the very old than we do in the very young because their tumors tend to present in more advanced stages probably due to delay in diagnosis (73, 79). We agree with Mettlin and associates that the tumors tend to behave about the same for each stage of presentation, regardless of the age, but that colon cancer in the very young patient and the very old patient is not recognized until late (80).

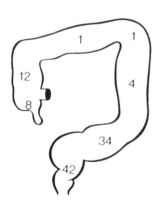

Figure 25.5. Anatomic distribution of the tumors. (Reproduced with permission from Wobbes TH: Carcinoma of colon and rectum in geriatric patients. *Age Aging* 14:321–326, 1985.)

Treatment

The surgical treatment for cancer of the colon and rectum does not differ from accepted surgical procedures for younger individuals. Cohen reports a resectability rate of 84.9% in patients aged 70 years and over in a prospective series of patients with large bowel cancer (81). Abdominoperineal resection is acceptable management for anorectal carcinoma in the elderly, but requires meticulous technique. Thomsen reports 52 patients over the age of 80 years who underwent abdominoperineal resection (82). Twenty-three percent (12/52) died before hospital discharge. Poor-risk patients and those unable to manage a colostomy may be better managed by radiation, cryosurgery, or cauterization for rectal cancer (83).

Hobler compared a series of GI patients aged 80 and over with a younger group of patients undergoing surgery for colon cancer (84). There was no difference in the 3-year survival curves. The risk of mortality could be predicted by stage of disease or type of operation required, but not by age group. The 80+ year old age group had a median length of hospital stay of 18 days versus 15 days for the younger group.

Carcinoma and Melanoma of the Anus

Basal cell carcinoma and Paget's squamous cell carcinoma of the anus occur in the elderly and can usually be treated by wide excision and skin graft. Melanoma of the anus tends to occur in older patients more often, and they have a poor prognosis (85, 86).

Preoperative chemotherapy and radiation have drastically reduced the need for surgical treatment of anal canal cancer. Flam reports that patients as old as 89 years with epidermoid carcinoma of the anus had complete regression of anal carcinoma following chemotherapy with 5-FU infusion and Mitomycin C with simultaneous whole pelvic radiation to 3000–4140 rads (89). Abdominoperineal resection is used only for treatment failures in the elderly patient.

Prognosis

Elderly patients with cancer of the colon and rectum have the same prognosis for the same stage of the tumor as do middle-aged and younger patients.

SUMMARY

Chronologic age is less important than physiologic age in determining survival in patients undergoing colon resection. Mortality most often results from cardiopulmonary problems or sepsis. Pre-existing disease and emergency procedures increase the morbidity and mortality rates in the elderly. Mortality may be decreased by performing early, elective operation in optimally prepared patients, rather than waiting until emergency laparotomy is necessary in the high-risk elderly patient. Elderly patients in good physio-

logic condition have operative risks similar to those of younger patients. Thorough preoperative determination of the elderly patient's physiologic condition is most important in determining the risk of operation. Age alone is a minor factor in determining operative risk if the patient's vital organs are physiologically intact and can handle the stress of a surgical procedure.

REFERENCES

1. Tucker JS: The ageing bowel. *The Pract* 225:1767–1771, 1981.
2. Pace JL: A detailed study of musculature of the human large intestine. PhD thesis, University of London, London.
3. Connell AM, Hilton C, Irvin G, Lennard-Jones JE, Misiewicz JJ: Variations in bowel habit in two population samples. *Br Med J* 2:1095–1099, 1965.
4. Milne JS, Williamson J: Bowel habit in older people. *Gerontologia Clinica* 14:55–60, 1972.
5. Brocklehurst JC: Colonic disease in the elderly. *Clin Gerontol* 14:725–747, 1985.
6. Avots-Avotins KV, Waugh DE: Colon volvulus and the geriatric patient. *Surg Clin N Am* 62:249–260, 1982.
7. Cathcart PMcD, Cathcart RS, Rambo WM: Management of massive lower gastrointestinal bleeding. *Am Surg* 43:217–219, 1977.
8. Boley SJ, Dibose A, Brandt LJ, Sammartano RJ: Lower intestinal bleeding in the elderly. *Am J Surg* 137:57–64, 1979.
9. Matolo NM, Link DP: Selective embolization for control of gastrointestinal hemorrhage. *Am J Surg* 138:840–844, 1980.
10. Schuster MM: Disorders of the aging GI system. *Hosp Pract* 11:95–103, 1976.
11. Shackleford RT, Zuidema GD: *Surgery of the Alimentary Tract.* Philadelphia, WB Saunders Co, 1982.
12. Parks TG: Natural history of diverticular disease of the colon. *Clin Gastroenterol* 4:53–69, 1975.
13. Segal I, Solomon A, Hunt JA: Emergence of diverticular disease in the urban South African black. *Gastroenterology* 72:215–219, 1977.
14. Whiteway J, Morson BC: Pathology of the ageing—diverticular disease. *Clin Gastroenterol* 14:829–846, 1985.
15. Kyle J, Davidson AI: The changing pattern of hospital admission for diverticular disease of the colon. *Br J Surg* 62:537–541, 1975.
16. Morson BC, Dawson IMP: *Gastrointestinal Pathology,* ed 2. Oxford, Blackwell Scientific Publications, 1979.
17. Almy TP, Howell DA: Diverticular disease of the colon. *N Engl J Med* 302:324–331, 1980.
18. Alexander J, Karl RC, Skinner DB: Results of changing trends in the surgical management of complications of diverticular disease. *Surgery* 94:683–690, 1983.
19. Morgenstern L, Weiner R, Michel SL: ''Malignant''

diverticulitis, a clinical entity. *Arch Surg* 114:1112–1116, 1979.

20. Gallagher JJ, Welch JP: Giant diverticula of the sigmoid colon. *Arch Surg* 114:1079–1083, 1979.

21. Arnold GJ, Nance FC: Volvulus of the sigmoid colon. *Ann Surg* 177:527–537, 1973.

22. Anderson MJ, Okike N, Spencer RJ: The colonoscopy in cecal volvulus. *Dis Colon Rect* 21:71–74, 1978.

23. Siroospour D, Berardi RS: Volvulus of the sigmoid colon: a ten-year study. *Dis Colon Rect* 19:535–541, 1976.

24. Starling JR: Initial treatment of sigmoid volvulus by colonoscopy. *Ann Surg* 190:36–39, 1979.

25. Ballantyne GH, Brandner MD, Beart RW, Ilstrup DM: Volvulus of the colon, incidence and mortality. *Ann Surg* 202:83–92, 1985.

26. Bak MP, Boley SJ: Sigmoid volvulus in elderly patients. *Am J Surg* 151:71–75, 1986.

27. Todd FJ, Forde KA: Volvulus of the cecum and colon, choice of operations. *Am J Surg* 138:632–634, 1979.

28. Kyle J: An epidemiological study of Crohn's disease in north east Scotland. *Gastroenterology* 61:826–833, 1971.

29. Fahrlander H, Baerlocher CH: Clinical features and epidemiological data on Crohn's disease in the Basel area. *Scand J Gastroenterol* 6:657–662, 1971.

30. Gupta S, Saverymuttu SH, Keshavarzian A, Hodgson HJF: Is the pattern of inflammatory bowel disease different in the elderly? *Age Aging* 14:366–370, 1985.

31. Mayberry JF, Dew MJ, Morris JS, Powell DB: An audit of Crohn's disease in a defined population. *J Roy Coll Phys Lond* 17:196–198, 1983.

32. Carr N, Schofield PF: Inflammatory bowel disease in the older patient. *Br J Surg* 69:223–225, 1982.

33. Altman DF: Gastrointestinal diseases in the elderly. *Med Clin N Am* 67:433–444, 1983.

34. DeDombal FT, Burton I, Goligher JC: Recurrence of Crohn's disease after primary excisional surgery. *Gut* 12:519–527, 1971.

35. Nugent FW, Veidenheimer MC, Meissner WA, Haggett RC: Prognosis after colonic resection for Crohn's disease of the colon. *Gastroenterology* 65:398–402, 1973.

36. Scott HW, Sawyers JL, Weaver FA, Fletcher JR, Adkins RB: Is ileoproctostomy a reasonable procedure after total abdominal colectomy? *Ann Surg* 203:583–589, 1986.

37. Block GE, Moossa AR, Simonowitz D, Hassan SZ: Emergency colectomy for inflammatory bowel disease. *Surgery* 82:531–536, 1977.

38. Albrechtsen D, Bergan A, Nygaard K, Gjone E, Flatmark A: Urgent surgery for ulcerative colitis: early colectomy in 132 patients. *World J Surg* 5:607–615, 1981.

39. Reiss R, Deutsch AA: Emergency abdominal procedures in patients above 70. *J Gastroenterol* 40:154–158, 1985.

40. Weedon DD, Shorter RG, Ilstrup DM, Huizenga KD, Taylor WF: Crohn's disease and cancer. *N Engl J Med* 289:1099–1103, 1973.

41. Gyde SN, Prior P, Macartney JC, Thompson H, Waterhouse JAH, Allan RN: Malignancy in Crohn's disease. *Gut* 21:1024–1029, 1980.

42. Levinson JD, Wall AJ, Kirsner JB: The problem of carcinoma in inflammatory disease of the bowel: selective base experiences. *South Med J* 65:209–214, 1972.

43. Lightdale CJ, Winawer SJ: Polyps and tumours of the large intestine. In Hellemans J, Vantrappen G (eds): *Gastro-intestinal Tract Disorders in the Elderly.* Edinburgh, Churchill Livingstone, 1984, pp 174–184.

44. Rosekrans PCM, Meijer CJLM, Vawal AM, Linderman J: Allergic proctitis: a clinical and immunopathological entity. *Gut* 21:1017–1023, 1980.

45. Ottinger J, Austen WG: A study of 136 patients with mesenteric infarction. *Surg Gynecol Obstet* 124:251–261, 1967.

46. Holt PR: The small intestine. *Clin Gastroenterol* 14:689–723, 1985.

47. Marston A: Ischaemia. *Clin Gastroenterol* 14:847–862, 1985.

48. Boley SJ, Sammartano R, Adams A, DiBiase A, Kleinhaus S, Sprayregen S: On the nature and etiology of vascular ectasias of the colon, degenerative lesions of aging. *Gastroenterology* 72:650–660, 1977.

49. Broden B, Snellman B: Procidentia of the rectum studied with cineradiography: a contribution to the discussion of causative mechanism. *Dis Colon Rectum* 11:330–347, 1968.

50. Ripstein CB: Procidentia: definitive corrective surgery. *Dis Colon Rectum* 15:334–336, 1972.

51. Altemeier WA: One stage perineal surgery for complete rectal prolapse. *Hosp Pract* 7:102–108, 1972.

52. Carter AE: Rectosacral suture fixation for complete rectal prolapse in the elderly, the frail, and the demented. *Br J Surg* 70:522–523, 1983.

53. Poole GV, Pennell TC, Myers RT, Hightower F: Modified Thiersch operation for rectal prolapse, technique and results. *Am Surg* 51:226–229, 1985.

54. Bomar RL, Sawyers JL: Trans-abdominal proctopexy for massive rectal prolapse. *Am Surg* 43:97–100, 1977.

55. Miller RL, Thomas J, O'Leary JP: Ripstein procedure for rectal prolapse. *Am Surg* 45:531–534, 1979.

56. Peltokallio P, Tykka H: Evolution of the age distribution and mortality of acute appendicitis. *Arch Surg* 116:153–156, 1981.

57. Hall A, Wright TM: Acute appendicitis in the geriatric patient. *Am Surg* 42:147–150, 1976.

58. Thorbjarnarson B, Loehr WJ: Appendicitis in patients over the age of 60. *Surg Gynecol Obstet* 125:1277–1280, 1967.

59. Santos A, Gelpesin A: Surgical mortality in the elderly. *J Am Geriatr Soc* 23:42–46, 1975.

60. Greenburg AG, Saik RP, Coyle JJ, Peskin GW: Mortality and gastrointestinal surgery in the aged. *Arch Surg* 116:788–791, 1981.

61. Greenburg AG, Saik RP, Pridham D: Influence of age on mortality of colon surgery. *Am J Surg* 150:65–70, 1985.

62. Boyd JB, Bradford B, Watne AL: Operative risk fac-

tors of colon resection in the elderly. *Ann Surg* 192:743–746, 1980.

63. Blake R, Lynn J: Emergency abdominal surgery in the aged. *Br J Surg* 63:956–960, 1976.

64. Cohen H, Willis I, Wallack M: Surgical experience of colon resection in the extreme elderly. *Am Surg* 52:214–217, 1986.

65. Cady B, Persson AV, Monson DO, Maunz DL: Changing patterns of colorectal carcinoma. *Cancer* 33:422–426, 1974.

66. Maglinte DDT, Keller KJ, Miller RE, Chernish SM: Colon and rectal carcinoma: spatial distribution and detection. *Radiology* 147:669–672, 1983.

67. Bernstein MA, Feczko PJ, Halpert RD, Simms SM, Ackerman LV: Distribution of colonic polyps: increased incidence of proximal lesions in older patients. *Radiology* 155:35–38, 1985.

68. Posner GL, Sharma DSN: Colon polyps: when are they malignant? *Geriatrics* 36:57–60, 1981.

69. Lane N, Kaplan H, Pascal PR: Minute adenomatous and hyperplastic polyps of the colon: divergent patterns of epithelial growth with specific associated mesenchymal changes. Contrasting roles in the pathogenesis of carcinoma. *Gastroenterology* 60:537–551, 1971.

70. Sweeney K, Petrelli N, Harrera L, Lopez C, Mittelman A: Cavernous hemangioma of the anus. *J Surg Oncol* 27:286–288, 1984.

71. Fernandez MJ, Davis RP, Nora PF: Gastrointestinal lipomas. *Arch Surg* 118:1081–1083, 1983.

72. Berg HK, Herrera L, Petrelli NJ, Lopez C, Mittelman A: Mixed juvenile-adenomatous polyp of the rectum in an elderly patient. *J Surg Oncol* 29:40–42, 1985.

73. Wobbes TH: Carcinoma of the colon and rectum in geriatric patients. *Age Aging* 14:321–326, 1985.

74. Silverberg E: Cancer statistics, 1983. *Ca* 33:9–25, 1983.

75. Hertz RE, Deddish MR, Day E: Value of periodic examination in detecting cancer of the rectum and colon.

76. Khan AH: Colorectal carcinoma: risk factors, screening, early detection. *Geriatrics* 39:42–47, 1984.

77. Adam YG, Calabrese C, Volk H: Colorectal cancer in patients over 80 years of age. *Surg Clin N Am* 52:883–889, 1972.

78. Jensen HE, Fenger HJ, Kragelund E, Nielson J: Carcinoma of the rectum in old age. *Acta Chir Scand* 139:536–567, 1973.

79. Adkins RB, DeLozier JB, McKnight WG, Waterhouse G: Carcinoma of the colon in patients 35 years of age and younger. *Am Surg* 53:141–145, 1987.

80. Mettlin C, Natarajan N, Mittelman A, Smart CR, Murphy CP: Management and survival of adenocarcinoma of the rectum in the United States: results of a national survery by the American College of Surgeons. *Oncology* 39:265–273, 1982.

81. Cohen JR, Theile DE, Holt J, David HC: Carcinoma of the large bowel in patients aged 70 years and over. *Aust NZ J Surg* 48:405–408, 1978.

82. Thomsen TA, Printen KJ: Abdominoperineal resection in the octogenarian. *J Am Geriatr Soc* 26:363–365, 1978.

83. Gingold BS: Local treatment (electrocoagulation) for carcinoma of the rectum in the elderly. *J Am Geriatr Soc* 29:10–13, 1981.

84. Hobler KE: Colon surgery for cancer in the very elderly. Cost and 3-year survival. *Ann Surg* 203:129–131, 1986.

85. Pyper PC, Parks TG: Melanoma of the anal canal. *Br J Surg* 71:671–672, 1984.

86. Wanebo HJ, Woodruff JM, Farr GH, Quan SH: Anorectal melanoma. *Cancer* 47:1891–1900, 1981.

89. Flam MS, John M, Lovalvo LJ, Mills RJ, Ramalho LD, Prather C, Mowry PA, Morgan DR, Lau BP: Definitive nonsurgical therapy of epithelial malignancies of the anal canal. *Cancer* 51:1378–1387, 1983.

Postgrad Med 27:290–294, 1960.

Chapter 26

Diseases of the Genitourinary System in the Elderly

Michael O. Koch, M.D., Fred K. Kirchner, Jr., M.D., F.A.C.S.

Many of the disease processes seen by general urologists occur more often in the elderly population. Benign enlargement of the prostate comes immediately to mind; however, most malignancies of the genitourinary system are also more frequent with advancing age. A number of neurologic conditions, such as sequela after strokes, senile dementia, and Parkinson's disease, may affect urinary bladder function. The urologic problems associated with these neurologic conditions are serious and may become a significant health threat to the individual. Incontinence, which is common in the elderly, is distressing both to the patient and to his or her family. In recent years a more enlightened attitude has developed toward sexual function in the elderly, and the urologist is now faced with increasing requests from elderly patients to aid in problems of erectile dysfunction. Finally, as in all organ systems of the body, the kidney itself undergoes slow but inexorable degenerative changes with advancing years. Knowledge of these alterations, which may represent a significant impairment to the renal function of the elderly patient, is important to the total care of the aged patient. It is especially important when caring for an elderly patient who is preparing to a undergo the stress of a surgical procedure.

RENAL PHYSIOLOGY IN THE ELDERLY

A number of morphologic and physiologic changes occur in the normal aging kidney. It is well to describe the morphologic changes, to dis-

cuss the alterations in glomerular and tubular function, and to consider their relevance to the surgical management of the elderly patient.

Dunnill and Halley (1) quantitatively examined the changes that occur in the morphology of the kidney during the process of aging. They examined 68 pairs of kidneys obtained at necropsy from both males and females all ages from birth to 90 years. All of their patients had suffered traumatic deaths, and none showed evidence of primary renal or cardiovascular disease. After excising the renal pelvis, renal volume was measured. Figure 26.1 is a graphic display of total renal parenchymal volume and renal cortical volume as a function of age. Both peak sometime after the age of 20, stay relatively constant until the age of 60, and steadily decline thereafter. Friedman and co-workers (2) studied the amount of functional renal tissue as it relates to age using radioisotopic renal scans. In a group of 35 elderly patients with a mean age of 75 years in their study, 71% were found to have abnormal renal scans. Forty-six percent (46%) of these patients showed focal areas of diminished renal uptake of the radioisotope. There appeared to be a discrepancy between the anatomic kidney size as determined by their excretory urograms and functional renal size as determined by isotopic scanning. They postulated that the deterioration in renal function seen with aging was unrelated to renal size and that some degree of vascular insufficiency might explain these defects.

Several studies have specifically analyzed the changes that occur in the glomerulus with aging. Kaplan and colleagues (3) examined histologic

370

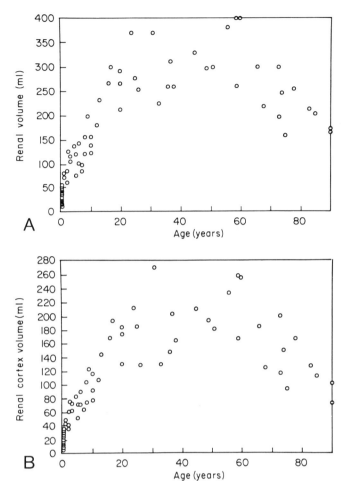

Figure 26.1. **A,** Total renal volume as a function of age. **B,** Renal cortical volume as a function of age. (From Dunnill MS, Halley W: Some observations on the quantitative anatomy of the kidney. *J Path* 110:113–121, 1972.)

kidney sections from 122 healthy patients for the presence of glomerular sclerosis. They quantitatively assessed the percentage of glomeruli in the kidney that were sclerotic in each of several age groups. After the age of 40, there is a continual and progressive increase in the percentage of sclerotic glomeruli. In patients over the age of 70, over 10% of glomeruli are sclerotic. Goyal (4) demonstrated a decreased number of glomerular cells, decreased number of tubular cells, and increased nuclear size with aging. Both the size and the number of cells in the glomerular tufts decreased progressively with aging.

Although it is uniformly accepted that there is progressive renal scarring and cortical loss with aging, there has been considerable controversy regarding whether these changes in the nephron units are a by-product of normal senescence or whether they are secondary to vascular

changes. McLachlan and colleagues (5) studied a group of kidneys from patients who had died of nonrenal diseases and who showed no evidence of intrinsic renal disease on postmortem pyelograms. They actually performed postmortem renal angiograms and attempted to correlate the evidence of any demonstrable renal vascular disease found on angiography with both renal weight and number of glomeruli per kidney. Glomerular numbers tended to decline with advancing age and the severity of age-related vascular changes increased, but the correlation between the two was poor. Glomerular involution in the senescent kidney appeared to be independent of the vascular effects. In a contrasting study, Griffiths et al. (6) studied 88 kidneys at necropsy from normal subjects aged over 80 years. These kidneys were also studied by postmortem pyelograms and arteriograms. They found moderate to severe calyceal scarring in 50% of the kidneys examined, and in 12-1/2% there was evidence of severe scarring. There was markedly decreased cortical area in patients aged over 65 years. In contrast to the Griffiths' work, the loss of renal cortex did appear to correlate with renal vascular changes more than with age. The majority of the vascular changes found on their study occurred in the interlobular arteries and in the arcuate arteries.

Takazakura et al. (7) examined the microvasculature in 63 autopsied kidneys ranging from 9 months to 92 years in age. They demonstrated that a percentage of afferent and efferent arterioles in the glomerulus directly communicate, thereby bypassing the glomerular capillary network. They coined the term to describe the percentage of capillaries in which the efferent and afferent arterioles directly communicated as the "continuity index." At ages less than 10 years, the "continuity index" is on the order of 10% or less. There is a linear increase in the "continuity index" until death. At the age of 80, it is approximately 90%-100%. This has a number of physiologic consequences. First, there is a gradual reduction in the circulation of blood through the cortical arteriolar-glomerular units with age. On the other hand, in the juxtamedullary nephrons, although the glomerular unit is bypassed, the blood shunts directly into the arteriolae rectae, thereby increasing blood flow to the medullary segments of the kidney. This tends to wash out the medullary osmotic gradient. In diseased kidneys with known glomerulonephritis, these investigators demonstrated that the continuity index far exceeded the percentage that would be expected to occur due to the aging process alone.

These microangiographic changes tend to be supported by studies that examine renal cortical blood flow. Hollenberg et al. (8) employed a xenon washout technique to assess renal blood flow in a group of 207 healthy human subjects ranging from the age of 17 to 76. Increasing age was associated with a significant and progressive reduction in every index of renal perfusion. Not only did overall blood flow fall with increasing age but also renal cortical blood flow fell to a disproportionate degree when compared to overall renal blood flow. This confirms the microvascular findings of shunting to juxtaglomerular

nephrons. Older subjects also demonstrated an inability to alter renal blood flow in response to salt loading or restriction.

These alterations in the renal parenchyma and the renal blood flow have a direct effect on both glomerular and tubular function. In a study of 884 subjects with no known renal or cardiovascular disease in the Baltimore longitudinal study on aging (9) there was a progressive decline in creatinine clearance from approximately 140 ml/min per 1.73 m² at age 30 to 97 ml/min per 1.73 m² at age 80. In a follow-up study from the same institution (10), 446 normal volunteers had serial creatinine clearances (between 5 and 14 studies were obtained from each subject between 1958 and 1981). These volunteers were subcategorized as being either normal or as having evidence of hypertension and/or edematous disorders. They have clearly demonstrated that in healthy subjects there was a decrease in creatinine clearance of .75 +/− .12 ml/min/yr. In patients having some evidence of hypertension or of an edematous disorder, there is a more rapid decrease in creatinine clearance of .92 +/− .32 ml/min/yr.

Cockroft and Gault (11) have given us a convenient formula for predicting creatinine clearance from serum creatinine. They reviewed the charts of 534 patients who had two or more 24-hour creatinine clearance studies determined at their hospital and demonstrated a number of interesting findings. First, creatinine excretion consistently declines with age. At age 20, between 20 and 25 mg/kg are excreted per 24 hours in the urine. By the age of 90–100, only 10–15 mg/kg are excreted in the same period. This is secondary to a decrease in muscle mass that is seen with aging, and it has an important implication in interpreting renal function from serum creatinine. An elderly patient with a given serum creatinine will have a lower creatinine clearance than a younger patient. Cockroft and Gault suggested the use of the formula: $Ccl = (140 - age) \times (weight\ in\ kg)/(72 \times serum\ Cr\ mg\%)$. This formula should be used with caution in those patients having a decreased percentage of lean body weight, such as in the cachectic person, paraplegics, and children, and in patients whose renal function is not in a steady state. A patient either developing or recovering from renal insufficiency cannot accurately be assessed

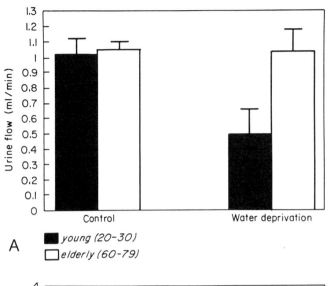

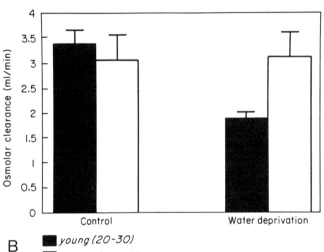

Figure 26.2. **A,** Age-related differences in ability to decrease urine flow with water deprivation. **B,** Age-related differences in ability to decrease osmolar clearance with water deprivation. (From Rowe JW, et al: The influence of age on the renal response to water deprivation in man. *Nephron* 17:270–278, 1976.

by the creatinine clearance prediction from this formula.

Alterations in tubular function are also seen with age. Epstein et al (12) examined the ability of patients to respond to a severe dietary restriction of sodium. They quantified the renal response to sodium restriction by studying the half-life in the reduction of urinary sodium excretion. The half-life for the reduction of renal sodium excretion in subjects aged under 30 years was 17.6 +/− .7 hours in contrast to the half-life of patients over 60 years of 30.9 +/− 2.8 hours. The mechanism responsible for this inability to conserve sodium was not clear from their studies. A decreased number of nephrons may

result in an increased filter load per nephron and therefore overload each nephron beyond its ability to conserve sodium effectively. Rowe and coworkers (13) examined the ability of patients of various ages to respond to water deprivation. In response to relatively short periods of water deprivation, subjects aged under 39 years were able to decrease urine flow and osmolar clearance quite effectively. In contrast, subjects aged between 60 and 79 demonstrated neither a decrease in urine flow nor a decrease in osmolar clearance. (Fig. 26.2A and B) These studies conclusively demonstrated an inability of the elderly patient to respond to acute alterations in both sodium and water homeostasis.

Weidmann et al. (14) examined elderly patients as compared to younger patients with respect to the renin and aldosterone system. Despite comparable body sodium and fluid balance in the younger and older age groups, serum renin concentration, plasma renin activity, and aldosterone concentrations are lower in the elderly. These differences become more pronounced when sodium intake is curtailed. These investigators also assessed the ability of the adrenal gland to produce aldosterone and cortisol in response to ACTH and found no difference between the two groups. Other investigators have examined the ability of the elderly to produce ADH in response to intravenous ethanol and saline loading (15). Osmoreceptor sensitivity in the elderly is significantly greater. It was the belief of these investigators that the increased ADH response in the elderly patient served to compensate for a degree of reduced renal ability to conserve salt and water.

The clinical significance of these morphologic and functional changes in the aging kidney is profound with respect to the care of the elderly patient, particularly in a surgical setting. Glomerular and tubular function progressively declines beginning around the age of 65. With diminished renal reserve it becomes increasingly important to be able to predict what renal function will be in a surgical setting. Because of decreased muscle mass in the elderly patient, serum creatinine tends to overestimate the true renal function. Assuming that the patient has a normal percentage of lean body weight and that renal function is stable, the formula given to us by Cockroft and Gault (11) should accurately predict renal function. If renal function is not stable, or lean body weight is questionable, then glomerular function is best assessed by a recent or current 24-hour creatinine clearance. Diminished tubular function in the elderly patient necessitates more accurate monitoring of salt and water balance. The inability to respond efficiently to acute alterations in salt and water balance makes the elderly patient much more prone to hyponatremia and hypernatremia. Both of these electrolyte abnormalities can result in profound alterations in the well-being of the patient. Because of the inability to conserve water and salt effectively in the elderly patient, urine output may not accurately reflect intravascular volume and renal perfusion.

Decreased glomerular function must also be taken into account in the elderly when prescribing pharmacologic agents that are cleared primarily by renal mechanisms. This is particularly important in the prescription of drugs that have nephrotoxicity, such as aminoglycosides. Concomitant disease processess that affect renal function, hypertension, diabetes, and a variety of urologic problems will all accelerate the processes that are seen with aging in the healthy kidney. These alterations in glomerular and tubular function in the elderly patient must be taken into account in order to manage these patients' fluid and electrolyte balance in a safe and effective manner.

IMPOTENCE IN THE ELDERLY MALE

It is estimated that ten million men are impotent in the United States and many of these men are elderly. It has also been estimated that 75% of men aged 70 and over are impotent (16, 17). This may be secondary to a number of physiologic changes that accompany the normal aging process.

Montague et al. (18) carefully evaluated 165 men who presented with complaints of sexual dysfunction. Approximately one-half of their patients were determined to have a functional etiology to their impotence, whereas the remainder had an unidentifiable organic cause. Twenty-seven percent (27%) of their patients were over 60 years old. Specific etiologies of organic im-

Table 26.1[a] Etiology in 77 Patients with Organic Impotence

Cause	Patients (percentage)
Diabetes mellitus	32 (41)
Vascular insufficiency	13 (16.8)
Peyronie's disease	12 (15.5)
Hypogonadism	10 (12.9)
Post-surgical	8 (10.3)
Neurologic	7 (9.0)
Traumatic	6 (7.7)
Pharmacologic	3 (3.8)
Post-priapism	2 (2.5)
Alcohol related	1 (1.2)
Undetermined	1 (1.2)

[a]Adapted from Montague DK, et al: Diagnostic evaluation, classification and treatment of men with sexual dysfunction. *Urology* 14:545–548, 1979.

potence from their study are given in Table 26.1. Two things are evident from their results. First, diabetes mellitus accounts for the largest precentage of men of all ages who have organic impotence. Second, a number of pathologic processes that are seen with increasing frequency in the elderly population can cause impotence, e.g.,diabetes, atherosclerosis, hypogonadism, and postsurgical changes.

A number of normal physiologic changes that occur with aging account for decreased sexual function in the elderly male. Mean serum total testosterone levels remain normal until about the age of 70; most investigators have shown a gradual decline thereafter (19, 20). In addition, there is a rise in estradiol and testosterone-binding globulin with old age. This causes a decreased serum-free testosterone, which is the physiologically active form of the male hormone, and an increased estradiol to testosterone ratio. This suggests that the primary pathophysiologic process seen with aging is one of Leydig cell failure in the testicle. These hormonal changes are reflected by noticeable morphologic changes in the elderly male, including decreased axillary, pubic, and facial hair and decreased testicular size. Penile size is unchanged.

Vascular changes are also seen in the penis in the aging male. There is fibrous proliferation in the intima, then medial fibrosis, calcification, and eventually thrombotic obliteration of the vascular channels in the cavernous bodies (21). These changes are particularly apparent in the diabetic patient.

Neurologic lesions can also affect erectile function. Many urologists believe that impotence in the diabetic patient is a consequence of the peripheral neuropathy seen in diabetes. Most diabetics with erectile dysfunction also demonstrate some evidence of neurogenic bladder disease on cystometric testing (22). Multiple sclerosis, spinal cord lesions, and peripheral neuropathies can also cause impotence.

A number of pharmacologic agents are associated with impotence; the antihypertensive medications and psychotropic drugs are the most commonly implicated.

Surgical causes of impotence are common in the elderly patient. Many of these procedures (e.g., prostatectomy, cystectomy, or abdominal perineal colon resections) disrupt the normal innervation to the corporal bodies. Other procedures (e.g., aortic grafting procedures) may cause impotence on a vascular basis.

Finally, a number of psychiatric disorders, in particular major depressive illness, are more common in the elderly and are associated with impotence.

Our primary approach to the elderly male with impotence has been one of education and reassurance. Many elderly patients with impotence will decline further evaluation after learning that erectile dysfunction is a normal part of the aging process. For the interested elderly male, further evaluation is in order. An important start in our routine evaluation is with a careful history and physical examination. The emphasis in the history is upon those aspects that would indicate a functional etiology versus an organic one. An abrupt onset of impotence associated with an emotionally traumatic event suggests a functional etiology. A slow onset accompanied by a strong desire for intercourse is typically seen with organic disease. Those aspects of the physical examination that would suggest an organic basis are most important. This would include decreased testicular size or stigmata of peripheral vascular disease in the extremities. Peripheral neuropathy may be present. Medication history is critical. Serum is routinely analyzed for fasting glucose, testosterone, and thyroid function. Penile blood pressure determination is made. Further investigations, including angiography, penile tumescence testing in a sleep lab setting, and detailed psychiatric testing, are then obtained according to the indications. It is almost certain that the percentage of patients with an organic basis for their impotence increases with advancing age. Many patients with impotence will obviously have elements of both an organic and a functional problem.

A number of treatment options are available to the impotent elderly male. Psychologic counseling can be expected to have satisfactory results for functional impotence. Revascularization procedures are rarely indicated in the elderly male, and penile prostheses are the most commonly employed form of therapy. Penile prostheses are essentially of two types: semi-rigid and inflatable. Semi-rigid penile prostheses are easy to implant, function well for intercourse, and have few complications (23). Concealment may be a problem for many patients. In general, however, results with semi-rigid penile prostheses have been quite satisfactory (8). Inflatable penile prostheses are more difficult to implant, and patients who have them suffer from a higher complication rate and need for replacement and revision (24, 25). Concealment is generally not a problem, however. Most recent results with the inflatable penile prostheses have yielded very satisfactory rates of device survivals and patient satisfaction.

Even more recently, intracavernous injection of vasoactive drugs has been utilized to produce pharmacologic erections (26). This has produced excellent results in some series; however, its efficacy in the elderly population is unknown. Prolonged erections and plaque formation at the injection site may be a problem with this form of therapy. Currently, long-term follow-up of this modality is not available, and FDA approval is lacking.

In summary, impotence is frequently a consequence of disease processes that affect the aging population. Multiple treatment modalities are available for the interested patient. We feel that these treatment modalities should be made available to the interested elderly male with the same degree of enthusiasm as they would be offered to a younger man. It is the responsibility of the physician to educate the elderly patient as to the common occurrence of this problem, the pathophysiologic mechanisms responsible, and the treatment modalities available.

URINARY INCONTINENCE

Urinary incontinence is a common and frustrating problem in the elderly patient. Reports on the incidence of urinary incontinence vary widely, depending on the definition for incontinence that is used, investigative technique employed, and the population being studied. In a study of the community-dwelling elderly in New Zealand, Campbell et al. (27) found a prevalence of urinary incontinence of 11.6% in those patients over age 65 and 21.7% in those over the age of 80. It has been estimated that the true prevalence of incontinence is even higher because many patients will not volunteer information on this subject, and physicians frequently fail to ask about it. In the institutionalized elderly

population the prevalence is higher still. The yearly cost of management of the elderly patient with urinary incontinence is enormous to our society. Ouslander et al. (28) have estimated that the yearly cost of managing urinary incontinence by catheter drainage is $2888 and between $2072 and $4532 without catheter drainage depending upon the alternative chosen. This translates into a cost of 0.5 to 1.5 billion dollars per year in the United States.

A discussion of the normal physiologic principles of urinary continence, those conditions that most commonly cause urinary incontinence in the elderly, and a proposal for a method of diagnosis and treatment is now in order. Emphasis will be placed on identifying the reversible causes of incontinence, and the discussion of the various collection devices and diapers will be limited.

Normal Micturition Physiology

The bladder is basically a storage organ. Normal micturition is dependent upon an adequate bladder capacity, the ability of the patient to empty the bladder, and normal sphincteric function. The bladder is composed of smooth muscle that has an intrinsic muscle tone, but this is modulated to a large extent by a sacral reflex arc. Afferent nerve fibers sensing wall tension leave the bladder and travel through the pelvic nerve to the detrusor nucleus, which is located in the intermediolateral column of the sacral segment of the spinal cord. There they synapse with preganglionic fibers that travel back to the detrusor muscle through the pelvic nerve and synapse with post-ganglionic autonomic fibers, which stimulate a release of acetylcholine. The bladder smooth muscle contraction is thus stimulated. This is called the sacral micturition reflex arc. The sacral detrusor nucleus also has connections with the pons, thalamus, hypothalamus, cerebellum, and cerebral cortex. The pontine micturition center is thought to coordinate urethral relaxation with detrusor contraction, whereas neuronal connections to centers above the pons are involved primarily with inhibition of the sacral reflex arc.

Normal urinary continence is dependent upon the urethral sphincter to resist relaxation and maintain a urethral pressure that exceeds bladder pressure. Alpha-adrenergic receptors are located in the internal urethral sphincter.

Stimulation of those receptors causes increased urethral contraction and increased tone. Conditions that reduce urethral resistance or increase bladder pressure will predispose to sphincter incompetence and urinary incontinence. Conversely, conditions that increase urethral resistance or decrease the pressure that the detrusor is capable of generating result in poor bladder emptying. Most of voiding dysfunction and essentially all types of urinary incontinence in the elderly can be understood and managed effectively with this limited knowledge of micturition physiology.

Specific Causes of Incontinence and their Management

Unstable Bladder

More than half of the elderly patients presenting to incontinence clinics have what has been termed the "unstable bladder" (29). Other terms for this entity include uninhibited bladder, irritable bladder, and detrusor instability or hyperreflexia. Viewed on a very simplistic level, this condition represents a loss of inhibition of the sacral micturition reflex arc by upper neuronal centers. This type of micturition difficulty is seen in a number of central nervous system disorders that are common to the elderly. Senile dementia, Parkinson's disease, and cerebrovascular disease are but a few. Loss of upper tract inhibition of the sacral micturition reflex arc results in increased detrusor tone, with clinical symptoms usually consisting of a desire to void at smaller volumes and a decreased ability to delay urination once the initial urge is felt. This type of incontinence is typically called "urge incontinence." It poses no threat to renal function, as bladder emptying is complete at normal intravesical pressures. It can be a major social inconvenience, however, particularly for the patient with decreased mobility who has to "go" frequently but who cannot reach facilities quickly.

Physical examination in these cases is generally unremarkable other than the sequelae of the underlying neurologic disease. Residual urine determinations are minimal or zero, and urinalysis is normal. Cystometric examination of the bladder will demonstrate an urge to void at 200 to 300 ml or less and an inability to inhibit detrusor contractions. Cystoscopic examination is un-

necessary. Treatment selection is dependent upon the overall cognitive impairment, and treatment is not absolutely necessary. Incontinence may best be managed with diapers. For the more alert and more cooperative patient a number of treatment modalitites are available. Behavior modification techniques have been used extensively in Europe with significant success; limited use and enthusiasm exist for these techniques in this country. These techniques generally consist first of an observation period during which the time of each incontinent episode is recorded. The patient is checked every hour or two to document the incontinence pattern. A number of incontinence devices, equipped with alarms, are available. Once the voiding and incontinence pattern is determined, a forced voiding regimen is instituted that allows the patient to void before incontinence supervenes. In the motivated and cognitively alert patient, the voiding interval may be slowly increased—so-called bladder training. A number of biofeedback techniques (30) and reward systems (31) have facilitated use of this approach. Simple measures, such as limiting fluid intake after a certain time at night, may be of benefit also.

Pharmacologic therapy with smooth muscle relaxants or anticholinergic medications is frequently helpful, particularly in the alert and cooperative patient. Propantheline (15 to 30 mg QID), oxybutinin (5 mg BID to QID), and imipramine (25 to 150 mg QHS) have all been used successfully. Caution should be used in the prescribing of all of these medications in the elderly, as side effects are definitely increased in this population (32).

Stress Incontinence

Stress incontinence refers to the transient and immediate loss of small amounts of urine following abrupt increases in intra-abdominal pressure. This condition is most commonly seen in multiparous females, but may also be seen in men following surgical procedures on the bladder neck or prostate. This accounts for only a small percentage of the cases of urinary incontinence in the institutionalized elderly, but a significant percentage of those in the community-dwelling population (27). Stress incontinence in women usually results from the anatomic changes in the bladder neck and urethra secondary to pelvic floor relaxation. This allows descent of the bladder and urethra, loss of the posterior urethrovesical angle, and loss of internal urethral sphincter tone. Mucosal atrophy in the post-menopausal female also decreases urethral resistance. Abrupt increases in intra-abdominal pressure are transmitted to the bladder but not to the urethra; consequently, bladder pressure exceeds urethral pressure and incontinence ensues. Stress incontinence in males generally results from surgical injuries to the bladder neck and external urethral sphincter that decrease urethral resistance.

These patients characteristically describe the loss of small amounts of urine with coughing, sneezing, laughing, or straining. These patients should be dry at night. The loss of large amounts of urine, a delay between straining and urine loss, or nighttime incontinence should make one very suspicious that there is another cause or at least some co-existing etiologic factor causing the incontinence. Many elderly women, for instance, will have a combination of an unstable bladder and stress incontinence.

Physical examination is critical to the establishment of this diagnosis. After the determination of post-void residual urine volume, the bladder is filled to near capacity. The catheter is removed and the patient is asked to cough or strain. The immediate leakage of small amounts of urine establishes the diagnosis. If no leakage occurs, the test is repeated in the 45 degree and upright position. Once leakage is demonstrated, one must decide if surgical correction will be of any benefit. Manual digital elevation of the bladder neck that re-establishes the normal posterior urethrovesical angle and the intra-abdominal position of the urethra should cause cessation of leakage with each cough.

A number of treatment modalities are available for this condition. Non-surgical methods consist of techniques for increasing urethral resistance. Estrogen administration, either topically or systemically, will reverse urethral mucosal atrophy in most post-menopausal women and thus increase urethral resistance. Pessaries are a simple technique that are particularly useful in patients with accompanying cystoceles, rectoceles, or uterine prolapse. Sympathomimetic drugs, such as ephedrine (25 to 50 mg TID) and phenylpropanolamine (50 mg TID), will usually be of significant benefit to many women. Up to two-thirds of women will be significantly improved with sympathomimetics, and about 25% will be cured (33). These agents increase internal urethral sphincter tone and thereby increase urinary outflow resistance. Caution should be utilized in the administration of these medications to patients with hypertension or ischemic cardiovascular disease. For patients with severe stress incontinence and/or failures of pharmacologic therapy, surgical correction offers very high success rates, even in the very elderly female (34). A variety of techniques have been used and described. They vary from open bladder neck suspension to needle urethropexy to anterior colporrhaphy. These are covered in some detail in Chapter 27. Success rates of approximately 90% are achieved with most of the commonly performed operations.

Overflow Incontinence

Overflow incontinence is seen in a wide variety of pathophysiologic processes. In essence, any condition that causes an imbalance between intravesical pressure and urethral resistance can cause ineffective bladder emptying and eventually bladder overdistention. Conditions that increase urethral resistance include urethral stricture and prostatic enlargement from benign hypertrophy or carcinoma. Conditions that decrease intravesical pressure include chronic bladder overdistention from obstructive processes and conditions that interrupt the sacral micturition reflex arc, such as abdominoperineal rectal resections, diabetic neuropathy, tabes dorsalis, and lesions involving the sacral segments of the spinal cord.

Patients who have overflow incontinence generally present with symptoms of frequent voidings of small amounts and an uncomfortable sensation of an inability to empty the bladder completely. In patients with an obstructive etiology to their overflow incontinence, the symptoms may also include straining to void and hesitancy. Many patients are remarkably asymptomatic, however, even with very large bladder residuals.

Physical examination will usually establish this diagnosis. Lower abdominal palpation and percussion will frequently reveal a distended bladder. Rectal examination may reveal prostatic enlargement, and this examination when done well remains the best method for screening for prostatic carcinoma. Patients who have a neurologic etiology for their urinary incontinence will generally demonstrate other stigmata of their neurologic disease. Diabetics with neurogenic bladders generally have a peripheral neuropathy and loss of pinprick sensation in their extremities. The local sacral reflex arcs are assessed by testing the cremasteric reflex, anal wink, and bulbocavernosus reflexes. The single hallmark of most importance in the diagnosis of overflow incontinence, however, is the demonstration of a markedly elevated post-void residual urine. Once this diagnosis is made, the specific etiology is ascertained by cystometry and cystoscopy. In the patient with an obstructive process, cystometry should demonstrate relatively normal or slightly elevated bladder capacity and moderately elevated bladder pressures. Cystoscopy will demonstrate the obstructing process, and the bladder should show some of the stigmata of chronic urinary obstruction, i.e., trabeculations and diverticula. Conversely, in the patient with a neurogenic etiology, cystometry will show bladder capacities that are significantly elevated and low bladder pressures. Cystoscopy in these cases should reveal no obstructive lesions.

Although these general rules are useful for the organizing of one's approach to this problem, many patients do not fit clearly into one category. For instance, patients with a long-standing obstructive process will develop a myogenic bladder from chronic overdistention. Relief of the obstruction after it has been present for a long time will not result in very effective voiding because the detrusor has become completely decompensated and is no longer able to generate an effective emptying contraction.

The management of this problem is very much dependent on the particular patient and his or her social situation. All types of overflow incontinence can be managed well with chronic intermittent clean catheterization, usually three or four times per day. Lapides et al. have conclusively shown that although about half of patients managed with this technique will have chronic bacteriuria, systemic illness is remarkably rare, and renal function is well preserved (35). In the patient with an obstructive process and one who could be considered as a surgical candidate, surgical relief of the obstruction will be of obvious

benefit, and referral to urologic care is recommended. A chronic indwelling Foley catheter should be considered the treatment of last resort and utilized only after all other reasonable avenues are exhausted.

Other Causes

Several other causes of urinary incontinence deserve mention. First, some patients will be incontinent solely on a functional basis. Although the overall contribution of this group to the incontinence problem is probably very small, it definitely appears to exist, particularly in the psychiatrically impaired or severely cognitively impaired individual. This is certainly a diagnosis of exclusion, however. The management of this type is probably best by some form of behavior modification therapy.

Iatrogenic components are present in many incontinent patients. Patients with modest degrees of obstructive uropathy are easily tipped over to the group of patients with overflow incontinence by medications that inhibit detrusor function. Anti-parkinsonian drugs, tricyclic antidepressants, and over-the-counter cold remedies can all do this. Diuretics can significantly exacerbate incontinence in patients with detrusor instability and in patients with decreased mobility. Sedatives create a decreased sensation of bladder fullness, particularly in patients with marginal mental facilities, and can result in incontinence.

The final form of urinary incontinence that should be mentioned is that of total urinary incontinence. This is a specific entity where there is continual leakage of urine, lack of bladder filling, and an absence of any voided volumes. This form of incontinence should be considered completely distinct from all other forms of incontinence; it always demands further investigation and, if possible, some form of surgical intervention.

Evaluation of Elderly Incontinent Patients

There has been a significant amount written recently advocating sophisticated urodynamic testing of all incontinent elderly patients (36–38). Our approach to the problem is born more out of pragmatism and represents an attempt to streamline the investigative and therapeutic process in these patients in whom both expense and mobility are important considerations. Sophisticated urodynamic testing has added very little to our ability to care for these patients.

Despite reports to the contrary, the history obtained from the patient is frequently of benefit in characterizing the type of incontinence. Of particular interest is the voiding pattern. The amounts voided, the intervals between voidings, when and how often the incontinent episodes occur, and how they relate to normal voidings are all important aspects that should be determined. A medication history should always be elicited. Physical examination should be complete and should include a brief mental status examination, neurologic examination with attention to the lower extremities and perineal reflexes, abdominal examination with bladder percussion, and a careful rectal examination. In patients with symptoms suggestive of stress incontinence, the bladder should be filled and the urethra observed for loss of urine with coughing and straining.

Routine laboratory studies obtained on the first office visit should include serum for BUN, creatinine, electrolytes, and glucose. Urine is always obtained for routine urinalysis and culture. A post-void residual determination is always made on the first visit as this gives the information that is the pivotal point for further management. Depending on the circumstances, patients with low post-void residual urine volumes may be either started empirically on anticholinergics or smooth muscle relaxants. The physician may choose to proceed with formal cystometric examination if he or she desires any further confirmation of the diagnosis of detrusor instability. Full urodynamic testing including urethral pressure profiles and sphincter electromyography has added very little to our ability to manage these patients and is not routinely used. In patients with elevated post-void urine volumes, cystometric examination of the bladder is always in order. In males we would also routinely perform cystoscopy. Obstructive lesions are managed surgically in all patients who are deemed to be surgical candidates. Patients with no obstruction or those not felt to be surgical candidates are managed by intermittent clean catheterization. Chronic indwelling Foley catheters are a last resort.

Finally, the presence of significant pyuria or hematuria should always make one suspicious of some underlying urinary pathology, such as stones or carcinoma of the prostate and bladder. An intravenous pyelogram or renal ultrasound should be obtained in all of these patients.

In summary, it is safe to say that urinary incontinence is a common problem in the elderly population. Physician ignorance of this problem remains significant. Incontinence frequently is the result of a significant underlying systemic, neurologic, or urologic pathology. A simplified diagnostic and management approach is presented to facilitate the management of these patients.

MALIGNANCIES OF THE GENITOURINARY SYSTEM

Carcinoma of the Prostate

Carcinoma of the prostate is one of the more common malignancies to affect men and has been mistakenly considered by some to be a relatively ''benign'' process in the elderly. However, prostate cancer is the third most common cause of cancer deaths in males in this country and is exceeded only by lung and colon rectal cancer. As with all other forms of cancer, earlier detection will increase rates of survival.

Unfortunately, most patients with carcinoma of the prostate present with either locally extensive disease or with metastatic disease. Only approximately 10% of patients present with an isolated palpable nodule and have normal acid phosphatase and bone scan (clinical stage B.) It is this group of patients who are potentially curable if treated with total removal of the prostate gland and seminal vesicles. Clinical stage B lesions are generally subdivided further, with B_1 lesions being defined as those with a nodule less than 1.5 cm to 2 cm and confined to a lobe of the prostate. B_2 lesions are larger and/or involve both lobes of the prostate, but are still felt to be confined to the prostate proper. This subdivision has clinical importance because the B_2 lesions have a higher incidence of pelvic lymph node metastases (29%–52%) (39, 40) versus the B_1 lesion (14%–21%) (41, 42).

About 40% of all patients with prostatic cancer will be stage C cancers at the time of their presentation. In these patients the malignancy has extended through the prostatic capsule, but there is no clinical evidence of distant metastasis. However, as evidenced in clinical stage B tumors, there is significant clinical understaging in these patients also. As many as 65% of patients with stage C tumors will be found to have pelvic node metastases (43).

It is unfortunate that stage D disease is a common stage of presentation, representing about 40% of all prostate cancers at the time of presentation. Stage D_1 disease represents those patients whose metastases are confined to pelvic lymph nodes. Therefore, this is almost always a pathologic staging. Within this classification are those cases that have been upstaged who were originally thought to have clinically lower stage disease. Stage D_2 disease includes all of those patients who had obvious clinical metastases at the time of the presentation. This is determined by bone scan or other evidence of soft tissue spread.

Stage A cancer of the prostate is never truly a "clinical stage." This is the cancer that is unexpected and is discovered only after histologic examination of prostatic curettings or of prostectomy specimens. The diagnosis is made after a surgical procedure has been performed for what was initially thought to be benign disease. This stage A classification represents approximately 10% of all patients with a carcinoma of the prostate, although the percentage of this stage in any one series may vary due to a number of contributing factors. Stage A carcinoma of the prostate is subdivided into A_1 and A_2. A_1 carcinomas of the prostate represent those instances when the total cancer volume is quite low and generally the cellular pattern is of low grade. On the other hand, stage A_2 disease consists of those patients who have a larger volume of carcinoma and/or high-grade disease. The dividing line between these two sub-stages varies somewhat from institution to institution.

Currently, there are a number of treatment options available that may either be used singularly or in combination for patients with carcinoma of the prostate. These options include radical prostatectomy; radiotherapy, either using external beam irradiation or interstitial irradiation; endocrine manipulation, either by administration of estrogens or antiandrogens or castration; and

finally no treatment.

Most, if not all, patients and especially the elderly with A_1 carcinoma of the prostate should be followed expectantly. All patients with stage A_2 disease or B_1 disease should be carefully considered to be candidates for radical prostatectomy. A reasonable argument for expectant observation may be made for patients who are still on the early part of the "growing curve" of their malignancy who are elderly or whose condition is frail.

Radical extirpation in patients with higher stage cancer of the prostate is generally not indicated. The chance for a cure of patients in this group is practically nil, and our attention for those patients should be directed toward alleviating symptoms. Radiotherapy using external beam mega-voltage radiation or interstitial radioactive seeds has been used in an attempt to control extensive local disease. However, follow-up studies from numerous series have shown a high incidence of persistent malignant cells in prostate biopsy specimens after radiotherapy. Also, postoperative complications after a staging pelvic lymphadenectomy and I-131 seed implantation are not always benign. Fowler and his co-workers (44) reported that 23% of their patients had postoperative complications, which included lymphoceles, hematomas, abscesses, and pulmonary emboli.

Finally, when to initiate endocrine therapy for disseminated or locally advanced cancer of the prostate is still an unanswered issue. Although endocrine therapy may delay progression of disease and symptoms, there are no convincing data to show that survival is prolonged. The choices of endocrine therapy for the most part include either bilateral orchiectomy or diethylstilbesterol, 1–3 mg a day. Higher doses of diethylstilbesterol are not warranted and in fact may lead to increased deaths from cardiovascular or thromboembolic disease. These potential cardiovascular complications can be avoided with orchiectomy. Also, painful gynecomastia, which occurs in many patients who are on estrogen therapy, is likewise avoided.

Although cancer of the prostate is not an innocuous tumor, when we are dealing with an elderly patient who may have a multitude of other medical problems, common sense must prevail. The caring physician should balance the risks of aggressive therapy with the natural history of the disease. Often he or she is in a position of ameliorating symptoms and not trying to achieve a cure.

Renal Cell Carcinoma

Renal cell carcinoma typically presents in the fifth through the seventh decades of life. It may present in a variety of ways. The so called classic triad for this tumor of pain, hematuria, and the presence of a flank mass is, in actuality, rarely the presenting complaint. The patient with renal cell carcinoma may present with one of the above stigmata or nonspecific complaints, such as weight loss, fever, loss of appetite, and malaise. A variety of paraneoplastic syndromes have been associated with renal cell carcinoma, including erythrocytosis, hypercalcemia, and hepatic dysfunction in the absence of liver metastasis.

Any mass lesion that is seen on excretory urography should be evaluated with renal ultrasound. If absolutely strict criteria for simple renal cysts are not met then one should proceed to either CT scan or arteriogram. Most of these tumors are hypervascular although certainly a solid hypovascular mass still could represent a renal cell carcinoma. Assessment of the renal vein and vena cava for tumor thrombosis should be vigorously pursued and evaluated. Whole lung tomograms or CT scans of the chest should be done to look for metastatic disease.

In the absence of metastatic disease, a radical nephrectomy done by the transabdominal approach with early ligation of the renal vessels is the treatment of choice. Extension of the tumor thrombosis into the vena cava does not appear to be as ominous a prognostic indicator as once thought when compared to the presence or the absence of capsular invasion or regional lymph node involvement (45).

In the presence of metastatic disease, nephrectomy is generally not indicated unless the patient has severe flank pain or there is life-threatening gross hematuria. In these instances, a palliative nephrectomy is justified.

In the elderly population, renal function may be seriously impaired either from surgical absence of one kidney or from bilateral parenchymal disease. In this situation, the surgeon is confronted with a difficult decision with regard to treatment options for the renal cell carcinoma. Certainly, split isotopic renal function studies should be obtained to assess the relative function from each of the kidneys if two are present. A decision then needs to be made as to whether the patient will have sufficient renal function after one diseased kidney is removed. If this is felt not to be the case or if the patient should have a solitary kidney, then serious consideration should be given to a partial nephrectomy. Although the wisdom of this approach has been questioned by some (46), others have felt that with proper patient selection this is a viable alternative (47, 48). In such patients, although the diagnosis may be made with reasonable assurance on CT scan, arteriography is usually helpful for outlining the tumor and blood supply and planning the surgical approach to these tumors. Surgical exploration can usually be done in situ, although occasionally a centrally located tumor may require ex vivo enucleation and auto-transplantation.

All of these decisions should be shared by the nephrology service in the event that surgical segmental excision is impossible and if the postoperative renal function is such that chronic dialysis will be needed.

Transitional Cell Carcinomas

Most transitional cell carcinomas of the urinary tract arise in the bladder although they can occur anywhere along the urothelial surface, including calices, renal pelvis, and ureter.

Patients with transitional cell carcinoma of the bladder may present with gross or microscopic hematuria. Signs and symptoms of bladder irritation, which are not explained by infection, should also cause suspicion. Likewise, patients with upper tract tumors may present with hematuria or, if the tumor is obstructive, with a dull flank ache. Upper tract tumors are usually seen as a subtle deformity or radiolucent filling defect in the upper collecting system. This always warrants further investigation. Tumors of the bladder are often missed on routine excretory urography and are usually seen only at the time of cystoscopic examination. Low grade, low stage, papillary transitional cell tumors of the bladder are best treated by transurethral resection and intensive follow-up. This follow-up includes a cystoscopy at 3-month intervals for

1 to 2 years. If there is no tumor recurrence at that point, the intervals may be increased to every 6 months. Should the patient have rapidly recurring tumors, consideration of intravesical chemotherapy using either thio-tepa or mitomycin C is advised.

If, on the other hand, invasive high grade cancer is found at the time of initial cystoscopy, the patient should be considered for total cystectomy with urinary diversion. There is only a very limited role for segmental cystectomy. Cystectomy with urinary diversion is a formidable operative procedure. There is a tendency among some to propose more conservative measures in the elderly patient. However, numerous reports would seem to indicate that, with proper patient selection, age per se should not be a contraindication to aggressive surgical treatment of this potentially lethal disease (49–53).

Transitional Cell Tumors of the Upper Urinary Tract

Evaluation of radiolucent filling defects or upper urinary tract bleeding can sometimes be a frustrating diagnostic exercise. Retrograde pylography, barbotage of suspicious lesions by ureteral catheters for cytologic analysis, and ureteroscopy all play a role in diagnosing transitional cell malignancies of the ureter and renal pelvis.

Although standard surgical therapy would dictate a total nephro-urectomy, which includes a cuff of bladder around the involved ureteral orifice, patients with low grade, low stage tumors might better be treated with a more conservative approach. Specifically, segmental resection of low grade, low stage tumors is certainly reasonable. It is obviously a less formidable procedure, and in the elderly patient it may also have the advantage of preserving total renal function (54, 55). Interestingly enough, a patient with a very undifferentiated tumor may have such a poor prognosis that even complete radical nephrectomy does not seem to affect survival. In this very small group, perhaps only palliative resection, especially in the face of renal insufiency, might be all that is indicated (56).

Testicular Carcinoma

Although germ cell testicular carcinoma is the most common malignancy of solid organs in young males, it is rare in the older age group. Lymphoma is the most common testicular tumor in the elderly. This usually represents a systemic disease although lymphoma confined to the testes is a remote possibility.

REFERENCES

1. Dunnill MS, Halley W: Some observations on the quantitive anatomy of the kidney. *J Path* 110: 113–121, 1972.
2. Friedman SA, Raizner AE, Rosen H, Solomon NA, Sy W: Functional defects in the aging kidney. *Ann Intern Med* 76: 41–45, 1972.
3. Kaplan C, Paternack B, Shah H, Gallo G: Age-related incidence of sclerotic glomeruli in human kidneys. *Am J Pathol* 80:227–234, 1975.
4. Goyal VK: Changes with age in the human kidneys. *Exp Gerontol* 17:321–331, 1982.
5. McLachlan MSF. Guthrie JC, Anderson CK, Fulker MJ: Vascular and glomerular changes in the aging kidney. *J Path* 121: 65–78, 1976.
6. Griffiths GJ, Robinson KB, Cartwright GO, McLachlan MSF: Loss of renal tissue in the elderly. *Br J Radiol* 49:111–117, 1976.
7. Takazakura E, Sawabu N, Handa A, Takada A, Shinoda A, Takeuchi J: Intrarenal vascular changes with age and disease. *Kidney Int* 2:224–230, 1972.
8. Hollenberg NK, Adams DF, Solomon HS, Rashid A, Abrams HL, Merrill JP. Senescence and the renal vasculature in normal man. *Circ Res* 34:309–316, 1974.
9. Rowe JW, Andres R, Tobin JD, Norris AH, Shock NW: The effect of age on creatinine clearance in men: a cross-sectional and longitudinal study. *J Gerontol* 31: 155–163, 1976.
10. Lindeman RD, Tobin J, Shock NW: Longitudinal studies on the rate of decline in renal function with age. *J Am Geriatr Soc* 33:278–285, 1985.
11. Cockroft DW, Gault MH: Prediction of creatinine clearance from serum creatinine. *Nephron* 16:31–41, 1976.
12. Epstein M, Hollenberg NK: Age as a determinant of renal sodium conservation in normal man. *J Lab Clin Med* 87:411–417, 1976.
13. Rowe JW, Shock NW, DeFronzo RA: The influence of age on the renal response to water deprivation in man. *Nephron* 17:270–278, 1976.
14. Weidmann P, DeMyttznaere-Bursztein S, Maxwell MH, Delima J: Effect of aging on plasma renin and aldosterone in normal man. *Kidney Int* 8: 325–333, 1975.
15. Helderman JH, Vestal RE, Rowe JW, Tobin JD, Andres R, Robertson GL: The responce of arginine vasopressin to intravenous ethanol and hypertonic saline in man: the impact of aging. *J Gerontol* 33:39–47, 1978.
16. Kinsey AC, Pomeroy WB, Martin CE, Gebhardt PH. *Sexual Behavior in the Human Male.* Philadelphia, WB Saunders, 1948, p 226.
17. Newman G, Nichols CR: Sexual activities and attitudes in older persons. *JAMA* 173:33–35, 1960.
18. Montague DK, James RE, deWolfe VG, Martin LM:

Diagnostic evaluation, classification and treatment of men with sexual dysfunction. *Urology* 14: 545-548, 1979.

19. Stearns EL, MacDonnell JA, Kaufman BJ, Padua R, Lucman TS, Winter JSD, Faiman C: Declining testicular function with age: hormonal and clinical correlates. *Am J Med* 57:761-766, 1974.

20. Baker HWG, Burger HG, deKretser DM, Hudson B, O'Connor S, Wang C, Mirovies A, Court J, Dunlop M, Rennie GC: Changes in the pituitary-testicular system with age. *Clin Endocrinol* 5:349-372, 1976.

21. Michal Ruzvarsky V: Morphologic changes in the arterial bed of the penis with aging. *Invest Med* 15:194-199, 1977.

22. Ellenberg M: Impotence in diabetes: the neurologic factor. *Ann Intern Med* 75:213, 1971.

23. Benson RC, Patterson DE, Barrett DM: Long-term results with Jones malleable penile prosthesis. *J Urol* 134:899-901, 1985.

24. Montague DK: Experience with semi-rigid rod and inflatable penile prostheses. *J Urol* 129:967-968, 1983.

25. Joesph DB, Bruskewitz RC, Benson RC: Long-term evaluation of the inflatable penile prosthesis. *J Urol* 131:670-673, 1984.

26. Zorniotti WA, Lefleur RS: Auto-injection of corpus cavernosum with vasoactive drug combination for vasculogenic impotence. *J Urol* 133:39-41, 1985.

27. Campbell JA, Reiken J, McCosh L: Incontinence in the elderly: prevalence and prognosis. *Age Aging* 14:65-70, 1985.

28. Ouslander JG, Kane RL, Abrass IB: Urinary incontinence in elderly nursing home patients. *JAMA* 248:1194-1198, 1982.

29. Weiss BD: Unstable bladder in elderly patients. *Am Fam Physician* 28: 243-247, 1983.

30. Cardozo L, Stanton SL, Hafner J, Allan V: Biofeedback in the treatment of detrusor instability. *Br J Urol* 50:250-254, 1978.

31. Carpenter HA, Simon R: The effect of several methods of training on long-term incontinent behaviorly regressed hospitalized psychiatric patients. *Nursing Res* 9:17, 1960.

32. Moisey CV, Stephenson TP, Brendler DK: The urodynamic and subjective results of detrusor instability with oxybutynin chloride. *Br J Urol* 52:472-475, 1980.

33. Stewart BH, Banowsky LH, Montague DK: Stress incontinence: conservative therapy with sympathomimetic drugs. *J Urol* 115:558-559, 1976.

34. Gillon G, Stanton SL: Long-term follow-up of surgery for urinary incontinence in elderly women. *Br J Urol* 56:478-481, 1984.

35. Lapides J, Diokno AC, Gould FR, Lowe BS: Further observations on self-catheterization. *J Urol* 116:169-171, 1976.

36. Pearson RM, Noe HN: Why urodynamic studies are important in urologic problems of the elderly. *Geriatrics* 34:43-53, 1979.

37. Castleden CM, Duffin HM, Asher MJ: Clinical and urodynamic studies in 100 elderly incontinent patients. *Br Med J* 282:1103-1105, 1981.

38. Fernie GR, Jewett MA, Halsall P, Zoritto ML: Urodynamic characterization of incontinence in the elderly by bladder volume. *J Urol* 129:772-774, 1983.

39. Grossman IC, Carpinillo V, Greenberg SH, Mollot TR, Wein AJ: Staging pelvic lymphadenectomy for carcinoma of the prostate: review of 91 cases. *J Urol* 124:632-634,1980.

40. Brendler CB, Cleeve LK, Anderson EE, Paulson DF: Staging pelvic lymphadenectomy for carcinoma of the prostate: risk versus benefit. *J Urol* 124:849-850, 1980.

41. Wilson CS, Dahl DS, Middleton RG: Pelvic lymphadenectomy for the staging of apparently localized prostatic cancer. *J Urol* 117:197-198, 1977.

42. McLaughlin AP, Saltzstein SL, McCullough DL, Gittes RF: Prostatic carcinoma: incidence and location of unsuspected lymphatic metastasis. *J Urol* 115:89-94, 1976.

43. Lieskovski G, Skinner DG, Weisenburger T: Pelvic lymphadenectomy in the management of carcinoma of the prostate. *J Urol* 124:635-638, 1980.

44. Fowler JE Jr, Barzell W, Hilaris BS, Whitmore WF Jr, Complications of ^{125}iodine implantation and pelvic lymphadenectomy in the treatment of prostatic cancer. *J Urol* 121:447-451, 1979.

45. Cherrie RJ, Goldman DG, Lindmer A, DeKermor JB: Prognostic implication of vena caval extension of renal cell carcinoma. *J Urol* 128:910-912, 1982.

46. Brannen GE, Correa RJ Jr, Gibbons RP: Renal cell carcinoma in solitary kidneys. *J Urol* 129:130-131, 1983.

47. Novick AC, Stewart BH, Straffon RA, Banowsky LH: Partial nephrectomy in the treatment of renal adenocarcinoma. *J Urol* 118:932-936, 1977.

48. Smith RB, DeKernion JB, Ehlich RM, Skinner DG, Kaufman JJ: Bilateral renal cell carcinoma and renal cell carcinoma in the solitary kidney. *J Urol* 132:450-454, 1984.

49. Ogawa A, Yanagisana Y, Nakamoto T, Wasiki M, Hirabayashi N, Nakama M: Treatment of bladder carcinoma in patients more than 80 years old. *J Urol* 134:889-891, 1985.

50. Zincke H: Cystectomy and urinary diversion in patients eighty years old or older. *Urology* 19:139-142, 1982.

51. Tachibana M, Deguchi N, Jitsukawa S, Murai M, Nakazono M, Tazaki H: One stage total cystectomy and ileal loop diversion in patients over eighty years old with bladder carcinoma. *Urology* 22:512-516, 1983.

52. Drago JR, Rohner TJ: Cystectomy and urinary diversion: a safe procedure for elderly patients. *Urology* 21:17-19, 1983.

53. Skinner EC, Lieskousky G, Skinner DG: Radical cystectomy in the elderly patient. *J Urol* 131:1065-1068, 1984.

54. Murphy DM, Zincke H, Furlow WL: Primary grade I transitional cell carcinoma of the renal pelvis and ureter. *J Urol* 123:629-631, 1980.

55. Zincke H, Neves RJ: Feasibility of conservative surgery for transitional cell cancer of the upper urinary tract. *Urol Clin N Am* 11:717-724, 1984.

56. Murphy DM, Zincke H, Furlow WL: Management of high grade transitional cell cancer of the upper urinary tract. *J Urol* 125:25-29, 1981.

Chapter 27

Gynecologic Diseases in the Elderly

Lonnie S. Burnett, M.D., F.A.C.O.G., Howard W. Jones, III, M.D., F.A.C.O.G.

Certain gynecologic conditions are more common among elderly women. Various types of pelvic relaxation with associated symptoms, such as stress urinary incontinence and malignant tumors, including those of the ovary, vulva, and endometrium, are the most common conditions requiring surgical treatment in the advanced age groups. Although the surgical techniques used for the treatment of these conditions are essentially the same in the aged as those in younger patients, the judgement required in selecting patients for the procedure may require considerable experience. In the patient who is a poor surgical candidate, alternative forms of therapy are often available, and the selection of the wrong candidate for surgical management may prove disastrous (1). On the other hand, we have seen many elderly women in whom an otherwise indicated surgical procedure was not recommended only because of concerns for the patient's age. Several years later many of these women will still be alive and reasonably well, yet they continue to suffer even worse symptoms from the gynecologic disease. It is then when she and her doctors suddenly realize that it would have been better to have done the operation sooner.

Elderly postmenopausal patients do not have the problems usually associated with pregnancy, such as infertility and endometriosis, and they rarely develop primary pelvic infections. Occasionally, uterine leiomyoma may become symptomatic causing pelvic pain or bleeding, although most leiomyomas regress and become less symptomatic following menopause.

PELVIC RELAXATIONS IN THE ELDERLY FEMALE

For most women the basic anatomic defects ultimately leading to pelvic relaxation begin with damage to the supporting ligaments and fasciae of the pelvis through the trauma of childbirth. Nevertheless, the development of many of these symptomatic relaxations as clinical entities may not occur until years later, often when the patient is elderly and additional support is lost through attenuation and atrophy associated with aging. All factors contributing to increased pressure on the pelvic floor (chronic cough, obesity, straining with defecation, etc.) increase the risk of symptomatic pelvic relaxation. Progressive pelvic relaxation, including total inversion of the vagina, may occur and first become apparent in the elderly patient following an upper respiratory tract infection that was associated with intense coughing. Occasionally after the institution of an exercise program that includes maneuvers that result in increases in intra-abdominal pressure, an especially active elderly women will first notice uterine descent.

Anatomic support for the vagina and its contiguous structures, such as the urethra, bladder, uterus, and rectum, is provided by the urogenital diaphragm, the pubourethrovaginal ligaments, the endopelvic fascia, the cardinal and uterosacral ligaments, and the levator ani muscles.

Urogenital diaphragm. Located within the pubic arch, this muscle and fascial layer provides support to the distal urethra and vagina. Defects in this structure contribute to the formation of a urethrocele with posterior rotation of the urethra and relaxed vaginal outlet.

Pubourethrovaginal ligaments. These extend from the posterior surface of the pubis to the distal urethra and vagina and when torn or damaged may result in urethrocele.

The endopelvic fascia. A well-defined layer of

condensed endopelvic fascia surrounds the genital tract and provides support to the vagina by its attachment to the pelvic walls in the region of the arcuate lines from the pubis to the ischial spine. Defects in this layer contribute to the formation of a wide variety of relaxation conditions, including cystourethrocele, uterovaginal prolapse, enterocele, and rectocele.

The cardinal ligaments. These represent condensations of endopelvic fascia around vessels and nerves. They extend from the cervix bilaterally to the pelvic sidewalls above the ischial spine. Laxity and attenuation of these ligaments contribute to uterovaginal prolapse.

Uterosacral ligaments. These highly important ligaments extend from the posterior lateral margin of the cervix and from the upper vagina to the anterior surface of the sacrum on each side of the rectum. Loss or attenuation of these strong supporting bands may result in vaginal prolapse or prolapse of the vaginal vault.

Levator muscles. That portion of the muscle in closest proximity to the genital tract (puborectalis) provides support to both the vagina and rectum. Attenuation, sagging and separation of the fibers of this structure contribute to both rectocele and prolapse.

Pelvic relaxations may involve multiple clinical entities, including urethrocele, cystocele, uterovaginal prolapse, enterocele, rectocele, and relaxed vaginal outlet. Although it is convenient to discuss these separately, in most instances the patient will present for evaluation with several problems and with multiple defects. When surgical repair is indicated, it is highly important to identify specifically each and every anatomic defect. Optimal surgical results and the avoidance of a high rate of recurrence require that each anatomic abnormality be taken into account and repaired when feasible.

Cystourethrocele

Although urethrocele and cystocele may occur independently, they are more frequently seen as a combined defect. Urethrocele refers to the sagging of the anterior vaginal wall and the underlying urethra. Because the external urethral orifice is fixed at the vestibule, urethrocele results in a posterior rotation and descent of the urethrovesicle junction from its normal position behind the symphysis. This is the anatomic defect

commonly (but not always) associated with stress urinary incontinence.

Cystocele refers to the sagging of the anterior vaginal wall underlying the bladder, and therefore it characteristically involves the entire upper vagina. When a urethrocele and a cystocele occur together (cystourethrocele), the sagging involves the entire anterior vaginal wall from the urethral orifice to the cervix, and the anterior wall may protrude well beyond the vaginal introitus, i.e., third degree. When a cystocele is present alone, especially in advanced degrees, urinary incontinence is rarely seen; in fact, the patient is more likely to experience incomplete bladder emptying and will sometimes have significant urinary retention.

Surgical Management of Cystourethrocele

Mild degrees of cystourethrocele are common in the elderly, and most need not be surgically corrected. The major indications for a surgical repair are symptoms that include stress urinary incontinence, discomfort associated with protrusion of a mass through the vaginal introitus, and chronic or acute urinary retention. Uterovaginal prolapse frequently accompanies this condition, and the surgical correction most commonly used includes removal of the uterus.

Anterior Vaginal Repair. This is accomplished by the vaginal route and involves a midline incision in the anterior vaginal wall overlying the area of defect. The vaginal wall is dissected away from the underlying urinary tract and endopelvic fascia, and the defect is corrected through plication of the fascia in the midline. This procedure is aimed at restoration of normal anatomy. The operation is simple and brief, is associated with minimal morbidity, and is well tolerated even in the elderly patient. When stress urinary incontinence is a prominent symptom, the surgical goal is to elevate the urethrovesicle junction to its normal retropubic position. Especially when the incontinence is severe, anterior vaginal repair has a significant failure rate especially with the passage of time. Other approaches are frequently preferable (2). These are discussed below.

Lateral Vaginal Repair. This operative approach is carried out retropubically and results in the reattachment of the paravaginal fascia to both pelvic sidewalls along the arcuate line extending from the pubis to the ischial spine. This technique is especially attractive because it restores normal anatomy and will result in correction of both the urethrocele and cystocele and in the relief of stress urinary incontinence. On the other hand, this operation requires an abdominal incision and a moderate amount of dissection in the retropubic space; recovery may therefore be less rapid than that associated with a vaginal approach.

Surgical Correction of Stress Urinary Incontinence

Urinary incontinence is a common symptom in the elderly female. Campbell et al. found a prevalence of 12% among women over 65 and 22% among women 80 year or older (3). Incontinence in this group frequently results from multiple factors, and decisions regarding management of the problem in a particular patient may require a very careful assessment of risks and benefits. Nevertheless, when genuine stress urinary incontinence is present as a single entity or as a contributing factor, a surgical approach should at least be considered and is often in the patient's best interest. Surgical procedures for this condition are rarely contraindicated on the basis of age alone. On the other hand, if senile dementia is present, the quality of life may only be very slightly affected by the correction of the incontinence. The convenience of the caretaker may be a factor, however.

Various operative procedures have been described, and all aim at the elevation of the urethrovesical junction back to its normal retropubic position.

Anterior Vaginal Repair

Performed entirely by the vaginal route, this procedure provides support to the urethrovesicle junction through plication of the perivaginal endopelvic fascia. Advantages include excellent tolerance by the elderly patient with little morbidity and a short hospital stay. Furthermore, the procedure can be done in conjunction with other vaginal procedures, such as vaginal hysterectomy and posterior vaginal repair; both of these procedures are commonly done in association with procedures for anterior relaxations. On the other

hand, there is increasing evidence that vaginal approaches are associated with an increased rate of recurrence of urinary incontinence, especially when follow-up extends over a period of 5 or more years.

Marshall-Marchetti-Krantz Procedure

This retropubic procedure elevates the urethrovesicle junction by suturing the attachment of the anterior vaginal wall to the periosteum of the posterior pubis (4). Overcorrection may occur, resulting in delayed voiding and urinary retention, and there is a small but definite risk of post-operative osteitis pubis.

Cooper Ligament Suspension

Originally described by Burch, this procedure and its modifications suspend the anterior vaginal wall in the area of the bladder neck by attachment to Cooper's ligament. The technique requires moderate retropubic dissection and when carried out alone is associated with an increased risk of subsequent enterocele. The modification by Stanton results in suspension not only of the urethra but also the bladder and therefore results in correction of any associated cystocele (5). Overcorrection may nevertheless result in urinary retention and delayed voiding.

Modified Pereya Technique

This combined abdominal vaginal approach begins vaginally with exposure of the pubocervical fascia in the area of the bladder neck. Utilizing a monofilament, nonabsorbable suture, a ligature carrier, and a small suprapubic incision, bilateral suspending sutures are attached to the perivaginal fascia, passed through the retropubic space, and tied over the fascia of the anterior abdominal wall. Elevation of the urethrovesicle junction to a retropubic position is the overall result. The procedure is brief, well tolerated even in the elderly patient, and is reported to be effective in about 90% of women. One special advantage is the option of carrying out other vaginal procedures when indicated without a change of position of the patient on the operating table.

The Stamey Procedure

This is a modification of the Pereya technique and results in elevation of the urethovesicle junction to a retropubic position utilizing bilateral nonabsorbable monafilament sutures that pass from a position lateral to the bladder neck through the retropubic space and are tied over the fascia of the anterior abdominal wall. As described by Stamey, the procedure is carried out utilizing endoscopic control with direct visualization of the bladder neck, thereby allowing a more accurate intraoperative assessment of the degree of suspension required for the relief of incontinence (6). The technique is simple and brief and is usually well tolerated even in the elderly patient. Stamey has reported highly successful results with relief of symptoms in about 90% of patients. A suprapubic catheter is usually left in place until the patient is able to void; in some instances spontaneous voiding may be delayed for several weeks.

Lateral Vaginal Repair

Described by Richardson and others, this technique aims at the restoration of normal anatomy through the reattachment of the paravaginal fascia to the arcuate line along the sidewalls of the pelvis (7). It results in restoration of the urethrovesicle junction to a retropubic position and in lengthening of the urethra itself. Although this technique is not yet widely used, Richardson and colleagues have reported highly successful results with minimal morbidity.

Uterovaginal Prolapse

Descent of the uterus through the vaginal canal may result in complete inversion of the vagina and is referred to as procidentia. Under these circumstances the bladder and even the ureters will follow the anterior vaginal wall downward and may be located outside of the vaginal introitus. Acute urinary retention and significant distal ureteral obstruction may be unexpected associated problems. When prolapse is early, incomplete, and accompanied by a cystourethrocele, incontinence is common. With a more complete prolapse, on the other hand, incontinence is rare, and urinary retention is much more likely. Relief of both the acute urinary retention and the distal ureteral obstruction can be achieved through the

replacement of the uterus into the pelvis.

Surgical correction of this dramatic appearing problem usually requires the removal of the uterus, resuspension of the vaginal canal, and the correction of many other defects, such as cystourethrocele, enterocele, and rectocele. The operative approach may be abdominal or vaginal. The choice of operation must take into account the patient's age and her general medical condition, the need to preserve vaginal function for intercourse, and those other factors that will influence the rate of recurrence, i.e., prolapse of the vaginal vault. In general, elderly patients tolerate vaginal procedures better than abdominal procedures, recovery is faster and serious morbidity is less frequent. If, after careful discussion with the patient, it becomes apparent that preservation of vaginal function is not important, the vaginal approach is especially suitable.

Vaginal Hysterectomy and Repair

For most elderly women, this is the procedure of choice for the management of uterovaginal prolapse. Following removal of the uterus through the vagina, the vaginal vault is suspended from the uterosacral ligaments utilizing a technique of culdoplasty, such as that described by McCall (8). A shelf is constructed from the uterosacral ligaments utilizing nonabsorbable sutures that are placed in such a way as to obliterate the cul-de-sac and eliminate the commonly present enterocele. The vaginal apex is then suspended from the uterosacral shelf. An anterior and posterior vaginal repair along with reapproximation of the levator muscles completes the procedure. This technique usually results in some shortening and narrowing of the vagina, which at times is sufficient to preclude satisfactory coitus.

LeFort Procedure

When the patient's age and medical condition make the risk of a major operation unacceptable, the LeFort procedure represents a compromise that may be acceptable and it should then be considered. A rectangular strip of vaginal mucosa is excised from both the anterior and posterior vaginal wall beginning about 2 cm distal to the cervix. The opposing defects are sutured together with consecutive rows of absorbable sutures resulting in closure of the vagina. A mucosal-lined tunnel on either side remains and permits the escape of cervical secretions or blood should the patient experience postmenopausal bleeding. The technique is generally very effective for correcting a prolapse, but causes the cervix and uterus to be inaccessible by the vaginal route. This technique should be considered only after exclusion of cancerous or precancerous lesions of the cervix or uterus and should probably be considered only when life expectancy is quite short. A significant disadvantage is the high rate of urinary incontinence that results from posterior rotation of the urethrovesicle angle, and it is commonly seen as a complication of this procedure.

Prolapse of the Vaginal Vault

Partial or complete prolapse of the vaginal vault is seen with increasing frequency among elderly woman who have previously undergone abdominal or vaginal hysterectomy. Defects of this nature are similar to those seen with uterovaginal prolapse; the inverted vagina carries with it the adjacent urinary tract and usually there is an associated enterocele. The problem is surgically complex because the uterosacral ligaments have been divided and are usually attenuated to the extent that they can no longer be utilized effectively for the resuspension of the vagina. Surgical correction can be achieved through the abdominal or the vaginal route. If preservation of normal vaginal function is a priority, an abdominal approach is usually preferable.

Vaginal Vault Sacropexy

Through an abdominal approach, the vaginal vault is identified and suspended to the presacral fascia, taking care to avoid injury to the sacral nerves or plexus. On occasion, the vagina will be of sufficient length to permit direct suturing to the sacrum, but more frequently there will be a requirement for an intervening bridge utilizing either synthetic or natural materials (9). Synthetic materials, such as Marlex or Dacron mesh, are highly effective, but on occasion chronic infection will require subsequent removal. Fascia lata taken from the lateral thigh through the use of a Masson fascia stripper has been widely used

with great success. During the operation the coexisting enterocele is repaired abdominally. If needed, a suspension of the vesicle neck can be achieved through a retropubic approach by one of the techniques described above.

Vaginal Repair of Vault Prolapse

Vaginal repair through the use of a modified Le Forte procedure (described above) or some other type of colpocleisis (closure of the vagina) may be effective, but results in loss of vaginal function and a risk of post-operative stress urinary incontinence.

If a vaginal approach is used with the aim of preserving vaginal function, the operative procedure usually includes an anterior and posterior colporrhaphy and an associated suspension of the vaginal vault through a culdoplasty utilizing the attenuated uterosacral ligaments. Although such a procedure is well tolerated in the elderly patient, disadvantages include compromise of vaginal function through narrowing and shortening of the canal and an increased rate of recurrence of the prolapse or the enterocele.

Enterocele

An enterocele results from extension and dissection of the cul-de-sac peritoneum through the fascia surrounding the posterior vaginal wall. The resulting hernia protrudes into the vaginal canal, may extend to and beyond the vaginal introitus, and is usually filled with small bowel and sometimes omentum. Although the condition usually accompanies one or more of the other forms of vaginal relaxation described earlier, it may occur alone. This condition is seen with the uterus in place and also after a prior hysterectomy. Repair may be accomplished by the abdominal or the vaginal route, but usually the latter is performed except under special circumstances. Repair, as with other herniae, requires dissection and removal of the sac followed by reconstruction of the posterior pelvic floor usually through plication of the uterosacral ligaments.

Rectocele and Relaxed Vaginal Outlet

A rectocele represents a protrusion or outpouching of the anterior rectal wall through the rectovaginal fascia. Protrusion occurs into the vaginal lumen, and it may be large enough to extend outside the vaginal introitus. Some degree of rectocele is common among the elderly, and most of these do not require surgical repair. It should be remembered that the defect begins with the damage resulting from childbirth, but the progression and enlargement that occur in the elderly come not only from the attenuation of connective tissue through aging but also from long-standing poor bowel habits associated with chronic constipation, habitual laxative use, and straining during defecation. Unless these underlying conditions are corrected, surgical repair is frequently followed by some degree of recurrence, and these are noticed to increase with time.

Relaxed vaginal outlet frequently accompanies a rectocele. The term, relaxed vaginal outlet, refers to a shortening and the attenuation of the perineal body resulting in the development of a close proximity between the vaginal introitus and the anal canal. The defect usually begins with damages sustained during childbirth. If the defect includes the anterior part of the anal sphincter, there may be no perineal body, and fecal incontinence may be a major symptom.

The surgical repair of a rectocele and relaxed vaginal outlet is usually accomplished simultaneously by utilizing a midline posterior vaginal wall incision that exposes both the anterior rectal wall and the attenuated and retracted fascia of the rectovaginal septum. The outpouching of the rectal wall is corrected through a series of mattress or purse-string sutures, and the perirectal fascia is reapproximated in the midline. Excessive vaginal mucosa is excised, and the posterior vaginal wall is closed. Reinforcement of the repair can be accomplished by the approximation of the levator muscles between the vagina and rectum. Although an aggressive reapproximation represents added insurance against recurrence, narrowing of the vaginal lumen may result, and this aspect requires constant evaluation during the operative procedure.

In repairing the relaxed vaginal outlet, the retracted muscles of the perineal body are identified laterally and reapproximated in the midline, resulting in reconstruction of the perineal body and the reforming of an appropriately wide separation between the vaginal introitus and the anal canal.

Alternatives to the Surgical Repair of Vaginal Relaxations

On occasion, the patient's advanced age, serious associated medical conditions, or impaired mental status will preclude the use of any of the described operative procedures. Under these circumstances and especially in patients with symptomatic relaxations involving prolapse of the uterus or vagina through the vaginal introitus, a compromise management can be achieved through the use of various vaginal pessaries (10). Such devices must be small enough to permit frequent changes by the patient or family and large enough to hold the prolapsed uterus or vagina in place and yet be retained in the upright or sitting position. Various types of "doughnut"-shaped pessaries (some inflatable) are most commonly effective and on occasion can be used for long periods.

Pressure necrosis from pessaries cause ulceration, and this is a common problem with their use. Good care of the elderly patient who has such a device requires frequent changes at weekly or, at the most, monthly intervals with cleansing douches and careful observation for pressure-induced ulcers. In some cases, a relaxed vaginal outlet prevents the retention of the pessary in the upright position.

MALIGNANT DISEASE

The common types of gynecologic malignancies all show an increased age-specific incidence rate, with increasing frequency for each year until approximately the ninth decade. Although the number of patients in each of the older decades is smaller, a higher percentage of women in those decades will have malignant tumors. Malignant gynecologic tumors are some of the more common indications for surgical procedures in the elderly female patient. The specific malignant diseases will be discussed, but a few generalizations about the subject are in order.

Although alternatives to surgical therapy, notably radiation therapy for cervical carcinoma, may provide similar results to surgical therapy in some diseases, the gynecologic surgeon should not be dissuaded from careful consideration of the surgical approach if this indeed provides the best chance of cure. Treatment alternatives should always be considered, but therapeutic compromises made with the idea that temporary palliation will "tide things over" until the elderly patient succumbs from her other medical diseases all too often result in a different and difficult dilemma in a few years to come. At that time, the patient, who has not died from old age, becomes increasingly symptomatic from her malignancy and is then often too fragile to be considered for surgical treatment (11). Lichtinger and co-workers reviewed a series of 89 patients who were more than 75 years of age and who underwent major gynecology operations for malignant tumors (12). With modern surgical intensive care and multisystems monitoring that have been available since 1976, hospital mortality in this group was reduced to 3.2%. Most of these surgical procedures were done for endometrial or vulvar carcinoma. When considering the management of gynecologic malignancy in the elderly patient with the double jeopardy of malignant disease and the general medical frailty of the usual aged patient, one may well decide that such a patient should be referred to a major medical center. There, the combined talents of multiple specialists who regularly deal with such problems will be available, and the success rate may well be improved (13).

The importance of a thorough and careful preoperative evaluation has been mentioned many times. Not only does this evaluation allow the physicians to identify the potential problems and assess the risks of the surgical procedure or other treatment modalities, but it will also provide reassurance to the patient and her family that the surgeon and the consultants are approaching her situation with care and thoughtful deliberation. It is not unusual that the most difficult person to convince of the advisability of the operation is the patient herself. Too often, elderly women have seen their friends die from cancer, and they may feel that the outcome of the procedure will be a brief and painful period and that death is inevitable. They may resist all forms of therapeutic intervention. We see this attitude often in family members of elderly patients and occasionally in the referring physician.

Endometrial Carcinoma

Adenocarcinoma of the endometrium is the most common invasive gynecologic malignancy in the United States today. Most patients with this disease are postmenopausal, with an average age of 59 at the time of diagnosis. The most common presenting complaint of a patient with endometrial cancer is postmenopausal bleeding. This occurs in over 90% of patients. High risk factors for endometrial carcinoma include estrogen therapy, obesity, nulliparity, and a previous history of endometrial hyperplasia. In the past, diabetes and hypertension have been cited as risk factors. Although these are common conditions among patient who have endometrial cancer, case control studies have demonstrated that there is no increased incidence of these conditions among endomentrial cancer patients when compared with women with benign causes of postmenopausal bleeding (14). Other causes for postmenopausal bleeding include hormonal therapy, atrophic vaginitis, endometrial polyps, and various types of endometrial hyperplasia.

Diagnosis and Staging

All women with postmenopausal bleeding should have a *dilatation of the cervix and fractional currettage* of the uterus and endocervix for a diagnosis. Hormonal therapy may indeed be the cause of bleeding, but it is also known to be associated with endometrial carcinoma, and therefore, merely discontinuing the medication without sampling the endometrium is not satisfactory management. In some patients with minimal uterine bleeding and with no high risk characteristics, an endometrial biopsy may be sufficient to rule out carcinoma. However, if any degree of hyperplasia is found on biopsy, a more thorough, formal fractional dilatation and curettage is certainly indicated. The importance of a *fractional* dilatation and curettage is emphasized because the proper staging of endometrial carcinoma requires an endocervical curettage to evaluate possible cervical involvement. Various other intra-uterine sampling techniques have been reviewed by Creasman and Weed, but most require special techniques or special equipment, and these techniques have not found wide acceptance (15).

The standard cervical Pap smear is not an adequate method of evaluating postmenopausal bleeding. Various estimates suggest that the Pap smear will be positive in only 35% to 50% of all patients with endometrial carcinoma.

Table 27.1 Definitions of the Clinical Stages in Carcinoma of the Corpus Uteri[a]

Stage 0	Atypical endometrial hyperplasia, carcinoma in situ. Histologic findings are suspicious of malignancy. (Cases of Stage 0 should not be included in any therapeutic statistics.)
Stage I	Carcinoma is confined to the corpus.
Stage Ia	Length of the uterine cavity is 8 cm or less.
Stage Ib	Length of the uterine cavity is more than 8 cm.
Stage II	Carcinoma has involved the corpus and the cervix, but has not extended outside the uterus.
Stage III	Carcinoma has extended outside the uterus, but not outside the true pelvis.
Stage IV	Carcinoma has extended outside the true pelvis or has obviously involved the mucosa of the bladder or rectum. A bullous edema as such does not permit a case to be allotted to Stage IV.
Stage IVa	Growth has spread to adjacent organs, such as urinary bladder, rectum, sigmoid, or small bowel.
Stage IVb	Growth has spread to distant organs.

[a]From *Annual Report on the Results of Treatment in Gynecological Cancer FIGO,* vol 19. Stockholm, Radium-hemmet, p 124.

Once a diagnosis of endometrial adenocarcinoma has been made, the tumor must be "staged" for therapeutic, prognostic, and statistical purposes. The classification system for cancer of the uterus that is generally accepted throughout the world is the one proposed by the International Federation of Gynecology and Obstetrics. This is shown in Table 27.1 (16). As with all gynecologic malignant tumors, except those involving the ovary, the classification system is a *clinical* one that does not permit the operative findings to influence staging. It is well recognized that this leads to a certain degree of staging inaccuracy. However, this is done with the purpose of standardization so that patients treated entirely with radiation therapy who never undergo laparotomy will have the same staging assignment as patients treated by hysterectomy.

It is important that patients with stage I disease, who constitute as many as 75% or 80% of all patients with endometrial carcinoma, must be further substaged on the basis of the uterine sounding depth and the degree of histologic differentiation of their cancer. Tumor grade is an especially important prognostic variable and

should always be taken into account when planning therapy. The incidence of lymph node metastasis varies greatly in patients with stage I disease depending on tumor differentiation. In addition, although the vast majority of patients with endometrial carcinoma have typical adenocarcinoma, special note should be made of the histologic findings of adenosquamous carcinoma or papillary adenocarcinoma, both of which have a poor prognosis (17, 18).

Lymph Node Metastases. Endometrial carcinoma spreads most commonly by lymphatic routes although direct extension and venous metastasis are not uncommon. Approximately 11% of patients with stage I endometrial carcinoma will have pelvic lymph node metastases. There is considerable variation in the extent and incidence of lymph node involvement depending upon the degree of differentiation of the tumor and depth of myometrial invasion (Table 27.2). In those cases where there is cervical involvement, stage II disease, the incidence of pelvic nodal metastases increases to 35% or 40%. In addition to pelvic lymph node metastases, the tumor may also have spread from the uterus along the ovarian lymphatics to involve the para-aortic nodes (19).

Therapy

Total abdominal hysterectomy with bilateral salpingo-oophorectomy is the cornerstone of treatment for patients with endometrial carcinoma. Because the disease frequently occurs in elderly patients, often in association with the common medical illnesses of obesity, diabetes, and hypertension, serious reservations concerning the surgical approach may be expressed by some elderly patients. Surgical removal of the

Table 27.2 Stage and Grade in Pelvic and Aortic Node Metastases[a]

Stage	Pelvic %	Aortic %
IA,G1	1.7	1.7
IA,G2	9.3	6.9
IA,G3	22.2	16.6
IB,G1	3.2	0.0
IB,G2	11.1	2.7
IB,G3	45.0	40.0

[a]From Diasia PJ, Creasman WT: *Clinical Gynecologic Oncology,* St. Louis, CV Mosby Co, 1981, p 139.

uterus significantly improves survival in most patients with endometrial carcinoma, and every effort should be made to accomplish this goal if at all possible.

For patients with stage I endometrial adenocarcinoma, most authorities in the United States would recommend initial total abdominal hysterectomy with bilateral salpingo-oophorectomy. This not only removes the primary cancer but also affords the opportunity for selective sampling of lymph nodes in the pelvic and aortic areas.

There continues to be active disagreement about the place of adjunctive radiation therapy in patients with stage I endometrial carcinoma. Some recommend either routine pre- or post-operative radiation (20), whereas others advocate selective use of radiation only for patients with positive lymph nodes or for those patients whose tumors show deep myometrial invasion (21). At Vanderbilt University, the protocols for the treatment of patients with stage I endometrial carcinoma all begin with primary hysterectomy with bilateral salpingo-oophorectomy for every patient. In women who have grade 2 and 3 tumors, pelvic and aortic lymph nodes are selectively removed for histologic examination. Peritoneal cytologic washings are routinely obtained from the pelvis and paracolic gutters and examined for malignant tumor cells. No further therapy is recommended for those patients who have no myometrial invasion. For patients with superficial myometrial invasion found at the time of hysterectomy an intravaginal cesium application delivering 6000 mGy to the vaginal surface is recommended from 3 to 6 weeks following hysterectomy. This has been shown to reduce the incidence of recurrence at the vaginal apex from about 10% to 2%. When the endometrial cancer has been found to penetrate more than 50% of the thickness of the myometrium, the risk of pelvic lymph node metastases approaches 40%, and even if the selective node sampling has been negative for metastatic disease, external whole pelvis radiation to 5000 mGy is adminstered. When pelvic or aortic lymph node metastases are demonstrated, therapy is individualized, but it almost always includes some form of extended field irradiation plus progestational therapy.

In patients with stage II disease the incidence of pelvic node metastases is approximately 35%,

and therefore, radiation is always included in the therapy plan. In most instances, external whole pelvis irradiation, intracavitary radioactive cesium, and hysterectomy are combined in one sequence or another. With gross involvement of the cervix, external radiation therapy is usually administered primarily, but there is an increasing trend toward hysterectomy before external radiation in many patients with microscopic cervical disease. Lymph node biopsies may be done for prognostic reasons, but pelvic irradiation therapy is always recommended in patients with gross or microscopic cervical involvement.

When the tumor is spread beyond the uterus in either stage III or stage IV disease, treatment is again individualized depending on the location and extent of the disease. However, total abdominal hysterectomy and bilateral salpingo-oopherectomy are recommended if the operation is technically feasible, if the patient has at least a 6-month life expectancy, and if she is otherwise a reasonable surgical candidate. The uterine bleeding associated with the progression of untreated tumor can be severe, and hysterectomy is felt to be extremely useful for palliation in these cases.

Vaginal hysterectomy has been recommended for patients with stage I endometrial cancer if they are grossly obese or if a vaginal approach might offer a rapid surgical procedure with less morbidity (22). This approach may be especially attractive in the elderly patient who will likely have some degree of pelvic relaxation and uterine prolapse and where simple vaginal hysterectomy (along with bilateral salpingo-oophorectomy if possible) would allow the skilled vaginal surgeon to complete the hysterectomy in 30 minutes or less. Rutledge has reviewed the indications for *radical abdominal hysterectomy* and pelvic lymphadenectomy in patients with endometrial carcinoma (23). This approach is generally not recommended for the elderly patient because of the prolonged operative time and associated blood loss. Because no real improvement in survival has been reported with this approach, we feel that the increased morbidity cannot be justified in the elderly patient.

Alternatives to Surgical Therapy

In the elderly patient with significant associated medical conditions, the risk of a surgical procedure may be a significant one, and alternative methods of therapy should be considered. As noted previously, radiation therapy alone has been widely used for treatment of endometrial adenocarcinoma. However, Bickenbach and his colleagues clearly outlined in a series of matched pairs of comparable cases that patients with even stage I cancers had worse 5-year survival when hysterectomy was not part of their management (24). The Stockholm method originally described by Heyman involves packing the endometrial cavity with multiple radioactive sources (25). This type of "Heyman packing" is rarely used in this country today because it is uncommon to find a patient whose uterus is sufficiently enlarged to accept multiple radioactive capsules. A general or regional anesthetic is required for this procedure. External irradiation is generally well tolerated even by debilitated patients, and using small fractions and small port sizes, doses of 5000 to 7000 mGy to the central pelvis can be achieved. However, even these large doses are generally inadequate to obtain the 80% to 90% cure rates that can be expected for stage I disease treated surgically.

Hormonal therapy with progestins has also been effective for palliation of endometrial carcinoma (26). This is usually not thought of as a curative treatment, although patients with well-differentiated tumors may respond quite well.

Results

The treatment results that can be expected for patients with endometrial adenocarcinoma are shown in Table 27.3. These are absolute 5-year survival reports collected from throughout the world by the International Federation of Gynecology and Obstetrics. Most published reports describe better 5-year survival statistics, but they usually represent more selected series and statistically "corrected" survival figures (16). It is important to note that age is a significant prognostic variable. Among 1509 patients with stage I and II endometrial carcinoma, the absolute 5-year survival rate was 64.8% for those patients under age 70, whereas those who were 70 or older had only a 43.5% survival. However, it is difficult to be sure of the true significance of age as a prognostic variable because advanced age may lead to treatment modifications that affect survival.

In the management of endometrical carcinoma, hysterectomy plays such an important role that a patient's age in and of itself should not be a contraindication to a treatment plan that provides the best chance of cure.

Ovarian Cancer

Carcinoma of the ovary is the fourth leading cause of death from cancer among women in the United States. The age-adjusted incidence rates show a steady increase in ovarian carcinoma each year until age 85. Over one-third of patients with ovarian cancer are 65 years or older.

One of the main reasons for the poor outcome in patients with ovarian carcinoma is the silent nature of this malignancy. Its intra-abdominal location makes it difficult to examine, and three-fourths of all patients with ovarian carcinoma will already have disease spread beyond the pelvis at the time of initial presentation. Until the disease has become widespread, symptoms are few and relatively nonspecific. Occasional vague pain, fullness, or bloating may be described. This vague pain is often transient in nature and not too severe and is attributed to something else. Quite often, these symptoms are elicited only in retrospect, but occasionally patients will have undergone a thorough gastrointestinal workup that will have been fruitless.

In a good review of the data from the Surveillance, Epidemiology, and End Results (SEER) Program of the National Cancer Institute, Yancik et al. found that older patients with ovarian cancer had more advanced disease (27). The median age for ovarian cancer was 54 years for stage I and 62 years for stages III and IV. Seventy-three and one-half percent of patients over age 75 who had ovarian cancer had stage

Table 27.3 Carcinoma of the Corpus Uteri, 1976–1978: Distribution by Stage and 5-Year Survival[a]

Stage	Patients Treated		5-Year Survival	
	No.	%	No.	%
I	10,285	75.7	7,729	75.1
II	1,885	13.9	1,089	57.8
III	844	6.2	253	30.0
IV	452	3.3	48	10.6

[a]From *Annual Report on the Results of Treatment in Gynecological Cancer*
FIGO, vol 19. Stockholm, Radiumhemmet, p 128.

Table 27.4 Ovarian Cancer: Clinical Staging

Stage I	Growth limited to the ovaries
Stage Ia	Growth limited to one ovary; no ascites
(i)	No tumor on the external surface; capsule intact
(ii)	Tumor present on the external surface and/or capsule ruptured
Stage Ib	Growth limited to both ovaries; no ascites
(i)	No tumor on the external surface; capsules intact
(ii)	Tumor present on the external surface and/or capsule(s) ruptured
Stage Ic	Tumor either Stage Ia or Stage Ib, but with ascites[a] present or positive peritoneal washings
Stage II	Growth involving one or both ovaries with pelvic extension
Stage IIa	Extension and/or metastases to the uterus and/or tubes
Stage IIb	Extension to other pelvic tissues
Stage IIc	Tumor either Stage IIa or Stage IIb, but with ascites present or positive peritoneal washings
Stage III	Growth involving one or both ovaries with intraperitoneal metastases outside the pelvis and/or positive retroperitoneal nodes; tumor limited to the true pelvis with histologically proven malignant extension to small bowel or omentum
Stage IV	Growth involving one or both ovaries with distant metastases; if pleural effusion is present there must be positive cytology to allot a case to Stage IV. Parenchymal liver metastases equals Stage IV
Special Category	Unexplored cases that are thought to be ovarian carcinoma

[a]Ascites is peritoneal effusion that in the opinion of the surgeon is pathologic and/or clearly exceeds normal amounts.

III and IV disease by the time the diagnosis was made, whereas only 47% of women under age 45 had such advanced disease. Surgical stage and tumor grade are far more important prognostic variables than patient age (28).

Diagnosis and Staging

Unlike all other gynecologic malignancies, ovarian cancer is a surgically staged disease (rather than clinically staged) because the diagnosis itself cannot be made with any certainty without a laparotomy. The FIGO staging system is shown in Table 27.4. Because ovarian carcinoma is a surgically staged disease, the need for an accurate evaluation of the extent of the disease at laparotomy should seem obvious. But, Young et al. have reported an alarmingly high incidence of inadequate staging, especially in women with early stage ovarian cancer (29). Patients with advanced disease present relatively little problem with staging and evaluation, but patients with stage I and II ovarian cancer may be inadequately staged unless a thorough evaluation of the abdomen is made, including washings for cytology, biopsy of the omentum, and careful inspection of the diaphragm, mesentery, and small bowel in addition to biopsy of the pelvic and aortic lymph nodes (30).

It is perhaps appropriate here to consider who should do the surgical procedure for patients with ovarian cancer. In cases where a small, mobile adnexal mass is present and the suspicion of ovarian cancer is low, any competent pelvic surgeon should be able to resect the tumor and do the proper staging evaluation that is necessary to decide on the appropriate postoperative therapy. However, when the masses are large and fixed and ascites is present, the chance of extensive tumor is great. Serious consideration should be given to referring these patients to an experienced gynecologic oncologist for the initial operation because extensive debulking surgery may be beneficial and the technical ability and judgement required for such procedures are not as highly developed in the surgeon who encounters extensive ovarian carcinoma only occasionally.

Indications for Surgical Therapy

In patients with ovarian carcinoma there are generally three main indications for operation. The first is for diagnosis and surgical removal of the tumor. The second is for "second look surgery," which is for the purpose of assessing the response to chemotherapy, and the third indication for the operative approach is to palliate patients with bowel obstruction from advanced ovarian carcinoma. Because these indications often require knowledge of the patient and the natural history of her disease, it is desirable for the patient to be followed by a single gynecologic oncologist who can perform the needed procedures, use the appropriate chemotherapy, and occasionally resort to radiation therapy when indicated.

Although recent studies by Hacker et al. (31)

suggest that aggressive *cytoreductive surgery* at the time of initial operation for ovarian cancer increased the length of survival, it is still not clear whether such an aggressive surgical approach actually increases the "cure" rate or only lengthens the time to symptomatic recurrence. It is widely believed that, when resection has been successful at reducing residual tumor volume to less than 2 cm, improved response to chemotherapy is observed. Whether the skill and aggressiveness of the surgeon are more important than the intrinsic malignancy of the tumor that allows or prevents extensive debulking is unknown, but the goal of primary surgical therapy for ovarian cancer should be to resect as much tumor as possible and yet allow the patient to recover promptly so that she will tolerate early postoperative chemotherapy satisfactorily. In the elderly patient superb clinical judgement is required to assess the extent of surgical resection that will prove beneficial to the patient without incurring too many complications or weakening the patient beyond her ability to tolerate chemotherapy. Advances in parenteral nutrition have made it possible to operate on debiliated patients, but the perioperative management of these patients often presents a difficult challenge.

The role of *"second look"* laparotomy to evaluate the results of chemotherapy in ovarian cancer is even more controversial. Several years ago it was widely believed that every patient who underwent chemotherapy should have a "second look" operation to assess the results of chemotherapy and provide guidance for future therapeutic decisions. However, it has become apparent that 15% to 59% of patients with no evidence of cancer on multiple biopsies at second look operation still develop recurrent disease, and the results of all types of treatment in patients found to have persistent cancer at second look have been extremely dismal. Therefore, the prognostic and therapeutic benefits of such an operation have been questioned recently, and "second look laparotomy" for ovarian cancer has become primarily a research protocol procedure and is not generally recommended for the average patient (32).

The natural history of ovarian carcinoma is a diffuse intra-abdominal spreading that frequently results in small bowel obstruction at multiple sites. In women with advanced disease the surgeon is often called upon to consider operating to relieve small bowel obstruction that has resulted from progressive cancer. Krebs and Goplerud have demonstrated that one operation on such patients is usually beneficial and results in prolonged survival (33). Nevertheless, it is important to realize that this is a palliative operation, and re-obstruction within 6 months is the usual course.

Alternatives to Surgical Therapy

Although the operative approach to ovarian carcinoma is very important, one will occasionally encounter patients whose medical condition or far advanced cancer makes the surgical approach difficult or of questionable benefit. In patients with advanced ascites and/or pleural effusion it is possible to make a presumptive diagnosis by cytologic examination of pleural or peritoneal fluid. Such patients may then be treated with several cycles of chemotherapy, with laparotomy being delayed to evaluate a response. If the effusions resolve and computed tomographic scans indicate a decrease in the size of the ovarian masses, resection may be reconsidered after several months. This is a very acceptable approach for selected patients. In general, thoracentesis prior to the initial operation will reduce the risk of pulmonary complications, but the removal of ascites can usually be accomplished at the same time as the exploratory laparotomy.

Radiation therapy has a limited role in patients with ovarian cancer, and it is usually applicable only in patients with very minimal or no residual disease.

Results

Surgical therapy alone is inadequate therapy for ovarian carcinoma except for patients with stage Ia, grade 1 tumors who have undergone adequate staging evaluation. The 5-year survival rates for patients with epithelial ovarian cancers are shown in Table 27.5. The overall survival rate for all patients is 29.9%. There is no doubt that newer combination chemotherapy has increased the length of survival, but the median survival for patients with stage III and IV disease is still only approximately 36 months. As noted in the beginning of this section, this is es-

Table 27.5. Treatment Results of Epithelial Carcinoma of the Ovary: Absolute 5-Year Survival from 83 Institutions around the World[a]

Stage	Number of Patients	5-Year Survival %
Ia	1122	72.3
b	286	56.1
c	217	58.1
IIa	277	47.7
b		
c	357	42.1
III	2660	13.5
IV	1258	4.5

[a]From *Annual Report on the Results of Treatment in Gynecological Cancer FIGO*, vol 19. Stockholm, Radiumhemmet, 1985, p 128.

pecially discouraging because the majority of patients with ovarian cancer already have stage III or IV disease at the time of their diagnosis. Patient age alone, however, should not eliminate the potential benefits of aggressive management.

Cervical Cancer

Although radical hysterectomy and pelvic lymphadenectomy are frequently used in the treatment of patients with early stage cervical carcinoma, radiation therapy is probably equally effective and is a very acceptable alternative in the older patient who is a poor surgical candidate. Occasionally, patients with recurrent cervical carcinoma will be candidates for total pelvic exenteration. In the past, age greater than 70 was a relative contraindication to this extensive surgical approach, but advances in perioperative management and medical therapy have made this contraindication less absolute. Patients with central pelvic recurrence following radiation therapy for cervical carcinoma who have no evidence of pelvic sidewall or distant metastasis are potential candidates for pelvic exenteration. Such procedures require close cooperation between the anesthesiologist, surgeon, and nursing personnel and should be done only in major medical centers where adequate staffing and experience are available.

Carcinoma of the Vulva

Carcinoma of the vulva is one of the least common of all gynecologic malignancies, accounting for only approximately 4% of female genital neoplasms. Surgical management with radical vulvectomy and bilateral inguinal-femoral lymphadenectomy continues to be the mainstay of treatment for vulvar carcinoma. The average age of patients with this diagnosis is 72, and it is not uncommon to find patients in the ninth or tenth decades of life with this disease.

The presenting symptoms are frequently bleeding, pain, or a mass. Elderly patients often exhibit considerable denial about symptoms and may delay seeing the physician for months or even years despite persistent symptoms. Although experienced physicians may be able to recognize various vulvar lesions by inspection, when there is any question about the possibility of malignancy, a biopsy should always be done using a small 4-mm Keyes biopsy punch with local anesthesia. There are several staging classifi-

Table 27.6. Definitions of the Clinical Stages in Carcinoma of the Vulva[a]

Stage 0	
TIS	Carcinoma in situ, intraepithelial carcinoma
Stage I	
T1 N0 M0	Tumor confined to the vulva; 2 cm or
T1 N1 M0	less in the larger diameter. Nodes are not palpable or are palpable in either groin, not enlarged, and mobile (not clinically suspicious of neoplasm).
Stage II	
T2 N0 M0	Tumor confined to the vulva; more than 2 cm in diameter.
T2 N1 M0	Nodes are not palpable or are palpable in either groin, not enlarged, and mobile (not clinically suspicious of neoplasm).
Stage III	
T3 N0 M0	Tumor of any size with
T3 N1 M0	(1) Adjacent spread to the lower urethera and/or the T3 N1 M0 vagina, the perineum, or the anus, and/or
T1 N2 M0	(2) nodes palpable in either one or
T2 N2 M0	both groins (enlarged, firm, and mobile, not fixed but clinically suspicious of noeplasm).
Stage IV	
T4 N0 M0	Tumor of any size
T4 N1 M0	
T4 N2nM0	(1) infiltrating the bladder mucosa
All conditions	and/or the upper part of the urethral
containing	mucosa and/or the rectal mucosa
N3 or	and/or (2) fixed to the bone or other
M1a or M1b	distant metastases. Fixed or ulcerated nodes in either one or both groins.

[a]From *Annual Report on the Results of Treatment in Gynecological Cancer FIGO*, vol 19. Stockholm, Radiumhemmet, p, 259.

Table 27.7 Results of Treatment for Invasive Cancer of the Vagina

		Survival				
Author	Total number of patients	Stage I %	Stage II %	Stage III %	Stage IV %	Overall %
Rubin (35)	68	79	52	54	0	49
Ball (36)	58	76	37	17	0	56
Benedet (37)	75	71	50	15	0	45
Pride (38)	43	66	41	25	0	37
Prempree (39)	71	83	65	40	0	56

cations used for vulvar carcinoma, but the clinical examination of tumor size and involvement of the vulva, vagina, and rectum is key (Table 27.6). The presence or absence of palpably suspicious lymph nodes is also used in the clinical staging, but this is notoriously inaccurate with approximately 30% false positives and false negatives.

Surgical Treatment

Despite the fact that this cancer commonly occurs in elderly patients, surgical therapy continues to be the main treatment modality and is usually well tolerated. Although radical vulvectomy with bilateral inguinal-femoral lymphadenectomy has been the treatment of choice for invasive vulvar carcinoma, in recent years various new approaches have been recommended for patients with very minimal disease. Morris has suggested the use of unilateral inguinal lympadenectomy for patients with primary tumors less than 2 cm in diameter confined to one side of the vulva without involvement of any midline structures (34). DeSaia and others have described a technique of selective superficial lymph node biopsy to evaluate the necessity for bilateral lymphadenectomy (40).

Alternatives to Surgical Therapy

Most patients can tolerate the procedure needed to remove vulvar carcinoma. This can be done under regional or even local anesthesia if necessary. Radiation therapy is not well tolerated on the vulva and is used infrequently for the primary treatment of vulvar carcinoma. However, radical vulvectomy or even simple excision of the tumor mass followed by radiation therapy to the inguinal nodes is a very effective alternative to lymphadenectomy. In most cases today when the inguinal nodes are positive, whole pelvic irradiation therapy is given, rather than surgical pelvic lymphadenectomy.

Results

Most vulvar carcinoma is diagnosed at a relatively early stage and results are excellent as illustrated in Table 27.7.

REFERENCES

1. Panayioyis G, Ellenbogen A, Grunstein S: Major gynecologic surgical procedures in the aged. *J Am Geriat Soc* 26:459–462, 1978.
2. Gillon G, Stanton SL: Long-term follow-up of surgery for urinary incontinence in elderly women. *Br J Urol* 56:478–481, 1984.
3. Campbell AJ, Reinken J, McCosh L: Incontinence in the elderly: prevalence and prognosis. *Age Aging* 14:65–70, 1985.
4. Krantz EK: The Marshall-Marchetti-Krantz procedure. In Stanton SL, Tanagho EA (eds): *Surgery of Female Incontinence.* New York, Springer-Verlag, 1986, p 87.
5. Stanton SL: Colposuspension. In Stanton SL, Tanagho EA (eds): *Surgery of Female Incontinence.* New York, Springer-Verlag, 1986, p 95.
6. Stamey TA: Endoscopic suspension of the vesicle neck. In Stanton SL, Tanagho EA (eds): *Surgery of Female Incontinence.* New York, Springer-Verlag, 1986, p 115.
7. Richardson AC, Edmonds PB, Williams NL: Treatment of stress urinary incontinence due to paravaginal fascial defect. *Am J Obstet Gynecol* 157:357–362, 1987.
8. Given JR FT: "Posterior culdeplasty": revisited. *Am J Obstet Gynecol* 153:135–139, 1985.
9. Addison WA, Livingood III CH, Sutton GP, Parker RT: Abdominal sacral culpopexy with mersilene mesh in the retroperitoneal position in the management of posthysterectomy vaginal vault prolapse and enterocele. *Am J Obstet Gynecol* 153:140–146, 1985.
10. Wingate MB: Geriatric gynecology. *Geriatr Med* 9:53–63, 1982.

11. Katz S, Branch LG, Branson MH, Papsidero JA, Beck JC, Greet DS: Active life expectancy. *N Engl J Med* 17:1218–1223, 1983.

12. Lichtinger M, Averette H, Penalver M, Sevin B: Major surgical procedures for gynecologic malignancy in elderly women. *South Med J* 79:1506–1510, 1986.

13. Djokovic JL, Hedley-Whyte J: Prediction of outcome of surgery and anesthesia in patients over 80. *JAMA* 242:2301–2306, 1979.

14. LaVecchia C, Franeschi S, Decarli A. Gallus G, Tognoni G: Risk factors for endometrial cancer at different ages. *JNCI* 73:667–671, 1984.

15. Creasman WT, Weed JR: Screening techniques in endometrial cancer. *Cancer* 38:436–440, 1976.

16. *Annual Report on the Results of Treatment in Gynecological Cancer FIGO,* vol 19. Stockholm, Radiumhemmet, 1985.

17. Ng ABP, Reagan JW, Storaasli JP, Wentz WB: Mixed adenosquamous carcinoma of the endometrium. *Am J Clin Pathol* 59:765–781, 1973.

18. Hendrickson M, Ross J, Eifel P, Martinez A, Kempson R: Uterine papillary serous carcinoma: a highly malignant form of endometrial adenocarcinoma. *Am J Surg Pathol* 6:93–108, 1982.

19. Burrell MO, Franklin EW, Powell JL: Endometrial cancer: evaluation of spread and followup in 189 patients with stage I or stage II disease. *Am J Obstet Gynecol* 144:181–185, 1982.

20. Aalders J, Abeler V, Kolstad P, Onsrud M: Postoperative external irradiation and prognostic parameters in stage I endometrial carcinoma: clinial and histopathologic study of 540 patients. *Obstet Gynecol* 56:419–426, 1980.

21. Bean HA, Bryant AJS, Carmichael JA, Mallick A: Carcinoma of the endometrium in Saskatchewan: 1966 to 1971. *Gynecol Oncol* 6:503–514, 1978.

22. Peters WA, Andersen WA, Thornton WN, Morley GW: The selective use of vaginal hysterectomy in the management of adenocarcinoma of the endometrium. *Am J Obstet Gynecol* 146:285–291, 1983.

23. Rutledge FN: Role of radical hysterectomy in adenocarcinoma of the endometrium. *Gynecol Oncol* 2:331–347, 1974.

24. Bickenbach W, Lochmuller H, Dirlich G, Ruland G, Thurmayr R: Factor analysis of endometrial carcinoma in relation to treatment. *Obstet Gynecol* 29:632–636, 1967.

25. Heyman J: The so-called Stockholm method and the results of treatment of uterine cancer at the Radiumhemmet. *Acta Radiol* 16:129–148, 1935.

26. Kohorn EI: Gastagens and endometrial carcinoma. *Gynecol Oncol* 4:398–411, 1976.

27. Yancik R, Ries LG, Yates JW: Ovarian cancer in the elderly: an analysis of surveillance, epidemiology, and end results program data. *Am J Obstet Gynecol* 154:639–647, 1986.

28. Schulz BO, Krebs D, Sellin D: The prognostic value of age for patients with common epithelial cancer. *J Cancer Res Clin Oncol* 109:152–155, 1985.

29. Young RC, Decker DG, Wharton JT, Piver S, Sindelar WF, Edwards BK, Smith JP: Staging laparotomy in early ovarian cancer. *JAMA* 250:3072–3076, 1983.

30. Buchsbaum HJ, Lifshitz S: Staging and surgical evaluation of ovarian cancer. *Semin Oncol* 11:227–237, 1984.

31. Hacker NF, Berek JS, Lagasse LD, Nieberg RK, Elashoff RM: Primary cytoreductive surgery for epithelial ovarian cancer. *Obstet Gynecol* 61:413–420, 1983.

32. Cain JM, Saigo PE, Pierce VK, Clark DG, Jones WB, Smith DH, Hakes TB, Ochoa M, Lewis JL: A review of second-look laparotomy for ovarian cancer. *Gynecol Oncol* 23:14–25, 1986.

33. Krebs HB, Goplerud DR: Surgical management of bowel obstruction in advanced ovarian carcinoma. *Obstet Gynecol* 61:327–330, 1983.

34. Morris JM: A formula for selective lymphadenectomy: its application to cancer of the vulva. *Obstet Gynecol* 61:327–330, 1983.

35. Rubin SC, Young J, Mikuta JJ: Squamous carcinoma of the vagina: treatment, complications, and long-term followup. *Gynecol Oncol* 20:346–353, 1985.

36. Ball HG, Berman ML: Management of primary vaginal carcinoma. *Gynecol Oncol* 14:154–163, 1982.

37. Benedet JL, Sanders BH: Carcinoma in situ of the vagina. *Am J Obstet Gynecol* 148:695–700, 1984.

38. Pride GL, Schultz AE, Chuprevich TW, Buchler DA: Primary invasive squamous carcinoma of the vagina. *Obstet Gynecol* 53:218–225, 1979.

39. Prempree T, Viravathana T, Slawson RG, Wizenberg MJ, Cuccia CA: Radiation management of primary carcinoma of the vagina. *Cancer* 40:109–118, 1977.

40. DiSaia PJ, Creasman WT, Rich WM: An alternate approach to early cancer of the vulva. *Am J Obstet Gynecol* 113:825–832, 1979.

Chapter 28

Sarcomas, Lymphomas, and Melanomas in the Elderly Patient

Anh H. Dao, M.D., R. Benton Adkins, Jr., M.D., F.A.C.S.

SOFT TISSUE SARCOMAS

General Considerations

The term "soft tissue" can be defined as the mass of extraskeletal connective tissue situated between the epidermis and the parenchymal organs. It constitutes more than half of the body weight and thus represents the single greatest amount of tissue in the human body. It connects, supports, and surrounds other anatomic structures and is present in every organ of the body. It consists of the voluntary muscles, fibrous connective tissue, and fat, along with the small vessels and peripheral nerves that supply these tissues. It derives embryologically from the mesoderm with contributions from the ectoderm.

Malignant tumors of the soft tissues are called sarcomas as opposed to carcinomas, which are tumors of epithelial tissue origin. This categorization of tumors appears somewhat arbitrary, because there are sarcoma-like tumors that develop from epithelium-like tissue. Two examples are the endothelium of blood vessels giving rise to angiosarcomas and the mesothelium of body cavities giving rise to mesotheliomas. These two tumors are included in the discussion of soft tissue tumors.

Incidence of Sarcomas

Sarcomas are relatively rare. According to the Third National Cancer Survey released by the National Cancer Institute in 1976, 4500 new cases of sarcomas occurred that year in the United States compared with 93,000 cases of lung cancer, 88,700 cases of breast cancer, and 29,000 cases of lymphoma. The annual age adjusted incidence rate is 2 per 100,000. There is no sex or racial predilection in the incidence (1).

The incidence of sarcomas decreases with age: Soft tissue sarcomas are more common in children and comprise 6.5% of all cancers in children under the age of 15 (1). In adults, they make up only 0.7% of all cancers. For unknown reasons, certain types of sarcomas show predilection for certain age groups. For example, embryonal rhabdomyosarcoma is almost exclusively seen in children, whereas malignant fibrous histiocytoma is predominantly a disease of adults.

Sites of Soft Tissue Sarcoma

Because connective tissue is present in every organ of the body, soft tissue sarcoma can arise almost anywhere. If one excludes the visceral sarcomas that are discussed elsewhere in appropriate chapters, then the lower extremities appear to be the major site for soft tissue tumors. Russell and co-workers in 1977 reviewed data on 1215 patients with sarcomas and found that 40% of the tumors occurred in the lower extremities, 32% in the trunk, 15% in the head and neck, and 13% in the upper extremity (2).

Classification of Soft Tissue Tumors

Earlier classifications based largely on the cellular configuration with such descriptive terms as round cell and spindle cell sarcomas have been abandoned.

400

Two recent classifications are winning wide acceptance by workers in the field of soft tissue pathology: one presented by Stout in 1957 (3) in the *Atlas of Tumor Pathology, Soft Tissue Fascicle,* later revised by Lattes in 1967 (4), and one proposed by the World Health Organization in 1969 (5). Both of these classifications are based on the histogenesis of the tumors. In general, sarcomas tend to reflect the morphologic appearance of the cell of origin. In the well-differentiated forms, it is often possible to classify these tumors according to the histogenetic type. In the poorly differentiated forms, difficulties arise. In the last few years, electron microscopic studies and tumor cell markers have helped considerably in categorizing these tumors. Table 28.1 presents a simplified version of Enzinger's classification containing only the malignant soft tissue tumors seen in adults and the elderly (6).

Relative Incidence of Sarcomas

The relative incidence of soft tissue tumor types varies widely from series to series. This is due in part to the disagreement between pathologists as to the exact histogenesis of a particular tumor. In addition, changes in classification with recognition of new tumor entities give rise to

Table 28.1. Soft Tissue Tumors of Adults and Elderly

Tissue of Origin	Malignant Tumor
Fibrous	Fibrosarcoma
Fibro-histiocytic	Malignant fibrous histiocytoma
Adipose	Liposarcoma
Smooth muscle	Leiomyosarcoma
Striated muscle	Rhabdomyosarcoma
Blood vessel	Hemangiosarcoma
Lymphatic vessel	Lymphangiosarcoma
Synovial	Synoviosarcoma
Mesothelial	Malignant mesothelioma
Peripheral nerve	Malignant schwannoma
Cartilage and bone	Extraskeletal chondrosarcoma
	Extraskeletal osteosarcoma
Mesenchymal	Malignant mesenchymoma
Unknown origin	Malignant granular cell tumor
	Alveolar soft part sarcoma
	Epithelioid sarcoma
	Clear cell sarcoma

Table 28.2. Incidence of Sarcoma

Type	Percentage
Fibrosarcoma	24.1
Liposarcoma	18.7
Rhabdomyosarcoma	14.8
Unclassified	12.5
Malignant fibrous histiocytoma	6.7
Synoviosarcoma	6.5
Leiomyosarcoma	4.8
Neurofibrosarcoma	4.5
Angiosarcoma	1.5

fluctuations in incidence.

Table 28.2 shows incidences as tabulated by (Rosenberg et al.) upon review of 3404 cases from 10 studies dates 1962 through 1978 (7).

Staging and Grading of Soft Tissue Tumors

The staging system designed by the Task Force of the American Joint Committee for Cancer Staging and End Results Reporting is now widely accepted and has proved useful (8). The system is based on four parameters: T for primary tumor, N for lymph node, M for distant metastases, and G for histologic grading. Details of this system are presented in Table 28.3.

The single most important prognostic factor in this system is the histologic grade of the primary tumor. The grade is determined by assessing several histologic parameters:

1. Degree of cellularity;
2. Nuclear atypia or pleomorphism;
3. Mitotic activity (number, abnormal figures);
4. Necrosis;
5. Capsulation and vascularity.

The number of grades is three in the AJC system but may vary in others from two to four. In grading soft tissue tumors, one must take into account the fact that the significance of different histologic parameters varies with the type of tumor. For example, the number of mitoses is important for grading fibrosarcoma and leiomyosarcoma, but much less so for malignant fibrous histiocytoma. Nuclear pleomorphism is minimal in highly malignant tumors, such as neuroblastoma and alveolar rhabdomyosarcoma. In addition, sarcomas may vary in morphologic

Table 28.3. Schema for Staging Soft Tissue Sarcomas by T N M G[a]

T	Primary tumor T_1 = Tumor less than 5 cm T_2 = Tumor 5 cm or greater T_3 = Tumor that grossly invades bone, major vessel, or major nerve
N	Regional lymph nodes N_0 = No histologically verified metastases to regional lymph nodes N_1 = Histologically verified regional lymph node metastasis
M	Distant metastasis M_0 = No distant metastasis M_1 = Distant metastasis
G	Histologic grade of malignancy G_1 = Low G_2 = Moderate G_3 = High
Stage I	Stage Ia, $G_1T_1N_0M_0$ = Grade 1 tumor less than 5 cm in diameter with no regional lymph nodes or distant metastases Stage Ib, $G_1T_2N_0M_0$ = Grade 1 tumor 5 cm or greater in diameter with no regional lymph nodes or distant metastases
Stage II	Stage IIa, $G_2T_1N_0M_0$ = Grade 2 tumor less than 5 cm in diameter with no regional lymph nodes or distant metastases Stage IIb, $G_2T_2N_0M_0$ = Grade 2 tumor 5 cm or greater in diameter with no regional lymph nodes or distant metastases
Stage III	Stage IIIa, $G_3T_1N_0M_0$ = Grade 3 tumor less than 5 cm in diameter with no regional lymph nodes or distant metastases Stage IIIb, $G_3T_2N_0M_0$ = Grade 3 tumor 5 cm or greater in diameter with no regional lymph nodes or distant metastases Stage IIIC, any $G_{1-3}T_{1-2}N_2M_0$ = Tumor of any grade or size (no invasion) with regional lymph nodes, but no distant metastases
Stage IV	Stage IVa, any $G_{1-3}T_3N_{0-1}M_0$ = Tumor of any grade that grossly invades bone, major vessel, or major nerve with or without regional lymph node metastases but without distant metastases Stage IVb, any $GTNM_1$ = Tumor with distant metastases

[a]From Russell WO, et al.: A clinical and pathological staging system for soft tissue sarcomas. *Cancer* 40:1562–1570, 1977.

appearance with well-differentiated areas mixed with poorly differentiated foci. In this case, the grade should be determined by the least differentiated areas.

Pathology of Soft Tissue Tumors in the Elderly

Malignant Fibrous Histiocytoma (MFH)

This is the most common soft tissue tumor of late adult life between 50 and 70 years of age. It presents as a painless, enlarging mass, most often involving the lower extremities. Several cases of MFH have been reported following radiation exposure (9). Hypoglycemia associated with large MFHs has been observed in a few instances.

Grossly, the tumor appears as fleshy, multilobulated masses located within skeletal muscles. (Fig. 28.1) Spreading along fascial planes is common, accounting for the high rate of local recurrence when it is incompletely excised. Microscopically, the tumor is composed of areas of spindle cells with a storiform pattern alternating with areas of marked pleomorphic elements. (Fig. 28.2) In these pleomorphic foci, giant tumor cells with bizarre nuclei and eosinophilic cytoplasm are numerous. Besides the typical storiform pleomorphic pattern, other histologic subtypes of MFH had been described. The myxoid MFH contains large areas of myxoid degeneration in the stroma. The giant cell type is so called because of the presence of numerous osteoclast-like giant cells. The inflammatory MFH shows infiltration of the tumor by dense inflammatory cells and foamy histiocytes. This particular type is commonly observed in the retroperitoneum of younger patients. Immunoperoxidase stains are helpful in identifying MFH because the cells of these tumors stain negative for keratin and positive for vimentin.

Fibrosarcoma

There was a time when fibrosarcoma was the most commonly encountered soft tissue tumor (10). Its incidence has declined noticeably since the acceptance of MFH as a separate entity and the separation of the fibromatoses from the bulk of fibrosarcomas (11). However, we still do not have rigid criteria set for this group of tumors,

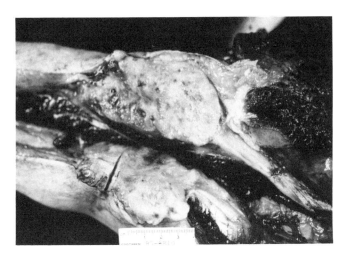

Figure 28.1. Malignant fibrous histiocytoma, present for 3 months, on the left shoulder of a 79-year-old man. The lesion, bisected, shows a slightly lobulated cut surface that is yellow with areas of hemorrhage. Note the general fusiform shape of the lesion, which appears to be confined to a single muscular unit.

and its separation from other spindle cell sarcomas remains difficult.

Clinically, fibrosarcoma presents as a slowly growing, painless mass, most commonly involving the lower extremities. It is rare in the head and neck. In older persons, squamous cell carcinomas of the head and neck present a predominantly spindly pattern that can be confused with fibrosarcomas. A number of cases of fibrosarcomas have been reported in patients exposed to radiation or in old burn scars (12, 13).

Microscopically, the pattern is rather uniform, with spindly cells arranged in fascicles that may intersect and give rise to the "herringbone" appearance. Nuclear size and shape vary but not markedly. (Fig. 28.3) As a result, bizarre tumor cells and anaplastic multinucleation are not observed. Mitotic activities are always present in variable number. Foci of heterologous elements, such as bone or cartilage, may be found. Electron microscopic examination shows tumor cells containing irregular nuclei, infrequent nucleoli, and prominent rough endoplasmic reticulum.

Liposarcoma

A common soft tissue tumor of adults, liposarcoma shows a peak incidence between 40 and 60 years of age. It has been observed, however, frequently in persons aged 70 and over, but is virtually unknown in children. It comprises up to 18% of all soft tissue tumors and is most frequently found in the thigh and retroperitoneum where it may reach a very large size (2).

Grossly the tumor appears well circumscribed with a lobulated surface. The cut surface varies from a pale yellow in well-differentiated tumor to myxoid or gelatinous appearance in other forms. Areas of hemorrhage and necrosis are fre-

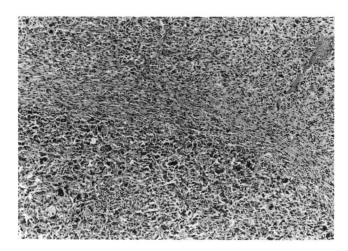

Figure 28.2. Microscopic features of malignant histiocytoma (same lesion as in Figure 28.1), depicting the storiform-pleomorphic type. A fascicular arrangement of spindly cells is shown in the center, running diagonally across the field. Numerous pleomorphic forms are seen in the lower left corner. (H&E, ×400)

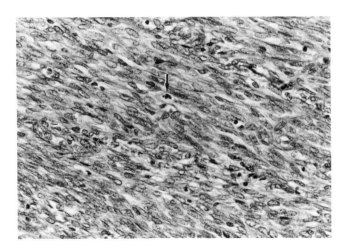

Figure 28.3. Fibrosarcoma displaying the fascicular pattern with scattered mitotic figures *(arrow)*. The nuclei, although large and hyperchromatic, show little pleomorphism. This lesion is from a chest wall recurrence of a primary pulmonary fibrosarcoma. (H&E, × 400)

quently seen. Microscopically, four different types of liposarcomas are described: well differentiated, myxoid, round cell, and pleomorphic liposarcoma. In the well-differentiated form, the tumor resembles a lipoma except for the slight variation in size and shape of the lipocytes and the presence of scattered lipoblasts with hyperchromatic nuclei. Areas of dense fibrosis as well as chronic inflammation exist, giving rise to the two sclerosing and inflammatory subtypes. Myxoid liposarcoma is the most common type encountered, comprising up to 40% of all liposarcomas. It is composed of masses of lipoblasts and a prominnet vascular network embedded in a myxoid stroma. The round cell liposarcoma is a poorly differentiated form of myxoid liposarcoma. The predominant cell type is the small, round lipoblast, and the capillary network is less prominent. Clinically, this is an aggressive tumor that tends to metastasize early. Pleomorphic liposarcoma is characterized by the presence of numerous giant tumor cells resembling those seen in malignant fibrous histiocytoma or pleomorphic rhabdomyosarcoma.

Leiomyosarcoma

Leiomyosarcomas of soft tissue are less common than liposarcoma and MFH. They are tumors of adults and can be divided into three clinical and anatomic groups: retroperitoneal and intra-abdominal leiomyosarcomas, leiomyosarcomas of skin and subcutaneous tissue, and vascular leiomyosarcomas (6). All three groups, however, show similar histologic appearance.

Retroperitoneal and intra-abdominal leio-

myosarcomas are found in later adult life, 60 years or older. Females predominate at the ratio of 2 to 1. The tumor is usually quite large at the time of resection, with a mean size of 16 cm (14). Adjacent organs, such as kidneys and pancreas, are often involved. Cutaneous and subcutaneous leiomyosarcomas are also tumors of late adult life. They are quite rare and present as solitary nodules on the extremities. Because of their location, they are readily palpable and usually are of small size (2 cm or less) at the time of removal. Pain is usually present. Vascular leiomyosarcoma is even more rare. It is found involving large veins more than arteries, with the inferior vena cava being the most common site. Symptoms vary with the location of the tumor, from Budd-Chiari syndrome when the hepatic vein is involved to nephrotic syndrome when the renal veins are affected.

Microscopically, leiomyosarcomas are composed of bundles of spindle cells with blunt-ended nuclei and abundant eosinophilic cytoplasm. In well-differentiated forms, the nuclei are regular in size and shape, and the cytoplasm contains myofibrils. In less differentiated forms, nuclei become more pleomorphic and the myofibrils less prominent. Multinucleated giant cells are not uncommon. Mitotic figures usually number 5 or more per 10 high power fields. Leiomyosarcoma cells are usually vimentin positive with immunoperoxidase stain.

Malignant Schwannoma

Malignant schwannomas constitute a poorly defined group with no accepted diagnostic criteria. Clinically, there is association between malignant schwannoma and von Reckling-hausen's disease. Up to 13% of patients with von Rechlinghausen's disease will develop malignant schwannoma after a latent period of 10 to 20 years (15). The lesion usually presents as a fu-siform mass growing along a major peripheral nerve or in a pre-existing neurofibroma.

Microscopically, it resembles fibrosarcoma with spindly cells arranged in more or less regu-lar fascicles. The nuclei are however more ir-regular with a wavy contour. The stroma con-tains myxoid zones. Occasionally, tumor cells may form vaguely nodular structures, suggestive of primitive tactile corpuscles. Malignant schwannoma cells are positive for S-100 protein and laminin, but negative for keratin. Heterolo-gous elements, such as bone or cartilage, are more frequently found than in fibrosarcomas. Electron microscopic study shows that the tumor cells possess branching cytoplasmic processes that form junctional complexes. Neurofilaments and microtubules are present, as well as basal lamina.

Rhabdomyosarcoma

The rhabdomyosarcomas are quite diverse in clinical presentation and histologic appearance. They, however, do have an uniform age inci-dence, mainly occurring in children and young adults. Of the three main types, embryonal, al-veolar, and pleomorphic, only the pleomorphic rhabdomyosarcoma is seen in older persons, the median age being 55 (16).

The incidence of pleomorphic rhabdomyosar-coma was high in the 1930s and 1940s. In per-sons in their fifties and sixties, its incidence has dropped dramatically, with much of the rhab-domyosarcomas reported being those found in children. This was due to the fact that many of the pleomorphic rhabdomyosarcomas reported in the past were actually sarcomas of some other types, such as MFH. At the same time, many cases of round cell sarcomas in children were reclassified as alveolar rhabdomyosarcoma.

Pleomorphic rhabdomyosarcoma is recognized histologically by the association of both round and pleomorphic cells that are haphazardly oriented. The cytoplasm is abundant and eo-sinophilic. Racquet cells and tadpole cells abound, but cross striation is very rarely demon-strated. On that basis, it is difficult to separate pleomorphic rhabdomyosarcoma from other pleomorphic sarcomas. Rhabdomyosarcoma cells contain glycogen. Immunoperoxidase stain for muscle-specific actin is positive, whereas my-oglobin stain is variable at best.

Angiosarcoma

These very rare tumors are primarily tumors of the elderly. There is predilection for the head and neck, especially the scalp. They affect mostly the skin and subcutaneous tissue and rarely arise from large vessels.

Angiosarcoma starts as small, single, or mul-tiple nodules of the skin that are asymptomatic at first. The nodules grow into papules and blisters that may bleed abundantly. Microscopi-cally, there are irregular vascular channels in-vading into fatty tissue and muscle. The tumor cells are large endothelial cells with hyperchro-matic nuclei. They form papillary projections into the vascular channels that are filled with blood. The stroma contains extravasated red cells. In poorly differentiated cases, vascular channels are not prominent, and it is difficult to separate these cases from other high grade sar-comas. Immunocytochemical methods identify Factor VIII in many of the tumor cells.

Kaposi's sarcoma is a form of angiosarcoma that deserves special attention. It has gained prominence with the spread of AIDS cases in the United States. This rare neoplasm possesses strong sexual and geographical distribution. Ninety percent occur in men. The disease can be divided into two geographical groups: those seen in Africa and those observed in other parts of the world (6).

In Africa, Kaposi's sarcoma is endemic. It af-fects younger patients and is characterized by a more aggressive behavior. In other parts of the world, except for the cases associated with AIDS, patients in the sixth and seventh decades are primarily affected. The disease is usually as-sociated with either another malignant neoplasm of the lymphoma-leukemia type or an altered im-munologic status (17). Clinically, Kaposi's sar-coma is manifested by multiple bluish nodules on the skin of the lower extremities that gradu-ally grow and coalesce into plaques and finally into polypoid masses. Ulceration and bleeding are frequently observed.

Microscopically, there are numerous capillary vessels invading the skin, lined by plump endothelial cells. The stroma contains heavy inflammatory infiltrates together with areas of hemorrhage and proliferating immature spindle cells. In more advanced lesions, the spindle cells become more prominent, forming densely cellular areas pushing the angiomatous foci more to the periphery. Metastases occur, as well as spontaneous regression of the lesions.

Lymphangiosarcoma

In 1948, Stewart and Treves reported six cases of lymphangiosarcoma in chronically edematous arms following radical mastectomy for carcinoma of the breast (18). Since then, several additional cases have been added, most of them arising in a setting of chronic lymphedema with the exception of tropical filariasis where chronic lymphedema does not appear to be a predisposing factor (6).

Clinically, the first sign of malignant degeneration is the appearance of macular lesions that grow and coalesce into papular confluent lesions that eventually ulcerate. The lesions progress to invade chest wall and metastasize to the lungs and viscera.

Although clinical observation strongly suggests lymphatic endothelial cells as the cell of origin, histologically it is always difficult to separate lymphangiosarcoma from other angiosarcomas. There are, as with other angiosarcomas, proliferating vascular spaces lined by plump, hyperchromatic endothelial cells. The vascular lumina as well as the stroma contain red blood cells. Hemangiosarcoma and Kaposi's sarcoma should always be considered in the differential diagnosis.

Treatment of Sarcomas

The treatment of soft tissue sarcomas in the elderly should not differ appreciably from that offered those in younger age groups. However, the recent emphasis on preserving limb and limb function and returning the individual to a high level of activity in our opinion should be reserved for the younger, more active patient. The multimodal approach of surgical resection, radiation treatment, and chemotherapy may be less appropriately used in the older age group than in the young. There will, of course, be exceptions to this rule. For those lesions located within the body cavities and upon the chest wall, abdominal wall, and back, some compromise in total resection of the tumor mass may be necessary, especially those in the retroperitoneal location.

Extremity Sarcoma

Radical local resection and/or amputation of those sarcomas occurring in the extremity offers the best chance for cure with the least amount of trauma and usually obviates the necessity for adjuvant irradiation or chemotherapy (19). There are several reasons to employ aggressive radical excision of extremity sarcomas in older patients in whom maintenance of limb function may not be critical. First of all, recurrence rates after radical, local resection that removes all of the tissue within the involved compartment or member without amputation ranges from 10%–20%; this improves to a rate as low as 5% after amputation. By contrast, the limb-saving operations are associated with local recurrence rates as high as 50%, thereby necessitating the use of radiation or chemotherapy (7). These adjuvant therapeutic measures are less well tolerated in older patients than in young age groups and are not very effective in treating soft tissue sarcomas. Second, elaborate muscle group, segmental bone, and extended function-saving resections are more traumatic and associated with a higher morbidity and mortality than extended wide local excisions or amputations. The need for lithesome agility is less critical, and the tolerance for reconstructive procedures, adjuvant therapy, and prolonged rehabitation programs is somewhat diminished in the elderly.

Truncal Sarcomas

For tumors of the thoracic or abdominal wall and back, wide radical excision with prosthetic material and flap reconstruction are well tolerated by the elderly. The unique situation of sarcomas of the retroperitoneal area offers a serious challenge to patient and surgeon alike (20–23).

In most elderly patients, we would not recommend extensive retroperitoneal dissection including kidneys and other abdominal organs for the removal of retroperitoneal sarcomas. Rather, a generous debulking of the tumor followed by postoperative radiation seems most appropriate.

Gastrointestinal tract sarcomas account for the second largest group of malignancies in the stomach and small bowel. These lesions should be treated surgically in all age groups because, unlike primary gastrointestinal tumors, they are not likely to be as responsive to radiation and chemotherapy. (See Chapters 20 and 23) Primary pulmonary sarcomas although rare do occur and should be treated surgically whenever possible. (See Chapter 16)

MESOTHELIOMA

Diffuse mesothelioma is a disease of late adult life, from 50 to 70 years of age. It arises most commonly from the pleural surface and less frequently from the peritoneum. There is a definite causal relationship between exposure to asbestos fibers and the occurrence of mesothelioma (24).

At the early stage, the disease is characterized by flat plaques or small nodules of firm yellow-white fibrous tissue covering the serosal surface. In more advanced cases, there is diffuse thickening of the pleura or peritoneum with compression of the lungs or viscera. Direct extension of pleural mesothelioma to the peritoneum is not rare.

Microscopically, most mesotheliomas exhibit a glandular and papillary appearance. The glandular elements are lined by cuboidal cells with vesicular nuclei and eosinophilic cytoplasm. Some mesotheliomas show sheets of mesothelial cells with little or no glandular differentiation.

Mesothelial cells stain positive for both keratin and vimentin. The asbestos fibers are recognized as "ferruginous bodies," golden-brown structures formed by deposits of mucopolysaccharides and hemosiderin pigments on an asbestos core.

Mesothelial tumors of the pleura and peritoneum are sarcomatous growths that arise from the serous lining of these cavities. They are sarcomas that spread by local invasion and are most often widely disseminated when diagnosed. Because of this, local control is rarely achieved by surgical resection, radiation treatment, or chemotherapy. The early localized lesion should be widely excised whenever possible. (See Chapter 16)

MALIGNANT GRANULAR CELL TUMOR

This is a rare tumor, accounting for 1%–2% of all granular cell tumors. First reported by Ravich and Stout (25), there are only about 25 cases so far reported (6).

Clinically, malignant granular cell tumors tend to be larger (average diameter of 4 cm or more). They are found only in adults. We have observed a case of a 7-cm granular cell tumor occurring in the chest wall of a 57-year-old woman. (Fig. 28.4) This tumor was resected but recurred 2 years later. There was also evidence of pulmonary metastasis, proven by needle biopsy (26).

Gross appearance of the tumor is that of an ill-defined, poorly circumscribed mass of pale yellow color. The malignant granular cell tumor

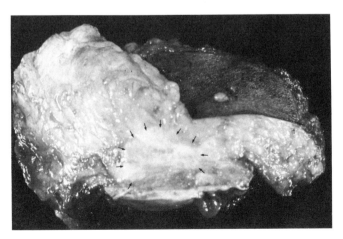

Figure 28.4. Malignant granular cell tumor from the chest wall of a 57-year-old woman. The cut surface shows an ill-defined, yellow-tan mass infiltrating subcutaneous tissue and intercostal muscles. This lesion recurred locally 2 years after resection, with pulmonary metastases demonstrated by x-ray and needle biopsy.

is very similar histologically to its benign counterpart, with nests of round to polygonal cells exhibiting small nuclei and abundant granular eosinophilic cytoplasm, lying in a fibrous stroma. The nuclei, however, show variation in size and shape in the malignant form, and mitotic figures are frequently seen. Granular cells are strongly positive for S100 protein. These poorly circumscribed lesions usually occur in the subcutaneous or submucosal layers. Wide excision is necessary to eradicate the malignant variant of this relatively rare lesion. All of these lesions should be treated as if they were malignant until they are proven otherwise in all age groups.

MALIGNANT MELANOMA

Every year, 14,000 new cases of cutaneous melanomas are diagnosed in the United States with an overall incidence of 4.5 in 100,000 Caucasians and 0.6 in 100,000 blacks (27, 28).

The incidence of malignant melanoma steadily increases with each decade of life so that in the 70–79 age group, there are 11.3 per 100,000 and at age 80 and above 16.1 per 100,000 have melanoma (12). The majority of melanomas are found between the third and sixth decades of life, with a median age of 46 (29, 30). There appears to be a better survival rate for women than for men under the age of 50 (30, 31). After menopause, there is no difference in survival between the two sexes.

Despite these large numbers, melanoma is still a relatively rare disease in the elderly. There is, however, an unexplainable worldwide rise in its overall incidence at the current rate of about 7% per year. This is an increase with an apparent doubling time of 10 to 17 years (28). The reason for this increase is unclear and cannot be accounted for by improved methods of diagnosing and reporting as there is also a parallel increase in mortality.

Pathology of Malignant Melanomas

Four major types of melanomas have been described: lentigo maligna melanoma, superficial spreading melanoma, nodular melanoma, and acral lentiginous melanoma.

Lentigo Maligna Melanoma (LMM)

Lentigo maligna melanoma (LMM) constitutes only a small proportion of all malignant melanomas, usually 4% to 10% (32). It is characterized by a long period of growth with most of the lesions noted to be present from 5 to 15 years. They are flat pigmented lesions located primarily on the face and neck of elderly patients (Hutchinson's freckle). It is uncommon in patients less than 50 years of age.

Clinically, the lesion has irregular borders with a flat surface showing various shades of brown. (Fig. 28.5) As the lesion becomes malignant, a portion of it may become nodular. As a rule, LMM does not have the same propensity for metastasis as the other three types of melanomas (33).

Microscopically, LMM is characterized by a proliferation of atypical melanocytes at the basal layers of the epidermis. The melanocytes are distributed individually or in nests and show retraction of the cytoplasm as a prominent feature. Nuclear atypia is mild to moderate. There is invasion of the epidermis by the same atypical melanocytes, as well as streaming of these cells down to the upper levels of the dermis. The latter also shows actinic degeneration and contains a band-like inflammatory infiltrate composed primarily of mononuclears and lymphocytes. The nodular melanoma that develops from a Hutchinson's freckle is often of the spindle cell type and exhibits limited aggressiveness. Another type of melanoma that may follow Huchinson's

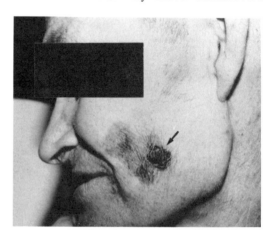

Figure 28.5. Lentigo meligna melanoma. The patient, a 57-year-old male, had a pigmented lesion on the cheek for several years. It had recently enlarged and showed a nodule near the posterior margin *(arrow)*. Photograph—courtesy of Dr. David L. Pase, Dept. Pathology Vanderbilt, Univer.

freckle is the desmoplastic melanoma, so called because of the extensive fibrosis in the stroma.

Superficial Spreading Melanoma (SSM)

This is the largest group of melanomas, constituting about 70% of all malignant melanomas (32). It has no age predilection and in about 30% of time develops from a pre-existing nevus. Typically, SSM shows a variegated surface, with colors ranging from jet black to grayish white. The borders are irregular with notching and indentation. A thin rim of pink-colored skin is often found at the periphery, representing host reaction to the lesion.

Histologically, SSM shows both vertical and horizontal growth phases. The vertical growth phase is characterized by irregular junctional activities with streaming of atypical melanocytes into the dermis. There is also upward spread of melanocytes, permeating the epidermis in single cells or small nests. At the dermoepidermal junction, the large clear melanocytes tend to form well-defined round nests reminiscent of tumor cells found in Paget's disease of the skin, hence the name of pagetoid spread. (Fig. 28.6A) The malignant melanocytes of SSM are one of two types: spindle or epithelioid. Usually one cell type predominates. Spindle cells tend to arrange in branching formations, whereas epithelioid cells lie in alveolar formations. The amount of pigment seen in this type of melanoma varies from abundant to almost non-existent. There is always a chronic inflammatory reaction in the adjacent stroma, consisting mostly of lymphocytes and mononuclears. The horizontal growth phase is manifested by the presence of pagetoid spread of malignant melanocytes in the basal layers of the epidermis at the edge of the lesion for 3 rete ridges or more.

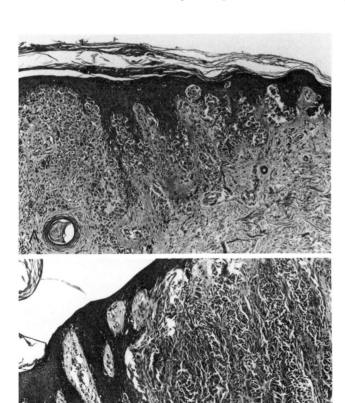

Figure 28.6. **A,** Superficial spreading melanoma: at the edge, there is pagetoid spread involving several rete ridges. Invasion of the dermis is shown at left. **B,** Nodular melanoma: No pagetoid nests of melanoma cells are found at the edges. Massive invasion of the dermis by melanoma cells is shown at right. (H&E, ×400)

Nodular Melanoma (NM)

This is the second most common type of melanoma, comprising 30% of cases. NM usually arises de novo without any pre-existing nevi. They are more common in middle-aged patients and tend to be more aggressive than SSM.

Clinically, NM is a raised, dome-shaped lesion with a blue-black color. A small number of NM are amelanotic and show a fleshy appearance. The borders are sharply demarcated. Larger lesions tend to ulcerate and bleed. NM usually has a much faster rate of growth than the other types.

Microscopically, only the vertical growth phase is present. (Fig. 28. 6B) There is downward growth of tumor cells that tend to form rounded nests or nodules. Cytology is variable, but in most cases, the tumor cells show large vesicular nuclei, prominent nucleoli, and amphophilic cytoplasm containing dusky pigment. At the base of the lesion, the tumor cell nests appear to push rather than invade the collagen bundles. Inflammation is minimal unless there is ulceration of the epidermis.

Acral Lentiginous Melanoma (ALM)

This type of melanoma is rare in Caucasians, but shows a much higher incidence in blacks, Hispanics, and Orientals (34). It typically occurs on the palm or sole or beneath the nail beds of older patients, 60 years of age and older. At the early stage, ALM resembles a LMM with irregular borders and various shades of brown. The surface is hyperkeratotic and may become ulcerated. ALM is much more aggressive than LMM, and metastases are not uncommon with this lesion (35). When it develops beneath nail beds it is usually the nail bed of a toe, and the toe nail is soon extruded leaving a black ulcerated nail bed. Fingers are rarely involved.

Microscopically, there is an increased number of atypical melanocytes at the dermoepidermal border. Melanocytes may be found scattered throughout the epidermis including the cornified layers. There is a tendency for nest formation, but large pagetoid nests are rare. (Fig. 28.7) A small number of melanocytes exhibit prominent branching of heavily pigmented dendritic processes. With the development of the vertical growth phase, invasion of the papillary dermis occurs. Chronic inflammation of the lichenoid types is often present. In fully developed lesions, nodules are found with invasion of deeper tissue.

Clinical Staging of Melanoma

A TNM staging system has been developed for melanomas, but it is rarely used because of its complexity (36). The system described in Table 28.4 is much simpler and preferred by clinicians.

Microscopic Staging and Tumor Thickness

Mehnert and Heard were the first to propose a histologic staging for melanomas (37). Clark further refined the staging to include five levels of microinvasion, which are described in Table 28.5 (38).

Generally speaking, the survival rate decreases

Figure 28.7. Acral lentiginous melanoma: This pigmented lesion of the plantar aspect of the foot shows invasion of the dermis by melanoma cells at lower left corner. Pagetoid involvement of the hyperkeratotic epidermis is demonstrated at right. (H&E, ×400)

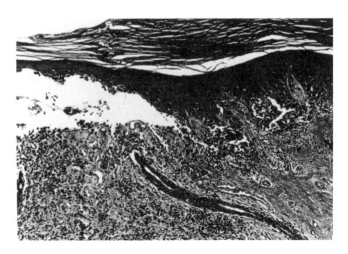

Table 28.4. Clinical Staging of Melanoma

I.   Local
     A.   Primary lesion alone
     B.   Primary and satellites within a 5 cm radius of the primary
     C.   Local recurrence within a 5 cm radius of a resected primary
     D.   Metastases located more than 5 cm from the primary site, but within the primary lymphatic drainage area

II. Regional node disease

III. Disseminated disease

with increasing level of invasion. However, there are circumstances in which level of invasion does not correlate well with survival. The thickness of skin varies from person to person and according to anatomic sites. Therefore levels are not comparable from different sites and from different persons. Furthermore, Clark's levels cannot be determined for nodular melanomas or for mucosal lesions where anatomic landmarks are absent. Balch and co-workers found that Clark's levels correlated well in patients with stage I disease, but no correlation was noted in patients with stage II disease (39).

Breslow was the first to correlate the thickness of the lesion with prognosis in melanomas: An inverse relationship between tumor thickness and survival was noted (40). Tumor thickness is measured from the top of the granular layers to the base of the tumor with an ocular micrometer (40). (See Table 28.6)

Breslow's data were confirmed by other studies (40–43). These studies also demonstrated that the most important indicator of prognosis in melanoma is the thickness of tumor (or depth of invasion). For that reason, it is important to include both Clark's level and tumor thickness in all pathology reports of excised melanomas.

Treatment

The hallmark of surgical treatment for all cutaneous malignant melanomas is wide local excision of the primary site and regional lymph node dissection for all melanomas beyond Clark's level III or for all of those primary lesions that have a tumor thickness beyond 1.5 mm. We would do regional node dissections for all acral lentiginous lesions no matter their thickness. This recommended therapeutic approach should be followed in all age groups. If regional nodes are palpable, we would do a regional node dissection regardless of Clark's level or Breslow's thickness of the primary tumor. In the elderly, only those most severe medical conditions that cannot be corrected or improved should be reason for deviation from this recommendation.

A special note should be made about those melanomas of the acral lentiginous variety where an extremely aggressive approach, including digital amputation, Ray amputation of fingers and toes, and sometimes much more extensive amputation of upper and lower extremities with regional lymph node dissection, will be necessary for the primary surgical approach to these lesions. Again, the age of the patient should not

Table 28.5 Clark's Levels of Invasion

Level I

All tumor cells confined to the epidermis with no invasion through the basement membrane (in situ melanoma)

Level II

Tumor cells penetrating through the basement membrane into the papillary dermis but not extending to the reticular dermis

Level III

Tumor cells filling the papillary dermis and abutting against the reticular dermis but not invading it

Level IV

Extension of tumor cells between the bundles of collagen characteristic of the reticular dermis

Level V

Invasion into the subcutaneous tissue

Table 28.6 Correlation of Tumor Thickness and Survival (Breslow)

Thickness mm	5-Year Survival %
0.75	100
0.75–1.5	74
1.51–2.25	80
2.26–3.00	27
3.00	25

alter the surgical approach for these particular lesions.

Chemotherapy and irradiation for metastatic or unresectable melanoma should be considered palliative only. Although there are sporadic reports of long-term disease-free intervals, systemic chemotherapy, radiation treatment, hormonal therapy, and immunotherapy have failed to show encouraging results. When an otherwise healthy elderly patient who has melanoma beyond the bounds of surgical resection presents for therapy, he or she should be considered a candidate for all of the forms of adjuvant therapy. Chemotherapy, radiation therapy, and secondary surgical procedures that would be offered a younger individual should be considered in the elderly. See Chapter 6 for the usual guidelines for the use of chemotherapy and radiation therapy in the elderly.

LYMPHOMAS

The lymphoid system (lymph nodes, spleen, thymus), together with the hematopoietic system (bone marrow) and the mononuclear phagocytic system (reticuloendothelial system), is responsible for the production of cellular elements of the blood and for the development of immunity. These three systems share the same origin, sites of action, and functions and often are affected by the same disease processes. It is therefore usually convenient to discuss neoplasms affecting these three systems in a unified fashion. However, because of the limited scope of this chapter, only neoplasms affecting the lymphoid system will be discussed. The reader is referred to textbooks on diseases of the bone marrow and reticuloendothelial system for a discussion of those neoplasms. Neoplasms of the mononuclear phagocytic system will be briefly reviewed when they involve lymph nodes, whereas neoplasms of the hematopoietic system, such as leukemias and myeloma, will not be considered in this chapter. (See Chapter 6)

Traditionally, lymphomas have been divided into two broad groups: Hodgkin's disease and non-Hodgkin's lymphoma. This arbitrary division has been very helpful both in clinical management and in understanding the biology of lymphomas, because the non-Hodgkin's lymphomas are actually composed of a variety of entities that differ from Hodgkin's disease in terms of their biology, pathology, and treatment.

Lymphomas that occur in the elderly are generally considered to have a poor prognosis because patients of this age group often present with advanced disease. Coexisting medical problems make aggressive management difficult and complicated. In addition, chemotherapy is usually less well tolerated. Certain anatomic sites, such as the upper airways and digestive tract, are predilection sites for the relatively frequent occurrence of primary lymphomas in the elderly (44). Surgical management of lymphomas in these local primary sites is rendered difficult, and in some of these areas, clinical staging is somewhat confusing because there is debate over whether involvement of the Waldeyer's ring or the thymus should be considered as extranodal involvement.

Approximately 30,000 new cases of lymphomas occurred in 1980 (45). Twenty-four percent of these cases were Hodgkin's disease. Although treatment for Hodgkin's disease has been fairly well standardized, it is not so for the non-Hodgkin's lymphomas. In the last 15 years, much improvement has been made with radiation therapy and chemotherapy. (See Chapter 6) Surgical management has been helpful in cases where the lesions are localized and there is no evidence of widespread disease. (See Chapter 20)

Hodgkin's Disease

Hodgkin's disease has been shown to display a bimodal age distribution with peaks at 30 and 70 years of age (46). Histologic differences between the two groups were demonstrated by Newell and Cole (47). The younger patients usually show a lymphocyte predominant histology, whereas older patients in the second peak usually belong to the lymphocyte depleted group.

The difference in histopathology coupled with the bimodal age distribution has led MacMahon to postulate that Hodgkin's disease has two etiologic processes: a biologic agent of low infectivity in young adults and a neoplastic process in older people (48). This theory has not been widely accepted because there is a possibility that the difference is due to variation of the host response to a single etiologic agent or mechanism.

Pathology of Hodgkin's Disease

The histologic classification of Hodgkin's disease proposed by Lukes and Butler in 1966 and subseqently modified by the Rye conference is currently in use (49). Basically, four histologic subtypes are recognized: lymphocyte predominance, nodular sclerosing, mixed cellularity, and lymphocyte depleted. The diagnosis of Hodgkin's disease depends on the finding of the characteristic Reed-Sternberg cell. In its classic form, the R-S cell shows a large polylobulated nucleus with a prominent, inclusion-like nucleolus. (Fig. 28.8) There is parachromatin clearing resulting in a perinucleolar halo. The cytoplasm is abundant and acidophilic or eosinophilic. Occasionally, the cell is binucleated and resembles an "owl's eye."

It should be pointed out that the presence of R-S cells by itself is not pathognomonic of Hodgkin's disease. Cells resembling R-S cells have been found in other conditions, such as mononucleosis, transformed cell lymphomas, and some carcinomas.

Lymphocyte predominant Hodgkin's disease is characterized by abundance of small lymphocytes. Lymph node architecture may be totally or partially destroyed. Typical R-S cells are hard to find, and those present are usually of the lymphocytic/histiocytic (L/H) variant. The L/H variant cells are large polyploid cells with folded, convoluted nuclei, unapparent nucleoli, and a variable amount of cytoplasm. This subtype is usually seen in young male patients and is the most favorable form prognostically.

Nodular sclerosing Hodgkin's disease is so called because of the presence of orderly bands of dense collagenous tissue dividing the node into nodules. The R-S cells are abundant in this subtype and belong to the "lacunar" variant: The cell appears to be situated in a lacuna, a phenomenon observed only in formalin-fixed tissue. The nuclei of lacunar cells are polylobated with lacy chromatin and with a small to intermediate nucleoli. These cells frequently occur in large numbers in semi-cohesive groups. The cytoplasm is water-clear or faintly eosinophilic. This form of Hodgkin's disease most commonly afflicts young female patients and usually has a favorable prognosis.

Mixed cellularity Hodgkin's disease is characterized by a mixed microscopic background with a variable proportion of plasma cells, eosinophils, lymphocytes, and histiocytes. R-S cells are in moderate numbers and are of either classic or mononuclear variants. This form of Hodgkin's disease frequently involves subdiaphragmatic organs and has a less favorable prognosis than the two previously described types.

Lymphocyte depleted Hodgkin's disease displays a microscopic picture of a depletion of cellular elements with an increase in the reticular framework. Two subtypes have been described: reticular and diffuse fibrosis. The R-S cells predominate the histologic picture with numerous anaplastic or sarcomatous forms. This type of Hodgkin's disease represents the most aggressive form, affecting mainly an older age group of patients who are frequently symptomatic with

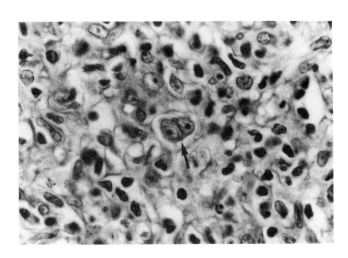

Figure 28.8. A binucleated Reed-Sternberg cell in a case of lymphocyte depleted Hodgkin's disease *(arrow)*. The nucleoli are large, and the cytoplasm shows perinuclear clearing. (H&E, ×400)

lymphadenopathy, hepato-splenomegaly, and bone marrow involvement.

Staging of Hodgkin's Disease

The first useful staging system for Hodgkin's disease was that proposed by Peters and colleagues in 1968 (50). This system was later modified at the Ann Arbor Staging Conferences in 1971 (51). Table 28.7 outlines this system.

In patients more than 50 years of age, Hodgkin's disease should be more carefully evaluated, not only because these patients have a higher proportion of lymphocyte depleted forms but also because they tend to have more advanced disease at the time of diagnosis, frequent extranodal involvement, poor response to therapy, and lower tolerance for radiotherapy and chemotherapy (52).

Treatment of Hodgkin's Disease

The surgeons's role in the treatment of localized Hodgkin's disease of the gastrointestinal tract, other abdominal viscera, mediastinum, and regional lymph node areas is traditionally reserved for diagnosis, debulking, and palliation. Staging of all forms of Hodgkin's disease and removing or debulking those tumor sites that cause symptoms or represent a large mass of tumor cell population should be done in patients of all age groups to offer relief of symptoms and palliation. As mentioned in Chapter 6, Hodgkin's disease in the second bimodal age peak tends to have slightly worse prognostic features and should possibly be approached more aggressively than would be required in a similarly staged disease in a younger age group.

Non-Hodgkin's Lymphomas

The term "non-Hodgkin's lymphoma" is used to designate a variety of different types of lymphomas for which we do not have an universally accepted classification. Until the 1960s, non-Hodgkin's lymphomas were divided into three major groups: lymphosarcoma, reticulum-cell sarcoma, and giant follicle lymphoma. Rappaport in 1966 proposed a classification that was later modified by other authors (53, 54). (See Table 28.8) The Rappaport classification was widely accepted by oncologists who found it useful in providing guidelines for prognosis and therapy. With the advances made in the field of immunology, other classifications were proposed. The Lukes and Collins classification proposed in 1974 was based primarily on immunologic subtypes (55). This system, outlined in Table 28.9, is gaining in popularity. The Kiel system proposed by Lennert et al. is primarily a morphologic system and is widely used in Europe (56). An international study, undertaken by the National Cancer Institute in 1976, culminated in a Working Formulation for clinical use (Table 28.10) that was regarded as a common lan-

Table 28.7. Ann Arbor Staging Classification for Hodgkin's Disease

Stage I
Involvement of a single lymph node region (I) or a single extralymphatic organ or site (IE)

Stage II
Involvement of two or more lymph node regions on the same side of the diaphragm (II) or localized involvement of an extralymphatic organ or site (IIE)

Stage III
Involvement of lymph node regions on both sides of the diaphragm (III) or localized involvement of an extralymphatic organ or site (IIIE) or spleen (IIIS) or both (IIISE)

Stage IV
Diffuse or disseminated involvement of one or more extralymphatic organs with or without associated lymph node involvement; the organ(s) involved should be identified by a symbol: A (asymptomatic) or B (symptomatic—fever, sweats, weight loss greater than 10% of body weight)

Table 28.8. Modified Rappaport Classification

Nodular
 Lymphocytic, poorly differentiated
 Mixed lymphocytic-histiocytic
 Histiocytic

Diffuse
 Lymphocytic, well differentiated
 Lymphocytic, intermediate differentiation
 Lymphocytic, poorly differentiated
 Mixed lymphocytic-histiocytic
 Undifferentiated, Burkitt's type
 Undifferentiated, non-Burkitt's type
 Histiocytic
 Lymphocytic

Table 28.9. Lukes & Collins Classification

Undefined cell types

T-cell types
  Small lymphocytic
  Mycosis fungoides/Sezarry syndrome
  Convoluted lymphocytic
  Immunoblastic sarcoma (T-cell)

B-cell types
  Small lymphocytic
  Plasmacytoid lymphocytic
  Follicular center cell
    Small cleaved
    Large cleaved
    Small noncleaved
    Large noncleaved
  Immunoblastic sarcoma (B-cell)

Histiocytic

Unclassifiable

guage for investigators to move from one classification to another (57). Equivalent terms in both Rappaport and Lukes and Collins classifications are given to facilitate comparison. (Table 28.10)

Pathology of Non-Hodgkin's Lymphomas in the Elderly

Nodular Lymphomas. Poorly differentiated lymphocytic lymphoma (NPDL) or follicular, small cleaved cell type is the most common form of nodular lymphoma, making up 30% to 40% of all lymphomas. It usually occurs in adults of 50 years of age or older and starts as an asymptomatic enlarged node in the cervical, axillary, or inguinal area. Following a prolonged indolent course, which may last up to 5 years, the disease is transformed to a more rapid progression with rapid enlargement of lymph nodes, appearance of systemic symptoms (fever, weight loss, etc.), infiltration of non-lymphoid organs, and worsening of the lymph node pathology. Histologically, the vast majority of the neoplastic cells are small lymphocytes with cleaved, indented nuclei. (Fig. 28.9) These cells usually contain surface immunoglobulins with kappa or lambda chains. Involvement of the bone marrow is frequent (up to 80% of cases) (58). Therefore, NPDL should be considered a systemic malignancy.

Table 28.10. Working Formulation Classification of Non-Hodgkin's Lymphoma with Equivalent Terms from Modified Rappaport and Lukes & Collins Classifications

Modified Rappaport	Working Formulation	Lukes & Collins
	Low Grade	
Well differentiated lymphocytic, diffuse	A. Diffuse, small cell lymphocytic	Small lymphocytic, diffuse
Poorly differentiated lymphocytic, nodular	B. Follicular, small cleaved cell	Small cleaved follicular center cell (FCC), nodular
Mixed lymphocytic and histiocytic nodular	C. Follicular, mixed small cleaved and large cell	Large FCC, cleaved or noncleaved nodular
	Intermediate Grade	
Histiocytic, nodular	D. Follicular, large cell	Large FCC, cleaved or noncleaved nodular
Poorly differentiated lymphocytic, diffuse	E. Diffuse, small cleaved cell	Small cleaved FCC, diffuse
Mixed lymphocytic and histiocytic, diffuse	F. Diffuse, mixed small and large cell	Large FCC, cleaved or noncleaved, diffuse
Histiocytic, diffuse	G. Diffuse, large cell, cleaved or noncleaved	Large FCC, cleaved or noncleaved, diffuse
	High Grade	
Histiocytic, diffuse	H. Immunoblastic	Immunoblastic sarcoma
Lymphoblastic, diffuse	I. Lymphoblastic, convoluted or non-convoluted	Convoluted lymphocytic
Undifferentiated, diffuse	J. Small noncleaved cell, diffuse Burkitt's or non-Burkitt's	Small noncleaved FCC

Figure 28.9. Malignant lymphoma, nodular, small cleaved cells; the neoplastic cells are slightly larger than normal lymphocytes with scanty cytoplasm. The nuclei show characteristic indentation and infoldings *(arrow)*. *(H&E, ×1000)*

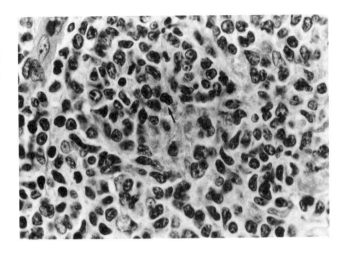

In mixed lymphocytic and histiocytic lymphoma (follicular, mixed small cleaved and large cell type), there is a mixture of small cleaved cells and large cells. The small cleaved cells are similar to those seen in NPDL. The large cells, which could be cleaved or noncleaved, are two to three times larger and show vesicular nuclei containing one to three nucleoli. The large cells should account for from 20% to 50% of the cell population within the actual tumor nodules.

Histiocytic lymphoma (follicular, large cell type) is the least common of all the types of nodular lymphomas. This type makes up only 10% to 15% of all cases. The tumor nodules are composed predominantly of large lymphoid cells with either round to oval nuclei or slightly irregular, indented nuclei. Mitoses are numerous. Despite the apparently limited stage of disease at the time of diagnosis, this type of lymphoma has the least favorable prognosis of all the nodular lymphomas due to frequent recurrences and progression to diffuse large cell lymphoma (59).

Diffuse Lymphoma. Diffuse well-differentiated lymphocytic lymphoma (DWDL) is a lymphoma of diffuse, small cell lymphocytic type. It is the solid counterpart of chronic lymphocytic leukemia and makes up about 5% of all non-Hodgkin's lymphomas. The neoplastic cells are usualy of B-cell origin and show a diffuse pattern of growth. Nuclei are small and round, surrounded by scanty cytoplasm. (Fig. 28.10) Nuclear chromatin is dense, and the nucleoli are indistinct. Mitotic activity is low. Bone marrow involvement is frequent, as well as involvement

Figure 28.10. Malignant lymphoma, diffuse, small, lymphocytic type: the cells are small with scanty cytoplasm. The nuclei are round with dense chromatin and indistinct nucleoli. (H&E, ×400)

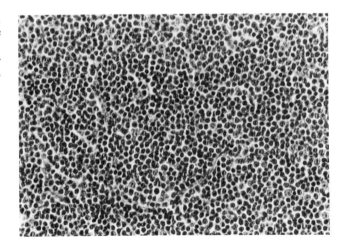

of liver and other non-lymphoid organs. The neoplastic cells may exhibit plasmocytic differentiation and become immunosecretory. Approximately 15% of patients with DWDL have monoclonal protein spikes, most often of the IgM kappa type (60).

Diffuse, mixed lymphocytic and histiocytic lymphoma (diffuse, mixed small and large cell type) occurs mainly in adults and is rarely seen in children. It makes up about 10% of lymphomas. The neoplastic cells are similar to those seen in nodular mixed lymphomas. Because there is no mixed type of lymphomas in the Lukes and Collins classification, this type of lymphoma is grouped under the heading of diffuse large cell lymphoma (cleaved or noncleaved cells). Some cases of diffuse lymphomas arise from a nodular precursor, and generous sampling usually reveals focal residual nodularity. B-cell markers may be demonstrated in these cells. The disease is often in advanced stage when diagnosed, and involvement of bone marrow, liver, and extranodal tissue is common.

Diffuse, poorly differentiated lymphocytic lymphoma (diffuse small cleaved cell; DPDL) consists of two subtypes. The subtype seen in adults is composed of cleaved cells with indented nuclei that are generally of B cell origin. B cell markers may be demonstrated in many of them. This type of lymphoma confers a poor prognosis. The second subtype, seen in children and young adults, is referred to as lymphoblastic lymphoma.

Diffuse, histiocytic lymphoma (diffuse, large cell type) is the most frequent of the diffuse lymphomas. This tumor accounts for approximately 30% of cases. It is, however, a heterogeneous group with about 60% being of B-cell origin and 40% of T-cell or null-cell origin. According to the Lukes-Collins classification, patients with follicular center cell lymphoma, cleaved or noncleaved large cell type, have a better prognosis than those with immunoblastic type. The neoplastic large noncleaved cells possess round to oval nuclei, sharp nuclear membranes, coarse chromatin network with one to four nucleoli, and pyroninophilic cytoplasm. (Fig. 28.11) The large cleaved cells show vesicular indented nuclei, marginated chromatin, and one to three nucleoli. Frequently, there is an admixture of small cleaved cells, making the distinction between large cell and mixed cell lymphomas difficult.

Immunoblastic sarcoma, formerly included in the diffuse histiocytic group, was only recently described by Lukes and Tindle (61). It can be of either B- or T-cell origin and often develops in a setting of abnormal immunologic conditions (organ transplant patients, autoimmune disease, etc.). The median age is 68 years. Histologically, the cellular infiltrate is composed of a mixture of small lymphocytes, plasma cells, and numerous immunoblasts. There is increased vascularity, and the background contains PAS-positive material.

Malignant Histiocytosis

A malignancy of the histiocyte macrophage

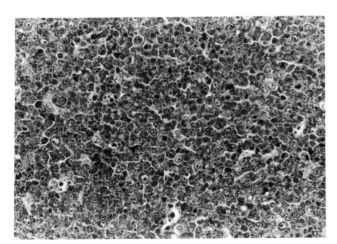

Figure 28.11. Malignant lymphoma, diffuse, large cell, noncleaved type: The neoplastic cells are large with round to oval nuclei exhibiting sharp nuclear membrane and one to four nucleoli. (H&E, ×400)

system, malignant histiocytosis represents the systemic form of the disease, whereas true histiocytic lymphoma is the localized form with nodal involvement and no systemic manifestation. In malignant histiocytosis, abrupt onset is noted with fever, hepato-splenomegaly, and progressive pancytopenia. Mild lymphadenopathy is noted in most cases. Microscopically, there is invasion of the sinusoids of lymph nodes, spleen, liver, and bone marrow by malignant cells of the monocyte macrophage system with large lobulated nuclei and abundant vacuolated cytoplasm. Multinucleation is frequent. Erythrophagocytosis is often observed in tumor cells. These tumor cells exhibit typical cytochemical reactions of the monocyte macrophage system: diffuse reactivity for non-specific esterase as well as acid phosphatast and beta glucuronidase.

Treatment of Non-Hodgkin's Lymphoma

When primary lymphomas of the lung, gastrointestinal tract, mediastinum, or retroperitoneum occur in the elderly, they should be treated surgically using the same indications that have been recommended for all persons with these types of tumors. For disseminated forms of lymphoma, radiation therapy and chemotherapy now offer dramatic and encouraging responses which have resulted in extremely long disease-free intervals and complete remissions or cure in many instances. See Chapter 6 for a detailed discussion of these forms of treatment.

SUMMARY

The occurrence of all of these special types of tumors in the elderly patient is becoming more and more apparent. As more of our population is reaching advanced age, more of these tumors will appear. As we have pointed out, sarcomas, lymphomas, and melanomas tend to appear in slightly different types and in slightly selected forms in the elderly. The fact that some of these tumors are actually more aggressive in the elderly may be somewhat surprising to those who have the mistaken idea that all tumors grow more slowly and behave in a more benign manner in elderly patients than they do in younger individuals. The surgical, radiotherapeutic, and chemo-

therapeutic approach to elderly patients with these special types of tumors must at times be more aggressive than the approach to a similar tumor in a younger patient. The intent of this chapter has been to point out those special incidences and situations in which the elderly patient's treatment should be carefully considered and those even more special situations in which the treatment should perhaps be different.

REFERENCES

1. *Cancer Patient Survival.* Washington, DC, US Department of Health, Education and Welfare. Publication No. (NIH) 77-792, 1976.
2. Russell WO, Cohen J, Enzinger FM, Hajdu SI, Heise H, Martin RG, Meissner W, Miller WT, Schmitz RL, Suit HD: A clinical and pathological staging system for soft tissue sarcomas. *Cancer* 40:1562-1570, 1977.
3. Stout AP: Tumors of the soft tissues. In *Atlas of Tumor Pathology.* Washington, DC, Armed Forces Institute of Pathology, 1957, Series 1, Fascicle 5.
4. Stout AP, Lattes R: Tumors of the soft tissues. In *Atlas of Tumor Pathology,* Washington, DC, Armed Forces Institute of Pathology, 1967, Series 2, Fascicle 1.
5. Enzinger FM, Lattes R, Torloni R: Histological typing of soft tissue tumours. *International Histological Classification of Tumours,* No. 3. Geneva, World Health Organization, 1969.
6. Enzinger FM, Weiss SW: *Soft Tissue Tumors.* St. Louis, The CV Mosby Co., 1983, pp 6-7.
7. Rosenberg SA, Suit HD, Baker LH, Rosen G: Sarcomas of the soft tissue and bone. In DeVita VT (ed): *Cancer: Principles and Practice of Oncology.* Philadelphia, JB Lippincott Co, 1982, pp 1039-1040.
8. Russell WO, Cohen J, Cutler S, Edmondson JH, Enzinger F, Hajdu SI, Heise H, Martin RG, Miller WT, Schmitz RL, Suit HD: Staging system for soft tissue sarcoma. *Semin Oncol* 8:156-159, 1981.
9. Angervall L, Johnson S, Kindblom LG, Save-Soverbergh J: Primary malignant fibrous histiocytoma of bone after radiation. *Acta Pathol Microbiol Scand* 87:437-446, 1979.
10. Meyerding HW, Broders AC, Hargrave RL: Clinical aspects of fibrosarcoma of the soft tissues of the extremities. *Surg Gynecol Obstet* 62:1010-1019, 1936.
11. Pritchard DJ, Soule EH, Taylor WF, Ivins JC: Fibrosarcoma: a clinicopathologic and statistical study of 199 tumors of the soft tissues of the extremities and trunk. *Cancer* 33:888-897, 1974.
12. Adam YG, Reif R: Radiation-induced fibrosarcoma following treatment for breast cancer. *Surgery* 81:421-425, 1977.
13. Fleming RM, Rezek PR: Sarcoma developing in an old burn scar. *Am J Surg* 54:457-465, 1941.
14. Ranchod M, Kempson RL: Smooth muscle tumors of the gastrointestinal tract and retroperitoneum. *Cancer* 39:255-262, 1977.

15. Guccion JG, Enzinger FM: Malignant schwannoma associated with von Recklinghausen's neurofibromatosis. *Virchows Arch Pathol Anat* 383:43–57, 1979.

16. Linscheid RL, Soule EH, Henderson ED: Pleomorphic rhabdomyosarcomata of the extremities and limb girdles. A clinicopathological study. *J Bone Joint Surg* 47A:715–726, 1965.

17. Reynolds WA, Winkelman RK, Soule EH: Kaposi's sarcoma. A clinicopathological study with particular reference to its relationship to the reticuloendothelial system. *Medicine* 44:419–443, 1965.

18. Stewart FW, Treves N: Lymphangiosarcoma in post mastectomy lymphedema: a report of 6 cases in elephantiasis chirurgica. *Cancer* 1:64–81, 1948.

19. Simon MA, Enneking WF: The management of soft-tissue sarcomas of the extremities. *J Bone Joint Surg* 58:317–327, 1976.

20. Karakousis CP, Velez AF, Emrich LJ: Management of retroperitoneal sarcomas and patient survival. *Am J Surg* 150:376–380, 1985.

21. Binder SC, Katz B, Sheridan B: Retroperitoneal liposarcoma. *Ann Surg* 187:257–261, 1978.

22. Kinne DW, Chu FCH, Huvos AG, Yagoda A, Fortner J: Treatment of primary and recurrent retroperitoneal liposarcoma. *Cancer* 31:53–64, 1973.

23. Braasch JW, Mon AB: Primary retroperitoneal tumors. *Surg Clin N Am* 47:663–678, 1967.

24. Selikoff IJ, Hammond EC, Seidman H: Mortality experience of insulation workers in the US and Canada. *Ann NY Acad Sci* 330:91–116, 1979.

25. Ravich A, Stout AP, Ravich RA: Malignant granular cell myoblastoma involving the urinary bladder. *Ann Surg* 121:361–372, 1945.

26. Morrison JG, Gray GF, Dao AH, Adkins RB: Granular cell tumors. *Am Surg* 53:153–160, 1987.

27. Silverberg E: Cancer statistics, 1985. *Cancer* 35:19–35, 1985.

28. Sober AJ, Fitzpatrick TB: Melanoma fact sheets. *Cancer* 29:276–279, 1979.

29. Elias EG, Didolkar MS, Goal IP, Formeister JF, Valenzuela LA, Pickren JL, Moore RH: A clinicopathologic study of prognostic factors in cutaneous malignant melanoma. *Surg Gynecol Obstet* 144:327–334, 1977.

30. Shaw HM, McGovern VJ, Milton GW, Farago GA, McCarthy WH: Malignant melanoma: influence of site of lesion and age of patient in the female superiority in survival. *Cancer* 46: 2731–2735, 1980.

31. Cutler SH, Young JL: Third National Cancer Survey: incidence data. *Natl Cancer Inst Mongr* 41:20–25, 1975.

32. Clark WH, From L, Bernardino EA, Milm MC: The histogenesis and biologic behavior of primary human malignant melanomas of the skin. *Cancer Res* 29:705–727, 1969.

33. McGovern VJ, Shaw HM, Milton GW, Farago GA: Is malignant melanoma arising in a Hutchinson's melanotic freckle a separate entity? *Histopathol* 4:235–242, 1980.

34. Reintgen DS, McCarty KM, Cox E, Seigler HF: Malignant melanoma in black American and white American

35. Balch CM, Milton GW: *Cutaneous Melanoma: Clinical Management and Treatment Results Worldwide.* Philadelphia, JB Lippincott, Co, 1985, pp 20–21.

36. Mastrangelo JM, Rosenberg SA, Baker AR, Katz HR: Cutaneous melanoma. In DeVita VT (ed): *Cancer; Principles and Practice of Oncology.* Philadelphia, JB Lippincott, Co, 1982, pp 1124–1170.

37. Mehnert JH, Heard JL: Staging of malignant melanomas by depth of invasion: a proposed index to prognosis. *Am J Surg* 110:168–175, 1965.

38. Clark WH: A classification of malignant melanoma in man correlated with histogenesis and biologic behavior. In Montagna W, Hu F (eds): *Advances in Biology of the Skin, Vol 8, The Pigmentary System.* London, Pergamon Press, 1967, pp 621–647.

39. Balch CM, Murad TM, Soong SJ, Ingalls AL, Halpern NB, Maddox WA: A multifactorial analysis of melanoma: prognostic histopathological features comparing Clark's and Breslow's staging methods. *Ann Surg* 118:732–742, 1978.

40. Breslow A: Thickness, cross-sectional area, and depth of invasion in prognosis of cutaneous melanoma. *Ann Surg* 172:902–908, 1970.

41. Balch CM, Murad TM, Soong SJ, Ingalls AL, Richards PC, Maddox NA: Tumor thickness as a guide to surgical management of clinical stage I melanoma patients. *Cancer* 43:883–888, 1979.

42. Wanebo HJ, Woodruff J, Fortner JG: Malignant melanoma of the extremities: a clinicopathologic study using levels of invasion (microstage). *Cancer* 35:666–676, 1975.

43. McGovern VJ, Shaw HM, Milton GW, Farago GA: Prognostic significance of the histological features of malignant melanoma. *Histopathol* 3:385–393, 1979.

44. Cobleigh MA, Kennedy JL: Non-Hodgkin's lymphomas of the upper aerodigestive tract and salivary gland. *Otolaryngol Clin N Amer* 19:685–710, 1986.

45. *Cancer Facts and Figures, 1980.* New York, American Cancer Society, 1980, p. 9.

46. MacMahon B: Epidemiology of Hodgkin's disease. *Cancer Res* 26:1189–1200, 1966.

47. Newell GR, Cole SR, Meittinen OS, MacMahon B: Age differences in the histology of Hodgkin's disease. *JNCI* 45:311–317, 1970.

48. MacMahon B: Epidemiological evidence of the nature of Hodgkin's disease. *Cancer* 10:1045–1054, 1957.

49. Lukes RJ, Butler JJ: The pathology and nomenclature of Hodgkin's disease. *Cancer Res* 26:1063–1081, 1966.

50. Peters MV: A study of survivals in Hodgkin's disease treated radiologically. *Am J Roentgenol* 63:299–311, 1950.

51. Carbone PP, Kaplan HS, Musshoff K, Smithers DW, Tubiana M: Report of the Committee on Hodgkin's Disease Staging. *Cancer Res* 31:1860–1861, 1971.

52. Lokich JJ, Pinkus GS, Moloney WC: Hodgkin's disease in the elderly. *Oncology* 19:484–500, 1974.

53. Berard CW, Dorfman RF: Histopathology of malignant

populations. A comparative review. *JAMA* 248:1856–1859, 1982.

lymphomas. *Clin Hematol* 3:39–76, 1974.

54. Berard CW: Reticuloendothelial system: an overview of neoplasia. In Rebuch JW, Berard CW, Abe MR (eds): *The Reticuloendothelial System*. Baltimore, Williams & Wilkins, 1975, pp 310–317.

55. Lukes RJ, Collins RD: Immunological characterization of human malignant lymphomsa. *Cancer* 34:1488–1503, 1974.

56. Lennert K, Mohri N, Stein H, Kaiserling F: The histopathology of malignant lymphoma. *Brit J Hematol* 31(suppl):193–203, 1974.

57. Rosenberg SA, Berard CW, Brown BW, Burke J, Dorfman RF, Glatstein E, Hoppe RT, Simon R: National Cancer Institute sponsored study of classification of non-Hodgkin's lymphomas: summary and description of a working formulation for clinical usage. *Cancer* 49:2112–2135, 1982.

58. Foucar K, McKenna R, Frizzera G, Brunning RD: Incidence and patterns of bone marrow and blood involvement of lymphoma in relationship to the Lukes-Collins classification. *Blood* 54:1417–1422, 1979.

59. DeVita VT, Hellman S: Hodgkin's disease and non-Hodgkin's lymphomas. In DeVita VT, Hellman S, Rosenberg SA (eds): *Cancer: Principle and Practice of Oncology*. Philadelphia, JB Lippincott, 1982, pp 1331–1401.

60. Mann RB, Jaffe ES, Berard CW: Malignant lymphomas—a conceptual understanding of morphologic diversity. A review. *Am J Pathol* 94:105–191, 1979.

61. Lukes RJ, Tindle BH: Immunoblastic lymphadenopathy, a hyperimmune entity resembling Hodgkin's disease. *N Engl J Med* 292:1–12, 1975.

Chapter 29

Management of the Elderly Atherosclerotic Patient

Patrick W. Meacham, M.D.

The age in life when the term "elderly" might be applied is debatable; however, for the purposes of this chapter we shall consider it to be over age 65. According to U.S. census statistics there are approximately 25 million people between the ages of 65 and 85 currently in the United States (1). It is projected that this number will increase to 58 million by the year 2025. Additionally, approximately 5 million people are currently in their ninth decade of life in the United States, and it is estimated that 40% of the current population will survive to reach age 80 (2). The current 80 year old should have an average life expectancy of between 5.6 and 8.2 years (2–5).

Although most vascular diseases have been reported in various age groups, the incidence of vascular disease gradually increases with age and is greatest in the elderly population. The most common significant vascular disease found in the elderly population is atherosclerosis. A progressive decline in the number and function of cells in most organs occurs with advancing age, causing an increased incidence of other major medical problems as the body ages (6). Although chronic medical problems, such as arthritis, diabetes, heart failure, and atherosclerosis, are more commonly found in the elderly population, the fact that an older age has been reached does not in itself constitute a contraindication to any form of specific therapy. "Physiologic age" is much more important in the consideration of a patient for treatment than is chronologic age. The severity of the risk factors have to be ascertained on an individual basis. Because atherosclerosis is believed to affect up to 30% of the American population over age 50 it may be assumed that by age 65 the average patient will have some degree of systemic atherosclerosis.

For the purpose of this text, we shall survey a sample of common atherosclerotic problems frequently seen in the elderly population.

THE ELDERLY ATHEROSCLEROTIC PATIENT

The elderly patient presenting with a complication or manifestation of atherosclerosis potentially carries several risk factors related to that same disease process. By far the most important risk factor is that of coronary occlusive disease. This is followed by cerebral vascular and renal disease, as well as lower extremity occlusive disease. Adult-onset diabetes mellitus is also very common in this population, and it may affect as many as one-fourth of the patients presenting with atherosclerotic processes. Degenerative joint diseases limiting mobility are also very common in this age group. Pulmonary function impairment, especially in long-term smokers, is another risk factor that is quite common, affecting 25% or more of the patients with atherosclerosis. The evaluation of these risk factors may be extremely important in determining the proper treatment of the elderly patient who has atherosclerotic disease with a surgical manifestation. Many of these risk factors may be elucidated by history and physical examination and simple blood and urine chemistries. If the patient has an atherosclerotic process that requires surgical intervention, especially if aortic cross clamping is to be necessary, more definitive screening tests should be considered.

WHO IS AN OPERATIVE CANDIDATE?

Advanced age by itself is not a contraindication to elective operation even for the more extensive aortic reconstructions, such as aneurysm repair. Many elderly patients, even in the ninth decade, will tolerate this procedure as well as their younger counterparts. For larger revascularization procedures, it should be remembered that the most important operative risk factor is that of ischemic heart disease. If an elderly patient has no history of myocardial infarction, angina, congestive heart failure, or serious arrhythmias and has no significant ECG abnormalities, then the patient *may* be in a low cardiac risk category despite the presence of other manifestations of systemic atherosclerosis. Evaluation of ventricular function by noninvasive means using radioisotopic ventriculography or real-time echocardiography both in the resting and exercise state (if possible) may reveal significant silent disease. Cardiac dysfunction may be revealed that may not be discernible on routine history and physical examination or with resting electrocardiography. Serious developing cardiac wall motion abnormalities or decreasing ejection fraction with stress should alert the physician to potentially lethal cardiac risk. If cardiac function appears to be stable on noninvasive testing, no further evaluation should be necessary and cardiac risk with the procedure should be low. If cardiac function is not stable during testing or if a history of angina, myocardial infarction, congestive heart failure, or serious arrhythmia is present, cardiologic consultation may be helpful for determining if further evaluation is warranted.

Pulmonary function should be evaluated, especially in patients with known pulmonary disease or in those who are smokers. For most patients, the ability to exercise adequately and a normal arterial blood gas determination on room air will suffice as evidence of adequate pulmonary function for operation. There are no absolute values in pulmonary function tests or arterial blood gases that serve as a contraindication to a major vascular procedure although the severe, poorly compensated states do carry significant risk and warrant careful scrutiny of the operative necessity. Cessation of smoking and treatment of chronic obstructive pulmonary diseases may improve the patient's overall pulmonary status and lower perioperative risks considerably. Patients with moderately severe

chronic obstructive pulmonary disease are usually managed successfully in the perioperative period if the physicians are alerted to the potential problem. Aggressive pulmonary toilet and judicious use of bronchodilators may thwart significant pulmonary complications.

The serum glucose aberrations of diabetes can usually be managed satisfactorily in the perioperative period, but because of the severity of the systematic arteriosclerosis that accompanies diabetes, this disease should be considered a major risk factor. Renal function is an important area of risk for major vascular procedures, as uremia (BUN greater than 30) adds significantly to overall risk. Decreased renal function, especially in the presence of diabetes, poses an increased risk of renal failure. This is true even with contrast-related diagnostic procedures. Careful attention to pre-study and preoperative hydration and monitoring of renal function is necessary in these patients.

Cerebral vascular disease should always be evaluated carefully by history and physical examination in all atherosclerotic patients. If prior history of stroke or transient cerebral ischemia is present and of recent occurrence, cerebral angiography is warranted prior to embarking on any surgical procedure. If the atherosclerotic elderly patient is asymptomatic but bruits are auscultated in the neck, noninvasive testing should be carried out to evaluate potentially severe lesions that could cause stroke or loss of life.

Hypertension is a primary risk factor in the development of atherosclerosis and is a perioperative risk factor as well. Good medical control of hypertension preoperatively is a prerequisite to a safe operative course.

ABDOMINAL AORTIC ANEURYSMS

The existence of aneurysms has been documented for at least 2,000 years. Aneurysms are most commonly found in the aged population and constitute one of the most dangerous of all manifestations of atherosclerosis. The incidence of aneurysms gradually increases with age along with the clinical presentation of other atherosclerotic manifestations. For our purposes we shall consider an aneurysm to be defined as aortic dilatation that has reached a diameter of twice the normal proximal or distal artery diameter in a given patient. Aneurysms carry several risks, including those of rupture, thrombosis, and distal embolism. The overwhelming risk with abdominal aortic aneurysms is that of rupture, causing severe internal hemorrhage leading to acute shock and death. Abdominal aortic aneurysms affect males three times more commonly than females, and they may have erratic growth rates, although the average rate of growth is approximately 0.4 cm per year (7).

Abdominal aortic aneurysm is a very common manifestation of atherosclerosis. Approximately 23,000 operations for abdominal aortic aneurysms were carried out in the year 1979 in the United States alone (8). Currently, almost all abdominal aortic aneurysms are atherosclerotic in etiology and, therefore, coexist with systemic atherosclerosis. The previously mentioned risk factors of systemic atherosclerosis are usually present in the elderly individual presenting with this diagnosis. Patients with aneurysms are at increased risk of death due to rupture, and the risk of rupture increases with the size of the aneurysm.

The diagnosis of abdominal aortic aneurysm is usually brought forth by an incidental finding, either by an examining physician or during radiologic testing for other potential disease processes. Thinner patients may themselves notice a pulsatile abdominal mass when lying supine. A skillful examining physician may palpate the mass and be able to evaluate the gross span by carefully palpating the lateral edges and measuring the distance between these. The diagnosis may be confirmed by the use of ultrasound or body scanners, such as computed tomography or magnetic resonance imaging. These modalities yield an accurate estimate of the diameter, as well as of the length of the proximal and distal aorta involved. Computed tomography and magnetic resonance imaging are especially accurate in this regard. Arteriography is helpful in delineating the exact anatomy, the presence of accessory renal arteries, and the extent of occlusive atherosclerotic disease in the neighboring and distal aortic branches in potential operative candidates. (Figure 29.1)

The presence of a tender, expansile, pulsating mass in a patient with acute onset of abdominal and/or back pain should be considered diag-

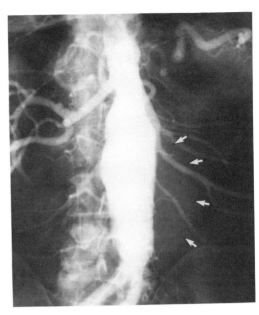

Figure 29.1. Aortogram of a 76-year-old male demonstrating a large abdominal aortic aneurysm (*arrows*) with laminated intraluminal thrombus. A congenitally absent left kidney is noted.

nostic for a ruptured abdominal aortic aneurysm. Patients with symptomatic aneurysm suggesting rupture or acute expansion with impending rupture should all be treated with emergent operative correction without any delay for "confirmatory studies." This should be carried out in any functional elderly individual despite the number of risk factors or age, as a ruptured aneurysm is almost universally fatal within a short period of time. It is clear that the mortality rate with treatment of ruptured aneurysms is high in most institutions, averaging approximately 50%; however, when untreated, the mortality approaches 100%.

Estes in 1950 reported the outcome of patients with abdominal aortic aneurysm who were followed conservatively (9). He noted a drastically reduced life expectancy in these patients. In his series of patients with aneurysms, 63.3% eventually died of aneurysm rupture. Reports of more recent series specifically concerned with elderly patients who had multiple medical problems and who did not undergo elective aneurysm repair indicate that approximately one-third of these patients died of rupture (10–12). In the patients whose aneurysms eventually ruptured, two-thirds of the aneurysms did so within the first 2 years after diagnosis (2, 5, 11, 13, 14). In one series 72% of the patients with abdominal aortic aneurysm and hypertension died of aneurysm rupture (10). The risk of operative mortality in dealing with the acutely ruptured abdominal aortic aneurysms in the older population varies from 57% to 74%, whereas the elective repair mortality rate is much lower (2, 5, 11–14). It is notable in most of these series that many of the patients who had untreated aneurysms had been denied treatment because of advanced age.

Petracek et al. polled 100 nonsurgeons regarding risk of elective repair of abdominal aortic aneurysms in patients 80 years or older (14). Fifty-one percent of the nonsurgeons responded that they would not recommend operative repair of an aneurysm in an 80-year-old patient. Ninety-four percent of these physicians believed that the elective mortality was greater than 10%, and 40% of the physicians polled believed that the mortality was greater than 20% (14).

Several series of older patients, including series of patients in their ninth decade of life, have been published (2, 4–6, 11, 13–16). In these combined series of patients older than 70 years of age there were 942 patients treated electively for repair of abdominal aortic aneurysm. The average mortality rate in these series was 8.9%, with a range of 0% to 13.5%. The risk of mortality related to elective resection is only slightly higher than that of the general population undergoing aneurysm repair; however, it is not statistically greater. Cooley reported a 5.3% mortality rate in 1460 patients (all ages) undergoing elective aneurysm repair (17). Patients in the ninth decade of life undergoing elective repair had mortality rates in different series varying between 2% and 12.5%. Most series note no statistically significant increase in mortality rate in the older age groups.

If the elderly population with aneurysms is studied for other risk factors, a reasonable evaluation of the individual's risk can be made. Because age by itself does not appear to be a highly significant risk factor the other associated risk factors have to be examined prior to recommending elective aneurysm repair. Hypertension was previously thought to be a significant risk factor that might negate proceeding with elective repair. In the patient with abdominal aortic aneurysm

and hypertension there is a threefold increased risk of rupture (10). The presence of hypertension coexisting with an aneurysm therefore creates a very strong indication to proceed with its resection after immediate preoperative blood pressure control has been established. The mortality risk of elective aneurysm repair is somewhat higher in the very elderly population; however, it is acceptable if other risk factors are few. The mortality risk will rise correspondingly as greater numbers of risk factors are added. In the elderly patient with an abdominal aortic aneurysm greater than 4 cm in diameter and no other notable risk factors, the risk of the elective procedure is much less than the projected risk of death due to rupture.

The elderly patient undergoing elective aneurysm repair is at increased risk of postoperative complications that may extend the period of hospitalization. Nonlethal complications are more likely in older patients, especially the over-80 age group. The risk of these complications again depends greatly on the degree and number of preoperative risk factors. Although more advanced multi-organ system degeneration may dictate a nonoperative approach, milder degrees of risk may be successfully managable surgically.

O'Donnell et al. noted that 45% of their elective aneurysm patients over age 80 had a history of atherosclerotic heart disease (5). Seven percent had a myocardial infarction history, 8% had congestive heart failure, and 43% had ECG abnormalities. Eleven percent of their patients had a history of renal disorders, and 25% had respiratory compromise. Seven percent had concomitant cerebral vascular disease. The mortality rate in their 44 octogenarians undergoing elective abdominal aortic aneurysm repair was 2%. Fifty-two percent, however, had nonlethal complications. Seven percent had myocardial infarction in the perioperative period, 9% congestive failure, 20% developed arrhythmias, 2% developed oliguric azotemia, 11% developed nonoliguric azotemia, 4.5% developed respiratory failure, 9% developed pneumonia, and 11% developed atelectasis.

Treiman et al. reported a 54% complication rate in their series of octogenarians undergoing elective aneurysm repair (2). One-third of the complications in their report were cardiac. The length of hospitalization required for elective repairs in octogenarians was from 13 to 22 days (2, 5). The quality of life following repair was judged as excellent in most cases. In one series 90% were ambulatory with a normal mental status examination at the time of discharge. Twenty percent required at least temporary nursing home placement (2). At 1 year postoperatively 80% had returned to preoperative functional status. In another series 93% had returned to their preoperative status 1 month postoperatively (5).

Pasch et al. projected the health care costs in the year 1979 due to aneurysm ruptures that could have been prevented by elective repair (8). If elective repair had been performed they estimated that $50 million could have been saved during that year because of the decreased need for hospitalization and intensive care unit utilization in elective repairs versus emergency repairs.

When assessing risks in a potential elderly preoperative candidate with an abdominal aortic aneurysm, Baker and Munns noted that patients with cardiac disease consisting of an abnormal ECG, history of myocardial infarction or angina, cardiomegaly, or clinical congestive heart failure demonstrated no significant increased risk in operative mortality (16). However, a history of myocardial infarction statistically decreased the overall 3-year survival. History of abnormal ECG or angina also decreased the 5-year survival. Patients with a history of stroke or transient cerebral ischemia tended to fare worse during and after aneurysm repair, although this difference was not statistically significant. Renal function impairment was a significant risk factor as survivors tended to have a lower preoperative BUN than nonsurvivors. Distal arterial occlusive disease and cigarette smoking were associated with a diminished 3-year survival. Chronic obstructive pulmonary disease was not a statistically significant risk factor in long-term survival.

From this data, it is evident that elective aneurysm repair can be performed in most elderly patients with acceptably low mortality risk, although careful medical preoperative preparation and postoperative care are mandatory due to a higher risk of nonlethal complications.

Evaluation and Treatment of the Elderly Patient with Abdominal Aortic Aneurysm

Once an aneurysm has been documented, a systematic workup to elucidate risk factors and operability should be undertaken. If there is any question about the size of the aneurysm or the linear extent of the aneurysm (i.e., involvement of the suprarenal or supraceliac aorta), a thoracoabdominal CT scan is advisable.

The most frequent cause of death in patients with aneurysms and the most important morbidity and mortality risk with repair is myocardial infarction. An evaluation of the heart is therefore very advisable. This is done most practically by obtaining a radionuclide ventriculogram (RVG) both in the resting and exercise state. An electrocardiographic tracing may be taken simultaneously. This study can give the physician a working knowledge of the cardiac reserve and an indication of developing myocardial ischemia with stress. Mural ischemia may be seen electrocardiographically or as a wall motion abnormality notable on scan. If the ejection fraction is adequate (i.e., greater than 50%) at rest but decreases with exercise, this may represent significant myocardial ischemia. Increased risk may be anticipated with the aortic clamping and unclamping required for aneurysm repair. A cardiology consultation is usually recommended for further evaluation of the heart if the RVG is positive for ischemia. A cardiac catheterization may be necessary if ischemia is felt to be severe. We feel that, in elective cases, if the aneurysm patient does have significant coronary artery disease, consideration for coronary revascularization should be given prior to abdominal aortic aneurysm repair. If coronary revascularization is needed, 6 to 12 weeks are then allowed between coronary revascularization and elective aneurysm repair.

A gross evaluation of pulmonary function is advisable. Full pulmonary function tests may be undertaken, and if severe chronic obstructive pulmonary disease is present, these tests can be repeated after placing the patient on bronchodilators. For practical purposes walking patients up and down stairs, noting their gross ventilatory ability, and checking arterial blood gas determinations on room air provide a baseline determination of pulmonary function.

A careful peripheral vascular examination may reveal other points of potential morbidity, including cerebrovascular disease and lower extremity occlusive disease. If carotid bruits are found and are asymptomatic, a duplex or real-time carotid ultrasound examiniation with waveform analysis may be helpful in separating highly significant from less significant lesions. Careful recording of pulses and Doppler examinations in the lower extremities may elucidate significant occlusive lesions of the lower extremity arteries. All of these aforementioned tests can be performed on the patient prior to hospitalization. If the patient appears to be a reasonable operative candidate, hospitalization and preoperative aortography are advisable, especially if there is abnormal renal function, hypertension, or significant occlusive disease in the lower extremity vessels. Arteriography is helpful in delineating the extent of the aneurysm and occlusive changes in the aortic branches near the aneurysm that may require operative therapy and in noting any accessory renal vessels that may come off the aneurysm itself.

When the decision is made to proceed with elective repair, overnight preoperative intravenous hydration is advisable to prevent sudden hypotension on anesthesia induction. Prior to anesthesia induction, placement of arterial and Swan-Ganz catheters is done in almost all elective aneurysm procedures. These monitoring catheters help intraoperatively and postoperatively in the management of blood pressure and in volume loading or unloading as required.

A full-length abdominal midline incision is utilized to provide adequate exposure for safely dealing with aortic aneurysm. During dissection care is taken to avoid any marked manipulation of the aneurysm to avoid dislodging a laminated thrombus or atherosclerotic debris from inside the aneurysm sac into the distal circulation. Aortic tube grafting is used whenever the occlusive and aneurysmal disease allows. If the aneurysmal disease extends out into the common iliac arteries, a bifurcation graft is utilized so that no portion of the aneurysm will remain and secure arterial anastomoses are ensured. Coordinating all operative maneuvers with the anesthesiologist allows for appropriate volume and pharmacologic maneuvers to be carried out so that the peripheral blood pressure and filling pressure remain as stable as possible.

Upon completion of the procedure the patient is monitored in the intensive care unit for 2 to 3 days with close surveillance of cardiac, renal, and pulmonary function. If the aneurysm had been extensive and the operative time has been lengthy, we prefer to allow the patient to awake gradually on the ventilator and be supported by the ventilator for the first 8–10 hours postoperatively. Routine electrocardiograms and CPK isoenzymes are obtained the operative day and for the following 2 days. If there is no indication of any myocardial damage and the patient is stable, he or she may then be transferred to a regular hospital room. As soon as the monitoring lines are discontinued, an aggressive ambulation program is begun, encouraging the patient to make short but frequent walks. This provides a good stimulus for lung, bowel, and bladder function and promotes better venous circulation in the lower extremities. The nasogastric tube inserted at the time of operation is generally removed at the same time or soon after the endotracheal tube is removed. The diet is advanced from ice chips and sips of water gradually through clear liquids to a regular diet as the bowel function returns. When patients are fully ambulatory and able to sustain themselves with an adequate oral intake, they are discharged from the hospital and are generally seen again within 1 week of the time of discharge. Patients with aneurysms or other forms of atherosclerotic disease need lifelong follow-up, as a continual surveillance of the arterial system is necessary. With a careful approach to preoperative evaluation, operative technique and monitoring, and postoperative care and long-term followup, the elderly aneurysm patient can usually expect a full return to preoperative functional status.

CEREBRAL VASCULAR DISEASE

In the past, "hardening of the arteries" was equated with advanced age and senility. In fact, atherosclerosis commonly targets the extracranial cerebral arteries and may cause stroke, which is currently a leading cause of death and disability, especially in the elderly population.

Many of the stroke-causing atherosclerotic lesions occur in the cervical arteries, which are amenable to premorbid diagnosis and preventive treatment. Cerebral vascular reconstructive procedures are prophylactic in nature, as revascularization to reverse completed strokes is no longer considered feasible or safe.

Because cerebral vascular occlusive disease so commonly coexists with other atherosclerotic lesions (i.e., coronary artery disease, aneurysms, aorto-iliac, and femoral occlusive disease) it is logical to screen carefully for the existence of common stroke-producing lesions when other forms of atherosclerosis are diagnosed. A careful vascular history and physical examination, checking all of the accessible target areas, should be performed.

Pathophysiology

The atherosclerotic occlusive lesion in the carotid artery may insidiously advance, growing inwardly by gradual lipid deposition in the subintimal and medial layers of the arterial wall. Relatively rapid growth of the lesion may be brought about by the hemorrhage within the plaque. A molten subintimal collection of atherosclerotic debris, complex lipids, and blood products may form, causing progressive luminal encroachment, turbulent blood flow, and increasing shear stress on the delicate intima. The formation of this complicated lesion is usually accompanied by a completely asyptomatic state. Symptoms are produced only when the arterial flow becomes severely compromised, or more commonly, when the overlying intimal cap of the lesion ulcerates, allowing exposure of the molten debris to the passing bloodstream. Micro-emboli may then be carried to the end organs, the brain, and the eye.

It is estimated that the vast majority of cerebral vascular symptoms are due to micro-embolism, causing transient ischemic attacks (TIAs) and strokes (18, 19). TIAs are manifested by contralateral sudden weakness, numbness, and sometimes dysphasia. If micro-embolism targets the ophthalmic branch of the internal carotid artery, a sudden, painless, ipsilateral monocular blindness may occur, "like a shade coming down." This is termed *amaurosis fugax*. These symptoms will generally last less than an hour. If the symptoms persist longer than 6 hours, a stroke or retinal infarction is likely. If symptoms last longer than 24 hours, infarction is considered

to have definitely occurred.

Non-lateralizing cerebral symptoms, such as generalized weakness, somnolence, personality changes, blackout spells, dizziness, etc., may occur secondary to gross overall blood flow diminution. They probably occur only in a very small subgroup of patients with severe occlusive involvement of the carotid and vertebral arteries. It is unlikely that single vessel occlusion would account for these symptoms. Posterior circulatory occlusive lesions causing vertebral basilar insufficiency are less common and may cause non-lateralizing symptoms, such as vertigo, drop attacks, weakness, and temporary paralysis of any combination of extremities.

If definite lateralizing symptoms are obtained by history, a thorough workup is indicated, even if no suspicious physical findings are present. Not all patients with a potential stroke-causing lesion will demonstrate a bruit or a diminished pulse. (Figure 29.2) For the lateralizing symptomatic group of patients, noninvasive testing may be performed, but should not preclude the use of arteriography, even if the noninvasive tests are unremarkable. Patients with lateralizing (micro-embolic) symptoms require a high resolution, clear arteriogram of both carotid arteries and preferably of all four cerebral arteries. Cervical and cerebral views in the anterior-

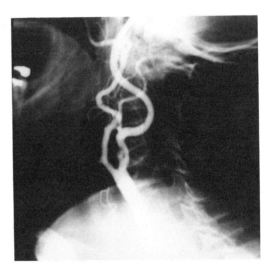

Figure 29.2. Carotid arteriogram of a 78-year-old male who presented with his second stroke and no carotid bruit. The small ulcerated area in the carotid bifurcation was missed by noninvasive evaluation.

posterior and lateral projections are necessary for a complete evaluation. Intravenous digital techniques usually do not supply the resolution necessary for accurate diagnosis of the symptomatic patient. We prefer standard biplane angiography of the carotid systems with arterial digital views of the arch and bilateral vertebral vessels. This very complete, high resolution study can be performed with approximately 100 cc of contrast.

The Asymptomatic Carotid Bruit

The functional elderly patient who is found to have carotid bruits and no elicited symptoms should be evaluated for the degree of stroke risk. If bruits are found to involve the full length of the cervical carotid artery, careful palpation of the arteries and recording of blood pressures in both arms should be performed. A weakened carotid pulse in the neck or discrepancy of arm blood pressure (greater than 20 mm Hg) indicates significant arch or great vessel occlusive lesions. Bruits in the midneck or higher suggest carotid bifurcation lesions. Bruits in the posterior triangle of the neck indicate vertebral orifice lesions.

Once the physical findings have been established, a noninvasive evaluation should be considered in any patient with focal bruits. A number of noninvasive techniques are available, including oculoplethysmography, Doppler scans, and newer techniques involving direct ultrasound. Probably the best means of noninvasive carotid evaluation is the duplex scan that combines real-time imaging with Doppler ultrasound (20). The artery and lesion can be seen and blood flow velocity information can be analyzed. Often the anatomy of the arterial plaque itself can be discerned. Intraplaque hemorrhage and ulceration may be notable on this noninvasive study. If lesions appear to be hemodynamically significant (i.e., greater than 75% stenotic) or if ulceration is suspected, arteriography may be indicated to evaluate the lesion further. If the lesions are less significant in appearance and there is little flow disturbance, conservative follow-up and interval repeat noninvasive study are preferable.

Arteriography should be considered in patients with hemodynamically significant stenosis by noninvasive testing. The type of contrast image may depend somewhat on the individual patient. Patients with diabetes or renal insufficiency should be studied with the smallest amount of contrast possible to avoid worsening their renal function. In these patients an intra-arterial digital technique may yield good resolution images of the carotid bifurcation lesions, and can be performed with less than 25 ccs of contrast. Additionally, these studies can be performed on an outpatient basis in low risk individuals. Intravenous digital angiography is a standard outpatient form of arteriography, but is preferable in non-diabetic patients with good renal function. The patient must be very cooperative during this form of long-exposure angiography, as the slightest motion or even a swallow may produce a noninterpretable image from which no meaningful information can be derived. Asymptomatic patients who have sonographically significant bilateral disease or findings consistent with arch, carotid, and vertebral involvement might be best served by standard arteriographic techniques so that the arch and all four vessels can be examined.

Which patients should be offered operation? This is still a very debatable question. The patients having lesions that cause less than 75% stenosis and contain no gross ulceration may probably be safely followed with serial examination and interval repeat noninvasive testing. The patients with serious symptomatic heart disease or other prohibitive risk factors may be better off followed conservatively for their asymptomatic carotid lesions unless lesions are tightly stenotic or severly ulcerated. Good risk elderly patients with stenosis greater than 75% or with gross ulceration should be considered for elective revascularization. In a general population of patients with asympomatic carotid stenosis, Thompson et al. demonstrated statistically reduced long-term rates of TIA and non-fatal stroke in patients treated by endarterectomy when compared with nonoperated patients (21).

Symptomatic patients with any degree of stenosis should be strongly considered for elective operative revascularization. Patients having repetitive (or crescendo) TIAs and severe complicated plaques should be considered for urgent operation. Patients with wavering neurologic symptoms and subtotal occlusion of the carotid artery angiographically should be considered for emergency anticoagulation and operation. These patients are at high risk for impending stroke.

Medical Therapy

Several multi-center studies have assessed the clinical treatment of patients with cerebral vascular disease using antiplatelet drugs (21–26). Although there are many unanswered questions remaining, these studies suggest that aspirin reduces the incidence and frequency of transient ischemic attacks. Additionally, there appears to be a beneficial effect from aspirin in reduction of death or stroke in males. The degree of significance of the beneficial effect of aspirin versus the beneficial effect of carotid revascularization has not yet been determined. The potential role of coumadin and other anticoagulants remains unclear.

Surgical Therapy

The commonly performed carotid artery revascularization by carotid endarterectomy was first attempted and reported in 1953 by Strully et al. (28). This first attempt, a carotid revascularization after acute stroke, was technically unsuccessful due to total internal carotid artery thrombosis. The first successful carotid reconstruction was performed the following year by H. H. Eastcott et al. by resection of a carotid bifurcation and direct carotid reanastomosis (29). Probably the first successful carotid endarterectomy was performed by DeBakey in 1953, although this was not reported until 1975 (30).

Direct carotid artery revascularization can be performed with low morbidity and mortality risks even in the elderly population. The endarterectomy procedure is prophylactic and is used to prevent the dreaded complication of stroke.

Edwards et al. reported a 4.7% mortality in 42 patients over the age of 80 years (bilateral operations in 10 patients) (4). There were no strokes in this group occurring on the operative side and one stroke occurring on the nonoperative side. Plecha et al. noted an increased mortality risk in patients over 75 years of age (1.5% in the less than 75-year group; 2.2%, 75–79 years; 3.3%, age 80–84 years), but interestingly found no mortality or perioperative strokes in their 42 patients who were 85 years or older (13). The leading cause of death in operative patients was myocardial infarction. In another large series, Benhamou et al. reported results on 183 patients over the age of 70 undergoing 220 cerebral

vascular operations (34 bilateral) (31). The mortality in the asymptomatic elderly patients undergoing carotid revascularization was 0.76%. The mortality rate for the patients with active symptoms undergoing operations was 4.3% for the entire 15-year period and was noted to be 3.2% during the last 3 years of the study. Ouriel et al. found no difference in the mortality and morbidity in the over-75 age group when compared with the under-75 year age group (32).

Technical Points

The occurrence of stroke is the most debilitating, isolating, and feared complication of atherosclerosis. Elderly patients with symptomatic cerebral vascular disease should be given a high priority for workup and treatment of that disease. When the decision is made to perform carotid revascularization, great care should be taken with other risk factors. We attempt to keep patients' blood pressure stable and at their normal level during anesthesia induction, throughout the surgical procedure, and in the immediate postoperative period. If the patient has a very tight stenosis, (i.e., greater than 95%) we prefer preanesthesia anticoagulation with intravenous heparin. The endarterectomy technique itself is standard and requires approximately 90 minutes of operating time. Attention to blood pressure control is stressed throughout the perioperative period. The head of the patient's bed is maintained at a 45° elevation postoperatively to minimize venous hemorrhage and wound edema. Cardiac and neurologic monitoring is carried out for 18–24 hours postoperatively. If the postoperative course is uncomplicated, even the elderly patient may be ready for discharge safely in 3 to 5 days postoperatively.

If the opposite carotid artery also will require revascularization, this may be performed when wound edema from the first reconstruction has resolved, generally in 3–6 weeks. If a recent stroke has occurred or been diagnosed or confirmed by CT scan, we prefer to delay cerebral revascularization for 4–6 weeks after the stroke to allow cerebral edema and local vasospasm to stabilize. With careful patient selection and attention to detail during the operation and perioperative period, even patients in their ninth decade of life may benefit from therapy to prevent a lethal or disabling stroke.

LOWER EXTREMITY ISCHEMIA

The aorta-iliac and femoral-popliteal arteries are a common target site for the development of atherosclerosis, as well as being a common target site for large cardiogenic emboli. The aged population is at risk for the development of these ischemic problems. It is appropriate when considering lower extremity ischemia to separate ischemia into two major groups—one group with mild to moderate ischemia causing exercise-related symptoms only (claudication) and the other, more severe ischemic group with limb jeopardy, causing rest pain, ulceration, or gangrene.

Claudication is a relatively mild ischemic state that does not portend immediate impending limb loss. The diagnosis of arterial claudication may be made by history and physical examination; its classical symptoms are muscular cramping or fatigue with exercise. The muscle groups affected generally indicate the supplying vessels involved with disease. Calf claudication is commonly caused by superficial femoral or popliteal artery occlusive disease. Calf and thigh claudication generally results from common femoral or external iliac artery occlusion. Calf, thigh, and buttock claudication is caused by common iliac or aortic occlusive disease. The historical findings may be confirmed by physical examination. This is done by recording the pulses and bruits both *at rest* and *immediately after exercise*. The postexercise examination is an important component of the arterial examination in a patient with exercise-related symptoms. The diagnosis may be further confirmed by resting and exercise arterial Doppler studies and waveform analysis. Selectivity in treatment is wise in the elderly patient with claudication, and a conservative approach may be safely tried before consideration of invasive treatment in this group of patients.

McCalister reported the natural history of claudicators and noted a greater than 50% improvement rate in those claudicating patients who could cease smoking and challenge symptoms with regular exercise (33). Approximately 25% of the patients remained stable, and another 25% worsened despite conservative therapy. No significant difference in ultimate limb loss was noted in claudicating patients between the conservative and surgically treated groups. Patients who either fail conservative management or who have significant disability from claudication should be considered for arteriography and revascularization by appropriate means.

Patients with severe degrees of ischemia causing true rest ischemic symptoms, such as burning or numbness in the toes or feet, ischemic ulcerations, or gangrenous changes in toes, demand a more aggressive approach early on to prevent limb loss. Impending limb loss should be considered an absolute indication for aggressive revascularization. Those patients in whom a functional recovery may be achieved with revascularization should be aggressively evaluated with arteriograms in order to detect the optimal means of revascularization. Patients who have a neurologically useless extremity that is unlikely to change with revascularization are best considered for primary amputation.

Aorta-Iliac Occlusive Disease

Reduced inflow to the lower extremities from aorta-iliac occlusive disease presents a challenge to the managing physician and may present several different treatment options. If the patient is found to have relatively few risk factors (determined by a similar workup as for patients with aneurysms) despite numerical age, a direct approach may be utilized in these good risk patients who may survive 10 years or more. A high patency rate with direct revascularization by aorta-femoral bypass grafting can be achieved (75% to 85% 10-year patency) (34). Plecha et al. noted a 2.9% mortality rate in patients less than 75 years old undergoing elective aortoiliac operations, whereas a 12%–15% mortality was reported in patients greater than 75 years of age (13). If the patient is at slightly higher risk and has unilateral disease, a unilateral direct approach may be utilized to afford high patency rates and a less physiologically challenging procedure. This may be accomplished by retroperitoneal ileofemoral bypass or endarterectomy. If the patient is poor risk, yet still demands operative revascularization due to severe ischemia, extra-anatomic bypassing may be the most optimal procedure as it does not require abdominal or retroperitoneal entry.

If the occlusion is unilateral, femoral-femoral bypass grafting may be carried out with general, regional, or even local anesthesia in the poorest risk patient. Femoral-femoral bypass is a procedure that poses a minimal challenge to the elderly high risk system and carries a 5-year patency rate of 44%–81% (35–38). If severe bilateral aorta-iliac occlusion is present axillo-bifemoral bypass grafting is an option that is not as physiologically challenging as direct approaches and carries acceptable patency rates, although thrombectomies may be required for continued patency over long periods of time. Five-year patency rates of 33%–77% have been reported (36, 39, 40). Thus, the patient with severe lower extremity, limb-threatening ischemia may be successfully managed by a variety of revascularization techniques. The technique used for inflow revascularization should depend on the individual elderly patient.

Femoral-Popliteal Occlusive Disease

Some patients with limb-threatening ischemia and occluded superficial femoral arterial segments may be found to have occluded or very stenotic profunda femoral arteries. In these elderly patients, a profunda femoral revascularization (profundaplasty) may be quite satisfactory in improving perfusion enough to alleviate rest pain or to heal smaller ischemic ulcers. Profundaplasty is performed by groin incision alone and can be done under local anesthesia if necessary. This procedure is a durable revascularization with a low morbidity and mortality rate (41).

Femoral-popliteal reconstruction, as is profundaplasty, is a less physiologically challenging revascularization in the elderly patient and is generally well tolerated. The decision to revascularize should be made depending on the significance of the degree of claudication, failure of conservative therapy, or the presence of limb-threatening ischemia. Femoral-popliteal reconstructions may be utilized using prosthetic grafts especially if above-the-knee popliteal artery patency is present; vein grafts may be used if below knee or tibial reconstruction is necessary. These reconstructions may be performed using general or regional anesthesia and offer 50%–80% 3-year patency rates.

Reinhold et al. reported their results with 63 elderly diabetic patients over the age of 70 treated for severe ischemia of the lower extremity with femoral-popliteal bypass (42). Sixty-nine bypasses were performed with no in-hospital deaths. The cumulative patency rates for the entire series was 68% for 1 year and 45% for 3 years. The patency rates were noted to be higher with saphenous vein grafts than with prosthetic grafts (72% 1 year, 56% 3 year). In patients with more favorable grafting criteria—that is, popliteal artery patency with two vessel run-off—the patency rates were much higher than with single vessel or isolated popliteal segment bypass. The combination of a favorable arterial reconstitution and use of autogenous vein grafts for the bypass yielded patency of 91% 1-year and 82% 3-year rates. Although there were no perioperative deaths in this series, there were 21 postoperative complications, most of which were cardiac.

Reichle et al. reported their results with femoral-popliteal bypass in 72 patients aged 70 or older (43). Initial limb salvage in these patients was 71.4%, with cumulative limb salvage at 5 years being 51%. Operative mortality in this series was 8.3% in patients over the age of 70, which contrasts with 1.7% in patients under the age of 70 years. This mortality did include bypass procedures and subsequent amputation procedures in those patients in whom limb salvage was not obtained.

More recently, Scher et al. report their experience with 168 consecutive patients over 80 years of age undergoing arterial reconstruction or percutaneous transluminal angioplasty (44). One hundred eighty-nine limbs were treated for limb salvage, and 182 operative procedures were performed. These consisted of 84 femoral-popliteal, 72 femoral-tibial, 12 axillo-femoral, 11 femoral-femoral, 2 axillo-popliteal, and 1 ileo-femoral bypass. The 30-day procedural mortality was 6%. The limb salvage rates were 84% 1-year, 74% 2-year, and 71% 3-year.

In the last 10 years, the availability of polytetrafluoroethylene grafts has been a significant advance in the armamentarium of the vascular surgeon. These grafts have a better patency rate than previous prosthetic grafts in femoral popliteal reconstructions, especially for above knee popliteal reconstructions. The use of these grafts may shorten operating time and dissection considerably. Ekman et al. reported their results using these grafts in lower extremity reconstructions in 68 elderly and high risk patients aged 70–88 years (45). Immediate postoperative mortality in this elderly and high risk group was 3%. Seventy-five percent of the limbs were intact 12 months after the operation, and 55% were intact 24 months postoperatively.

Under most circumstances, when an acceptable vein is present, autogenous vein is the bypass graft of choice for long-term patency, especially for below knee popliteal and tibial reconstructions. However, the availability of better prosthetic grafts has allowed vascular surgeons to opt for a shorter procedure with less dissection in elderly and high risk patients with acceptable patency and limb salvage rates.

Embolism and Embolectomy

As is evident from the previous discussion, the incidence of heart disease causing myocardial ischemia, congestive heart failure, and arrhythmias is quite high in the elderly population. Often the most aged and least stable patients will present with acute lower extremity ischemia secondary to cardiogenic embolus. This condition can usually be diagnosed readily by the history of acute onset of severe symptoms with no prior symptoms. Physical examination may be all that is necessary to confirm the diagnosis in someone with no prior ischemic symptoms and in whom the other extremity maintains normal pulses. The abrupt loss of pulsation below the site of embolus impaction is associated with marked ischemic changes in the distal extremity. In a majority of patients presenting with lower extremity embolus, cardiac arrhythmia, congestive heart failure, or myocardial infarction will precede the embolic event. Coldness, pain, paresthesias, pallor, mottling of the distal skin, and loss of distal neurologic function are the cardinal signs. If the pulse examination in the opposite extremity is normal, the diagnosis of embolus is highly likely and arteriography is usually not necessary. If severe vascular occlusive changes are present elsewhere, arteriography may be necessary to confirm the diagnosis and delineate the extent of other points of occlusive disease. This subgroup of the elderly population with acute limb ischemia is made up of generally very unstable patients with varying degrees of cardiac insufficiency and ischemia. In the face of an acute lower extremity embolus, immediate limb jeopardy is present, and if the severe ischemic changes cannot be reversed

quickly, limb loss is imminent.

Complete anticoagulation with heparin is necessary to control clot propagation in the already ischemic extremity and to prevent any further emboli from occurring. Fortunately, these unstable elderly patients in acute limb jeopardy can be treated expeditiously with balloon catheter embolectomy. Femoral artery exposure and embolectomy under local anesthesia are usually very well tolerated even by the most unstable elderly patient. Anticoagulation with heparin should be continued postoperatively until oral anticoagulation with warfarin is therapeutic. The oral anticoagulation should be continued indefinitely. Additionally, aggressive medical treatment and cardiac arrhythmia control are mandatory.

Allermand et al. reported a series of 56 patients aged 80 years or greater presenting with acute lower extremity embolus (46). They found an overall mortality rate of 32%. In patients presenting with lower extremity ischemia and a simultaneous myocardial infarction, the mortality rate was 100%. Thirty-eight patients survived the embolectomy procedure under local anesthesia, and 29 of these patients avoided amputation. The high mortality rate in these patients is indicative of the cardiac instability that is already present. Furthermore, recurrent or simultaneous emboli to brain, viscera, etc, account for the high mortality with this condition. Lower extremity embolectomy under local anesthesia is a less physiologically challenging procedure than primary amputation and should be considered even in the extremely aged patient with multiple associated medical problems.

Percutaneous Transluminal Angioplasty

Percutaneous transluminal angioplasty is a relatively new interventional treatment modality in occlusive arterial disease. Although long-term results in prospective randomized studies have not yet become available, this procedure does appear to be a promising addition to the treatment armamentarium in arterial occlusive disease. It may be especially important in elderly and debilitated patients with higher associated surgical and anesthetic risks. It is especially applicable in the treatment of lower extremity occlusive disease both in the iliac and femoral-popliteal regions. The technique is appealing in that only

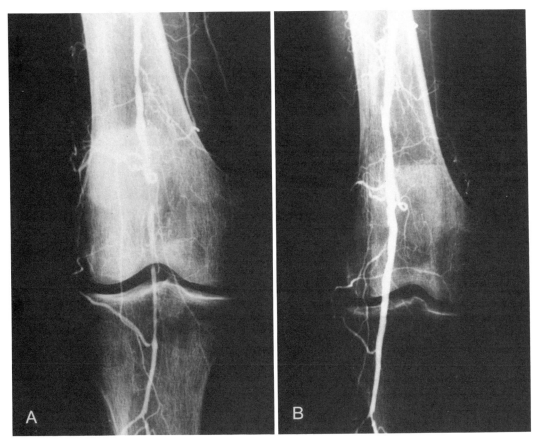

Figure 29.3. Popliteal arteriogram of an 89-year-old female in poor health who presented with toe-tip necrosis and an ankle pressure of 30. The sequential stenoses were successfully dilated by balloon catheter, allowing uneventful healing of a simple toe amputation.

a local anesthetic is required, and with a successful procedure, the hospital stay may be very short.

Selection of appropriate patients for this procedure is important as all occlusive lesions are not amenable to this technique. Although totally occluded segments have been successfully dilated and reported, it is preferable and safer to restrict its usage to hemodynamically significant but not totally occlusive lesions. The preferable atherosclerotic lesion for angioplasty is a midtrunk arterial lesion that is not at a major branch point and is relatively short. Gruntzig, who is credited with the modern balloon angioplasty technique development, reported an 83% 2-year patency rate of iliac-arterial occlusive lesions (46). Kumpe and Jones in 1982 also reported an 86% 2-year patency rate of iliac lesion angioplasty (48). Waltman et al. the same year reported a 92% 2½-year patency rate for iliac dilatation (49).

In the femoral-popliteal area, lesions may also be successfully dilated with appropriate patient selection. Although patency rates are lower in the more distal, slower-flow arteries, temporary patency and flow improvement may allow healing of ulcers or toe amputations to occur. (Figure 29.3) Two-year patency rates of 56%–75% have been reported (47–49).

Although this technique is still evolving and undergoing careful scrutiny, it has been shown to be a valuable addition to the armamentarium and can be utilized alone or along with surgical revascularization. For example, the elderly patient presenting with severe lower extremity ischemia and found to have an isolated external iliac stenosis and superficial femoral artery occlusion can be treated with femoral-popliteal bypass and simultaneous iliac arterial dilatation. When used appropriately, the technique offers at least short-term palliation with minimal anesthesia requirements and a low complication rate.

CONCLUSION

Although it is clear that the elderly patient carries at least a slightly higher mortality risk and a significantly higher risk of nonlethal complications, individualized evaluation for significant risk factors and appropriate selection of treatment should be carried out, as many of these patients may be offered significant palliation and even increased life expectancy. The elderly patient even in the ninth decade of life may have sufficient physiologic reserve to tolerate even large arterial reconstructive procedures and may benefit significantly from such procedures. It is clear that the elderly patient should not be denied life-saving or limb-saving procedures purely on the basis of numerical age only. In many cases the elderly patient with atherosclerosis may even be a better risk than some younger patients with a more accelerated form of atherosclerosis. Individual evaluation is mandatory, and life-long follow-up following either aggressive interventional or conservative treatment should be employed.

REFERENCES

1. U. S. Bureau of the Census: *Current Population Reports*, Vol. 922, 1980, pp 25–28.
2. Treiman RL, Levine KA, Cohen JL, Cossman DV, Foran RF, Levin PM: Aneurysmectomy in the octogenarian. A study of morbidity and quality of survival. *Am J Surg* 144:194–197, 1982.
3. Edmunds, LH Jr: Resection of abdominal aortic aneurysms in octogenarians. *Ann Surg* 165:453–457, 1967.
4 Edwards WH, Mulherin JL Jr, Rogers DM: Vascular reconstruction in the octogenarian. *South Med J* 75:648–652, 1982.
5. O'Donnell TF Jr, Darling RC, Linton RR: Is 80 years too old for aneurysmectomy? *Arch Surg* 111:1250–1257, 1976.
6. Harbrecht PJ, Ahmad W, Garrison N, Fry DE: Influence of age on the management of abdominal aortic aneurysm. *Am Surg* 48:93–97, 1982.
7. Bernstein EF, Dilley RB, Goldberger LE, Gosink BB, Leopold GR: Growth rates of small abdominal aortic

aneurysm. *Surgery* 80:765–773, 1976. 8. Pasch AR, Ricotta JJ, May AG, Green RM, DeWeese JE: Abdominal aortic aneurysm: the case for elective resection. *Circulation* 70(suppl I):I-1-I-4, 1984.
9. Estes JE Jr: Abdominal aortic aneurysm: A study of one hundred and two cases. *Circulation* 11:258–264, 1950.
10. Szilagyi DE, Elliott JP, Smith RF: Clinical fate of the patient with asymptomatic abdominal aortic aneurysm and unfit for surgical treatment. *Arch Surg* 104:600–606, 1972.
11. Esselstyn CB Jr, Humphries AW, Young JR, Beven EG, deWolfe VG: Aneurysmectomy in the aged? *Surgery* 67:34–39, 1970.
12. Foster JH, Bolasny BL, Gobbel WG Jr, Scott HW Jr: Comparative study of elective resection and expectant treatment of abdominal aortic aneurysm. 129:1–9, 1969.
13. Plecha FR, Bertin VJ, Plecha EJ, Avellone JC, Farrell CH, Hertzer NR, Mayda J II, Rhodes RS: The early results of vascular surgery in patients 75 years of age and older: an analysis of 3259 cases. *J Vasc Surg* 6:769–774, 1985.
14. Petracek MR, Lawson JD, Rhea WG Jr, Richie RE, Dean RH: Resection of abdominal aortic aneurysms in the over-80 age group. *South Med J* 73:579–581, 1980.
15. DeBakey ME, Crawford ES, Cooley DA, Morris GC Jr, Royster TS, Abbott WP: Aneurysm of the abdominal aorta. *Ann Surg* 160:622–639, 1964.
16. Baker WH, Munns JR: Aneurysmectomy in the aged. *Arch Surg* 110:513–517, 1975.
17. Cooley DA, Carmichael MJ: Abdominal aortic aneurysm. *Circulation* 70 (suppl I):I-5-I-6, 1984.
18. McDowell FF: Transient cerebral ischemia: diagnostic considerations. *Prog Cerebrovasc Dis* 22:309–324, 1980.
19. Schmidley JW, Caronna JJ: Transient cerebral ischemia: pathophysiology. *Prog Cerebrovasc Dis* 22:325–342, 1980.
20. Wetzner SM, Kiser LC, Bezreh JS: Duplex ultrasound imaging: vascular implications. *Radiology* 150:507–514, 1984.
21. Thompson JE, Patman RD, Takington CM: A symptomatic carotid bruit: long-term outcome of patients having endarterectomy compared with unoperated controls. *Ann Surg* 188:308–316, 1978.
22. Canadian Cooperative Study Group: A randomized trial of aspirin and sulfinpyrazone in threatened stroke. *N Engl J Med* 229:53–59, 1978.
23. Evans G: The effect of drugs that suppress platelet surface interaction on incidence of amorosis fujaques and transient cerebral ischemia. *Surg Forum* 23:239–241, 1972.
24. Fields WS, Lenak NA, Frankowsk RF: Controlled trial of aspirin in cerebral ischemia. *Stroke* 8:301–316, 1977.
25. Fields WS, Lenak NA, Frankowski RF, Hardy RJ: Controlled trial of aspirin in cerebral ischemia. Part II. *Stroke* 9:309–319, 1978.
26. Olsson JE, Brechter C, Backlund H, Krook H, Muller R, Nitelius E, Olssen O, Tornberg A: Anti-coagulant

versus anti-platelet therapy as prophylactis against cerebral infarction in transient ischemic attacks. *Stroke* 11:4–9, 1980.

27. Fields WS, Lemak NA, Frankowski RF, Hardy RJ, Bigelow RH: Controlled trial of aspirin in cerebral ischemia. *Circulation* 62(suppl V):90, 1980.

28. Strully KJ, Hurwitt ES, Blankenburg HW: Thromboendarterectomy for thrombosis of the internal carotid artery in the neck. *J Neurosurg* 10:474–482, 1953.

29. Eastcott HHG, Pickering GW, Robb CG: Reconstruction of the internal carotid artery. *Lancet* 2:994–996, 1954.

30. DeBakey ME: Successful cartoid endarterectomy for cerebrovascular insufficiency—19 year followup. *JAMA* 233:1083–1085, 1975.

31. Benhamou AC, Kieffer E, Tricot JF, Maraval M, Lethoai H, Benhamou M, Boespflug O: Carotid artery surgery in patients over 70 years of age. *Int Surg* 66:199–202, 1981.

32. Ouriel K, Penn TE, Ricotta JJ, May AG, Green RM, DeWeese JA: Carotid endarterectomy in the elderly patient. *Surg Gynecol Obstet* 162:334–336, 1986.

33. McAllister FF: The fate of patients with intermittent claudication managed non-operatively. *Am J Surg* 132:593–595, 1976.

34. Brewster DC, Darling RC: Optimal methods of aortic-iliac reconstruction. *Surgery* 84:739–748, 1978.

35. Brief DK, Brener B, Alpert J, Parsonnet V: Crossover femoral femoral grafts followed up five years or more: an analysis. *Arch Surg* 110:1294–1299, 1975.

36. Eugene J, Goldstone J, Moore WS: Fifteen year experience with subcutaneous bypass grafts for lower extremity ischemia. *Ann Surg* 186:177–183, 1976.

37. Flanigan P, Pratt DG, Goodreau JJ, Burnham SJ, Yao JST, Bergan JJ: Hemodynamic and angiographic guidelines in selection of patients for femoro-femoral bypass. *Arch Surg* 113:1257–1262, 1978.

38. Livesay JJ, Atkinson JB, Baker JD, Busuttil RW, Barker WF, Machleder HI: Late results of extra-anatomic bypass. *Arch Surg* 114:1260–1267, 1979.

39. Johnson WC, LoGerfo FW, Vollman RW, Carson JD,

O'Hara ET, Mannick JA, Nabseth DC: Is axillo bilateral femoral graft an effective substitute for aorto bilateral iliac femoral graft? *Ann Surg* 186:123–129, 1976.

40. Ray LI, O'Connor JB, Davis CC, Hall DG, Mansfield PB, Rittenhause EA, Smith JC, Wood SJ, Sauvage LR: Axillo femoral bypass: a critical appraisal of its role in the management of aortoiliac occlusive disease. *Am J Surg* 138:117–128, 1979.

41. Bernhard VM: Profundaplasty. In Rutherford RB (ed): *Vascular Surgery* ed 2. Philadelphia, WB Saunders, 1984, pp 590–596.

42. Reinhold RB, Gibbons GW, Wheelock FC, Hoar CS: Femoro-popliteal bypass in elderly diabetic patients. *Am J Surg* 137:549–555, 1979.

43. Reichle FA, Rankin KP, Tyson RR, Shuman CR, Finestone AJ: The elderly patient with severe arterial insufficiency of the lower extremity, limb salvage by femoro-popliteal reconstruction. *Circulation* 60 (Suppl I): I124–I126, 1979.

44. Scher LA, Veith FJ, Ascer E, White RA, Samson RH, Sprayregen S, Gupta SK: Limb salvage in octogenerians in nonogenerians. *Surgery* 99:160–165, 1986.

45. Ekman CA, Claes G, Carlsson I: Use of polytetrafluoroethylene grafts in elderly and high-risk patients. *South Med J* 75:1553–1555, 1982.

46. Allermand H, Westergaard-Nielsen J, Nielsen OS: Lower extremity embolectomy in old age. *J Cardiovasc Surg* 27:440–442, 1986.

47. Gruntzig A: Die percutane transluminale Rekanalisation chronischer Arterienverschlusse mit einer neuen Dilatationstechnik. 24 Verlag Gerhard Witzstrock, Baden-Baden, 1977.

48. Kumpe DA, Jones DN: Percutaneous transluminal angioplasty: radiologic viewpoint. *Vasc Diag Ther* 3:19, 1982.

49. Waltman AC, Greenfield AJ, Novelline RA, Abbott WM, Brewster DC, Darling RC, Moncure AC, Ottinger LW, Athanasoulis CA: Transluminal angioplasty of the iliac and femoral popliteal arteries, current status. *Arch Surg* 117:1218–1221, 1982.

Chapter 30

Musculoskeletal Diseases in the Elderly

Ronald E. Rosenthal, M.D., F.A.C.S.

This chapter will deal with those musculoskeletal diseases that are secondary to demineralization, inflammation, infection, degenerative processes, trauma, malignancy, and peripheral vascular diseases and in particular those conditions that are problems in elderly patients. Surgical conditions resulting from these processes and their management in the elderly patient will be emphasized. The impact of the increasing numbers of elderly people is particularly felt by those who deal with diseases of the musculoskeletal system. Certain disease patterns are characteristically seen in the elderly. Demineralization of the skeletal system, whether from disuse or osteoporosis, will predispose the elderly patient to significant fractures after minimal trauma. Degenerative arthritis of the hip and knee are examples of musculoskeletal problems that are characteristic for elderly people. The extent of an elderly person's disability from such an arthritic joint may be more a function of that person's lifestyle than the actual radiographically demonstrated extent of the disease. Malignancies affect the skeleton of the elderly, mostly from metastatic adenocarcinomas or malignancies of the blood-forming organs. Peripheral vascular disease of the lower extremities in the elderly patient frequently leads to gangrene, which then will require an amputation. Excellent prosthetic rehabilitation can be accomplished in many elderly patients for whom a below-the-knee amputation was necessary.

An elderly person with a fracture can expect the fracture to unite and to have good, although not normal, function of the part. Major elective, semi urgent, and emergency orthopaedic procedures can be performed in most elderly patients with a reasonably high level of safety. Ambulatory patients who sustain fractures about the hip can be expected to be ambulatory after timely surgical correction of the fracture, although they may not always move with the same stamina and gait pattern as before. A patient with metastatic breast carcinoma who sustains a pathologic fracture secondary to a metastatic lesion in the femur should be treated surgically with the expectation that she may again become ambulatory. Although the natural history of her underlying carcinoma will not be altered, she may have many months, even years, of quality life. The patient with a displaced Colles' wrist fracture may benefit from the use of an external fixator so that her wrist may have a better cosmetic appearance as well as good function after the fracture heals. The elderly patient with peripheral gangrene of the foot requiring amputation should be approached from the rehabilitative, not the ablative, standpoint. "Amputation" is only half of the appropriate concept. The full concept is "amputation and prosthetic fitting."

The result of successful care of the elderly patient with a musculoskeletal disease or injury can be extremely gratifying. Fractures or arthritic conditions in the elderly should be approached as aggressively and optimistically as one does the younger patient. Elderly patients with degenerative joint conditions should be considered for reconstructive procedures if their activity level is being severely compromised by the condition. An elderly patient with a major fracture should be evaluated with the idea that he or she can be returned to the same functional level as before the injury if the fracture can be successfully treated.

FACTORS INFLUENCING ORTHOPAEDIC TREATMENT OF THE ELDERLY

It is the functional state of the patient, not his or her age, that is the prime consideration affecting orthopaedic treatment. Many different functional levels can be found among patients of the same chronologic age. Senile, debilitated, nonambulatory patients from nursing homes may not be considered for any orthopaedic procedures, whereas functional, alert, patients, even though much older, may tolerate surgical procedures well and make excellent rehabilitation patients. Patients over the age of 100 have had successful repair of hip fractures and left the hospital ambulatory. Elective total joint replacements have been done for patients in their eighties when their functional states have warranted it (1). (See Figure 30.1)

The patient's general condition affects the decision regarding treatment. Many elderly patients have chronic, but stable, medical conditions. Very few absolute contraindications to emergency orthopaedic procedures exist. Acute myocardial infarction, acute pulmonary edema, overwhelming sepsis, or the terminal stage of an incurable disease are the most common. Decisions regarding elective operations of all types must be individualized. A patient who is nonambulatory and not functioning independently is a poor candidate for reconstructive surgery. The rehabilitation following most major orthopaedic procedures may be and often is quite vigorous; patients who cannot cooperate in their own rehabilitation program because they cannot understand it will not benefit from the major reconstructive effort that initiated the need for rehabilitation. Massively obese patients generally are poor surgical risks and poor rehabilitation candidates at all ages. Patients with incoordination may also do poorly after reconstructive procedures. Patients with uncontrolled infections usually should not undergo elective orthopaedic procedures, the risk of surgical wound infection being too great. A wound infection following orthopaedic operations in any patient is serious; in the elderly patient, it is usually catastrophic. Patients with severe skeletal demineralization, from whatever cause, require different surgical procedures and present with a different set of potential complications. The activity level

of the patient is a major factor in the quality of his or her bone stock.

Patients are never made "normal" by the orthopaedic procedure or by most other operations. The goals of the procedure must be realistic: to return the patient to as near a functional state as he or she was at prior to the injury or prior to the onset of the degenerative process. Patients, or their families, may believe what they read in the lay press about "miracle" joint replacement operations and that these devices will make them normal. An elderly person usually requires a cane, or even crutches, and walks with a limp years after a successful surgical procedure on a hip or knee. Some stiffness and deformity of the wrist, elbow, or shoulder follow fractures in these areas. No surgical procedure will alter the natural history of systemic osteoporosis. Surgical treatment of a pathologic fracture will not cure the patient's metastatic carcinoma or multiple myeloma. Below-the-knee amputation and prosthetic fitting of a patient with diabetic gangrene of the foot will not alter systemic cardiovascular disease.

The socio-economic impact in the United States of the care of musculoskeletal trauma and

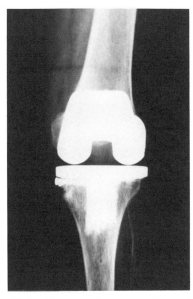

Figure 30.1. Postoperative x-ray of a total knee replacement (TKR) in an 82-year-old woman. The patient had severe degenerative disease and was disabled by pain. Postoperatively, she walked with a cane and resumed her previous lifestyle.

disease in the elderly is massive. The cost of the acute care of fractures secondary to osteoporosis is estimated at over 2 billion dollars a year (2). There are approximately 210,000 fractures about the hip yearly, representing a cost of over 1 billion dollars. The average age of these patients, three-fourths of whom are women, is 75 (3). Approximately 25% will be discharged to long term nursing home care and will rarely leave such a facility alive. The cost of nursing home residence is usually borne by the state through its Medicaid program; Medicaid covers 90% of all patients in long term nursing homes in New York. Welfare, which includes Medicaid, is the largest item in the budget of most states.

Elderly patients who are discharged home following hospitalization for orthopaedic problems usually need home health nursing and/or physical therapy assistance for months after their operation or injury. The elderly person may not deteriorate solely as a direct result of his or her injury, but rather the injury may hasten the progress of a process already underway. The family may have been contemplating a major change for the elderly person, such as a move from an independent apartment to a protected environment, at the time when a major accident and fracture occurred. Such an event will usually precipitate the decision. The family and the patient must always be prepared for some change in the elderly individual's lifestyle after a major fracture or operative procedure.

In calculating the risk-benefit ratio of the elderly patient, the consequences of non-operative treatment of the condition must be understood and considered. A senile, fragile, non-ambulatory patient in a nursing home who sustains a fracture about the hip may not benefit from surgical correction, and his or her lifestyle will not be altered if the hip remains essentially untreated (4). In such a patient, the risks of a major surgical procedure will outweigh the benefits. However, with this and few other exceptions, most patients should be offered surgical stabilization of a fracture about the hip unless there is a dire, absolute, surgical contraindication (5).

Not all treatment decisions in the elderly patient are matters of life and death; the benefits of an enhanced lifestyle, improved ambulation, and greater independence are desirable goals in the elderly, as well as in younger patients. The risks and costs of hospitalization and surgical care and of disruption of the patient's life to allow rehabilitation are greater in the elderly, but such obstacles need not be overwhelming.

SPECIFIC DISEASE CONSIDERATIONS

Six general categories of musculoskeletal diseases will be discussed in this section: osteoporosis and demineralization, inflammatory disease and infection, degenerative joint disease, fractures and trauma, malignant lesions of the skeleton, and peripheral vascular disease and amputations.

Osteoporosis and Demineralization

Demineralization, whether from postmenopausal osteoporosis, disuse, or chronic illness, is probably the most important factor in managing skeletal diseases in the elderly. Bony demineralization is often obvious radiologically. However, subtle differences in x-ray technique may give a false impression of skeletal mineralization. The Singh index, which is the technique of measuring bone mineralization as a function of the femoral trabecular pattern, gives a rough but not entirely accurate measure of the extent of demineralization (6). Clinically, demineralization most often becomes a problem in the spine, femur, radius, and ankle. Osteoporosis does not affect the skeleton uniformly; it is much more profound in the femur than in the tibia (7). Progressive compression deformities of the thoracic vertebrae result in kyphosis and shortening of stature. The osteoporotic bones may be painful even without fracture.

In the early stages of development, compression fractures of the vertebrae may be barely detectable radiologically and may take several weeks to become apparent. Malignancies of the spine also may be difficult to diagnose in the early stages before the characteristic radiologic features appear. Clues to the early diagnosis of these conditions are found in the history, which will characteristically reveal the onset of and a fairly rapid increase in localized pain, with or without obvious trauma. Routine blood chemistries are normal in osteoporosis although abnormalities of some values may suggest an underlying systemic disease that affects the patient's activity level.

There is no reliable, effective treatment for post-menopausal osteoporosis. Current concepts deal with prevention or attempts to arrest progression of the disease. Much is written in the lay press about calcium, but calcium is just one part of what we know to be a complex biochemical disorder. Increasing the calcium intake of an elderly person has not been shown to restore bone mass. Adding exogenous estrogens may retard osteoporosis, but will not reverse it. Treatment with calcitonin, or fluoride, has been attempted in the past and abandoned as ineffective or harmful (8). Physical activity is an important factor in predicting and managing osteoporosis, as is racial and ethnic background. Post-menopausal osteoporosis is largely a disease of white women. The goal of treatment is pain relief and, equally important, maintenance of a reasonable level of physical activity. Occasionally, a thoraco-lumbar or lumbo-sacral orthosis is necessary for severe back pain that is secondary to osteoporosis. Many elderly patients will not tolerate anti-inflammatory drugs. Narcotics should be used with extreme caution—even an elderly person can become habituated to codeine.

We rarely use estrogens or anti-inflammatory drugs in the treatment of osteoporosis, but often recommend mechanical devices, such as a lightweight orthosis and/or a cane, and very mild, over-the-counter analgesics, such as acetaminophen.

Inflammatory Diseases and Infection

Elderly people may develop inflammatory or infectious diseases of the bones and/or joints. Some of these conditions are easily managed; others are not. Surgical treatment is not often indicated in most inflammatory conditions, but is usually necessary to manage most infections.

Paget's disease of the bone is a specific, inflammatory disease of bone characteristically seen in the elderly. It may involve the shaft or articular surface of a bone or several bones. Somewhere between 20% and 40% of patients with radiologically demonstrable Paget's disease will have symptoms. These symptoms may range from mild aching to disabling pain and may include associated complications of pathologic fractures and malignant degeneration. Medications currently in use for these problems are calcitonins and diphosphonates. These drugs may provide symptomatic relief, but to date no medication has been shown to reverse the skeletal changes of Paget's disease (9).

Pagetoid involvement of the hip or knee may produce disabling symptoms. Fractures may occur through involved long bones. The quality of pagetoid bone is variable and unpredictable. It may be hard, brittle, soft, avascular, or highly vascular. The surgical treatment of pagetoid joints by the use of arthroplasty may be a relatively straightforward procedure, or it may be associated with massive bleeding. Fracture fixation may be impossible due to brittle bone, or it may proceed normally. Non-unions of fractures are more common in Paget's disease. The surgeon must be aware of the likelihood of technical difficulties when dealing with patients who have this abnormal bone condition.

Malignant degeneration occurs in about 1% of patients with Paget's disease. This neoplastic change usually takes the form of osteosarcoma or fibrosarcoma. The patient with this complication will usually complain of increasing pain, and x-rays will show progressive bone destruction. Treatment is usually by amputation, primarily to eliminate a painful, useless, extremity. These are serious and highly malignant tumors; the 5-year survival rate is less than 10%.

Crystal-induced arthropathy may be a cause of inflammatory joint disease in the elderly due to crystals of urates or pyrophosphates. Early detection and modern treatment of gout have eliminated the majority of the irreparably destroyed joints that were formerly described. Occasionally, an attack of acute, gouty arthritis may occur in a post-operative or post-trauma patient. It may mimic an acute, septic arthritis clinically. Identification of urate crystals in the joint fluid and the finding of an elevated serum uric acid level will help identify the disease. X-rays in acute gouty arthritis usually are normal; the characteristic changes of gout only appear after several attacks.

Pyrophosphate arthropathy, or pseudogout, usually is superimposed on a joint with some degree of pre-existing degenerative changes. The joint is warm; there is effusion but no infection. X-rays show a characteristic chondrocalcinosis; when the knee is involved, these changes can be seen in the menisci, as well as the articular cartilage. Treatment for this condition is with anti-inflammatory medications.

Rheumatoid arthritis may occur in the elderly. It affects men and women equally in this age group (10). The onset may be acute or insidious. The characteristic appearance of fusiform swelling in the metacarpo-phalangeal joints of the hand and wrist may be present, or the joint changes may be so non-specific that the disease is confused with acute gout or pseudogout. Treatment may be difficult because of the elderly person's intolerance to gold or potent anti-inflammatory drugs. Late sequelae of rheumatoid disease may be managed with total joint replacement, arthroplasties of the hands, or tendon transfers as indicated.

Septic arthritis occurring primarily in an elderly patient is an ominous sign. The synovial membrane is normally resistant to infection; intact joints usually do not develop infection unless there is widespread sepsis or underlying disease. Septic arthritis in the elderly may not be acute; the patient may show little systemic signs of infection. Any swollen joint, without an obvious cause, should be aspirated and the fluid examined for cells and crystals and cultured for bacteria. Protein and glucose determinations are helpful. The protein content of the fluid is elevated and the glucose depressed in septic arthritis, but the final diagnosis usually rests on the identification of the infective organism. A markedly elevated white cell count, predominantly of PMNs, is a further clue.

The treatment of septic arthritis includes antibiotics, mechanical debridement, and immobilization. Virtually all antibiotics cross the synovium, so that local injections into the joint are not necessary. Surgical drainage is done to remove a fibrinous plug mechanically and break up intra-articular locules so that systemic antibiotics can be effective. This usually cannot be accomplished by repeated aspirations alone. Immobilization of the joint should be continued until the acute symptoms have subsided. The treatment of infection of a joint is cause to deviate from the principle of re-establishing motion. Control of the infection is a greater priority, and this cannot be achieved in the presence of motion. The exact duration of antibiotics necessary for adequate treatment is controversial; most authors recommend a 3-week course. The underlying cause for the development of infection in a joint should always be sought and eliminated.

Osteomyelitis in the elderly rarely occurs from hematogenous spread. Bone infection is usually secondary to an infected open fracture, joint implant, or open reduction of a closed fracture. Antibiotics alone are not adequate; surgical treatment is necessary. Usually, a joint implant must be removed and the joint debrided. Under carefully controlled conditions, another implant may be re-implanted several months later with some likelihood of success (11). Infection following fracture usually cannot be controlled until the fracture has united. Fixation devices are left in place until that time, and then removed. Some infections will then become quiescent. Systemic antibiotics are usually administered for a total of 6 weeks. Osteomyelitis in the elderly, as in younger patients, is not cured. But, as long as a walled-off pocket does not develop, an elderly patient can lead a normal life even with a focus of chronic drainage. Osteomyelitis associated with ischemic ulcers is dealt with later in this chapter.

Degenerative Joint Disease

The incidence of degenerative joint disease increases with age. Arthritis of the knee is more common in women than men. There may be little correlation between a patient's x-ray findings and his or her symptoms. The initial treatment of degenerative joint disease is with moderate exercise and anti-inflammatory medications, provided that there are no medical contraindications to their use. If the patient's disability becomes such that activity is curtailed, then he or she should be seriously considered for surgical reconstruction.

Arthroplasty is now a common procedure for disabling degenerative joint disease even in the advanced age group.

Total hip replacement, which has been in common use in the United States since about 1970, has proven to be one of the most successful pain relief operations devised for painful hips. Thousands are performed yearly. Relief of pain and improvement in motion are dramatic. Rehabilitation is straightforward, and most patients can resume a quality lifestyle. Like all operations, however, total hip replacement carries risks. Urinary tract and pulmonary infections, thromboembolic episodes, late loosening, and breakage of components of the prosthesis, although not common, are serious complications. Infection, either immediate or late, remains the most feared complication of total joint replacement and virtually ensures failure.

Total knee replacement has not achieved the widespread use and satisfaction that total hip replacement has, but in carefully selected patients with severe, disabling, degenerative arthritis of the knee, it may successfully rehabilitate an otherwise disabled patient. Successful total knee replacement is a more exacting surgical procedure than total hip replacement, although the risks and complications are similar.

Arthroplasties of the shoulder and elbow are limited to a few, carefully selected patients. In general, degenerative arthritis is a much more disabling disease in the elderly when it involves the lower extremities than when it involves the upper. Attempts have been made to develop a satisfactory ankle arthroplasty with little success. For the rare patient with disabling degenerative or post-traumatic arthritis of the ankle who cannot be managed with non-operative means, arthrodesis of the ankle may be indicated. With that exception, arthrodesis is rarely indicated in managing arthritis in the elderly.

Arthritis of the spine is frequently diagnosed in the elderly. Many radiologic changes in the elderly spine—osteophyte formation, disc space narrowing, or facet joint sclerosis—do not correlate with symptoms. Degenerative changes that may be significant include spinal stenosis, a narrowing of the anteroposterior diameter of the spinal canal secondary to hypertrophic changes in the pedicles and laminae. This condition may require a decompressive laminectomy. Another condition exists and is known as disseminated, idiopathic, skeletal hyperostosis (DISH). In this disorder, there is hypertrophic interbody ankylosis with progressive restriction of motion. Surgical procedures have little to offer the patient with DISH.

Fractures and Trauma

As mentioned above, fractures constitute major and common problems in the elderly. Fractures in elderly patients tend to result from falls, rather than from major industrial or transportational trauma, although elderly people are occasionally involved in motor vehicular accidents. Fractures of the aged long bones may be comminuted although they are often not widely displaced. The porotic bone of the elderly often predisposes to compression or impacted fractures from minimal trauma. The common serious fractures in elderly patients involve the wrist, shoulder, hip, knee, ankle, and the spine.

Colles' fractures of the distal radius of the elderly patient unite readily but often with residual stiffness and/or deformity. The exact best method of managing a Colles' fracture is controversial; no one method is ideal. The characteristic appearance of the wrist at the time of injury is the "silver fork" deformity. The wrist is angulated dorsally, deformed, and swollen. The fracture can be reduced either by manipulation or by traction and then casted. Over a period of weeks, however, the precise reduction may be lost, and the fracture then heals with radial deviation of the wrist and with prominence of the ulnar styloid. Although this may be an excellent functioning wrist, its cosmetic appearance may be unsatisfactory. Many different techniques have been suggested over the years for fixation of these fractures. These suggestions include crossed wires, pins and plaster, and open reduction. Currently, the external fixator is the preferred method to maintain length during the healing process if closed manipulation is not satisfactory (12). This technique requires an anesthetic and the use of the operating room. Threaded pins are placed in the second or third metacarpal and the radial shaft and connected with the fixator frame. This is worn for 6 to 8 weeks. No cast is used. This technique will result in a better appearing wrist, but one that is stiffer. The personal preference of the author is to treat a Colles' fracture by manipulation and follow the patient closely. If significant reduction is lost in the first week, then the use of the external fixator is considered. If used, the fixator is left on for 6 weeks.

Fractures about the shoulder usually involve

the proximal humerus and occur through the surgical neck. Most of these can be treated with a sling and with early motion. Union of the fracture occurs within a few weeks; the major concern is shoulder stiffness. A great deal of deformity at the fracture site can be accepted with the anticipation that a functioning, pain-free, though stiff, shoulder will result. Occasionally, a fracture is completely displaced and needs manipulative reduction. Open reduction should be reserved for those widely displaced fractures involving the tuberosities, or for fracture-dislocations. Fixation of multiple, comminuted fragments in the elderly shoulder is often impossible; in fractures or fracture-dislocations where the head of the humerus is sheared off at the anatomic neck, the use of a primary humeral head prosthesis may be indicated. Regardless of the treatment, early motion, in the form of pendulum exercises, should be started within the first week or two. The exercises can be done in the sling. The sling should be discontinued at the earliest possible moment and exercises to the elbow and wrist added.

Fractures about the hip constitute the most important group of fractures in the elderly. The goal of treatment is stabilization of the fracture so that the patient may be mobilized very soon, ideally be ambulatory, but at least out of bed into a sitting position. This can rarely be accomplished without a surgical procedure. This operation should be carried out within the first 24 hours, if possible, as the patient's medical condition is likely to deteriorate progressively from the pain and forced immobility secondary to the untreated fracture. The usual medical conditions found in the elderly can be adequately evaluated and corrected during that period of time. Some acute or concomitant problems are contraindications to surgical repair: acute myocardial infarction, pulmonary edema, or decubiti in the area of the proposed procedure. Fractures about the hip are classified into three categories: femoral neck (or intracapsular), intertrochanteric, and subtrochanteric. Dislocations and fracture-dislocations of the hip are rare in the elderly.

Most femoral neck fractures will not unite without surgical treatment. The ideal treatment is surgical stabilization of the fracture with multiple pins. In elderly patients with impacted or non-displaced fractures, fixation may be accomplished in situ with multiple, cannulated screws. This can be accomplished rapidly with minimal blood loss and surgical exposure and allows prompt post-operative mobilization and weight bearing. Displaced fractures require manipulative reduction and may be more difficult to hold with screws. Full weight bearing after these fractures may not be safe for 3 months. Even after successful union of the fracture, late aseptic necrosis of the femoral head may occur, resulting in an unsatisfactorily functioning hip and mandating a secondary, reconstructive arthroplasty. Multiple pin or screw fixation of the fractured hip does require a special fracture table and operating room image-intensification x-ray equipment. Although the actual operating time may be less than 1 hour, the total anesthetic time may exceed 2 hours because of the necessary time spent in the accurate positioning of the patient and in the reduction of the fracture.

Because in many elderly patients who have displaced femoral neck fractures initial attempts at fixation of the fracture are likely to fail, primary replacement of the femoral head with an endoprosthesis has become the treatment of choice. This is a definitive procedure that is rapidly carried out on a regular operating table with a minimum of eqiupment. It allows for prompt postoperative weight bearing and rapid rehabilitation of the elderly patient. It does not result in a normal hip. This repair requires more extensive surgical exposure, and although the initial results are gratifying, loosening and settling of the prosthesis may eventually result in a painful hip.

Patients who are active, have good bone stock, can cooperate in a rehabilitation program, and can protect their hip are probably best treated with internal fixation. The cannulated lag screw system is recommended, using a minimum of three screws across the fracture site. In general, patients under age 70 will fall into this category. Patients who are not candidates for internal fixation are treated with primary endoprosthesis. The Austin Moore prosthesis has been used for over 30 years and remains the most widely used device today. Newer two-and three-piece devices with different shaft, neck, and head sizes may allow a better fit and may last longer. The author's current preference is to use the Austin Moore prosthesis in the very elderly or severely impaired patient and to use a press fit system,

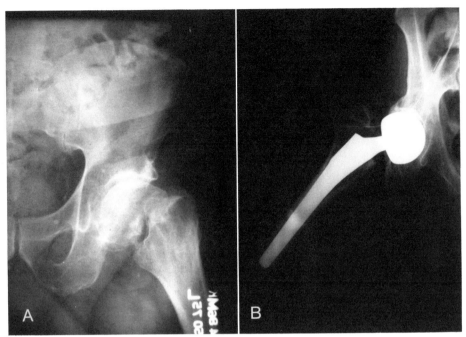

Figure 30.2. A femoral neck fracture in an otherwise healthy 78-year-old woman. This was treated with primary prosthetic replacement of the femoral head with a bipolar prosthesis that allowed early weight bearing. **A,** Preoperative x-ray, showing the displaced femoral head. **B,** Postoperative x-ray, showing the prosthesis has been press-fit into the femoral shaft, allowing a rigid fixation.

such as the Biofit (R), on the more vigorous patients who are not candidates for primary internal fixation. The posterolateral exposure is most preferred, and the patient should be mobilized out of bed the next day (13). (Figure 30.2)

Intertrochanteric fractures in the elderly patient present a special challenge. Comminution and osteoporosis may prevent anatomic reduction and rigid fixation. Bleeding from the extensive open bone surfaces adds to the surgical and anesthetic risk. These patients tend to be older and more fragile than those with femoral neck fractures. Surgical treatment requires a fracture table and image intensification x-ray equipment. Non-comminuted or stable fractures are reduced into position by traction and internal rotation. The femur is exposed surgically, and a lag screw is placed under x-ray control up the femoral neck and attached to a side plate that is held to the femoral shaft with screws. In order to achieve a stable reduction in a comminuted fracture, an osteotomy to allow the major fragments to impact into each other may be necessary. This often will result in shortening and external rotation,

but it may be the only way to achieve firm fixation. Failure to recognize an inherently unstable intertrochanteric fracture will result in postoperative loss of good reduction and the cutting out and displacement of the fixation devices (14). The use of a medial displacement osteotomy on comminuted fractures is recommended by the author.

The patient is mobilized out of bed on the first postoperative day and then into a standing position a day or two after that. Fixation must be secure enough to tolerate early weight bearing. Many elderly people cannot partially bear weight. They either bear full weight, or they do not walk. Often, a patient can walk with minimal assistance within a week after the hip fracture is repaired. Patients usually begin with a walker and graduate to crutches and then to a cane. Most elderly patients will then require some sort of ambulatory support indefinitely.

Subtrochanteric and femoral shaft fractures are less common in elderly patients than fractures about the hip. Surgical stabilization of these fractures is necessary to mobilize the patient. Subtrochanteric fractures may be treated with a hip compression screw and long side plate or with specialized intramedullary nails. The femoral shaft in an elderly patient may have a wide medullary canal and not grip a standard intramedullary nail well. The interlocking nail, which provides fixation at the proximal and distal ends, has been used successfully in elderly patients (15).

The proper method of prevention of pulmonary embolism in the elderly fracture patient is a controversial subject. Mobilization, rather than anticoagulation, may be the key to the prophylaxis of thromboembolic complications (16). The risks of anticoagulation are considerable in the elderly. If anticoagulation is used, it is generally begun with a loading dose of coumadin the night following the operation. The dosage is adjusted by daily prothrombin determinations and discontinued when the patient is ambulatory. The author does not routinely anticoagulate elderly fracture patients unless they have a history of previous thrombophlebitis or pulmonary embolism. (See Chapter 3)

Discharge planning begins upon or soon after admission to the hospital. Patients who will require a great deal of support and assistance to ambulate or whose mental state precludes independent living will require placement into a rehabilitation facility, and some will require long term nursing home placement. Others who are alert and have a supportive home environment may return to it and should be encouraged to do so. Although the decision to return a patient to his or her home situation or to consider nursing home placement cannot always be made until after the necessary operation is done, initial evaluation by social services is vital in starting what may be a complicated bureaucratic process. The social worker is usually as important to the patient's recovery and rehabilitation as the physical therapist.

Fractures about the knee are ideally treated by open reduction and internal fixation with specialized plates and screws. (Fig. 30.3) However, in elderly people, a supracondylar femur or tibial plateau fracture may be so comminuted that rigid surgical fixation is impossible. For those patients, supracondylar or tibial plateau fractures may be treated in traction and with a cast brace. In very fragile patients who must be mobilized,

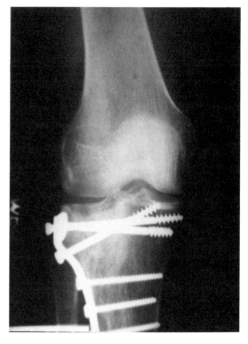

Figure 30.3. Postoperative x-ray of a comminuted fracture of the lateral tibial plateau in a 68-year-old man. Rigid fixation with a buttress plate and multiple screws was possible, so that early motion could be started. The fracture healed well.

primary casting although it will not allow anatomic repositioning of the fracture will permit the patient to get out of bed early. In demented, uncooperative patients, primary amputation at the site of a distal femoral or proximal tibial fracture may be the only treatment possible.

Fractures about the ankle may be particularly difficult to treat in the elderly. The ideal treatment is to restore the ankle joint surfaces to anatomic position. A few displaced fractures can be reduced, closed, and held with a cast. This allows the patient to get out of bed, but does not allow him or her to ambulate immediately (17). Most fractures, however, are unstable and require internal fixation. Conventional techniques may fail when applied to the elderly. The porotic bone may not hold standard plates and screws, and fixation is then lost. Any significant displacement of an ankle fracture places the overlying skin at great risk and may result in a catastrophic skin slough. These patients can be managed with an external fixator. Pins are placed in the distal tibia, the calcaneus, and the metatarsals;

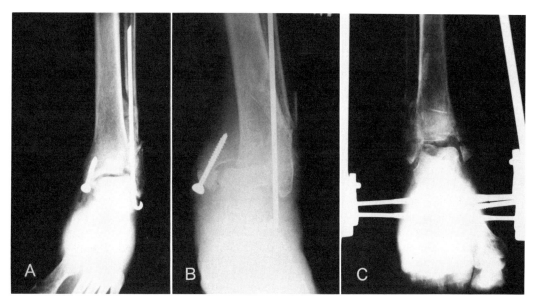

Figure 30.4. An 81-year-old woman sustained a trimalleolar fracture-dislocation of her ankle. An attempt was made to fixate it with standard techniques. **A,** Operating room x-ray immediately after fixation with a screw and intramedullary rod. **B,** X-ray made 10 days later, showing complete disruption of the repair and redislocation of the ankle. **C,** X-ray showing application of the external fixator. The porotic bone would not hold any fixation device so the fixator was applied. The dislocation has been reduced. After 4 months, the fixator was removed and the patient allowed to bear weight in an orthosis.

the fracture is reduced and the frame constructed. This arrangement is less than ideal as it often does not accomplish anatomic reduction and leaves the patient with a cumbersome, fearsome appearing frame. However, this technique may allow union with a fairly good ankle when conventional fixation methods cannot be used. This will also prevent potentially catastrophic skin breakdown. The frame should stay on until some radiologic evidence of union is seen. This may take up to 3 months. (Fig. 30.4)

Multiple trauma may occur in elderly patients from automobile accidents or severe falls. The principles of managing fractures in the elderly polytrauma patient are essentially the same as for a younger patient. Elderly patients usually tolerate traction poorly so there is even greater urgency in mobilization. Early, sometimes primary, sleketal fixation may be even more important in an elderly patient than in a younger one. Multiple trauma in the elderly is more fully discussed in Chapter 31.

Malignant Lesions

Primary or metastatic malignancies may oc-

cur in any bone in the body. The most common skeletal malignancies are metastatic carcinomas of the breast, prostate, and lung and are usually seen in the spine, femur, and pelvis. Multiple myeloma is the most common primary malignancy of bone seen in the elderly. If the patient has a known primary carcinoma that has a known propensity for skeletal metastases, the diagnosis of the cause of a skeletal complaint may be apparent. Occasionally, the appearance of a skeletal metastasis is the first indication that the underlying malignant disease exists. Metastatic lesions usually present with progressive pain, local tenderness, and symptoms suggestive of chronic disease, i.e., weight loss, weakness, anorexia. The patient may have ignored the symptoms until a pathologic fracture or paraplegia occurs. Physical examination of the site usually discloses local tenderness, and sometimes induration or peripheral edema will be present. The radiologic appearance of skeletal malignancy may vary from no obvious x-ray changes at all to a large, irregular, lytic lesion with an obvious fracture through it.

Metastatic disease in the skeleton is treated to

relieve pain and to restore function. Restoration of stability to the affected part is necessary to mobilize the patient. In short, the goals of treating pathologic fractures are no different from the goals of treating non-pathologic fractures in the aged. The common lesions that metastasize to the skeleton are relatively resistant to local radiation or chemotherapy. Pathologic fractures, once they occur, should be treated aggressively. Although these fractures may occur from minimal trauma and be minimally displaced, they are often extremely painful and may prevent the patient from getting out of bed. Prompt surgical stabilization with appropriate fixation devices, augmented with methylmethacrylate cement if necessary, will allow immediate stability and ambulation. A large number of these patients will have far advanced disease, and their survival may be measured in months, not years. Ultimate union of the fracture, which may be compromised by the presence of the malignant tumor and by the surgeon's use of cement, is not necessarily the goal; immediate stability is. Unless a patient is in an obviously terminal state, a pathologic fracture of a long bone should be stabilized.

A malignant lesion that is at risk for fracture should be identified and stabilized prophylactically. Lesions that involve over one-third of the diameter of the bone or that involve the calcar femorale, lesser trochanter, or femoral neck fall into this category (18). However, it is not always obvious that a lesion is at risk for fracture, and multiple x-rays, CT scans, and radionuclide imaging may all be necessary to delineate the extent of the lesion accurately. Prior to attempting surgical stabilization, complete studies of the entire involved bone are necessary in order to identify any distal lesions that might interfere with proper seating of the fixation device. Surgical stabilization might not be possible in a bone that is riddled with osteolytic lesions. In addition, careful clinical examination must be made to rule out metastases in other bones, such as the spine, so that further fractures do not occur in the course of the surgical procedure.

For lesions in the proximal femur that either have fractured or are at risk for fracture, the author's preference is the Zickel or Brooker-Wills Nail, depending on whether the lesion is near the lesser or greater trochanter. At the time of the operation, the lesion may or may not be exposed, but tissue samples for histologic study can usually be obtained to confirm the tissue diagnosis. If there is an obvious primary lesion, or the diagnosis of metastatic disease has already been confirmed, then extending the surgical procedure just for the purpose of obtaining tissue may not be necessary. However, tissue samples are mandatory when a primary lesion is not obvious. Lesions involving the femoral neck are best managed by primary hemiarthroplasty. If the implant cannot be firmly fixated into the bone, then methacrylate cement is added. (Fig. 30.5)

Postoperatively, the patient is mobilized as rapidly as possible. Adjuvant chemotherapy can be started as soon as the patient has recovered from the procedure; radiation therapy can be effectively administered to the affected bone in the presence of metal. A great advantage of closed over open nailing is that it avoids a wound directly over the radiation field so that treatment can be started early. If fixation is firm, then the patient can resume protected weight bearing.

Malignant lesions of the vertebrae are more difficult to treat, and the approach is more controversial. Compression fractures of the spine are common sequelae to malignant disease. In general, if there is no neurologic involvement and the posterior elements are not involved, then nonoperative treatment may be adequate. Patients with impending or complete paraplegia may require surgical decompression and stabilization. Newer surgical techniques using Harrington Rods or segmental interlaminar wiring offer some advantages when there is interest in stabilizing the spine posteriorly. However, the usual spinal cord encroachment is from an anteriorly located lesion in the vertebral body, and these lesions can only be decompressed by an anterior exposure. This is a major surgical procedure and should be reserved for those patients with neurologic involvement whose lesions cannot be expected to respond to radiation or to chemotherapy (19).

Malignancies involving the humerus often mandate surgical fixation; a painful humerus cannot be stabilized adequately by non-operative means. Metastatic malignancies to the tibia or forearm are quite rare, but the principles of treatment are the same: stabilization to allow mobilization with minimal pain. The rare malignancy involving a digit, if sufficiently painful, is usually

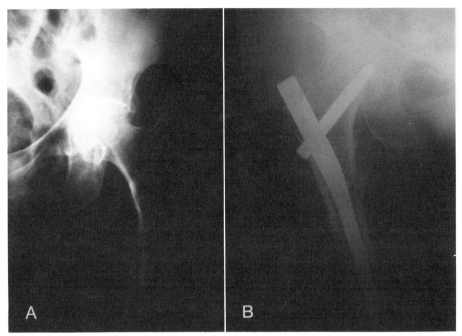

Figure 30.5. Metastatic carcinoma of the breast to the proximal femur in a 79-year-old woman. **A,** Preoperative x-ray: The lytic area is visible just distal to the lesser trochanter. **B,** Postoperative x-ray: The lesion was stabilized with a Zickel Nail. Fixation was sufficiently firm so that cement augmentation was not necessary. The patient was ambulated and given radiation therapy.

best managed by primary amputation.

Primary malignancy in the elderly skeleton is usually from multiple myeloma. Although this is a radiosensitive lesion, impending or obvious pathologic fractures should usually be treated surgically, using the same principles as used for metastatic disease. Primary malignant tumors arising from skeletal elements are extremely rare in the eldery, except for those that arise in previously irradiated or pagetoid bone. Amputation is the usual treatment.

Peripheral Vascular Disease and Amputation

Vascular insufficiency, a common condition in the elderly, often affects the lower extremities. Surgical attempts at revascularization may be unsuccessful, and in the elderly patient with vascular insufficiency and ulceration of a foot, healing of an ischemic ulcer may not occur. Deep infection commonly is associated with ischemic ulcers of the foot. If the infection involves bone, the ulcer will not heal no matter how effectively the extremity can be revascularized until the in-

fected bone is surgically removed. The dysvascular patient with gangrene of the foot should be approached aggressively. Once a determination of underlying bone involvement is made, then amputation must be considered. Long term antibiotic therapy will not cure this kind of osteomyelitis. Some patients are willing to live with a chronic, draining ulcer and will refuse amputation, but the majority can and should be rehabilitated with amputation and prosthetic fitting.

Foot amputations should be considered when a toe only is involved. Amputation or disarticulation of the toe may be adequate in this situation. If the infection involves one metatarsal, a resection of that ray may heal, but that is a rare situation. The infection usually involves adjacent bones. In those cases, no operation short of foot amputation will heal. The transmetatarsal amputation has limited value in cases of peripheral gangrene and will only succeed when the entire plantar surface up to the toe creases is intact and the metatarsals can be resected through their middle thirds. It is unlikely that a transmetatarsal or any forefoot amputation will succeed in a vascularly impaired foot. Successful Symes amputations have been reported when done in carefully selected cases. The infection must be limited to the foot, and there must be good blood supply to the leg. All infection must be controlled before the definitive procedure is carried out. Wagner has advocated a two-stage procedure, where the primary procedure is an open amputation and definitive closure is done secondarily (20).

Below-the-knee amputation is the best procedure for most vascularly impaired elderly patients who require lower extremity amputation. The patient with this amputation can be rehabilitated very well with the use of a modern prosthesis that will allow early ambulation on a pain-free limb. An above-knee amputation is rarely necessary and should only be considered after obvious failure to heal of a below-knee amputation, when the disease process extends into the calf, or in a non-ambulatory patient. The dysvascular elderly patient almost never walks again with an above-knee prosthesis, whereas he or she has an excellent chance of walking with a below-knee prosthesis. Many different laboratory tests have been suggested as predictors of the survival and healing of a below-knee amputation stump, but it is the surgical and postoperative technique more than anything else that will determine the success of the amputation. A detailed description of the technique is beyond the scope of this book, but a few principles of amputation bear repeating. If there is obvious bleeding at the amputation site, it should heal. Infection in the amputation stump usually means failure, so there should be no residual infection in the extremity. This may necessitate a two-stage procedure where the first procedure is a rapid, open amputation through the distal leg and the second procedure is a formal below-knee amputation of correct shape and length. Improper postoperative care will cause failure. A plaster cast, extending up to the knee, will hold the knee in full extension and facilitate wound healing. Anything less, such as a posterior plaster splint, is inadequate. Careful postoperative wrapping of the stump, first by the physical therapist and then by the patient, will contour the stump to allow prosthetic fitting. The patient should be mobilized on crutches rapidly. The wound must be allowed to heal fully; skin sutures or staples can

be left in for weeks. Premature removal of skin sutures will virtually guarantee failure (21). The prosthetist must be involved early in the patient's care; the elderly patient must be made to realize that amputation is not the "end of the world" and that he or she may have a satisfactory or even an excellent gait pattern and lifestyle afterwards.

CONCLUSIONS

Elderly patients are becoming the major patient population group being seen by the general orthopaedic surgeon. As with other surgical disciplines, chronologic age alone is not a contraindication or a deterrent to many orthopaedic surgical procedures. Degenerative disease of the weight bearing joints can be addressed surgically in patients well into their advanced years. Advances in medical care for the elderly have enabled large numbers of these patients to come to the point where elective, major, reconstructive orthopaedic procedures may be expected to improve quality of life with a minimum of risk. Fractures in the elderly remain a major challenge; the treatment of the fracture is often dictated by the patient's age and general condition. A major fracture in an elderly patient, however, unless it is accompanied by a significant medical illness need not mean the end of a person's life. The injury might, however, mean a change in lifestyle. Elderly patients with skeletal malignancies can be kept comfortable and functional by surgical stabilization of impending or actual pathologic fractures.

Aggressive surgical treatment of many common orthopaedic conditions in the aged is actually the more conservative approach. The goals of early mobilization and rapid return to function are often best served by operative treatment. Elderly people tolerate orthopaedic as well as other operations surprisingly well.

Surgical advances are being made in fracture fixation and in arthroplasty techniques. It must be anticipated that new concepts in joint replacement and implant fixation will allow an increasing number of elderly patients to benefit from arthroplasty. New techniques of fracture fixation can be used to mobilize more rapidly these elderly patients and to improve function. New knowledge about the causes and treatment of osteoporosis may radically alter the scope of geriatric orthopaedics if this one overwhelming cause for skeletal complications can be addressed.

The major concern of orthopaedic surgery in the elderly is to return the patient as nearly as possible to the same functional state that he or she had prior to the orthopaedic procedure. Some elderly patients sustain injuries and never recover. Others live for many years after a major fracture or reconstructive procedure. Some require orthopaedic care as part of the care of an incurable disease. The orthopaedic surgeon must work closely with the family and social service agencies. Improvement in or maintenance of a worthwhile lifestyle and not increasing longevity is the major goal of the orthopaedic surgeon in the care of the elderly patient.

REFERENCES

1. Adkins RB Jr, Scott HW Jr: Surgical procedures in patients aged 90 years and older. *South Med J* 77:1357–1364, 1984.
2. Barker SB, Harvey AH: Fall injuries in the elderly. *Clin Geriatr Med* 1:501–512, 1985.
3. Kenzora JE, McCarthy RE, Lowell JD, Sledge CB: Hip fracture mortality. Relation to age, treatment, preoperative illness, time of surgery, and complications. *Clin Orthop Rel Res* 186:45–56, 1984.
4. Lyon LJ, Nevins MA: Nontreatment of hip fractures in senile patients. *JAMA* 238:1175–1176, 1977.
5. Devas M: Orthopaedics. In Steinberg FU (ed): *Cowdry's The Care Of The Geriatric Patient,* ed 5. St Louis, CV Mosby, 1976, pp 258–274.
6. Singh M, Nagrath AR, Maini PS: Changes in trabecular patterns in the upper end of the femur as an index of osteoporosis. *J Bone Joint Surg* 52-A: 457–467, 1970.
7. Burstein AH. Reilly DT, Martens M: Aging of bone tissue: mechanical properties. *J Bone Joint Surg* 58-A: 82–86, 1976.
8. Specht EE: Hip fractures, skeletal fragility, osteoporosis, and hormonal deprivation in elderly women. *West J Med* 133:297–303, 1980.
9. Ouslander JG, Beck JC: Paget's disease of bone. *J Am Geriatr Soc* 30:410–414, 1982.
10. Ziminski CM: Treating Joint inflammation in the elderly: an update. *Geriatrics* 40: 73–88, 1985.
11. Calandruccio RA: Arthroplasty of the hip. In Crenshaw AH (ed): *Campbell's Operative Orthopaedics,* ed 7. St Louis, CV Mosby, 1986, pp 1444–1456.
12 Cooney WP: External fixation of distal radial fractures.

Clin Orthop Rel Res 180:44–51, 1983.
13. DeLee JC: Fractures and dislocations of the hip. In Rockwood CA Jr, Green DP (eds): *Fractures in Adults,* ed 2. Philadelphia, JB Lippincott, 1984, pp 1234–1240.
14. Dimon, JH III, Hughston, JC: Unstable intertrochanteric fractures of the hip. *J Bone Joint Surg* 49-A:440–451, 1967.
15. White GH, Healy WL, Brumback RT, Burgess AL, Brooker AF Jr: The treatment of fractures of the femoral shaft with the Brooker-Wills distal interlocking intramedullary nail. *J Bone Joint Surg* 68(A):868–876, 1986.
16. Day, L: Pulmonary embolism and deep vein thrombosis in patients with hip fractures. In Meyers, MH (ed): *Fractures of the Hip.* Chicago, Year Book, 1985, pp 320–342.
17. Beauchamp CG, Clay NR, Thexton PW: Displaced ankle fractures in patients over 50 years of age. *J Bone Joint Surg* 65-B:329–332, 1983.
18. Behr JT, Dobozi WR, Badrinath K: The treatment of pathologic and impending pathologic fractures of the proximal femur in the elderly. *Clin Orthop Rel Res* 198:173–178, 1985.
19. Errico TJ, Kostiuk JP: Diagnosis and treatment of metastatic disease of the spinal column: a review. *Contemp Orthop* 13:15–26, 1986.
20. Wagner, FW: Amputations of the foot and ankle: current status. *Clin Orthop Rel Res* 122:62–68, 1977.
21. Burgess EM, Romano RL, Zette JH, Schrock RD: Amputations of the leg for peripheral vascular insufficiency. *J Bone Joint Surg* 53-A:874–884, 1971.

Chapter 31

Trauma in the Aged

Gerald B. Demarest, M.D., F.A.C.S., Kenneth L. Mattox, M.D., F.A.C.S.

Currently, trauma is the fifth leading cause of death in the elderly. Although this group represents 11% of the population, it accounts for 25% of trauma fatalities or 24,000 deaths per year (1). Until recently, knowledge regarding trauma care of this group has been sparse. The advent of geriatric care, the rapid growth of this group, and their disproportionate demands on health care and other social services have made it increasingly important to gain an understanding of the age-related factors involved in injury. On the average, elderly accident victims remain in the hospital twice as long as younger patients. Most of these events are the result of a complex interaction between changes of aging and hazards of the environment, particularly in the home, on the streets, and in hospitals or institutions (2).

A significant accidental injury in a frail, elderly patient often leads to functional dependency, a decline in multiple organ systems, and, ultimately, institutionalization or death. For these reasons, prevention of accidents in elderly patients and optimal care of those who suffer accidental injury are important responsibilities of the physician (2).

Persons aged 65 or older are less likely than persons in other age groups to be injured at all, but more likely to have a fatal outcome from those injuries that do occur (3, 4). For all injuries combined, population death rates are the highest in this group at 166 deaths per 100,000 population for people aged 75–84 years, compared with 64 deaths per 100,000 for people aged 15–24 years. This is a reflection of this population's overall reduced intrinsic reserve and high risk for complications (1).

Reported causes of injury and death in the elderly group have remained fixed over the last two decades and are listed on Table 31.1. Falls are the leading cause of injury and death, ac-

counting for 40% of fatalities in this group (5). Motor vehicle accidents cause 22% of elderly fatalities, and one-third of these are accounted for by injuries to elderly pedestrians. House fires or ignition of clothing causes the majority of burn deaths seen in the elderly. Firearms, suffocation, and poisoning make up the majority of the remaining fatalities in descending order (1).

ETIOLOGY

Falls

Falls represent the second leading cause of unintentional injury deaths in the United States and are exceeded only by motor vehicle related deaths. As a result of falls in and around the home, ten thousand individuals die annually and seven million persons are injured (6). In the elderly, falls are the largest cause of injury mortality and account for approximately 40% of injury deaths. Most deaths from falls occur in persons aged 65 or greater (7). Both the incidence and severity of complications as a result

Table 31.1 Accidental Fatalities of Persons Aged 65 Years or Older by Etiology[a]

Cause	Number	Percentage
Falls	9600	40%
Motor vehicle accidents	6000	25%
Driver/passenger	4000	
Pedestrian	2000	
Fire, burns	1700	6%
Firearms	1200	
Suffocation, ingested objects	1200	
Suffocation, mechanical	600	
Poisoning (solid, liquid)	400	
Poisoning (gas)	300	
Other	3000	
Total	24,000	

[a]From *Accident Facts*. Chicago, National Safety Council, 1981.

450

of falls rise steadily with age, though a decline in mortality rates for falls has been ongoing since 1978 (1). The majority of elderly persons who fall do not die. As a result of the falls, however, a large number of emergency room visits and subsequent hospital admissions occur.

In the elderly, falls most commonly are a result of the accumulated effects of age and environmental hazards. Studies evaluating falls in the home reveal three times as many women as men are involved in falls that occur in the home (7). Older people are stiffer and less coordinated and have gaits that are unstable. Impairments in vision, hearing, and memory place these people at high risk even in the home environment, with its inherent hazards that can cause falls (8).

Acute changes in cardiac status account for as many as 25% of falls in the elderly. A relative decrease in cerebral blood flow is an important cause of falls. Orthostatic hypotension as a result of hypovolemic venous pooling, loss of muscle mass in lower extremities, and autonomic dysfunction are likely to induce this condition and thereby increase the risk of fall. Syncope, the sudden unexpected loss of consciousness, is an important cause of serious falls. The causes of syncope include decreased cerebral blood flow from a variety of conditions, as well as from metabolic derangements including hypoglycemia, hypoxia, and acid base disturbances. "Drop attacks" are defined as sudden, unexpected falls without associated loss of consciousness or dizziness. This condition usually presents as a sudden flaccid weakness in the lower extremities, and its cause is usually attributed to transient vertebral-basilar artery insufficiency. This etiologic possibility should be considered if an elderly patient falls when reaching for an object or when hyperextending the head. Falls from dizziness or vertigo are extremely common. These symptoms are usually a reflection of one of the above-mentioned underlying etiologies, as well as a result of vestibular dysfunction or from the use of various drugs.

Drugs, including alcohol, are a cause or contributing factor in many falls. Especially important are sedatives, antihypertensives, diuretics, and hypoglycemic agents. Anemia, occult blood loss, transient ischemic attacks (TIA), hypothyroidism, unstable joints, severe osteoporosis with spontaneous fracture, epilepsy, and electrolyte imbalance are other important causes of falls in the elderly.

Motor Vehicle Accidents

Each year some 4,000 individuals aged 65 years or older are killed as drivers or passengers in motor vehicles. An additional 2,000 aged persons are killed as pedestrians (9).

The elderly do not have higher crash rates than other age groups, but do have a substantially higher crash experience per miles traveled when compared to middle-aged drivers if reported highway crashes per 100 drivers are examined (10, 11). Although the young driver is more likely to be involved in a serious single-vehicle crash of danger to him- or herself and any other passengers, the elderly driver more often has a two-vehicle collision (12, 13). Furthermore, the very elderly are as likely to be involved in fatal crashes as young drivers, and this incidence substantially exceeds the fatality experience of middle-aged drivers (9). Once injured, the elderly driver is obviously less likely to survive the injury.

There can be little doubt that the elderly pedestrian is ill equipped to deal with the hazards of the streets and highways (3). Studies show that pedestrian fatalities are comprised of three groups: preschool and elementary school-aged children, middle-aged alcoholics, and the elderly (14, 15).

The effect of the aging process appears to have a major influence on the likelihood of occurrence, the risk of injury, and the cause of death in the elderly who are involved in motor vehicle accidents. Reduced ability to see and hear are two examples of factors in the aged that increase those risks. Several parameters of visual ability decrease markedly with age, including daylight acuity, glare resistance, and night vision (3). Occurrence of medical conditions that alter attention and consciousness are of major importance (3), as well as minor alterations of judgement because of the onset of senile changes in the brain. Finally, there is often decreased ability to implement appropriate actions once decided upon by the elderly because of agility-impairing medical conditions, including severe arthritis, emphysema, heart disease, decrease in muscle mass, and other less common physical impairments (3).

Burns

Exposure to fire or burns from contact with hot substances are the third leading cause of trauma deaths in the elderly, accounting for some 1700 deaths annually (9). One-third of these elderly individuals are fatally injured secondary to alcohol ingestion and smoking in bed or by being caught in a building fire with exposure to heat and to the toxic products of combustion. The majority of the remainder who sustain injury and death are burned by the ignition of clothing or by prolonged contact with hot substances (3). Factors associated with degenerative disease and the physical impairments that accompany aging appear to contribute substantially to the over-representation of the elderly (16). The elderly are more likely to get into trouble initially because of falls against hot surfaces, inability to hold things without spilling them, and because of a lesser sensitivity of nerve endings to substances that may be too hot. Because of these physical infirmities and limitations, the elderly person who comes into contact with a hot surface or who is exposed to fire often is not able to remove him- or herself until extensive damage has occurred. Once burned, pre-existing cardiovascular, respiratory, and renal disease often make it impossible for the elderly to overcome a serious but otherwise possibly survivable injury (3). (See also Chapter 2)

UNIQUE ANATOMIC CHARACTERISTICS OF THE ELDERLY TRAUMATIZED PATIENT

Cardiovascular Disease

Cardiovascular diseases in the elderly are complex, arising from a combination of changes associated with age-related disorders, acquired cardiovascular disease, and pathologic conditions unique to old age. Prolonged hemodynamic stresses and the biologic changes of aging over a lifetime produce anatomic, histologic, biochemical, and electrophysiologic changes that impair cardiovascular function and diminish cardiac reserve (17).

The aged heart manifests a decrease in strength of contraction, cardiac output, speed and force of contraction, stroke volume, ventricular ejec-tion fraction, left ventricle diastolic compliance and filling, and increased impedance to left ventricular ejection (17).

Acquired cardiovascular diseases in the aged include ischemic heart disease usually secondary to atherosclerosis, orthostatic hypotension, cardiac dysrhythmias, TIAs, and congestive heart failure. The decreased inotropic response of the aged heart to catecholamines prolongs contraction, as well as chronotropic and vasodilation capacity. As a result, sudden major stress can precipitate cardiac dysrhythmias, heart failure, and sudden death (17).

Osteoporosis

Osteoporosis affects an estimated fifteen million persons, one-third of whom have severe demineralization with vertebral fractures. Postmenopausal osteoporosis in women and senile osteoporosis in men are insidious in onset and generally follow a protracted course (18). Most investigators now believe that increased bone resorption is the primary mechanism of osteoporosis and that a gradual and progressive increase in bone resorption over prolonged periods of time leads to calcium loss and the development of osteoporosis. Risk factors, in addition to bone changes due to the aging process, include sex hormone deficiencies related either to aging or to pathology, other hormonal imbalances, low calcium intake for prolonged periods of time, vitamin deficiencies, metabolic anomalies involving vitamin D, protein deficiency in the diet, and physical immobilization (18).

The morbidity associated with osteoporosis is frequently disabling and sometimes devastating. In the United States, 80% of patients who sustain hip fractures have pre-existing osteoporosis. This fact accounts for many of the 160,000 of these injuries that occur each year. Annually, 2% of women and 1% of men aged 85 or older sustain femoral fractures (19). Vertebral compression or crush fractures of the spine are a common disabling feature of advanced osteoporosis caused by collapse of demineralized vertebral bodies. These can occur in association with common activities, such as bending and lifting, or may be a consequence of the long term effect of carrying the weight of the body upright. The overall effect of progressive osteoporosis in the elderly is unknown, but probably is a significant factor in the occurrence and severity of fractures secondary to trauma. It must certainly add to the morbidity and mortality associated with injuries (18).

Pulmonary Disorders

In old age, the lung has lost much of its elasticity due to losses of elastin. With this, a significant degree of alveolar dilatation occurs, specifically in the lung periphery, resulting in the so-called senile emphysema (20). Additionally, changes in the composition of collagen occur, with an increased number of cross links between subunits of collagen resulting in increased rigidity of structural tissue in the lung. This effect leads to an alteration in lung compliance and gas exchange.

Aging has been related to a decrease in vital capacity (VC) and forced expiratory volume in 1 second (FEV_1), as well as a progressive reduction in arterial oxygen tension (PaO_2). Residual volume (RV), functional residual capacity (FRC), and closing volume (CV) all increase with age. The total lung capacity (TLC) and arterial CO_2 tension ($PaCO_2$) remain constant throughout life (20).

With increasing age, a number of respiratory-dependent systems undergo alteration consistent with the aging process. Disordered patterns of breathing, including primary alveolar hypoventilation, sleep apnea syndromes, and Cheyne-Stokes breathing, may be a result of a combination of endocrine, neurologic, and circulatory disturbances with aging that predisposes to these conditions (20).

With increased age, reduced levels of consciousness, dysphagia, and dysfunction of the lower esophageal sphincter occur. With this, a tendency to gastro-esophageal reflux occurs with increased frequency, predisposing elderly patients to aspiration and its consequences. Dyspnea is a subjective phenomenon and is related to an awareness of the need for increased respiratory effort. In aging, the progressive worsening of chronic heart disease, cardiomyopathies, and hypertensive states are all associated with left ventricular dysfunction, which can also lead to dyspnea (20).

The incidence of pneumonia in elderly patients is increased, and when it develops, they tend to have more serious complications, debilitation, and associated illness than younger patients with pneumonia. The actual frequency of pneumococcal pneumonia in the elderly is reported to be five to six times higher than in younger patients (21). The occurrence of other gram positive and gram negative pneumonias in the elderly appears to be increased in hospitalized patients. *Klebsiella, Pseudomonas, Haemophilus,* and *Escherichia coli* are found more frequently in the elderly in nosocomial infection (21). Lung diseases, other systemic illness, use of antibiotics, and debilitation with increased age have all been implicated as factors responsible for the increased incidence of infection by these organisms.

UNIQUE PHYSIOLOGIC CHARACTERISTICS OF THE TRAUMATIZED ELDERLY PATIENT

Nutrition/Metabolism

One of the most significant factors influencing the successful response to trauma in spite of age is nutrition. An elderly person's ability to obtain adequate nutrition may be impaired due to losses of income, mobility, relatives, friends, or even self-esteem (22). Protein-caloric malnutrition is recognized more frequently among all hospitalized patients. Increased numbers of inpatient referrals for nutritional support services are for persons over age 60 (23).

Nutritional assessment tests, including percent ideal body weight, somatic protein mass, creatinine/height index (CHI), visceral proteins, absolute lymphocyte count, and measurements of cellular mediated immunity, have been described for a younger population. Many measurements commonly performed in nutritional assessment may be unreliable in the elderly due to the various effects of the aging process. In developing nutritional status norms for the elderly, careful subject selection will be necessary in order to exclude the presence of any acute or chronic disease state. Also, consideration must be given to the specific physiologic effects of the aging process (24). The various effects of disease on blood proteins, including hepatic dysfunction, renal disease, and congestive heart failure, must be considered in nutritional assessment of the elderly. In addition, the acute stress of trauma, hypoxia, burns, and various carcinomas each can alter albumin synthesis. Finally, large numbers of immunologic abnormalities described in association with malnutrition have been documented in the elderly and have also been ascribed to the effects of aging (25).

The caloric needs of men and women decline with age as related to decreased metabolic rate, decreased activity levels, and, in some degree, reduction in the total mass of metabolically active cells (22). Aged persons require fewer total calories but not less protein, vitamins, or minerals. Stressful environments and increased physical demands in trauma, infection, chronic disease, and the altered gastrointestinal function of aging may impair dietary nitrogen utilization. Clinical protein deficiencies can be correlated with fatigue, muscle weakness, tissue wasting, poor wound healing, and lack of energy (22). The current recommended daily allowance for protein is 0.8 g/kg of body weight. Studies have shown that this may not be an entirely accurate figure and that, in conditions of stress, higher levels of protein intake may be necessary (26). It seems probable that the elderly may require even more protein than younger patients to maintain nitrogen balance when their caloric intake is reduced. This nitrogen need looms even larger when one considers that most illnesses common to the elderly can cause transient losses of body protein that will need to be replaced (27).

Infectious Diseases in the Elderly and the Senescence of the Immune System

The incidence of and mortality rates from most types of bacterial infections are higher in the elderly. The explanation for this is two-fold: associated predisposing illnesses and immunologic senescence. Bacterial pathogens, such as gram negative bacilli, are more likely to occur in older patients than younger patients. In addition, the diagnosis of bacterial infection in the elderly patient may be more difficult than in the younger patient. Finally, the underlying pathogenesis of a bacterial infection may differ in the elderly population compared to a younger group (28).

The treatment of bacterial infection in the elderly must include and allow for the consideration of several factors. These include (1) the

particular toxicity of some antibiotics in the elderly, (2) the fact that dosage based on creatinine clearance changes with age, (3) the existence of a larger variety of potential bacterial pathogens for most disease, making empiric therapy more difficult, and (4) the more fulminant course of many bacterial infections in the elderly patient (28).

The immune system changes with age. The increased susceptibility of elderly patients to infections, neoplastic disease, and perhaps to vascular injuries may be a consequence of immune senescence (29). With aging, cell mediated and humoral immune response to foreign antigens is decreased, whereas the response to autologous antigens is increased. It has been suggested that autoantibodies and circulating immunocomplexes, which can damage tissues and organs, contribute to many of the pathologic changes that occur with age (29). In the last decade, many of the changes in the immune system that accompany aging have been defined and related to the involution of the thymus gland. Whether immune senescence is a primary or secondary contributor to the pathology of aging, it is likely that increased knowledge of immune senescence and the increasing ability to correct immune defects that occur in the elderly will offer considerable promise for future control of diseases of aging (29).

DIAGNOSIS AND TREATMENT

History and Physical Examination

As with all trauma patients, the principles of evaluation and treatment of the geriatric trauma victim include an initial evaluation of patient status regarding maintenance of the airway, breathing, and circulation. This is followed by management of acute, life-threatening conditions and then by performing an in-depth history and physical examination. In the field or upon arrival in the emergency room, initial management principles should first focus on patency of the airway, adequacy and quality of breathing, and a rapid evaluation of intravascular volume status. Close, continuous monitoring of vital signs should be high on the list of priorities because of the elderly person's relative intolerance to shock and its effect. The establishment of large bore intravenous catheters as a means of obtaining blood for diagnostic laboratory evaluation and type and cross-matching is important early on in the management of traumatic illness. This manuever also allows access to a port for fluid resuscitation and transfusion access, as well as serving as a means of rapid medication administration.

Along with the physical evaluation of the patient, an in-depth history should encompass pertinent information regarding the particulars of the injuring event, significant past medical history, medications, previous hospitalizations and operations, allergies, immunization status, and the time of the patient's last meal.

The neurologic evaluation in the form of level of consciousness and assessment according to the Glasgow Coma Scale should be determined and recorded. This evaluation should be repeated at frequent intervals as a means of documentation in the evolution of a changing neurologic injury.

The importance of maintaining a high index of suspicion for the risk of a cervical spine injury in any patient who sustains head or maxillofacial trauma should be emphasized. Radiographic studies routinely performed in the emergency room remain the same for the elderly patient as for all patients sustaining trauma and include a cross-table lateral cervical spine film that will allow the visualization of all seven cervical and the first thoracic vertebrae. This film should be taken in all patients who sustain injury to the head or neck. Hyperextension injuries are significantly common in the elderly patient who falls forward and sustains injury to the forehead or face. Such hyperextension can "pinch" the cervical cord between the ligamentum flavum and posterior osteophytes that are especially common in the elderly population (30). The patient who is comatose, or who is alert but has positive cervical spine findings, must be immobilized with a rigid collar or with sand bags until a cross-table lateral radiograph can be interpreted as demonstrating no injury.

Patients who manifest airway compromise and who are at risk for potential cervical spine injury should undergo airway control by intubation. This is accomplished through blind nasotracheal or oral intubation with an assistant holding axial traction and limiting head extension or flexion. When this is not possible, cervical crycothyroidotomy should be done if airway obstruction is imminent.

Head Injuries

Although elderly patients have a higher incidence of subdural and intraparenchymal hematomas from head trauma, they sustain relatively fewer severe cerebral contusions than do the younger patients (31). Subdural hematomas are nearly three times as frequent in the elderly as they are in younger groups, but the development of epidural hematomas is extremely rare (31). It is important to note that a subdural hematoma may present in an elderly patient as the cause of a gradual, neurologic decline. In fact, the cause of a fall for which a physician is examining the patient may be the result of an earlier fall in the remote past (31).

Except for specific indications, the routine use of head computed tomography (CT) scans has supplanted routine skull x-rays for patients with head injury. This modality provides rapid, accurate, sequential cuts and gives detailed information on structural damage of the brain and supporting elements. Indications for CT scan generally include those individuals who present with loss of consciousness for periods of time greater than 5 minutes, patients who present with changes in level of consciousness, or those who have lateralizing neurologic findings.

Chest Trauma

For the elderly patient who sustains significant blunt chest trauma, management principles remain the same as for patients of any age. Normal workup of the elderly patient sustaining blunt chest trauma includes a routine AP chest x-ray. Because of the less elastic chest wall of the older person, blunt trauma is more likely to fracture several ribs or the sternum. These elderly patients will frequently present with soft tissue injury manifested by ecchymosis or hematoma formation. Crepitation or grating at the fracture site is a common finding. Too frequently, trauma from a fall or from an apparently insignificant blow will result in chest wall pain and will be associated with an occult hemo- or pneumothorax. The history of a rapid deceleration during the accident should alert one to the risk of a thoracic aortic injury and to the consideration of diagnostic aortography, even without the findings of a widening of the mediastinum on the AP chest film or the other constellation of x-ray findings usually described in this clinical syndrome.

With superimposed medical disease and underlying intolerance to respiratory compromise in many elderly patients, early arterial blood gas evaluation may give early indication of respiratory compromise in the high risk elderly patient. Low dose supplemental oxygen by nasal cannula or by face mask is frequently of benefit for the elderly patient with minimal respiratory compromise, but it may be contraindicated in the patient with chronic obstructive pulmonary disease (COPD) and decreased CO_2 ventilatory drive. Early endotracheal intubation should be considered for those patients manifesting respiratory distress demonstrated by more than 40 breaths per minute, PaO_2 levels less than 60 torr, and $PaCO_2$ levels above 50 torr.

Abdominal Trauma

The determination of significant intra-abdominal injury in the elderly patient following blunt or penetrating trauma frequently presents a diagnostic dilemma for the attending surgeon, especially in the decision whether or not to operate. The frailty of this population group and their intolerance to hypovolemic shock allow little margin for error in the determination of intra-abdominal injury. Therefore, a high index of suspicion should always be accompanied by an aggressive approach in order to reduce the high morbidity and mortality rates in this population.

With blunt trauma, the most likely organs to be injured include liver, spleen, bladder, and kidney. Operative exploration is mandated by the following: (1) signs and symptoms of intravascular volume depletion without other obvious sites of ongoing blood loss outside the peritoneal cavity or retroperitoneal space, (2) obvious peritoneal irritation manifested by involuntary guarding, and (3) fractures of the pelvis and/or lower rib cage in patients in whom intra-abdominal injury is strongly suspected (32). For those patients in whom less obvious signs and indications are present, diagnostic peritoneal lavage and abdominal CT scan have proven to be excellent adjunctive diagnostic measures for the determination of significant bleeding or organ injury. These studies, along with an intravenous pyelogram (IVP), a cystourethrogram, and on occasion an abdominal arteriogram, will be beneficial in elucidating the presence of abdominal injury in the difficult-to-evaluate but otherwise stable patient.

When evaluating patients with penetrating abdominal injuries, a similar approach should be followed. Those patients with obvious ongoing blood loss, evisceration, or positive findings suggestive of peritoneal irritation require abdominal exploration. Patients with less obvious signs and symptoms who have sustained a head injury and decreased level of consciousness, who have paralysis, or who are under the influence of alcohol or drugs are best managed in the following way. Wounds of the anterior abdomen, nipple to pubis between anterioraxillary lines, are explored locally. Patients with hemothorax or pneumothorax on AP chest x-ray or patients with penetration of the anterior abdominal wall fascia should undergo diagnostic peritoneal lavage. The precaution of stomach and bladder decompression by the placement of a nasogastric tube and Foley catheter, respectively, should be performed prior to placement of the lavage catheter in order to prevent injury to these structures. Five to 10 cc of nonclotting blood returned in the lavage catheter mandates operative exploration. If no blood is returned on aspiration, 1000 cc of Ringer's lactate solution is infused, and the returned fluid is examined. Currently there are controversies as to the absolute number of red cells in the returned lavage fluid that warrants exploration. Most centers utilizing this technique will explore patients with absolute red cell counts of 50,000 RBCs/mm³ or greater (33). Spun lavage fluid hematocrits of greater than 2%, absolute white cell counts of 500 WBC/mm³, evidence of bile, elevated amylase, bacteria, or food particles on laboratory evaluation also are all indications for operative exploration.

Previous abdominal operative procedures represent an absolute contraindication to peritoneal lavage. Under these circumstances, consideration should be given to the use of a double contrast abdominal CT scan for evaluation of the abdomen as an alternative diagnostic modality.

The retroperitoneal abdominal structures continue to present a difficult anatomic area to evaluate for the site of injury. The genitourinary and vascular structures as well as the duodenum and pancreas may be evaluated by various adjunctive diagnostic studies, including IVP, cystourethrogram, abdominal arteriography, ultrasonography, and abdominal CT scan. Each of these studies may play a significant role in elucidating injuries that may have occurred in this region.

Fractures

Osteoporosis that occurs with increasing age is a condition that significantly increases the risk of fracture in the elderly patient. This risk mandates a careful examination of the bony structures of the extremities in all elderly patients who have sustained trauma. A careful history will lead to a high index of suspicion regarding the likelihood of fractures of the hip, shoulder, upper arm, and wrists. Careful examination of these areas, including neurovascular structures, will frequently lead to an early diagnosis of the specific injury. The principle of early splinting and stabilization of the fracture for prevention of further injury should be adhered to and will lead to reduction in morbidity and a more favorable final result in the aged patient.

Colles' Fracture

The Colles' fracture is usually the result of a fall on the outstretched dorsiflexed hand. This fracture of the distal radius occurs in the metaphyseal area. It is accompanied by the classic fracture at the base of the ulnar styloid process approximately 60% of the time (34). The typical "dinner fork" deformity is usually obvious with swelling at the volar wrist and a dorsal depression deformity.

Evaluation of this fracture should include careful testing of the median nerve and the motor function of the finger flexors. Lateral and AP wrist films are mandatory and should visualize all carpal bones to rule out a more complex injury. Thought should always be given to the risk of a concomitant injury at the elbow because of the nature of the fall or forces involved that caused the wrist fracture. These fractures represent potentially complex injuries, and various degrees of malunion are common.

Fractures of the Humerus

Fractures of the humerus are the result of inadvertent falls with absorption of the force on the deltoid area. The resultant injury is commonly a fracture of the surgical neck of the humerus (Fig 31.1). A similar fracture can occur due to a transmitted force through the humeral shaft when the blow is absorbed by an outstretched hand. Presentation is usually characterized by pain and tenderness in the shoulder or upper humeral area, and a large ecchymosis may accompany the injury. Significant with these injuries is the frequent finding of a concomitant shoulder dislocation. These injuries should be confirmed by appropriate upper arm and shoulder x-rays.

Of major importance in the evaluation of the surgical neck of the humerus is the determination of whether the fracture is impacted or disimpacted. First, with impacted fractures, no fracture segment can be displaced more than 1.0

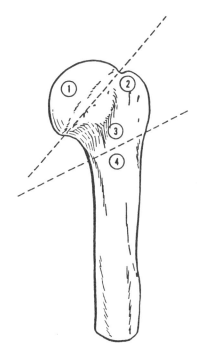

Figure 31.1. Humeral neck fractures occur between two or more segments: (**1**) head, (**2**) lesser tuberosity, (**3**) greater tuberosity, (**4**) shaft. (Reproduced with permission from Chipman C: Falls and their consequences. In Bosker G, Schwartz G (eds): *Geriatric Emergencies.* Englewood Cliffs, NJ, Brady Comm Co, 1984, p 189.)

cm or angulated more than 45°. Second, with impacted fractures, the arm can be moved gently hanging from the shoulder, the waist bent 20°–30°, without evidence of pain. Patients with disimpacted fractures will generally experience pain on such movement. Impacted fractures demonstrate no false motion of the humerus when the shoulder is rotated gently from a flexed elbow. Treatment of an impacted fracture is that of shoulder sling and progressive range of motion. In general, disimpacted fractures require hospitalization for surgical fixation.

In the elderly, early mobilization with movement of the affected joint is important for the prevention of long term joint stiffness and limitation in joint range of motion. Questions regarding the diagnosis of humeral fractures should be addressed by the orthopaedic consultant.

Fractures of the Hip

The most common hip fracture seen in the elderly are those of the proximal femur. In general, individuals with these injuries are unable to walk. Because of significant pain, patients prefer not to be moved and are usually unwilling to sit even in a partially upright position. Pain from these injuries is usually localized to the area of the greater trochanter or anterior pelvis. Occasionally, hip fractures can present as pain referred to the knee (35).

Isolated hip fractures do not usually present with hypovolemic shock, but determination of the patient's intravascular volume status should be made early with institution of an intravenous catheter for fluid administration. Early determination of intactness of neurovascular structures should be assessed and compared with those of the opposite extremity. Following initial management, appropriate x-ray evaluation should include the affected hip and pelvis and both femoral necks and trochanters.

Fractures of the hip occur in one of four areas: subcapital, transcervical, intertrochanteric, and subtrochanteric. (Fig 31.2) Intertrochanteric fractures are the most common followed by transcervical fractures (36). The majority of these require operative fixation, and early orthopaedic consultation is mandatory. (See Chapter 30)

SPECIAL OPERATIVE CONSIDERATIONS

Monitoring

Operative monitoring of body temperature has become routine. The elderly trauma patient is particularly susceptible to the deleterious effects of hypothermia, especially during long operative procedures when large volumes of fluid and blood are being given intravenously. Under these circumstances, the use of blood warmers for infused fluids, warming blankets, and external heat lamps in those severely injured patients when there is a drop in core temperature below 35° centigrade is mandatory.

Intra-arterial pressure monitoring is currently in general use for all patients undergoing surgical treatment for major trauma. The benefits of this monitoring are to provide a continuous evaluation of systolic and diastolic pressure measurements and to serve as a port for access to arterial blood samples for the measurement of arterial blood gas parameters.

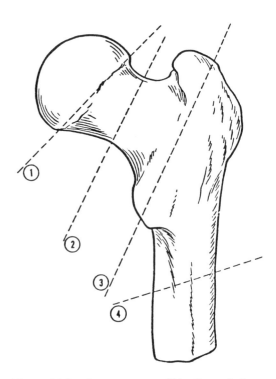

Figure 31.2. Common areas of hip (femoral) fracture in the elderly: (**1**) subcapital, (**2**) transcervical, (**3**) intertrochanteric, (**4**) subtrochanteric.

In the surgical management of the geriatric trauma patient, the frequent presence of a variety of superimposed disease states makes careful fluid resuscitation and accurate monitoring mandatory, especially in those cases of acute intravascular volume loss and shock. In addition to measurement of blood pressure, pulse, respiratory rate, ECG, and urine output, preparations for the monitoring of central venous pressure (CVP) to be measured at frequent intervals should be considered, especially for those patients receiving large volumes of fluid or for those with a history of heart disease. The progressive CVP response to a fluid challenge is much more significant than that of a series of isolated readings. A sharp rise in CVP with rapid infusion of fluids indicates that the right heart cannot handle the load and that infusion rates should be slowed. Those patients with low CVPs and hypotension should be considered hypovolemic, and the fluid challenge and blood replacement should be continued. Although usually accurate for fluid resuscitation, the response of CVP to fluid challenge becomes much less reliable in the face of sepsis, acute respiratory failure requiring positive pressure ventilation, or when pre-existing cardiac and pulmonary disease is present (37).

For patients with severe coronary artery disease or for those undergoing major operative procedures, consideration of the placement of a Swan-Ganz pulmonary artery catheter for measurement of pulmonary wedge pressure (PWP) should be given. The pressure, thus measured, is that of the back pressure in the blood vessels in the lungs via a balloon occluded artery and is a reflection of left ventricular function. A PWP reading of less than 10 torr suggests hypovolemia, whereas readings greater than 20 torr may indicate intravascular overload or left ventricular failure. As with the CVP, the progressive response of the PWP to a fluid challenge is more revealing than isolated readings.

Fluid Requirements

The geriatric trauma patient requires fluid and electrolyte replacement preoperatively and intraoperatively in amounts similar to those used for younger patients; however, several important considerations should be noted. These older individuals have a blood volume requirement that

is similar to that of younger individuals, but even in mild disease states, hemoglobin content decreases, and red cell fragility increases. Compensatory anemia should be considered one of the most common disorders of blood volume encountered among geriatric patients. In addition, chronic hypovolemia is frequently found in this group of patients in which disease states of malnutrition, chronic infection, malignancies of the GI tract, and metastatic disease are common.

With aging, there is a progressive diminution in renal plasma flow and in glomerular filtration, with a consequent decrease in renal function. Tubular function is decreased more than glomerular function, and the ability of the kidney to concentrate urine diminishes. These changes are often aggravated by chronic passive congestion secondary to myocardial insufficiency and result in impaired renal function and azotemia. The utilization of diuretics for the control of hypertension or for the removal of intravascular volume in patients with congestive heart failure results in a depletion of serum potassium and in other electrolyte abnormalities and should be monitored closely with frequent laboratory evaluation.

Initial Fluid Therapy

Isotonic electrolyte solutions are used for initial resuscitation. This type of fluid provides transient intravascular expansion and further stabilizes the vascular volume by replacement of accompanying interstitial fluid losses. Ringer's lactate solution is the initial fluid of choice followed by normal saline. Although normal saline is a satisfactory replacement for many conditions, it has the potential for predisposing to hyperchloremic acidosis when used in the volumes usually administered to injured patients. This potential hazard is more critical in the face of impaired renal function. The initial fluid bolus is given as rapidly as possible. The usual dose is 1 to 2 liters. The patient's response is observed during this initial fluid administration, and further therapeutic and diagnostic decisions are based on the observed response (38).

A small group of patients will respond rapidly to the inital fluid bolus and will remain stable. Such patients have generally lost less than 25% of their blood volume. No further fluid bolus or immediate blood administration is indicated in this small group of patients, but typed and cross-matched blood should be kept available for them. The largest group of patients will respond to the initial fluid bolus; however, as initial fluids are slowed, these patients will begin to show deterioration in circulatory perfusion indices. Continued fluid administration and the initiation of blood administration are indicated. The response to blood administration should identify the patients who are still bleeding and who will require rapid surgical intervention. For those patients who show minimal or no response to initial fluid administration, the surgeon is faced with a serious dilemma. Either the initial diagnosis of hypovolemic shock is correct and rapid blood administration and surgical intervention are needed for exsanguinating hemorrhage or the initial diagnosis of shock was incorrect and an alternative therapy should be undertaken. The central venous pressure is a very useful tool in differentiating between these two groups of patients. Those with exsanguinating hemorrhage should have a very low central venous pressure, and those with other causes for their hypotension should have a normal or a high central venous pressure.

Patients with a transient response to the initial fluid administration, or who have a minimal or no response, and who have obvious active ongoing blood loss should be considered for immediate blood transfusion. In these cases, fully cross-matched blood is preferable. Type-specific saline cross-matched blood can be provided by most blood banks within 10 minutes. Such blood is compatible within ABO and RH blood types. Incompatibilities of minor antibodies may exist. Such blood is appropriate for patients with life-threatening shock situations. If type-specific blood is unavailable, Type O blood should be given to patients with exsanguinating hemorrhage. Cold blood is associated with a high incidence of myocardial dysrhythmias and paradoxical hypotension. Blood should always be warmed before and during massive transfusions especially in elderly patients (38).

Length of Operation

As with all operative procedures, morbidity and mortality are directly related to the length of the procedure done for traumatic injuries. Though age, physical condition, injury type, and extent of operation represent important variables, the duration of an operative procedure in the injured geriatric patient should reflect only the time it takes to control the acute condition that threatens life (39). Prolonged anesthesia linked with a significant amount of blood loss in a debilitated elderly patient predisposes him or her to a state of shock that may become irreversible (39). As with all procedures done for trauma, rapidity of control of blood loss, correction of life-threatening conditions, and meticulous attention to detail of technique, all done in as short a time interval as possible, will lead to a better outcome with less risk of complications.

Indications for Non-Interventional Therapy

The moral and ethical issues of when to withhold operative therapy in the elderly trauma patient are complex and are based on several factors including survivability, return of function, and quality of life. Although an important consideration, the allocation of resources should remain in the political realm and should not influence our surgical judgement. Decisions regarding operative intervention and postoperative care ideally should include the patient, medical team, and family members or other responsible parties. These deliberations and decisions in such cases will serve several valuable functions: (1) to ensure that the patient's self-determination is being respected, (2) to guarantee that medical intervention is serving the patient's best interest, (3) to allow adequate resource allocation and equity considerations, and (4) to reduce physician-nurse-family misunderstandings and discontent about resuscitation and support practices (40).

For those patients who are competent, the decisions for care are usually clear and easily determined providing the patient has received comprehensive information regarding the nature of the injury and a reasonable assessment of survivability. Unfortunately, in many cases, neurologic injury or a constellation of injuries has rendered the patient such that he or she is no longer an active participant. In these cases, the use of a "Living Will," protocols for "do not resuscitate" (DNR), and the determination of brain death have been instituted in an effort to deal with these issues. Imbus and Zawacki (41) have utilized this approach in burn patients who have such severe injuries that "survival is unprecedented." This protocol has been used with success in burn units, stands as a model in dealing with these issues, and underscores the importance with the elderly of preservation of dignity and quality of life and a concerted effort for self-determination.

SPECIAL POSTOPERATIVE CONSIDERATIONS

Intensive Care Unit

With the advent of more complex postoperative monitoring, the use of the intensive care unit (ICU) as a mode and site for therapy has gained widespread acceptance. The high technological aspect of the care provided in this setting has allowed a much closer evaluation of different systems status on a minute-to-minute basis and has improved patient outcomes. This has not occurred without a price. Recent studies have reviewed the cost of outcomes of intensive care for ICU admissions of the elderly. In a 2-year study conducted between 1977 and 1979, 44% of admissions to ICUs were for patients over 65 years of age and 21% were above 75 years (42). Major interventions (i.e, endotracheal intubation and mechanical ventilation) were more likely to occur in the elderly and occurred more frequently as the age increased. In medical ICUs, the 1-year accumulated mortality for patients over 75 years old was 44%. The average cost of hospitalization did not differ significantly in the survival groups of elderly at different age levels compared to non-survivors of the same age groups (42).

Surgical intensive care unit (SICU) admissions for geriatric patients sustaining traumatic illness reflect an overall mortality of 15%. Oreskovich (43) found that the Injury Severity Score (ISS) was not as reliable and as predictive of survival in the elderly injured. Major predictors were that of hypovolemic shock and central nervous system injury (43). Osler and co-workers, in 1987, examined a cohort of 100 injured elderly retrospectively and were able to predict the ultimate demise of the injured elderly correctly 72.5% of the time with a sensitivity of 50% and within specificity of 97.5% using a model derived through regression analysis. In this study, only age, presence of shock, and Glascow Coma scale

were required for this level of predictive accuracy. (Osler TM, unpublished data)

In general, the ICU environment provides the opportunity for the close observation of the elderly trauma patient in the critical postoperative period with the monitoring and the care for those systems at most risk for acute change as a result of their traumatic illness, pre-existing disease, or more appropriately, the salubrious effects of operative intervention.

Pulmonary Considerations

Respiratory complications are the most common and in many respects the most severe problems experienced in the postoperative geriatric patient. Risk factors that predispose these patients to respiratory complications include pre-existing pulmonary disease, emphysema, COPD, history of heavy tobacco use, and the chronic effects of aging. In addition to ventilatory support, early mobilization, vigorous pulmonary toilet, chest physical therapy with coughing and deep breathing, postural drainage, and the use of incentive spirometry all help reduce the risks of atelectasis and pneumonia. An early sputum culture will frequently give a clue to an impending pneumonia and may serve as a guide to future antibiotic therapy. The judicious use of narcotics, careful splinting with coughing, and nasogastric decompression all aid in reducing risks of pulmonary complications in the elderly patient.

Mobility

There is no question that the early mobilization of the geriatric patient is of major importance in the reduction of risk of pulmonary consequences in the postoperative period, including the risks of atelectasis, pneumonia, pulmonary embolus, and vascular problems. Early mobilization is also beneficial for the reduction and prevention of skin breakdown and for the avoidance of the development of pressure sores and decubiti. Not enough can be said for the benefits of early mobilization in terms of the psychologic lift and in the promotion of the "will to live" that are so important in this age group. The fact that the patient is out of bed reinforces the idea that he or she is alive, recovering, and moving toward normal patterns of daily activity, and it is therefore critical in improving the mental status and attitude of elderly patients.

Nutrition

It can be said that, of the major advances in surgical care in the past 20 years, the ability to provide adequate nutritional input to surgical patients has had a major effect upon the reduction of morbidity and mortality. The provision of calories in the form of balanced substrates including carbohydrates, proteins, lipids, vitamins, and trace elements has resulted in a dramatic overall reduction of mortality and complications in the geriatric trauma patient. The determination of increased energy requirements is of major importance following the initial period of stress in the postoperative period. Increased energy expenditure is accompanied by humoral changes that serve both as mediators of the stress response and, in part, controllers of the flow of energy and protein substrate to preserve effective circulating volume, critical organ function, and wound repair (44). Whether nutrition is given enterally, peripherally, or in the form of central venous total parenteral nutrition will depend on the condition of the patient, ability to feed, severity of injury, and the patient's previous nutritional status. The consideration of and the use of a nutritional assessment consult can be of major benefit early in the patient's postoperative course. The calculation of the energy requirements and the determination of the patient's overall nutritional status are vital to the success of many surgical procedures.

OUTCOMES

Return to Functional Levels

Studies concerning return to functional levels following recovery from trauma and its care in the elderly provide data that are controversial and varied. In a 1984 study of elderly injured in whom 96% were independent in their activities of daily living at the time of injury, only 7% of these patients were independent at 1 year following injury and 72% required maintenance in a facility with full nursing care (43). This is in contrast to the reports of DeMaria who studied a similarly injured elderly population and found that 89% returned to home by 1 year and that 57% returned to independent living at the pre-injury functional level (45). Osler and his associ-

ates have shown that the 1-year mortality in surviving elderly patients was 20%, not significantly different from that predicted by actuarial tables for this group, and only 30% experienced a decrease in functional status. (Osler TM, unpublished data)

It is likely that the differences in these studies represent variables of individual patient populations, types of injuries sustained, and modes of therapy instituted. It would seem, however, that of elderly survivors of traumatic injury, there are significant numbers who sustain long term impairment as a result of their injuries and who require the services of health care maintenance facilities, and this number far exceeds that of their younger, healthier counterparts.

Predictors of Outcome

Very little has been written to date regarding those markers or indices that can be used to determine outcome expectations of the traumatized elderly. The recent development of trauma scoring systems has added little toward determining those individuals who are likely not to survive. A national conference designed to evaluate the usefulness of various measures of severity of injury emphasized the limitation of these indices when they are applied to the elderly (46), and this was confirmed by the studies of both Oreskovich (43) and Osler (Osler TM, unpublished data). Markers of survival may be those aspects of previous medical illness. Though no specific studies have shown a correlation of survival with a history of pre-existing diseases, one cannot help but believe that there exists a direct relationship between major pre-existing medical illness and the likelihood of complications and increased risk for mortality with associated major trauma. Other predictors of outcome are likely to be the type and severity of trauma sustained, major neurologic injury, multiple system injury, presence of shock, respiratory compromise, and injury-promoting sepsis. All are likely to increase the risk for mortality in the elderly, as they do in all age groups of trauma patients.

REFERENCES

1. *Accident Facts.* Chicago, National Safety Council, 1981.
2. Snipes GA: Accidents in the elderly. *Am Fam Physician* 26:117–122, 1982.

3. Waller JA: Injury in the aged: clinical and epidemiological complications. *NY State J Med* 74:2200–2208, 1974.
4. Hogue CC: Injury in late life: Part I epidemiology. *J Am Geriatr Soc* 30:183–190, 1982.
5. Chipman C: Falls and their consequences, part I. In Bosker G, Schwartz G (eds): *Geriatric Emergencies*. Englewood Cliffs, NJ, Brady Comm Co, 1984, pp 189–193.
6. Perry BC: Falls among the elderly: a review of the methods and conclusions of epidemiologic studies. *J Am Geriatr Soc* 30:367–371, 1982.
7. Chipman C, Sarant G: Falls and their consequences, part II. In Bosker G, Schwartz G (eds): *Geriatric Emergencies*. Englewood Cliffs, NJ, Brady Comm Co, 1984, pp 195–205.
8. Rubenstein LZ: Falls in the elderly: a clinical approach. *West J Med* 138:273–275, 1983.
9. *Accident Facts*. Chicago, National Safety Council, 1983.
10. Laur AR: Age and sex in relationship to accidents. *Traffic Safety Res Rev* 3:21, 1959.
11. McFarland RA, Junc GS, Welford AT: On the driving of automobiles by older people. *J Gerontol* 19:190–197, 1964.
12. Waller JA, Goo JT: Highway crash and citation patterns and chronic medical conditions. *J Safety Res* 1:13, 1969.
13. Baker SP, Spitz WU: Age effects and autopsy evidence of disease in fatally injured drivers. *JAMA* 214:1079–1088, 1970.
14. Haddon W, Valien P, McCarroll JR, Umberger CJ: A controlled investigation of the characteristics of adult pedestrians fatally injured by motor vehicles in Manhattan. *J Chronic Dis* 14:655–678, 1961.
15. Gerber SR: Cuyahoga court corner's statistical reports, 1960–1970. Cleveland, Ohio.
16. Barancik JI, Shapiro MA: *Pittsburgh Burn Study*. Pittsburgh and Alleghancy City, Pennsylvania Environmental Health Program, Graduate School of Public Health, University of Pittsburgh, Pennsylvania, 1972.
17. Harris R: Cardiovascular diseases in the elderly. *Med Clin N Am* 67:379–394, 1983.
18. Spencer H: Osteoporosis: goals of therapy. *Hosp Pract* 17:131–148, 1982.
19. Brocklehurst JC, Exton-Smith AN, Lempert Barber SM, Hunt LP, Palmer MK: Fracture of the femur in old age: a two-centre study of associated clinical factors and the cause of the fall. *Age Ageing* 7:7–15, 1978.
20. Bradstetter RD, Kazemi H: Aging and the respiratory system. *Med Clin N Am* 67:419–429, 1983.
21. Tillotson JR, Lerner AM: Pneumonias caused by gram negative bacilli. *Medicine* 45:65–76, 1966.
22. Reed LC, Eckert C: Enteral and paraenteral nutritional support. In *Handbook of Geriatric Emergency Care*. Baltimore, University Park Press, 1984, pp 158–163.
23. Young EA: Nutrition, aging, and the aged. *Med Clin N Am* 67:295–313, 1983.
24. Mitchell CO, Lipschitz DA: Detection of protein-calorie malnutrition in the elderly. *Am J Clin Nutr* 35:398–406, 1982.
25. Chandra RK: Rosette-forming T lymphocytes and cell-mediated immunity in malnutrition. *Br Med J* 3:608–609, 1974.
26. Gersovitz M, Motil K, Munro HN, Scrimshaw NS, Young VR: Human protein requirements: assessment of the adequacy of the current recommended dietary allowance for the dietary protein in elderly men and women. *Am J Clin Nutr* 35:6–14, 1982.
27. Munro HN: Nutritional requirements in the elderly. *Hosp Pract* 17:143–154, 1982.
28. Berk SL, Smith JK: Infectious disease in the elderly. *Med Clin N Am* 67:273–293, 1983.
29. Weksler ME: Senescence of the immune system. *Med Clin N Am* 67:263–272, 1983.
30. Cloward RB: Acute cervical spine injuries. *Clin Symp* 32:2–32, 1980.
31. Kirkpatrick JB, Pearson J: Fatal cerebral injury in the elderly. *J Am Geriatr Soc* 25:489–497, 1978.
32. Trunkey DD: Abdominal Trauma. In Trunkey DD, Lewis FR (eds): *Current Therapy in Trauma 1984–1985*. Burlington, Ontario, BC Decker Inc, 1985.
33. Galbraith TA, Oreskovich MR, Heimbach DM, Herman CM, Carrico CJ: The role of peritoneal lavage in the management of stab wounds of the abdomen. *Am J Surg* 140:60–64, 1980.
34. Dobyns JH, Linscheid ZL: Fractures and dislocations of the wrist. In Rockwood CA, Green DP (eds): *Fractures*. Philadelphia, JB Lippincott Co, 1975, pp 358–372.
35. Devas M: Orthopaedics. In Steinberg FU (ed): *Cowdry's Care of the Geriatric Patient*, St. Louis, CV Mosby, Co, 1976, pp 258–274.
36. Laskin RS, Gruber MA, Zimmerman AJ: Intertrochanteric fractures of the hip in the elderly. *Clin Orthop* 141:188–195, 1979.
37. Tousaint GPM, Burgess JH, Hampson LG: Central venous pressure and pulmonary wedge pressure in cited surgical illness: a comparison. *Arch Surg* 109:265–269, 1974.
38. Shock. In *Advanced Trauma Life Support Course Instructor's Manual*. Chicago, American College of Surgeons 1984, pp 179–191.
39. Glenn F: Pre- and postoperative management of elderly surgical patients. *J Am Geriatr Soc* 9:385–393, 1973.
40. President's Commission for Study of Ethical Problems in Medicine and Biomedical and Behavioral Research: *Deciding to Forego Sustaining Treatment*. Washington DC, US Government Printing Office, 1983.
41. Imbus SH, Zawacki BE: Automony for burned patients when survival is unprecedented. *N Engl J Med* 297:308–311, 1977.
42. Campion EW, Mulley AG, Goldstein RL, Barnett GO, Thibault GE: Medical intensive care for the elderly: a study of current use, costs, and outcomes. *JAMA* 246:2052–2056, 1981.
43. Oreskovich MR, Howard JD, Compass MK, Carrico CJ: Geriatric trauma injury patterns and outcome. *J Trauma* 24:565–572, 1984.
44. Wilmore DW, Long JM, Mason AD, Skreen RW, Pruitt BA: Catecholamines: mediator of the hypermetabolic

response to thermal injury. *Ann Surg* 180:653–669, 1974.

45. DeMaria EJ, Kenney PR, Merriam MA, Casanova LA, Gann DS: Aggressive trauma care benefits the elderly.

J Trauma (In Press).

46. Trunkey DD, Siegel J, Baker SP, Gennarelli TA: Panel: current status of trauma severity indices. *J Trauma* 23:185–201, 1983.

Chapter 32

Thermal Injuries in the Elderly[a]

Anne E. Missavage, M.D., Major MC, Basil A. Pruitt, Jr., M.D., Colonel MC, F.A.C.S.

CAUSES OF BURNS

A burn is a common traumatic event that most people will experience during a lifetime. Elderly individuals appear to suffer more burn injuries than others due to decreased mobility and decreased awareness of danger. The ability to survive burn injury is influenced by age, so that elderly individuals with even a small burn are at more risk for a fatal outcome than younger adults. Slater and Gaisford in 1981 reported that the number of elderly burn patients was increasing. Twenty percent of their patients were aged 65 or older, and the mortality rate of these patients was 63%. Pre-existing pulmonary and cardiac disease seemed to contribute to the mortality (1). In 1980, Linn reviewed hospitalized burn patients in Florida. He found that patients aged 65 or greater presented with larger, more severe burns, suffered more complications, and had decreased survival (2).

Data from patients admitted to the U.S. Army Institute of Surgical Research allow the construction of a predictor model for mortality based on age and burn size. Figure 32.1 indicates that in adults, mortality for a given sized burn increases as age increases. The figure also displays the LD_{50} (that size burn associated with a 50% mortality), which has increased to its present level as a result of advances in burn care and general care. The increased mortality of burn injury in the elderly is a consequence of both age-related deterioration of organ function and the presence of chronic diseases. Because of the increased likelihood of an adverse outcome, all elderly persons suffering burns should be considered for in-hospital care, and burn unit care should be considered for all those with burns associated with an anticipated mortality of 20% or more (Table 32.1). Even if a patient is to be transferred to a burn unit for definitive care, treatment should be initiated at the facility in which the patient is first seen.

The hospital course and outcome of 432 burn patients 50 or more years of age who were admitted to the U.S. Army Institute of Surgical Research between January 1976 and December 1985 have been reviewed. (Table 32.2) The average burn covered 34% of the total body surface with an average estimated full thickness injury of 19% of the total body surface. Two hundred twenty patients survived, 209 patients expired, and 3 patients were transferred early in their care. Autopsy examination was carried out on 129 patients, 62% of deaths. The most common cause of burn injury in these patients was mishandling of gasoline and other flammable fuels; many of these accidents were contributed to by dementia or mobility problems. Other causes of burns in this group appeared to be related to decreased awareness of hazards and decreased mobility; these involved cooking accidents, explosions of natural gas stoves, accidental ignition of clothes, and smoking in bed. Housefires were responsible for 65 burns, automobile and recreational vehicle accidents in 32 patients. Twenty-six patients were burned by explosions while working on oil rigs, gas lines, transformers, electrical units, and welding jobs.

GENERAL CONSIDERATIONS

Skin Changes with Burn and Age

With aging, the skin becomes more suscepti-

---

[a]The opinions or assertions contained herein are the private views of the authors and are not to be construed as official or reflecting the views of the Department of the Army or the Department of Defense.

465

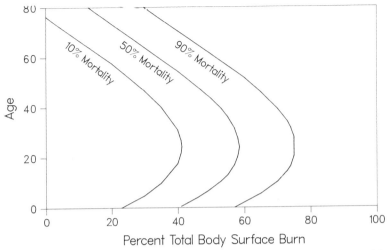

Figure 32.1. Burn mortality 1980–1984. Mortality statistics from the US Army Institute of Surgical Research for a recent period are shown. For any size burn, increased age is associated with a decrease in survival.

ble to burn injury. Depth of injury is determined by the temperature of the heat source and the length of time applied. The decrease in skin thickness and elasticity that occurs with age will increase the depth of burn resulting from application of a given amount of heat. Histologic changes in aging skin include dermal atrophy, fewer fibroblasts, blood vessels, and capillary loops, fewer sweat and oil glands, loss of hair

and flattening of the dermoepidermal junction. These changes lead to irregular thinning of the skin, decreased resistance to shearing, and decreased nutrient transfer to epidermis (3). All of these changes as well as age-associated decreases in epidermal turnover and repair slow the rate of healing of burns in the elderly and decrease the resistance of the epidermis to infection. Diminution of skin blood flow due to atherosclerotic changes in the vessels of an elderly patient also influences burn depth by limiting heat removal in the area of injury and

Table 32.1   Triage Criteria for Burn Patients[a]

Minor Burn Injury—can be treated as outpatient
  Second-degree burn less than 15% of body surface in adult, 10% of body surface in child
  Third-degree burn less than 2% of body surface
Moderate Burn Injury—requires hospitalization
  Second-degree burn of 15%–25% of body surface in adult, 10%–20% of body surface in child
  Third-degree burn up to 10% of body surface
Major Burn Injury—requires treatment in a specialized burn center
  Second-degree burn more than 25% of body surface in adult, 20% of body surface in child
  Third-degree burn more than 10% of body surface
  Any complication conditions
    Age less than 5 or more than 60 years
    Burns of hands, feet, face, perineum
    Inhalation injury
    Significant pre-existing disease
    Associated trauma

[a]From American Burn Association recommendations.

Table 32.2   Elderly Burn Patients at the US Army Institute of Surgical Research: January 1976–December 1985

	Average Age	Average Total Burn	Average Full Thickness Burn
	years	*% of body surface*	
432 patients	62 (50–97)	34 (1–100)	19 (0–97)
220 survivors	59 (50–97)	20 (1–64)	8 (0–49)
209 non-survivors	65 (50–93)	49 (1–100)	31 (0–97)

permitting the tissues to be exposed to higher temperatures for a longer time. Hypotension during resuscitation may further impair skin blood flow to the extent that partial thickness injury converts to full thickness injury. Hypotension or infection later in the post burn course may also decrease local blood flow and result in conversion of partial thickness injury to full thickness necrosis. (Fig. 32.2)

Separation of eschar and maturation of the burn wound proceed more slowly in the elderly patient. Delayed formation of granulation tissue in wound beds and delayed healing of burns occur in the elderly patient. Decreased perfusion, decreased metabolic reserves, and alteration in neuroendocrine control of tissue synthesis probably all contribute to impaired healing and response to injury.

RESUSCITATION—EARLY PHASE

Fluids

The early burn care is focused on maintenance of circulation and oxygenation. During the initial period of fluid sequestration, manifested by a transcapillary fluid loss into the interstitium proportional to the extent of the burn, the plasma volume deficit must be replaced by the administration of electrolyte-containing fluids. Various formulae for fluid administration during resuscitation have been found to be effective, which suggests that the majority of burn patients have enough physiologic reserve to tolerate imprecision in volume, electrolyte, or protein administration. Elderly patients do not have the same tolerance of stress and are more difficult to manage. In view of the sensitivity of the elderly patient to volume overload, the authors use the Modified Brooke formula for resuscitation, which recommends 2 ml of lactated Ringer's solution/kg/percent burn for the first 24 hours postburn, 25% albumin diluted to physiologic concentration in normal saline at 0.3–0.5cc/kg/percent burn to replace the plasma volume deficit, plus 5% dextrose in water to maintain urinary output in the second 24 hours. (Table 32.3) Urinary output is measured hourly, with adjustment of the infusion rate to obtain a urine output of 30–50 ml per hour. The rate of fluid administration with any of the resuscitation formulae must be adjusted according to the patient's response.

Early hemodynamic responses to the increase in capillary permeability in the burn patient

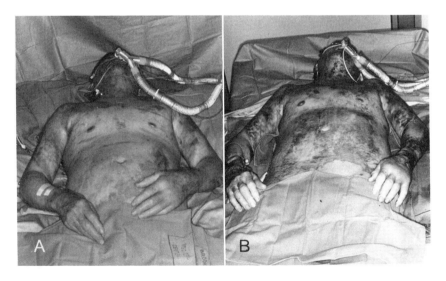

Figure 32.2. **A**, This 82-year-old man with a 46% burn experienced hemodynamic instability on the third post-burn day due to the development of pulmonary edema. **B**, Conversion of his originally partial thickness burns to full thickness injury was evident on the fifth post-burn day. Note the patchy dark discoloration of the wounds, particularly those of the neck and arms. Burn wound biopsies later revealed fungal microinvasion of the wounds in these areas of change.

Table 32.3 Modified Brooke Resuscitation Formula

First 24 hours
Adult: Lactated Ringer's solution 2 ml/kg/percent burn
   Urine output 30–50 ml/hour[a]

Second 24 hours
5% albumin-containing plasma substitute
   0.3 ml/kg/percent burn for 25–50% burn
   0.4 ml/kg/percent burn for 50–70% burn
   0.5 ml/kg/percent burn for greater than 70% burn

5% dextrose in water to maintain urinary output
   0.5–1.0 ml/kg/hour

[a]75–100 ml/hour in patients with significant urinary hemochromagen concentrations.

include vasoconstriction and decreased cardiac output as blood and plasma volumes are lost. Vasoconstriction that helps to maintain perfusion pressure is produced in response to the loss of fluid through the injured capillaries and gradually relents as fluids are replaced. Cardiac output initially falls, but in resuscitated patients by the end of the first 24 hours after thermal injury, it returns to near normal levels, despite the fact that blood and plasma volumes are only incompletely corrected. This increase in cardiac output is produced through increases in heart rate and contractility, despite the decrease in circulating blood and plasma volume. The maximum heart rate that can be sustained decreases with age, and this mechanism for support of cardiac output is further impaired by any pre-existing cardiac disease.

Prior myocardial infarctions, ischemia, or arrhythmias may not permit the elderly heart to respond appropriately to the demand invoked by the thermal injury. A history of cardiac-related disease (hypertension, congestive heart failure, or myocardial infarction) was obtained in more than one-fourth of the 432 patients studied. Arrhythmias, myocardial infarctions, and cardiac failure were prominent events in 20 patients dying within 7 days of injury. Vasoconstriction in response to hypovolemia in the elderly patient may add to any fixed atherosclerotic lesions and further depress cardiac function, increase prerenal azotemia, impair cerebral circulation, or produce thrombotic arterial occlusion in peripheral vessels. Renal failure, manifested by low urine output and increasing blood urea nitrogen and creatinine levels, occurred in most of the pa-

tients who expired shortly after their injury. Impairment of peripheral circulation and extremity ischemia were documented in three patients who expired early post burn; one patient required amputation. In nine other patients surviving more than 48 hours, amputations of extremities were required, and ten patients required amputations of digits late in their hospital course. In the latter patients, the burns of the digits that appeared initially to be deep partial thickness were later found to involve deeper tissue.

Airway

The status of the airway and the adequacy of ventilation should be evaluated immediately in the thermally injured elderly patient. Depth of respirations and flow of air in the upper airway are immediately assessed. Patients with apnea or stridor require immediate intubation. The nasal route of endotracheal intubation is preferred as the tube is more easily secured. Most other patients brought from the scene of burn injury should have oxygen applied by mask. Arterial blood gases and carboxyhemoglobin levels are checked as soon as possible in patients with significant facial burns or those who were burned in a closed space. The results are used to determine the need for continued oxygen therapy. Carbon monoxide inhalation can occur in any patient who is injured in a fire. Inhaled carbon monoxide is avidly bound to hemoglobin and inhibits the normal oxygen-hemoglobin binding and oxygen release. Levels of carboxyhemoglobin greater than 40% may be associated with collapse or coma due to tissue hypoxia; elderly patients with pre-existing pulmonary or cardiac disease may be particularly sensitive to a reduction in arterial oxygen carrying capacity. Because the dissociation of carbon monoxide from hemoglobin is proportional to the partial pressure of oxygen in the blood, treatment with 100% oxygen administered using a well-fitting nonrebreathing mask accelerates the reduction of carboxyhemoglobin levels. Treatment with oxygen in a hyperbaric chamber may be useful in patients who are comatose due to carbon monoxide poisoning.

Some patients with very severe encircling burns of the truck may require escharotomy to improve ventilation. The unyielding eschar overlying the thorax prevents adequate respiratory excursions, and high positive pressure ventilation is required to produce adequate air flow. In patients receiving oxygen-enriched air, a respiratory acidosis caused by such burns may be identified by arterial blood gas sampling. To relieve the limitation of the chest wall motion the eschar is incised along the anterior axillary lines. If the eschar involves a significant portion of the anterior abdominal wall, the anterior axillary line escharotomies should be connected by an escharotomy along the costal margin, which allows improvement in diaphragm motion and air movement. Peak inspiratory pressure on the ventilator will decrease after successful chest escharotomy.

Hyperventilation begins on the second post-burn day and characteristically peaks at levels of 2 to 2 1/2 times normal rate in the first postburn week. This has been attributed to the increased oxygen consumption that characterizes the hypermetabolic response to injury (4). The use of a topical agent containing mafenide acetate, a carbonic anhydrase inhibitor, may further accentuate the hyperventilation. Carbon dioxide production is an end product of carbohydrate metabolism, and a high carbohydrate intake can increase ventilatory requirements. Respiratory failure and a requirement for mechanical ventilation due to excess carbohydrate feeding were not identified in these elderly patients. Elderly patients with limited pulmonary reserve may be unable to ventilate spontaneously at the level required to meet these needs and more often require mechanical ventilatory assistance than do younger patients.

Pulmonary edema is another cause of respiratory insufficiency for which mechanical ventilatory support may be necessary. Pulmonary edema most commonly develops following resuscitation on the third to fifth post-burn day, when edema fluid is being reserved and the intravascular volume expanded. (Figure 32.3) Pulmonary edema is rare during resuscitation, but may occur in the elderly burn patient with limited cardiac reserve. Later in the post-burn course, pulmonary edema may occur if evaporative water loss is reduced by grafting and fluid replacement is not proportionately reduced. Pulmonary edema has also occurred when a large volume of fluid has been administered subcutaneously to facilitate autograft harvest and that fluid is resorbed. The amount of fluid infused for such purpose should be limited to a maximum of one blood volume, and the minimum amount for successful harvesting should be used in the patient with any limitation of cardiac reserve.

Inhalation injury should be suspected in patients with a history of being burned in a closed space, being burned by ignition of petroleum products, or having inhaled fire or smoke. Findings of singed nasal vibrissae, pharyngeal burns, carbonaceous sputum, or stridor also suggest in-

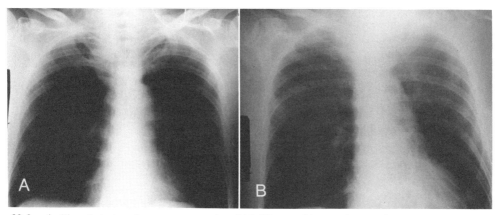

Figure 32.3. **A**, The admission chest roentgenogram of this 82-year-old man who sustained a 46% burn (Figure 32.2) was unremarkable. **B**, A repeat roentgenogram obtained on the third post-burn day demonstrates the development of pulmonary edema as intravascular volume is expanded by resorption of edema fluid. The increase in lung markings and cephalization are indicative of an increase in lung water. Deterioration of oxygenation (PaO_2 decreased from 150 to 100 torr on 35% FIO_2) and hemodynamic instability were noted at this time.

halation injury. These patients should all be evaluated by fiberoptic bronchoscopic examination and/or [133]Xenon ventilation perfusion scintiphotographic scan. Bronchoscopy will identify laryngeal edema, mucosal edema, erythema, ulcerations, and particulate carbonaceous deposits in the bronchial tree. A [133]Xenon lung scan may demonstrate trapping of inhaled gas, but may be falsely positive in patients with chronic obstructive pulmonary disease. Evidence of inhalation injury requires that the patient be carefully watched for the early development of laryngeal edema and airway compromise. Inhalation injury also predisposes a patient to the later development of pneumonia. One hundred fifty-six elderly patients (44 survivors, 112 non-survivors) were diagnosed as having inhalation injury by bronchoscopic examination or by [133]Xenon lung scan, and pneumonia developed in 97. Early intubation in patients with inhalation injury may prevent respiratory arrest from laryngeal edema that may develop during fluid resuscitation. The endotracheal tube also facilitates suctioning to remove secretions and sloughing, necrotic tracheal mucosa. Continuous positive airway pressure (CPAP) at low respiratory rates will help intubated patients maintain expansion of alveoli and clearance of secretions. Other supportive care of the patient with inhalation injury includes administration of humidified oxygen and aerosolized saline to improve mobilization of secretions, as well as encouragement of coughing and deep breathing. Prophylactic antibiotics or steroids are not effective in the patient with inhalation injury, and their use may only promote the development of resistant bacterial pneumonias (5).

Endotracheal intubation of the burn patient is the preferred route of access to the airway, and early tracheostomy is not usually required, unless secretions and debris cannot be cleared through the endotracheal tube. Tracheostomy is performed in patients requiring prolonged intubation who are not able to be weaned easily from ventilatory support due to pulmonary failure or copious secretions. Tracheostomy may also be useful in patients with extensive facial burns because it eliminates the need for the endotracheal tube and securing ties and makes it easier to maintain facial and oral hygiene. When the facial burn is ready for grafting, a tracheostomy will permit anesthetic administration that does not encumber the operative field. Tracheostomy may also enable the patient requiring ventilatory support to consume an oral diet. During the past 10 years, 57 elderly patients required tracheostomy at the USAISR, of whom 13 survived and 44 died. Only one of five patients who underwent tracheostomy in the first week because of inability to clear secretions and debris survived. Four of 27 patients who had tracheostomies performed during the second week after burn injury lived, as did 8 of 25 patients who had tracheostomies after the second week. A tracheostomy should be performed only if the translaryngeal route of intubation is not feasible or if adequate airway toilet cannot be maintained through an endotracheal tube. If prolonged access to the lower airway is required for respiratory failure, there is little benefit of changing from a translaryngeal tube to a tracheostomy before the second to third week of intubation (6). Tracheal stenosis and tracheal malacia have been associated with both tracheostomy and endotracheal intubation, but were not seen in this group of patients, and appear to have become less frequent with the use of low-pressure cuffed tubes. Although tracheo-esophageal fistula formation may occur in patients with prolonged intubation, probably from erosion of the tissues between the endotracheal and nasogastric tubes, this complication was not identified in this group of elderly burn patients.

Circulation

The fluids administered to maintain blood flow to the viscera and carcass may produce sufficient edema beneath the eschar in limbs with circumferential full thickness burns to impair blood flow to distal (or underlying) tissues. The pulses in all burned extremities must be checked on admission to the hospital and rechecked at least hourly for the first 48–72 hours after the burn. All burned extremities should be elevated continuously and actively exercised to improve venous and lymphatic return. Hourly monitoring of the pulses in the palmar arch vessels and the posterior tibial artery enables one to assess the adequacy of the circulation of the limbs. Diminution or loss of pulses is an indication for escharotomy to relieve tissue pressure and restore circulation to the limb. In the elderly patient with pre-existing atherosclerotic lesions, relatively minor amounts of edema may be sufficient to impair perfusion and necessitate escharotomy.

Direct measurement of muscle compartment pressure is best avoided because penetration of the invariably contaminated eschar would seed the deep tissues and increase the risk of subfascial infection. Fasciotomy has been required only in cases of electrical injury, deep burns involving muscle, or burns with associated trauma—conditions characterized by edema beneath the investing fascia. When the mechanism of injury suggests the possibility of muscle injury, and the palpation of the extremity confirms increased pressure within a muscle compartment, fasciotomy is performed.

Monitoring

The goal of monitoring in the elderly burn patient is to anticipate, prevent, or modify complications. In all but minimally burned patients, cardiac monitoring is used to detect arrhythmias. Hourly monitoring of urine output is used to guide the administration of fluids in the resuscitation period, but in elderly patients with pre-existing cardiac or renal disease it may be necessary to measure central venous pressure, pulmonary artery wedge pressure, and cardiac output to optimize fluid resuscitation. Decreased cardiac filling as indicated by decreased central venous pressure and pulmonary wedge pressure is initially treated by increasing the rate of fluid administration. If cardiac output and urine output are not improved in response to fluids, colloids are added to the resuscitation regimen to limit total amount of sodium and water required for resuscitation.

Elderly patients with diminished cardiac reserve can rapidly develop heart failure during resuscitation. Profound hypotension and cardiac arrest occurred in six patients who died in less than 24 hours after the burn, and pre-existing heart disease or acute myocardial infarction was implicated. Elevation of pulmonary artery wedge pressure with inadequate increases in cardiac output in response to administered fluids suggests the need for inotropic support during resuscitation. Dopamine is started at 5 mcg/kg/min, and the dosage is adjusted according to the response of the cardiac output. Patients previously treated

for hypertension may have low systemic blood pressure due to excessive increases in systemic vascular resistance and increased afterload and may require small doses of vasodilators for afterload reduction to improve blood flow and organ perfusion. Hydralazine (0.5 mg/kg) or nitroprusside (0.01 mg/min) can be used with extreme caution when adequate volume loading has been achieved. Such treatment requires frequent monitoring of arterial pressure and cardiac output.

Sepsis may produce hypotension and require rapid infusion of fluid to correct a plasma volume deficit. Additional monitoring by pulmonary arterial catheterization to guide fluid administration is useful in the elderly patient with sepsis. Typically, pulmonary artery pressure in a patient with sepsis is low, whereas cardiac output is elevated and peripheral resistance decreased. An increased rate of fluid administration is the initial treatment response to such physiologic instability. In the elderly patient with acute cardiac disease, the heart may not be able to respond with adequate output, and inotropic support should be added.

Because the incidence of suppurative thrombophlebitis increases as the duration of cannula residence increases, all intravenous cannulae should be changed every 3 days. The incidence of infection in cannulated peripheral arteries has been nil, reflecting the higher blood flow and customarily limited duration of cannulation. The need for invasive monitoring for elderly patients must be continually reassessed to allow removal of the device as soon as practical and to limit its duration of contact with tissues and blood.

LATER CARE

Nutrition

Metabolic responses in thermally injured patients are proportional to the magnitude of the injury. The acute effects of injury produce hypometabolism, which is succeeded by hypermetabolism on the second or third post-burn day. In patients with extensive burns (greater than 45% of the total body surface) the hypermetabolism peaks at 2-2½ times normal energy requirements late in the first post-burn week and thereafter gradually recedes to normal levels as the burns heal or are grafted. The increased metabolic demands if unmet by nutritional support result in erosion of lean body mass, increased nitrogen loss, and weight loss. Cold stress may exaggerate the metabolic rate increase and should be avoided. Increased heat loss due to exaggeration of evaporative water loss from the burn wound can further contribute to cold stress. The elderly patient has impaired thermoregulatory responses and is more susceptible than younger patients to hypothermia as a result of accelerated heat loss in a cool environment (7). In order to minimize thermal stress, burn patients should be nursed in an environment in which the temperature is maintained at 30 °C, with supplemental external heating if body temperature is not maintained.

Immediate post-burn ileus occurs in most burn patients with burns of more than 20% of the total body surface. As soon as gastrointestinal motility returns, oral alimentation is begun to ameliorate tissue wasting and weight loss due to the hypermetabolism. Protein and calorie needs can be approximated from nomograms that estimate burn-size related increases in metabolic rate above the basal metabolic rate, which decreases with advancing age. (Table 32.4) The patient, if able to consume adequate protein and calories to satisfy the calculated needs, is provided the appropriate oral diet with high calorie and protein supplements. Poor appetite is common, and spontaneous intake can only be slightly increased, so tube feedings may be necessary to supplement or replace oral diet and satisfy metabolic needs. Nasogastric or nasoenteric tube feedings can be used; however, impaired gastric emptying that occurs with exposure to

Table 32.4 Nutritional Needs in an Elderly Patient[a]

Age: 92 years	Sex:male	Total burn: 46%
Height: 188 cm	Pre-burn weight: 86.9 kg	
Body surface area: 2.13 square meters		

Basal metabolic rate: 28.05 Kcal/m²/hour (unburned)[b]
Estimated metabolic rate: 54.2 Kcal/m²/hour (burned)[b]

Estimated caloric needs: 3475 Kcal/day
Estimated protein needs: 145 gm/day

[a]Patient in Figure 32.2.
[b]Due to age, number of calories required decreased by 15%.

anesthetics or with sepsis may cause emesis that may result in aspiration. To avoid this complication, gastric residuals should be aspirated prior to each bolus gastric feeding and continously with small bowel feeding, and the quantity of liquid supplement administered should be decreased when the majority of the previous feeding is aspirated back from the stomach. Hiatal hernia and supine positioning may allow regurgitation and are relative contraindications to this mode of nutrition. Operative placement of tubes for jejunal feeding should be avoided because separation of the bowel from the abdominal wall has been common in burn patients.

In patients who cannot tolerate enteral nutrition, intravenous alimentation by central vein is begun with solutions containing hypertonic glucose, amino acids, and emulsified fats. Glucose tolerance is present in patients with diabetes and is more likely to occur in elderly patients than in young adults. The sudden appearance of glucose intolerance is an early sign of infection and should prompt a search for the site of infection. Hyperglycemia is treated by adding insulin to the parenteral alimentation fluids; if that does not control the hyperglycemia, the rate of glucose administration is decreased to avoid hyperglycemic coma as a consequence of osmotic diuresis.

BURN WOUND CARE

Control of bacterial density, debridement of nonviable tissue, maintenance of mobility and function, and timely operative closure are the goals of wound care in burn patients, especially the elderly who have less tolerance to prolonged stress. After the admission assessment and stabilization of the burn patient, attention is turned to the care of the wound. The burn wounds are gently cleansed with an antiseptic soap, and bullae are carefully debrided to remove surface contamination and loose nonviable tissue. Control of bacterial proliferation then becomes important and is achieved by the use of topical antimicrobial therapy.

Wound cleansing with a surgical detergent disinfectant, such as chlorhexidine solution, is carried out daily. Iodine-containing disinfectants should be avoided as significant absorption of iodine through denuded tissues has been documented to produce suppression of lymphocyte activity (8), and may produce hypothyroidism by the Wolff-Chaikoff effect (9). Immersion of these patients at the time of cleansing is avoided to prevent exposure of the entire wound to the enteric flora. Ambulatory patients can cleanse themselves in a shower, and non-ambulatory patients can be cleansed in bed or cleansed with a water spray while lying on a plinth suspended above a Hubbard tank. Anesthesia is not used for daily debridement of loose, nonviable tissue, which is carried only to the point of pain or bleeding, but analgesia should be used to reduce the pain associated with cleansing and debridement.

There are three available topical agents of documented effectiveness: 11.1% mafenide acetate burn cream, 1% silver sulfadiazine burn cream, and 0.5% silver nitrate soaks. All appear to be capable of limiting microbial proliferation in burn wounds when application is begun in the immediate post-burn period, but only mafenide acetate contains an active component that can diffuse into the nonviable eschar and exert a bacteriostatic effect on the bacteria in an already heavily colonized wound. Each of the three topical agents has advantages and limitations (Table 32.5), a knowledge of which permits one to employ the agents with the flexibility needed to meet the wound care needs of a given patient. To minimize agent-related limitations and complications, the authors presently alternate application of mafenide acetate and silver sulfadiazine burn creams on a 12-hour basis. Mafenide acetate burn cream is applied after the morning wound cleansing, and silver sulfadiazine is applied 12 hours later in the evening. Hypersensitivity to either or both of those agents mandates the use of 0.5% silver nitrate soaks that are changed twice or thrice daily and periodically moistened with additional 0.5% silver nitrate solution to prevent evaporation from increasing the concentration of silver nitrate to cytotoxic levels.

Topical antimicrobial agents do not sterilize the burn wound. Topical chemotherapy limits microbial proliferation and maintains the bacterial density at levels below 10^5 organisms per gram of tissue, which are seldom associated with invasive infection. In patients in whom the topical therapy is ineffective in controlling microbial proliferation or those with severe immunologic compromise, the dreaded complication of

Table 32.5 Topical Antimicrobial Burn Wound Agents

	Advantages	Limitations
Mafenide acetate (Sulfamylon cream) 11.1% cream	Penetrates eschar Wound visible Associated injuries visible No gram-negative resistance Motion of joints maintained	Painful for 20–30 minutes after application to second-degree burns; Inhibition of carbonic anhydrase activity may predispose to metabolic acidosis Hypersensitivity (7%) Delays eschar separation
Silver nitrate 0.5% occlusive dressings	No hypersensitivity Painless except for dressing change No gram-negative resistance Decreases heat loss	No eschar penetration Loss of Na+, K+, Cl−, Ca++, Dressings limit motion, Discolors unburned skin of patient, skin of personnel, and environment
Silver sulfadiazine (Silvadene cream) 1% cream	Painless Wound visible when used without dressings Associated injuries visible Motion of joints maintained	Poor eschar penetration Bone marrow suppression Hypersensitivity (rare) Resistance of many *Enterobacter cloacae* and *Pseudomonas* sp. Plasmid mediated resistance to multiple antibiotics

invasive burn wound infection can occur. Early detection of burn wound infection is accomplished by daily complete examination of the entire burn surface for signs of burn wound invasion. (Table 32.6)

If any of the clinical signs of burn wound infection are present, a burn wound biopsy of that area showing the most prominent changes must be performed to assess the microbial status of the wound. (Fig. 32.4) The biopsy is obtained from that area of the wound showing the most pronounced changes and must include underlying viable subcutaneous tissue, as well as the eschar. (Fig. 32.5) The specimen is divided for histologic examination and quantitative culture. Neither surface culture monitoring nor qualitative burn wound culturing is reliable in making a diagnosis of invasive bacterial infection of the burn wound (10). The results of the culture identify the inhabitants of the burn wound and the predominant organism for which antibiotic sensitivities should be determined. The specimen for histologic examination can be processed by either the frozen section technique in one half hour or by the rapid technique in 4 hours. The pathologist examines the prepared section to identify the microscopic criteria of burn wound invasion (Table 32.7) and make the critical differentiation between burn wound colonization and invasive burn wound infection. (Fig. 32.6)

A diagnosis of burn wound infection mandates a change in wound care. Subeschar antibiotic clysis and administration of systemic antibiotics followed by excision of the burn wound and definitive autografting are the optimum management. If autograft donor sites are not available or one is uncertain about the removal of all infected tissue, temporary coverage of the excised

Table 32.6 Clinical Signs of Burn Wound Infection

Focal black, dark brown, or violaceous areas of discoloration

Conversion of second-degree burn to full thickness necrosis

Hemorrhagic discoloration of subeschar fat

Unexpectedly rapid eschar separation and/or marked subeschar suppuration

Edema, violaceous discoloration, or superficial ulceration of unburned skin at wound margins

Erythematous nodular lesions in unburned skin (may ulcerate or escharify in time)

Vesicular lesions in healing or healed second-degree burn[a]

[a]Characteristic of herpes simplex virus infection.

wound bed can be obtained by application of cutaneous allografts or another biologic membrane. Spread of infection to the local blood vessels is a harbinger of systemic blood-borne infection. If microvascular involvement in the septic process has permitted blood-borne dissemination of the causative organism, hematogenous pneumonia or acute bacterial endocarditis may eventuate. If the primary and secondary septic foci cannot be controlled, systemic sepsis may evoke multiple organ failure leading to death.

Operative excision of eschar has been increasingly utilized to effect early closure of burn wounds. The elderly, who have delayed epithelialization and delayed separation of eschar, were previously managed with daily debridement and prolonged application of topical agents, until granulation tissue adequate for skin grafting eventually appeared. This method allowed continued fluid and protein losses from the wound and prolonged the exposure of the patient to the risk of burn wound infection. The work of Deitch

Figure 32.4. A 72-year-old man with a 68% burn and inhalation injury became hypotensive on the 12th post-burn day. Careful examination of the full thickness burn wound of the right leg demonstrated focal areas that had become darkly discolored; a biopsy was performed on one such area on the anterolateral aspect of the leg just proximal to the inferior margin of the wound *(arrow)*. Despite appropriate systemic antibiotics and clysis of the invaded wounds, the patient expired on post-burn day 14 with burn wound sepsis.

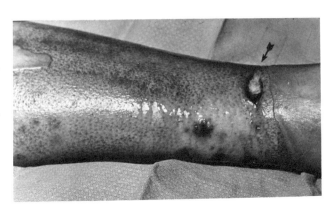

Figure 32.5. A burn wound biopsy specimen is excised from an area of hemorrhagic color change in a 59-year-old man. The biopsy must include bleeding, viable subeschar tissue as shown here. Histologic evaluation revealed microinvasion of aspergillus into viable tissue.

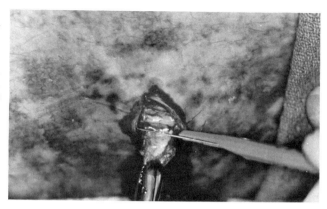

suggests that even elderly patients can tolerate early excision and grafting of burn wounds and that early definitive closure of burns decreases the risk of infection in the wound, decreasing hospital stay and promoting survival in this group, compared to historical controls (11, 12). On the other hand, Housinger et al. advocate conservative treatment of the elderly burn patient with moderate-sized burns up to 40% of the total body surface and significant underlying illness or disability. Emphasis on meticulous burn wound care, adequate nutrition, early return to normal activities, and close outpatient supervision resulted in fewer complications, shorter hospital stays, and equivalent functional results in elderly physically ill burn patients as compared to a similar group that was subjected to excision and grafting (13).

In the treatment of an elderly patient with extensive burns excision may be precluded by hemodynamic instability or respiratory complications, and the timing of excision is often dictated by the patient's general condition. One hundred fifty-seven patients (36.6%) of the 432 elderly patients reviewed could not be stabilized

sufficiently for surgery and sucumbed to their injury without excision having been performed. Fifty-one (11.9%) of the elderly patients healed their burns without grafting and were discharged. The remaining 221 (51.1%) patients (169 survivors with average burns of 22%, 52 nonsurvivors with average burns of 34%) underwent debridement and grafting; 125 of these within 3 weeks of injury. The post-burn day (PBD) excision decreased during the period reported. In 1976, the average time of the first grafting was 32nd PBD, whereas in 1985, the average time of the first grafting was the 18th PBD. By the end of the decade encompassed by the review, few patients were being allowed to separate spontaneously the eschar from their burn wound prior to skin grafting. Although burn wound excision is being carried out more frequently and at an earlier time, no decrease in duration of hospital stay has been observed in the survivors. (Fig. 32.7)

When preparing the elderly patient for the operation, adequate ventilation must be established and an adequate blood volume maintained. When serum sodium, urea nitrogen, and creatinine are all within normal ranges and weight loss is appropriate for the time post-burn, adequate hydration of a patient with good cardiac and renal reserve is likely. Administration of fluids or conversely a diuretic may be necessary in patients who have lost water too rapidly or too slowly, respectively. Prior use of antihypertensives and cardiac drugs may affect the retention of fluid, and these medications may need readjustment. In pre-existing disease, adequate monitoring may require placement and use of central venous, arterial, or pulmonary arterial catheters. These

Table 32.7 Histologic Classification of Burn Wound Infection

Stage I: Colonization in nonviable tissue
(I,a): Superficial colonization
(I,b): Penetration of nonviable tissue
(I,c): Proliferation at the viable-nonviable tissue interface

Stage II: Invasion into viable tissue
(II,a): Microinvasion
(II,b): Generalized invasion
(II,c): Microvascular involvement

Figure 32.6. This histologic specimen from a burn wound biopsy demonstrates the perivascular "cuffing" typical of *Pseudomonas* burn wound invasion. (Stage II, c) This specimen was prepared by the rapid technique.

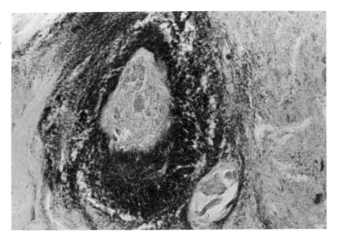

may be placed preoperatively and used to guide necessary corrections of cardiac and renal function prior to and during the operation.

The elderly patient should be carefully evaluated by the anesthesiologist prior to operation. Pre-existing disease may influence the choice of anesthetic agents, such as the preference for narcotic agents in the elderly with cardiac disease. Impaired pulmonary function may require modification of ventilatory support intra-operatively or continuation of support postoperatively. The technique of induction of anesthesia should also be considered. Inasmuch as succinylcholine has been reported to cause massive release of potassium in burn patients when administered between the 18th and 66th post-burn days, it is best avoided at all times lest life-threatening arrhythmias be produced. Adequate amounts of cross-matched blood products should be ordered and be available prior to operation. In general, blood loss is replaced with packed red cells and crystalloid solutions; however, patients with deficiencies of coagulation factors and clinical bleeding may require supplemental fresh frozen plasma. Thrombocytopenia with a platelet count less than $50,000/mm^3$ should be corrected by administration of platelets preoperatively, and additional platelets should be transfused during the operation if bleeding becomes significant.

Perioperative antibiotic therapy is used in all patients. Manipulation of the burn wound often produces bacteremia that may result in hemato-

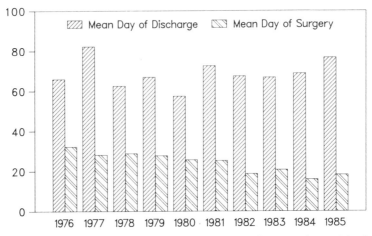

Figure 32.7. Operation and discharge day. The post-burn day of the first operative excision is seen to decrease during the period shown. However, the day of discharge in survivors shows no change during the same period, despite increased use of operative excision of eschar.

genous infections of tissues remote from the wound. Perioperative antibiotics should be chosen on the basis of the predominant flora as determined by the institution's microbial surveillance program. In this group of patients reviewed, those having excision of extensive burns were customarily treated with vancomycin and amikacin to provide protection against *Staphylococcus aureus* and gram-negative bacilli, which were the common bacteria isolated from the burn wound. Patients who have smaller, usually less heavily colonized burns are treated with perioperative penicillin to prevent streptococcal graft infection. Perioperative antibiotics are continued for only 24 hours in patients with no concurrent infection. Such a brief duration of treatment reduces the risk of inducing antibiotic resistance in the resident bacteria and the risk of yeasts and fungi supplanting the bacterial flora of the burn wound.

The elderly patient tolerates excision and grafting of burn wound well when the surgical procedure is carefully conducted. The length of the procedure should be limited so that blood loss and heat loss are not excessive. In general, the operative procedure per se should not exceed 2 hours, blood loss should not exceed one blood volume, and no more than 20% of the body surface should be excised at a single sitting. Physiologic instability may require intraoperative resuscitative efforts or even early termination of the procedure. Excision of the eschar is carried out rapidly with prompt control of blood loss from the excised areas by application of topical thrombin and pressure, followed by electrocautery as needed to obtain hemostasis. If two surgical teams are used to decrease operative time, special attention must be given to control of blood loss and prompt replacement of the combined blood loss. Tourniquets are generally avoided in the elderly because the tourniquet may damage atherosclerotic vessels and induce subsequent thrombosis.

The depth of the excision depends on the depth of the burn. Tangential excision in which the final cut surface is intradermal is generally associated with excellent skin graft take and good cosmetic and functional results as one would anticipate because burns treatable in this fashion are only partial thickness. Full thickness burns can be excised by the tangential technique with the plane of excision being the investing fascia. The use of a hemostatic scalpel permits simultaneous division and coagulation of vessels. Bleeding is least when excision is carried out at the level of the investing fascia where the perforating vessels are readily identified prior to arborization and easily controlled. Excisions into the subcutaneous fat must be carefully performed to ensure removal of all marginally perfused, relatively avascular fat; this hypovascular fat may have the color of normal viable adipose tissue, but will commonly dessicate and necrose under newly placed skin grafts.

Selection of donor sites in the elderly patient should take into account their postoperative problems with positioning and mobility. Posteriorly placed donor sites may receive too much pressure and develop full thickness skin loss. Air drying of donor sites is preferred, and dependent donor sites are elevated to permit exposure to air. The air-fluidized bed has been used for some elderly patients to decrease focal pressure on the posterior surfaces and improve the drying of donor sites. As the skin thins with age, removal of thick autografts may produce a deep dermal or full thickness skin loss, which will itself require grafting for closure. Consequently, undue pressure that can increase the thickness of a skin graft independent of dermatome setting must be avoided while harvesting skin grafts from elderly patients.

The positioning of the elderly patient is of great importance to the ultimate graft take. Immobilization of the cutaneous autografts is necessary to prevent mechanical displacement and permit vascularization. However, prolonged immobilization of the postoperative patient may result in limitation of joint motion, promote the development of decubitis ulcers, accentuate dependent edema, foster the development of atelectasis and pneumonia, and increase confusion and disorientation by reducing visual stimuli. In general, the grafted areas are immobilized in a functional position only until the skin grafts are vascularized (about 7 days). The newly grafted areas are then exercised daily by the physical therapist to regain any lost mobility, and protective dressings or splints are used to avoid damage to the fragile grafts.

The use of topical burn wound chemotherapy has decreased the incidence of invasive burn wound infection since its introduction in the mid-1960s. In the past 10 years, only 24 of the 432 elderly patients were identified as having burn wound sepsis. Twenty cases occurred in the first 5 years encompassed by this review, and only 1 patient of the 24 survived. The reason for the decreased incidence of burn wound sepsis in this group is uncertain, but earlier excision of the burned tissue and closure of the burn wound may have contributed to it.

COMPLICATIONS

Pneumonia

The reduction in burn wound infection has been accompanied by an emergence of pneumonia as the most common form of infection occurring in the burn patient. Most pneumonia occurs as a complication of inhalation injury that impairs ciliary function, and decreases surfactant production. These patients commonly develop atelectasis, which may progress to pneumonia involving variable amounts of lung parenchyma. Bronchoscopy commonly reveals viscid endobronchial exudates, mucosal ulcerations, and sloughing respiratory mucosa that may cause mechanical obstruction of large bronchi. When pneumonia occurs, initial systemic antibiotic therapy is based on a gram stain of the sensitivities of the organisms recovered by culture. Frequent suctioning or bronchoscopy may be needed to clear the exudate and endobronchial debris if the patient is unable to cough adequately. Inhalation injury and pneumonia are responsible for increases in mortality that are age and burn size related. Inhalation injury will increase the mortality of a given sized burn by up to 20%, and pneumonia will increase the mortality by up to 40%. The mortality-enhancing effects are independent and additive and if both conditions are present (pneumonia is a frequent sequela of inhalation injury) mortality is increased by a maximum of 60% depending on the age and extent of burn (14). Because of this, the mortality-enhancing effects of inhalation injury and pneumonia are evident in elderly patients even when the burns are of limited extent.

Elderly patients who are immobilized following surgical procedures by the tethering necessary for monitoring catheters, ventilators, or treatment of associated injuries are apt to develop this complication. Deterioration of pulmonary function and development of bronchopneumonia are most common in patients with posteriorly situated grafts who require prone positioning in the post-grafting period; atelectasis secondary to the impairment of chest wall excursion and impaired clearance of airway secretions appear to be the causes. Consequently, prone positioning should be avoided if possible and be of as limited duration as possible if unavoidable. Pulmonary function of any patient requiring prone positioning must be monitored on a frequently scheduled basis and the patient repositioned if significant compromise is identified.

Other pneumonias are of hematogenous origin. These present with single, usually rounded, peripheral infiltrates and are a consequence of bacteremia from a site of suppurative thrombophelitis, an infected burn wound, an intra-abdominal abscess, a soft tissue abscess, or rarely a urinary tract infection. With their decreased tolerance to infection, the elderly may not be able to clear bacteremias as effectively as younger persons, and their lungs serve as both a microbial filter and culture medium for bacterial proliferation. When such an infiltrate appears, the source of infection must be identified and controlled and the pulmonary infection treated.

In the 10 years covered by this review, 153 patients were diagnosed as having pneumonia during their hospitalization. Twenty-nine of these patients survived and 124 died. The pneumonia occurred in association with inhalation injury in 97 patients (21 survivors, 76 non-survivors). Fifty-six patients (8 survivors, 48 non-survivors) who had no inhalation injury developed pneumonia; most of these had other sites of infection including the burn wound, suppurative thrombophlebitis, and urinary tract identified. Because the development of pneumonia in elderly burn patients is associated with increased mortality, prompt identification and treatment of inhalation injury, prevention of aspiration, and effective treatment of infections prior to hematogenous dissemination will be associated with increased survival in this group.

Gastrointestinal Complications

Previous generations of burn surgeons have

feared Curling's ulcer as the most common life-threatening gastrointestinal complication in burn patients, occurring in 11% of elderly patients in a previous review (15). Since 1976, antacid and H_2 receptor antagonist prophylaxis has been routinely employed, and only one elderly patient has developed bleeding from an acute duodenal ulcer that required surgical intervention. Current management of the elderly burn patient includes administration of cimetidine beginning on admission and pH monitoring of the gastric aspirate above 5.0.

Ileus of the small and large bowel is a more common gastrointestinal tract complication. This is evident immediately post-burn in virtually all patients with burns of 25% or more of the body surface and commonly relents by the third or fourth post-burn day. Later in the post-burn period ileus is a common early sign of sepsis. In mild cases ileus may impair gastric emptying and prevent successful enteral feeding. With more severe ileus, gastric distension, regurgitation, and aspiration can occur. This may have contributed to the deaths of seven patients who succumbed to pneumonia following aspiration. Persistent or recurrent impairment of gastrointestinal motility, at times accompanied by some degree of distension, was documented in eight other elderly patients. The diagnosis of the intra-abdominal pathology was difficult in these elderly burn patients, all of whom had pneumonia. At autopsy unsuspected perforation of the small bowel was found in one patient, and a perforation of the sigmoid colon in one. A celiotomy was performed in the other six patients at which time a bowel perforation was identified in two patients and distension of the cecum in four. The patients with perforation had resection or closure and neither survived. Three patients had a cecostomy performed and one survived, and the fourth patient who survived had no pathology identified at operation and decompression was not required. Burn wound of the anterior abdominal wall can mask peritoneal signs, and impairment of immune function in burn patients decreases local reaction to and containment of infection. Confusion or obtundation in the elderly patient will make cooperation with examination impossible. Intra-abdominal infection should be suspected in the elderly burn patient who deteri-

orates despite appropriate treatment for known sources of sepsis.

Liver failure manifested by jaundice was commonly seen in critically ill elderly patients. In 1975, Czaja prospectively reviewed a group of non-pediatric burn patients without prior history of liver disease and found clinical and laboratory evidence of hepatic disease in many of the patients with large burns. Abnormal transaminase values were consistent with the autopsy findings of hepatocellular injury occurring early in the post-burn course. Hyperbilirubinemia occurred later after burn injury and was typically associated with intrahepatic cholestasis (16). Seventy-five of the elderly patients had a history of heavy ethanol intake or delirium tremens on admission. Five patients with a history of cirrhosis and three others with prior porto-caval shunts all expired. Four of these patients with severe liver failure died with ascites and jaundice, and two died with bleeding varices. The pre-existing liver disease in many of these patients made the differential diagnosis of jaundice quite difficult. Acalculous cholecystitis and necrosis of the gallbladder wall that were identified in two patients can be attributed to shock, sepsis, hemolysis, ileus, and dehydration. Ultrasonic or computed tomographic demonstration of enlargement of the gallbladder with thickening of the wall suggests the possibility of acalculous cholecystitis. Radiolabeled autogenous white cell scintigraphic scanning may be more specific for making the diagnosis of acalculous cholecystitis, but is not applicable to patients with open wounds overlying the gallbladder. This diagnosis was made in only two patients who underwent cholecystectomy and survived. In septic patients with hyperbilirubinemia, abnormalities of liver function should be sought and treatable intra-abdominal pathology such as cholecystitis excluded.

Thrombophlebitis

Suppurative thrombophlebitis is an intravenous infection that in burn patients most commonly occurs at a site of intravenous cannulation. This is manifested by signs of systemic infection, and less than half of the patients will have local signs of infection even when the infection involves a peripheral vein. The diagnosis is confirmed by biopsy of the infected vein and identification of intraluminal purulence, an intraluminal thrombus infiltrated by inflammatory cells and bacteria, or an intraluminal thrombus from which bacteria are recovered on culture. Excision of the involved peripheral veins with prolonged antibiotic treatment for involved central veins is necessary for treatment after identification of suppurative thrombophlebitis. Unfortunately, many cases are first identified only at autopsy. The incidence of suppurative thrombophlebitis is minimized by changing the site of intravenous cannulation every 72 hours and meticulously aseptic handling of intravenous lines and infusates, particularly those containing glucose.

Suppurative thrombophlebitis was identified in 16 of 432 elderly patients (3.7%) during the last 10 years. The average burn size in these sixteen patients was 35.8% with 22.4% full thickness burn, similar to that of the entire elderly burn population. Seven patients had suppurative thrombophlebitis diagnosed only at autopsy. Nine patients underwent biopsy, excision of involved veins, and treatment with systemic antibiotics, and five of them survived. Associated complications included pneumonia in 13 of these patients, and heart failure in 5, as well as renal failure, respiratory failure, and gastrointestinal complications in others. The need for prolonged intravenous cannulation (more than 1 month in nine patients) and the need for invasive monitoring devices occasioned by the complications that occurred in these elderly patients predisposed them to the development of intravenous infection. The benefits derived from the use of any intravenous device should be weighed against the attendant increased risk of suppurative thrombophlebitis.

PREVENTION OF BURNS

Because the elderly patient suffers so greatly from the effects of thermal injury, prevention of burn injury is an important means of decreasing death due to burns in the aged. Careless handling of cigarettes and matches was recorded in 48 patients (11%). These patients with pre-existing smoking history frequently also had pulmonary disease and tolerated burn injury poorly. Cessation of smoking would have been of great health importance. Seventy-nine patients (18%) had a history of heavy alcohol intake documented on admission. In many of the cases, acute intoxication contributed to faulty judgement and the accidental injury. Accidents while cooking accounted for 39 injuries (9%) that occurred when clothing ignited from contact with a hot stove or overturned protruding hot objects on the stove. Elderly persons need to exercise great care while cooking and should not wear loose, hanging clothing. Hot water scalds from tap water that was excessively heated occurred in eight elderly persons (2%). These injuries can be avoided by keeping hot water heaters set below 120°F (49°C), which extends the time needed to cause full thickness burns to 10 minutes (17). If the elderly recognize their developing infirmities and increase their awareness of surrounding dangers, many burn injuries will be avoided. Warning devices may be used to alert the elderly person to unsuspected fires and allow more time to escape.

Care of the elderly burn patient is best provided in a burn center where a multidisciplinary team approach can be used to address the special problems of these patients. The elderly patient presents much the same concerns as a younger burn patient, but will not tolerate the same degree of expected complications of burn injury as the younger patient because of the consequences of aging and disease. Cardiovascular instability during resuscitation, pulmonary compromise from inhalation injury and pneumonia, fragility of skin and poor healing, and nutritional needs for healing require early, skilled intervention that is best provided in a burn center. Attention to the impaired physiologic responses of the elderly patient and prompt institution of the treatment modifications necessary to maintain or restore organ function and effect timely wound closure will prevent the development of complications, ensure optimal functional results, and maximize survival.

REFERENCES

1. Slater H, Gaisford JC: Burns in older patients. *J Am Geriatr Soc* 29:74–76, 1982.
2. Linn BS: Age differences in the severity and outcome of burns. *J Am Geriatr Soc* 28(3):118–123, 1980.
3. Gilchrest BA: Age-associated changes in the skin. *J Am Geriatr Soc* 30:139–143, 1982.

4. Petroff PA, Hander EW, Mason AD: Ventilatory patterns following burn injury and effect of sulfamylon. *J Trauma* 15:650–656, 1975.

5. Levine BA, Petroff PA, Slade CL, Pruitt BA: Prospective trials of dexamethasone and aerosolized gentamicin in the treatment of inhalation injury in the burned patient. *J Trauma* 18:188–192, 1978.

6. Lund T, Goodwin CW, McManus WF, Shirani KZ, Stallings RJ, Mason AD, Pruitt BA: Upper airway sequelae in burn patients requiring endotracheal intubation or tracheostomy. *Ann Surg* 201:374–382, 1985.

7. Wagner JA, Horvath SM: Influences of age and gender on human thermo-regulatory responses to cold exposures. *J Appl Physiol* 58:180–186, 1985.

8. Ninnemann JL, Stein MD: Suppressor cell induction by Povidone-Iodine: in vitro demonstration of a consequence of clinical burn treatment with betadine. *J Immunol* 125:1905–1908, 1981.

9. Zamora JL: Chemical and microbiologic characteristics and toxicity of Povidone-Iodine solutions. *Am J Surg* 151:400–406, 1986.

10. McManus AT, Kim SH, McManus WF, Mason AD, Pruitt BA: Comparison of quantitative microbiology and histopathology in divided burn-wound biopsy specimens. *Arch Surg* 122:74–76, 1987.

11. Deitch EA, Clothier J: Burns in the elderly: an early surgical approach. *J Trauma* 23:891–894, 1983.

12. Deitch EA: A policy of early excision and grafting in elderly burn patients shortens the hospital stay and improves survival. *Burns* 12:109–114, 1985.

13. Housinger T, Saffle J, Ward S, Warden G: Conservative approach to the elderly patient with burns. *Am J Surg* 140:817–820, 1984.

14. Shirani KZ, Pruitt BA, Mason AD: The influence of inhalation injury and pneumonia on burn mortality. *Ann Surg* 205:82–87, 1987.

15. Pruitt BA, Mason AD, Hunt JL: Burn injury in the aged or high-risk patient. In Siegel J, Chodoff P (eds): *The Aged and High Risk Surgical Patient.* New York, Grune & Stratton, 1976, pp 523–546.

16. Czaja AJ, Rizzo TA, Smith WR, Pruitt BA: Acute liver disease after cutaneous thermal injury. *J Trauma* 15:887–893, 1975.

17. Katcher ML: Scald burns from hot tap water. *JAMA* 246:1219–1222, 1981.

Chapter 33

Ophthalmic Diseases in the Elderly

James H. Elliott, M.D., F.A.C.S., Stephen S. Feman, M.D., F.A.C.S.

The surgical diseases of the eye can be divided into two main areas. It is convenient, first, to consider surgical aspects of the anterior segment of the eye and in the second section to deal with the problems related to the posterior segment of the eye.

A few general principles about surgical diseases of the eye in the elderly are appropriate to consider. Two decades ago, when one considered eye procedures in the elderly, the age of the patient and the status of his or her general health were the most paramount considerations in the decision to operate. This applied equally to elective, urgent, and emergency eye operations. Today, this has changed; the patient's age or systemic disease status remains a factor, but at a much lower level of importance in surgical decisions. Now, elective surgical procedures are common in patients who are renal transplant recipients, those who have end-stage renal disease, and in those who require dialysis. Patients with the severest and most fragile forms of insulin-dependent diabetes mellitus (IDDM) are operated upon frequently.

The principal reasons for this change are the low mortality and low morbidity figures that have resulted from improved general anesthesia and local anesthetic techniques. The primary improvement in the use of local anesthesia for eye procedures has been the development of longer acting infiltrative anesthetics that do not require supplemental use of epinephrine compounds to achieve satisfactory durations of anesthesia, e.g., bupivicaine (marcaine). The standard local anesthetic agents used at this time for eye procedures consist of 0.75% marcaine and 2% xylocaine mixed 50:50; to this is added Wydase to facilitate dispersion. Usually a total of 5 cc of this mixture is used for akinesia and 3 cc for retrobulbar anesthesia. There are many variations to this local anesthesia method currently in use in the United States today. With these local anesthetic blocks, one can achieve anesthesia and akinesia of the eye and the periorbital tissues for periods up to 3 hours. Surgical procedures for hypertensive patients and those patients with cardiovascular disease who have a risk of hypertensive crises or severe arrhythmias are no longer cancelled for fear of some impending disaster.

Another factor that positively affects the surgical approach to older patients is the increased longevity and better general health and nutrition of our elderly. Elderly patients have gradually developed a philosophy of responsibility for their own health. In the decade of the 1960s, the average age of a patient needing a cataract extraction for restoration of vision that would enable the patient to be responsible for his or her own hygiene and health care and a degree of independence was 64 to 65. Today the average age of a patient needing cataract extraction for occupational indications or to improve or maintain a desirable lifestyle is 76–78 years of age. Many patients are obviously much older.

Today, surgical procedures on the eye are considered so safe that the Health Care Financing Administration, which develops regulations implemented by Medicare and the Peer Review Organization (PRO), has mandated that all cataract extractions will be done on a same day or on an ambulatory basis. Failure to "comply" or failure to obtain prior approval for hospitalization for such procedures results in nonpayment of covered services by the Medicare carriers. In our community, a full 90% of patients with cataracts have their surgical procedures done on an ambulatory basis; at the same time, there are many situations in which patients in a tertiary care facility, such as the Vanderbilt University Medical Center (VUMC), will require hospitalization for cataract and/or other surgical procedures on the eye. These include renal transplant recipients who are on immuno-suppressant drugs, those who have brittle diabetes, patients on chronic or acute renal dialysis, and other patients with similar severe, disabling, systemic medical conditions. In spite of many systemic diseases, advancing age, and ever-increasing financial and social pressures, the elderly patient continues to deserve our special efforts to maintain the valuable sense of sight.

SURGICAL PROCEDURES OF THE ANTERIOR SEGMENT OF THE EYE IN THE ELDERLY

Surgical Diseases of the Eyelid

Chalazion is a pyogenic granuloma that forms in the meibomian glands of the eyelid. It is an infectious process within the tarsus of the upper and lower eyelids and is caused by the obstruction and subsequent infection of the meibomian gland openings. It is not necessarily age related and can be treated successfully by surgical means if conservative medical therapy fails.

Essential blepharospasm is a morbid and disabling condition characterized by involuntary spasms of the orbicularis muscle in the periorbital area. It occurs principally in the population over age 50, and it is usually bilateral.

The cause of blepharospasm is unknown and may be functional, or it may be the result of repetitive involuntary discharges from the higher cortical centers of the central nervous system. When ocular, psychological, and neurologic causes have been ruled out and conservative treatment regimens of muscle relaxants, neurologic drugs, or facial nerve blocks have failed, invasive surgical intervention is then indicated. Many surgical procedures are used; they include differential section of the seventh cranial nerve, total avulsion of the roots of the seventh nerve where it exits in the preauricular area, and the coronal flap method for extirpation of segments of the orbicularis muscle. Each of these techniques is associated with considerable complications and, even in the best surgeon's hands, with variable results. The 5-year success rate for all of these operations is less than 50% in eliminating the condition for which the procedure was done (1, 2).

Ectropion may be cicatricial and non-cicatricial. The non-cicatricial form (senile) is the most common lid condition that occurs in the elderly and with few exceptions occurs universally on the lower lids. It is caused by an excessive horizontal length of the tarsal plate. It occurs as an eversion of the lid mainly during sleep or at the time of tight lid closure.

The correction is nearly always surgical and may be performed on an ambulatory basis. The most common method of correction is the Kuhnt-Szymanowski procedure or one of its modifications (2). A neglected ectropion of the lower lid results in a chronic blepharo-conjunctivitis, constant tearing requiring an ever-present handful of Kleenex or some other absorbent material, drying and keratinization of the usually moist palpebral conjunctival mucous membranes, and eventual corneal ulceration (exposure keratitis). This last complication occurs because of chronic exposure to air and drying of the lower third of the cornea during sleep, and it may result in corneal perforations and loss of the eye.

Occasionally an elderly person will develop an ectropion that involves only the punctum of the lower lid (nasal one-third of the lower lid). The rotation of the punctum away from the lacrimal lake results in epiphora. The surgical correction requires a different approach than does the senile ectropion procedures. The usual methods for this condition are the "Lazy T" procedure described by Byron Smith and the Z-T plasty, which is basically a modification of the "Lazy T" procedure. Another method used for correction of medial ectropion is effected by use of the medial canthal ligament for suture plication. All of these procedures turn the eyelid back to a near normal postion.

Cicatricial ectropion is caused by secondary scarring of the lids following trauma, infection, irradiation, tumor, or previous eyelid procedures. Removal of all the scar tissue and replacing the skin by the use of grafting procedures are usually required.

Surgical Treatment of Glaucoma

Glaucoma is a blinding eye disease that is progressive, insidious, and relentless. There are many forms of glaucoma, and all forms tend to be most severe in the elderly.

For convenience of discussion and for therapeutic reasons glaucoma is divided into narrow angle and open angle types. This is an anatomic classification that is based on the width of the anterior chamber angle, which is measured with a gonioscopic contact lens examination. There are many secondary types of glaucoma under the above primary types, and on occasion, some patients suffer from a combination of both primary narrow angle and open angle glaucoma.

The most common type of glaucoma in the elderly is the primary chronic open angle glaucoma. The onset of this type of glaucoma is very insidious; the patient is almost totally asymptomatic until it is far advanced. It affects 2% of all patients aged 40 years and over and fully 8%–10% of all patients who have insulin-dependent diabetes mellitus (3). It is a genetically inherited disease with autosomal recessive transmission. It has a multifactorial inheritance pattern as judged by human lymphocytic antigen (HLA) studies and family studies done by using topical corticosteroid responsiveness (4–6).

Primary open angle glaucoma (POAG) is principally a medically treatable, chronic, incurable disease. The principal methods of medical treatment are topical drops with beta-blocker, epinephrine compounds, various miotics, and acetylcholinesterase inhibitors, along with a variety of orally administered carbonic anhydrase inhibitors. Unfortunately, each and every one of these medications can cause multiple and predictable side effects in a significant percentage of elderly patients. When this occurs, one needs to compare the risk-to-benefit ratio of such medical therapy to alternative surgical procedures.

The indications for the surgical correction of patients with POAG are those of progression of the disease as judged by repeated visual field examinations. These progressive changes can be measured also by the volume of pathologic cupping of the optic nerve. This progression must be documented to exist when the patient is compliant and using maximum *tolerated* medical therapy. This medical therapy includes the combined use of a beta-blocker, miotic, and adrenalin compound topical and a carbonic anhydrase inhibitor orally, e.g., Diamox.

At this stage, a patient with significant changes from POAG will need to be evaluated for some surgical procedures.

Non-Invasive Surgical Procedures for Glaucoma

Argon laser trabeculoplasty (ALTP) was popularized and evaluated by James Wise of Oklahoma City, Oklahoma, as a non-invasive ambulatory procedure. It has high efficacy with few complications and with relatively few side effects (7, 8). It is now the procedure of choice for a patient who has progressive POAG in spite of maximum tolerated medical therapy. It consists of placing 50 micron argon laser burns through a slit lamp delivery system with the use of a gonioscopic contact lens along the anterior border of the trabecular pigment band in the anterior chamber angle. The mechanism of action by which intraocular pressure is lowered is thought to be an increase in the rigidity of the wall of the trabecular spaces, which increases the size of the porous outflow channels. Approximately 140 individual spot burns are placed and evenly distributed throughout the 360° circumference of each eye for optimal therapy. According to most studies and in our experience, this produces a predictable lowering of the intraocular pressure (IOP) by 8–12 mm Hg in 85% of eyes, no change in pressure in 12% of eyes, and in 3% of eyes the pressure may be increased slightly (7–10).

The beneficial effect of argon laser trabeculoplasty (ALTP) on POAG has been shown in clinical studies to last an average of 5 years. Repeat ALTP above the optimal amount stated is of questionable value.

The complications include synechia formation from the peripheral iris to the cornea in areas of the burns, short-term corneal abrasion from the contact lens, mild inflammation (iritis), and a short-term increase of intraocular pressure to high levels (for 24–48 hours).

Laser iridotomy may be done with either the YAG or argon laser or by a combination of the two. Not every YAG laser has a thermal mode to control microscopic hemorrhage during the performance of a laser iridotomy. Laser iridotomy is the treatment of choice in any patient with acute or potential angle closure glaucoma. This technique has permitted the surgeon to avoid the many complications previously seen with surgical (invasive) peripheral iridectomy, which was the treatment of choice prior to the development of laser techniques (11, 12).

Cyclocryotherapy is also a non-invasive method used to destroy or ablate the ciliary body by freezing the tissue. A cryoprobe is centered approximately 3 mm posterior to the limbus, and applications are made for 50 to 60 seconds after the probe tip temperature reaches −79 °C. This results in some pain and discomfort postoperatively and requires lid akinesia and retrobulbar anesthesia for the procedure. It is indicated in various far advanced and difficult cases, in cases of chronic open angle and angle closure types of glaucoma, or when a combination of the two types exists that has failed to respond to the usual conventional medical and surgical procedures (13–15).

Argon laser of ciliary processes is also used to destroy ciliary body (CB) processes by a physical, rather than a chemical, method. The problem so far has been in the ability to focus the laser beam optically onto the CB processes because of the difficulty, even with the maximally dilated pupil, of visualizing the CB processes. They remain hidden from view even when all the various mirrored contact lens currently available are used. Under special conditions (e.g., a patient with a full iridectomy) this technique has a place in the overall management of difficult cases. It also has the appeal of being a noninvasive method. Another term for this procedure is "transpupillary argon cyclophotocoagulation" (16, 17). This method has largely fallen into disuse, but may be a modality to use in special circumstances.

Neodynium: YAG cyclophotocoagulation is another technique to destroy the ciliary body noninvasively when aqueous humor is produced. It requires use of a long-pulse YAG laser, which is used in the thermal mode. It is applied on the surface of the sclera 3 mm posterior to the limbus at 32 spots circumferentially 360°. In contrast to the transpupillary argon cyclophotocoagulation method, this technique may be used to destroy the ciliary body without dilatation of the pupil and even in the presence of corneal scarring or in the face of a dense cataract. This method is still under investigation, and there has been insufficient experience with it to determine its true role in the overall approach to the treatment of glaucoma by non-invasive methods. Certainly at the present time it is much more expensive to perform than cyclocryotherapy, which accomplishes the same result with less cost and less sophisticated technology (18).

Therapeutic transcleral ultrasound oblation of the ciliary body is another expensive high-tech method that makes use of sophisticated instrumentation to destroy ciliary processes of the eye where the aqueous is produced. Therefore, it is similar to cyclocryothermy, but utilizes a different physical method to accomplish the destruction of tissue that produces aqueous humor in the eye. The clinical efficacy of this method has not been ascertained. It does have the advantage of being non-invasive and can be used when the media of the eye is opaque, e.g., with dense cataract or corneal scarring. It is applied with an appropriate ultrasound probe transsclerally. In 1986, the instrument used for this procedure cost $65,000 (19).

All of the above procedures may be complicated by uveitis, hypotomy, blindness, transient but rapid and very high rise in the intraocular pressure, phthisis bulbi, flat anterior chamber, and/or vitreous, choroidal detachment, cystoid macular edema of the retina, and scleral thinning. The transpupillary argon cyclophotocoagulation technique is probably associated with the fewest complications of all the procedures, but it also has the most limited clinical indications and the least effectiveness.

Invasive Surgical Procedures for Glaucoma

Cyclodiathermy has largely been abandoned, but at one time was principally indicated for treatment of glaucoma in patients who had had previous cataract extraction. The procedure consists of reflecting a conjunctival flap in one quadrant of the eye to expose the bare sclera. Then, fine penetrating diathermy needles are passed through the sclera into the ciliary body. The appropriate amount of radiofrequency diathermy is applied to destroy the ciliary body. Multiple puncture sites are required and must be made under sterile operating room conditions. It has largely fallen into disuse, but may still be useful in rare selected cases or in underdeveloped countries (20, 21).

Trabeculectomy is the most popular, widely used method for the treatment of medically uncontrolled glaucoma. It creates an opening and pathway for aqueous humor to drain from the anterior chamber to an area beneath the conjunctiva (filtering bleb). All procedures of this type are called filtering procedures.

The goal of *filtering procedures* is to create

a pathway for the aqueous humor to flow from the anterior chamber into the subconjunctival and sub-Tenon's spaces. In the past, this path was created by burning, trephining, or punching a hole through the full thickness of the sclera. The advantage of such procedures is that they allow rapid and constantly maintained lowering of the intraocular pressure. The disadvantage is that they may lower the pressure too much and result in hypotomy, flat anterior chamber, and cataract. In more recent years, the trabeculectomy operation has become popular because it serves all the desired filtering activities while leaving a partial thickness of sclera as a residual tissue to restrain the aqueous outflow. For this reason, although its pressure-lowering activity is less than a full-thickness filter, it has significantly reduced the surgical complication rate, especially late-onset bacterial endophthalmitis.

The trabeculectomy procedure consists of reflecting an outer scleral flap, which is reflected over the cornea under a conjunctival flap. Then an inner scleral flap that is usually rectangular in shape is mobilized and excised and includes a 3 mm arc of trabecular meshwork anterior to the scleral spur. The outer scleral flap is then resutured at the posterior corners with fine sutures, and the conjunctival mucous membrane is resutured in its normal anatomic position. Aqueous humor then flows from the anterior chamber, through the opening in the excised inner scleral flap, through the three sides of the rectangle of the outer scleral flap that covers the "trap door" to be absorbed beneath the conjunctiva. A "filtering bleb" is then formed. Other glaucoma-filtering procedures are based on the same basic principles and tenents just described. Each of the alternative methods has it advocates. These methods include the sclera iridectomy with scleral lip cautery, trephination procedures, iridencleisis, and posterior lip or anterior lip scleral punch procedures (22).

In difficult and resistant cases of glaucoma, filtrating procedures utilizing setons, implants, or valves may be necessary. Several ophthalmic centers in the United States are using alloplastic materials fabricated to create permanent lumens or canals for aqueous humor to drain out of the anterior chamber to beneath the conjunctiva. These setons are sutured in place. They have limited usefulness, and many complications are associated with their use. Their failure rate is high because the lumen in the silicone tubing obstructs easily and frequently. The two principal implants in current use are the Denver-Krupin valve and the Malteno implant (23–25).

Several invasive filtering procedures used in congenital glaucoma but not indicated in the treatment of glaucoma in the elderly are goniotomy, goniopuncture, and trabeculotomy.

Another invasive filtering procedure that was frequently used during the 1930s, 1940s, and 1950s but since discarded is the cyclodialysis procedure. This is an internal, rather than an external, filtration procedure used in glaucoma occurring in aphakia (patients with previous cataract extraction) (26).

Surgical Treatment of Cataract

A cataract is any opacity in the lens. Although cataracts may be classified as to time of development (congenital or age related) or as to anatomic location within the lens (cortical or nuclear), it is most effective to classify cataracts as to whether or not they influence vision. There are many cataracts that do not interfere with visual function and do not require extraction; in others, the clinical judgement of the surgeon is needed to determine if the visual impairment is enough to warrant the associated surgical risks. In such a situation, the surgeon needs to ask two major questions. The first is whether the patient's functional ability is reduced by the cataract to a level that satisfies the risk-to-benefit ratio. The second is whether or not the visual function can be sufficiently improved by the operation. In dealing with an elderly population, this latter question becomes more important. The coexistence of cataract with glaucoma and retinal degeneration becomes more common with increasing age. A successful cataract operation is of no value to a patient who has a coexisting disorder that prohibits visual improvement. The evaluation of the visual potential of an eye in the presence of a cataract may be extremely difficult. In such a situation, a series of tests to evaluate physiologic responses may be needed. Such tests will allow one to establish the percentage of visual impairment caused by coexisting optic nerve disease, glaucoma, retinal degeneration, and cataract. It is only with this knowledge that one can determine if the planned procedure will offer enough benefit to overcome the surgical risks.

Cataract Extraction Procedures

The cataract operations to restore visual acuity have become highly skilled and safe invasive procedures at the current state-of-the-art level. These procedures are usually divided into two distinct types: intra-capsular cataract extraction (ICCE) and extra-capsular cataract extraction (ECCE). Engineering achievements in the past 20 years have made ECCE a procedure with a high success rate, a low complication rate, and such superb technical control that over 95% of all cataract extractions in the United States are now of this variety.

The extra-capsular operation involves the removal of the lens nucleus and cortex through an opening in the anterior lens capsule. This leaves the posterior capsule in place, which eliminates complications associated with vitreous adherence to the iris, cornea, and incision. It also provides for fixation of an artificial intraocular lens if the surgeon plans to add that step to the operation. The posterior capsule acts as a barrier to the exchange of molecules between aqueous and vitreous; studies have suggested that this will lower the incidence of macular edema, retinal detachment, and corneal edema.

Extra-capsular extraction is best performed in the presence of a dilated pupil. An anterior capsulotomy less than 7 mm wide is performed. At the same time, the anterior chamber is kept from collapsing by the infusion of a visco-elastic substance, such as sodium hyaluronate. The lens nucleus can be removed manually or emulsified through an incision of 3 mm in length. Successful extra-capsular extraction requires the use of an operating microscope with co-axial illumination. With the use of recent technical refinements, the procedure can be performed under local anesthesia in an ambulatory surgical center in less than 1 hour of operating room time.

The most common problem of extracapsular extraction is late opacification of the residual posterior capsule. This is reported to occur in more than 25% of cases within 1–3 years. However, the YAG laser can be used to manage the opacified posterior capsule without repeated surgical invasion of the eye. The YAG laser shock wave, produced by optical breakdown, results in a predictable and controlled disruption of the opaque posterior capsule.

Posterior Chamber Lens Implantation Technique

This commonly used technique of extracapsular cataract extraction allows for posterior chamber lens implantation. The posterior chamber lens has developed with time and modification into a very safe and effective device for use in humans. There are countless models and styles, all of which are equivalent in safety and effectiveness. The procedure, which is performed always under an operating microscope, consists of elevating a conjunctival flap in the superior 180° of the eye. A small incision is made to introduce a bent 25-gauge needle attached to a continuous irrigating cannula. The needle is used to perform a circular 6.5–7.0 mm diameter anterior capsulotomy in "can-opener" style. The irrigation solution contains "balanced salt solution" with added glutathione and 0.5 cc of 1:1000 aqueous solution of adrenalin per 500 cc of finished irrigating solution. The adrenalin is vital to maintaining the dilatations of the pupil during the procedure. After the anterior capsulotomy is completed the cornea-scleral incision is enlarged to 11.5 mm in length (chord tangent of a circle). The nucleus of the lens is then delivered after installation of Healon (sodium hyaluronate) to protect the corneal endothelium (posterior layer of cornea). The nucleus is usually delivered by pressure on the globe inferiorly at the limbus and counterpressure superiorly on the globe 4 mm posteriorly to the corneal-scleral incision.

There are four stages or elements to the planned extra-capsular cataract extraction and posterior chamber lens implant: (1) the anterior capsulotomy, (2) the delivery of the nucleus of the lens, (3) the clean-up of the cortex of the lens, and (4) implantation of the posterior chamber lens.

Following delivery of the nucleus, the cortical clean-up can be done with either automated or manual techniques. At our institution, we favor the automated technique for irrigation and aspiration of the residual lens material that remains after delivery of the nucleus of the lens. With the automated technique, almost 100% of the residual lens cortex fibers can be removed. The irrigation solution attached to the irrigation-aspiration unit is the same one used for the anterior capsulotomy.

After completion of the cortical lens clean-up, the posterior capsular bag that is left behind is distended with Healon. This distension of the bag creates a "cocoon" or pocket into which the posterior chamber lens is inserted. When in the bag, the new artificial lens floats inside the eye. One of the reasons the posterior chamber lens has been so well tolerated by human eye tissues is that it does not touch or attach to any moving part of the eye, e.g., the iris.

Approximately 1 to 3 years following a planned extra-capsular cataract extraction and posterior chamber lens implant some 25% of patients will experience reduction of visual acuity that is due to clouding of the posterior capsular membrane. This is easily diagnosed by the ophthalmologist, and the vision can be restored by a simple, safe, effective non-invasive method. It is for this indication that a YAG laser is used as a "cold knife" to cut through the posterior capsule membrane and create a new opening to allow for clear vision. A YAG ABRAHAM contact lens applied to the eye facilitates the procedure (28).

Anterior Chamber Lens Implantation

Because of late postoperative complications, the anterior chamber lens is used almost exclusively today for back-up purposes. In 5% of cases, it is technically impossible to remove all of the cortical lens material without rupturing the posterior capsule. In these situations, if the patient wants an intra-ocular lens implant, it has to be of the anterior chamber lens style, which fits anterior to the iris. This is because with rupture of the posterior capsule there is no support for the posterior chamber lens implant. Complications that occur late after anterior chamber lens implant include hyphema, glaucoma, loss of clarity of the cornea (corneal edema), and uveitis (sterile inflammation of the eye).

The incidence of post-cataract extraction bacterial endophthalmitis is now only one case per thousand operations. This is a low incidence, but this complication destroys all useful vision in over 50% of the cases.

With the current highly skilled and refined cataract extraction procedure described an elderly patient can reasonably expect better vision after the operation in more than 95% of the cases.

If the vision is not better after the procedure, it is almost always because there is some underlying retinal pathology (macular degeneration) (27).

Other Cataract Procedures

There are occasional instances when the older standard procedure of intra-capsular cataract extraction might be the procedure of choice. In this technique all the lens is removed with a cryoextractor after the zonules are lyzed with alpha-chymotrypsin (29).

There are other instances where a retinal surgeon may remove a cataract during a vitrectomy procedure through the pars plana of the eye. This is called a pars plana vitrectomy-lensectomy procedure.

Some surgeons still prefer using the Kelman phacoemulsification technique for removal of the lens nucleus and cortex. It has however largely fallen into disfavor, although it was very popular in the late 1960s and 1970s. There are rare instances where a secondary anterior or posterior chamber lens implant is performed. A secondary lens implant procedure is one in which there is an interval of 6-8 months to years between the cataract extraction and the lens implant procedure (29).

Also in selected rare instances an intra-ocular lens implant may be exchanged for another one. This is called a lens exchange procedure.

Surgical Correction of Corneal Conditions

Certain corneal procedures are performed in the elderly. The most common of these is the penetrating keratoplasty procedure (PKP). This procedure needs to be differentiated from a lamellar keratoplasty where only a partial thickness corneal transplant is done.

The most common sizes for a penetrating keratoplasty are an 8.0 mm donor into a 7.5 mm diameter recipient bed. Also a 8.5 mm donor into an 8.0 mm diameter host cornea is common.

The main indication for PKP is to restore visual acuity. This decrease in visual acuity is usually a result of corneal scarring or edema or a combination of the two. If this opacification of the cornea cannot be corrected by medical or a simpler surgical operation then PKP is indicated. The diseases that result in opacification and vascularization of the cornea and that are amenable to surgical correction by PKP are herpes keratitis, corneal dystrophies, keratoconus, trauma, aphakic and pseudophakic bullous keratopathy, and corneal degenerations.

The PKP procedure is always done under the operating microscope, and the most common suture is a 10–0 monofilament nylon. After trephination of the diseased corneal button from the recipient, the new donor button is sutured onto the host. The donor button is placed on a bed of Healon during the suturing. This protects the vital layer of donor corneal endothelium from damage caused by rubbing the iris or cornea of the host. At one time a 360° continuous running suture was favored to anchor the donor to the host cornea. More recently, surgeons are returning to the use of 16–24 direct radial sutures. By cutting the sutures at selected times during the postoperative period, the development and prevention of corneal astigmastism can be regulated during the postoperative period. All knots are buried in the corneal tissue so they will not irritate the upper lids and the patient will be more comfortable. Overall, the PKP procedure has about a 90% chance of success as judged by an optically clear and functioning donor cornea. Approximately 75% of these patients will obtain a Snellen visual acuity of 20/40 or better (30).

When a PKP is combined with a planned ECCE and posterior chamber lens implant it is called a triple procedure (31). Sometimes a trabeculectomy is performed for control of glaucoma with either or both of the PKP and cataract procedures (32, 33).

Another corneal procedure done in the elderly as an alternative to a secondary lens implant is a procedure called epikeratophakia (EKP). The main indications for this procedure in the elderly is for patients who do not like or tolerate thick cataract glasses or contact lenses and in whom a secondary intraocular lens implant procedure is contraindicated.

In this situation a donor-lyophilized human donor lenticule is sutured on top of the patient's cornea. This "donor lenticule" is of a precise optical power for the recipient patient, although the recipient will need a spectacle lens to refine his or her vision at distance, as well as a bifocal for reading at near distances.

Some people have referred to this EKP as having a "living contact lens" sutured onto the eye. This is not quite correct because the human corneal tissue is allostatic and not allovital. Many patients who have had this procedure performed for adult aphakia have obtained a good visual result with Snellen visual acuity in the 20/30–20/40 range (34).

DISORDERS AND SURGICAL TREATMENT OF THE POSTERIOR EYE IN THE OLDER PATIENT

Surgical Procedures of the Vitreous

Vitreous procedures are necessary for many different eye disorders. In the older population, these procedures are most often used to remove vitreous opacities that are not clearing on their own. The majority of such situations are caused by vitreous hemorrhages secondary to diabetes mellitus. In most individuals, there is a history of insulin-dependent diabetes mellitus for over 20 years before the diabetic retinopathy progresses to a level that can produce such hemorrhage (35).

The general principles of such procedures have become well established in the past decade. In most situations, a closed system to maintain the ocular volume is required; this prevents the collapse of the globe and anatomic distortion. Such an operation is performed usually by penetrating the eye at the level of the pars plana. Several microscopic instruments can be inserted into the eye through this region while infusing an optically clear solution into the eye to maintain the ocular volume. At the same time, the opaque vitreous gel can be removed by dissection under the microscope. Current surgical techniques use instruments that are less than 1.5 mm in diameter and that are designed to cut vitreous free from attachments and remove it from the eye. In addition, bleeding sites within the eye can be coagulated, and retinal breaks may be identified and closed. Current research is evaluating the use of artificial agents, such as gases and silicone oil, in the vitreous cavity. The gas-fluid interface, or the silicone oil-fluid interface, has a surface tension that can close temporarily retinal breaks to prevent retinal detachment. In this manner, the surgeon has time to use additional intraocular instruments to create a permanent repair of the retina.

In recent years, refinements in surgical techniques have improved visualization of the intraocular contents during the operation. In many situations, fibrous bands across the vitreous and along the retinal surfaces can be identified and removed by microscopic dissection. With the removal of such bands, the opaque vitreous can be cleared, and the distortion of the retinal surface corrected, to result in better postoperative vision (36).

Retinal Detachment

There are many different kinds of retinal detachments. The variety that occurs most often in the older population, and for which corrective procedures are of greatest benefit, is the rhegmatogenous retinal detachment. This term is derived from the Greek word "rhegma," which means "a break"; this type of retinal detachment is characterized by a break in the continuity of retina that allows fluid vitreous to pass into the sub-retinal space. The surgical correction of this disorder is devoted to the closure of such a break.

Over one-third of all patients who are operated upon for retinal detachment repair are in the decade between 60 and 70 years of age; in addition, more than half of all such patients are over 60 years of age. Sixty percent of such problems occur in male patients; this high incidence is thought to represent a preexisting history of trauma. Many patients appear to have a predilection for this disorder; almost 20% of individuals who have a detachment in one eye will develop a detachment in the fellow eye at some future time. Over one-third of retinal detachments occur in individuals who have had some other type of previous eye operation. Newer techniques of cataract extractions are thought to reduce this association; however, a statistically valid study has not proven this reduction yet (37).

The concept that a retinal break causes a retinal detachment was emphasized first by the work of Jules Gonin (38). However, it was not until the development of the binocular stereoscopic indirect ophthalmoscope and methods for microscopic evaluation of the human retinal surface in vivo that this observation could be extended into clinical practice. Now, each of the breaks in the detached retina can be identified before initiating surgical correction. A surgical technique that produces closure of the breaks in the retina will allow the retina to re-attach itself. Although the retinal pigment epithelium will remove the fluid remaining in the sub-retinal space, surgical techniques to enhance this activity are used in many cases. Various means of creating an inflammatory response surrounding the retinal break, such as diathermy, cryotherapy, and photocoagulation, can result in a scar that seals the defect and results in a permanent re-attachment (39).

Age-Related Macular Degeneration

Age-related macular degeneration is one of the major causes of new blindness in the United States. Of all varieties of new blindness reported each year in the United States, 14 percent can be accounted for by this disorder (40).

Age-related macular degeneration is believed to originate from pre-existing disorders of the retinal pigment epithelium. These start out as small retinal pigment epithelial detachments and drusen. With time, these progress to develop three additional problems: areas of geographic atrophy of the retinal pigment epithelium, serous fluid detachments of the retinal pigment epithelium, and choroidal neovascularization growing under the retina. Several independent studies indicate that the majority of individuals who become blind from age-related macular degeneration do so from the neovascular variety (41–43). It is estimated that more than 90% of the individuals who become legally blind from age-related macular degeneration have choriodal neovascular changes associated with it.

Several epidemiologic studies have demonstrated important features associated with the blinding changes of age-related macular degeneration. This disorder reaches its peak of influence in the decade between age 75 and 85; almost a third of individuals within this age range have some manifestation of this disorder, but only a few progress to blindness (41). There does not appear to be a sex predilection for this problem (44, 45). Although epidemiologic surveys have failed to show a difference between racial groups, several studies have reported that decreased pigmentation of the eye, such as reduced iris color, and chronic photic exposure are associated with an increased risk of blindness (42).

Surgical procedures to prevent this visual loss have been proven to be of benefit in select cases. A nationwide treatment trial has found that many eyes can maintain vision by use of laser photocoagulation; although visual improvement is not achieved in all cases, the prevention of additional visual loss is of great significance (46). The nationwide trial, however, was limited to eyes that had choroidal neovascular membranes greater than 200 microns from the center of the fovea and had visual acuities better than 20/100. In the trial, treatment consisted of bichromatic argon blue-green laser lesions of 200 microns each, placed in a contiguous manner, and extending more than 125 microns beyond the edge of the neovascular membrane. This treatment resulted in complete obliteration of the neovascular complex. In all patients in this study, untreated eyes were twice as likely to have progressive visual loss as were the treated eyes.

Although the beneficial effect of such treatment was documented by this research, this was only demonstrated in eyes meeting the study's select criteria. For eyes that have other aspects of age-related macular degeneration, treatment may be of value, but a detailed risk to benefit analysis is not available. In addition, photocoagulation using other types of lasers, such as monochromatic argon-green, krypton-red, or other wave lengths, needs to be evaluated.

Malignant Melanoma of the Choroid

The malignant melanoma of the choroid is the most common malignancy of the eye. In the United States, it is found at a frequency of 1 new case per 200,000 population each year. Although the average age of a patient with such a tumor is in the sixth decade, the peak incidence of this tumor is at age 70 (47).

The size of a choroidal melanoma is the single most important criterion for making a judgment regarding therapy. Lesions measuring less than 2 mm in thickness, with a base diameter of under 10 mm, are difficult to differentiate in a clinical manner from benign lesions in this area. For this reason, these are usually followed carefully to demonstrate growth before any form of therapy is recommended. It has been found that there is a critical threshold of tumor size; when the total volume of such a tumor is greater than 1400 cubic mm, there is a great risk of metastatic disease. It is estimated that the typical choroidal melanoma has a slow growth pattern and takes almost 5 years to double in volume. For this reason, it is safe, in most cases, to follow suspicious lesions before recommending any form of intervention. The prognosis for this tumor is related to the tumor size and cell type. For tumors less than 10 mm in greatest diameter that contain predominantly spindle cells, there is a 95% survival rate for 5 years or more. With an increase in the percent of epithelioid cells in the tumor, the survival rate drops to 80%. The larger the tumor and the greater frequency of epithelioid cells within the tumor the poorer the survival. The cytologic finding of 5% or more cells with the epithelioid cell type implies a poor prognosis (47).

For centuries, surgeons have believed that removing a cancer can prolong the life expectancy of the patient. Controversy regarding this concept was produced in 1979 by reports that the standard surgical procedure of enucleation may increase mortality by promoting metastasis (48). Although this controversy has not been resolved completely, this has prompted research in the treatment techniques that do not require enucleation of the eye. Current research compares radiation treatment to enucleation; one project, the Collaborative Ocular Melanoma Study involves over 30 major eye centers throughout the United States. Preliminary reports from similar studies have not demonstrated which therapy is best (49, 50).

REFERENCES

1. Wesley RE: Coronal flap in treatment of blepharospasm. In: *Techniques in Ophthalmic Plastic Surgery.* New York, John Wiley, 1986, pp 413–416.
2. Leone CR Jr: Plastic surgery. In Spaeth GL (ed): *Ophthalmic Surgery: Principles and Practice.* Philadelphia, WB Saunders Co, 1982, pp 547–652.
3. Epstein DL: Primary open angle glaucoma. In: *Chandler and Grant's Glaucoma,* ed 3. Philadelphia, Lea & Febiger, 1986, pp 129–180.
4. Becker B: The genetic problem of chronic simple glaucoma. *Ann Ophthalmol* 3:351, 1971.
5. Damgaard-Jensen L, Kissmeyer-Nielsen F: HLA histocompatibility antigens in open-angle glaucoma. *Acta Ophthalmol* (Copen) 56:384–388, 1978.
6. Ritch R, Podos SM, Henley W, Moss A, Southern AL, Fotino M: Lack of association of histocompatibility antigens with primary open angle glaucoma. *Arch Ophthalmol* 96:2204–2006, 1978.

7. Wise JB, Witter SL: Argon laser therapy for open angle glaucoma, a pilot study. *Arch Ophthalmol* 97:319–322, 1979.

8. Wise JB: Long-term control of adult open angle glaucoma by argon laser treatment. *Ophthalmology* 88:197–202, 1981.

9. Wilensky JT, Lampol LM: Laser therapy for open angle glaucoma. *Ophthalmology* 88:213–217, 1981.

10. Schwartz AL, Whitten ME, Bleiman B, Martin D: Argon laser trabecular surgery in uncontrolled phakic open angle glaucoma. *Ophthalmology* 88:203–212, 1981.

11. Moster MR, Schwartz LW, Spaeth GL, Wilson RP, McAllister JA, Poryzees EM: Laser iridectomy, a controlled study comparing argon and Neodynium:YAG. *Ophthalmology* 93:20–24, 1986.

12. Robin AL, Pollack IP: A comparison of Neodynium:YAG and argon laser iridotomies. *Ophthalmology* 91:1011–1016, 1984.

13. Bellows AR, Grant WM: Cyclocryotherapy in advanced inadequately-treated glaucoma. *Am J Ophthalmol* 75:679–684, 1973.

14. DeRoetth A Jr: Cryosurgery for the treatment of advanced chronic simple glaucoma. *Am J Ophthalmol* 66:1034–1041, 1968.

15. Burton TC: Cyclocryotherapy. In: *Current Concepts in Ophthalmology.* St. Louis, CV Mosby, Co, 1974.

16. Zimmerman TJ, Worthen DM, Wickham G: Argon laser photocoagulation of ciliary process and pigmented pupillary membrane in man. *Invest Ophthalmol* 12:622–623, 1973.

17. Lee PF: Argon laser photocoagulation of the ciliary processes in cases of aphakic glaucoma. *Arch Ophthalmol* 97:2135–2138, 1979.

18. Klapper RM, Wandel T, Donnenfeld ED: Neodynium:YAG laser by clocoagulation in treatment of glaucoma. *Ophthalmology* 93:80, 1986.

19. Burgess SE, Silverman RH, Coleman DJ, Yablonski ME, Lizzi FL, Driller J, Rosado A, Dennis PH: Treatment of glaucoma with high-intensity focused ultrasound. *Ophthalmology* 93:831–838, 1986.

20. Stocker FW: Response of chronic simple glaucoma to treatment with cyclodiathermy puncture. *Arch Ophthalmol* 34:181, 1985.

21. Walton DS, Grand WM: Penetrating cyclodiathermy for filtration. *Arch Ophthalmol* 83:47, 1970.

22. Shields MB: *Textbook of Glaucoma,* ed 2. Baltimore, Williams & Wilkins, 1987.

23. Krupin T, Kaufman P, Mandell A, Ritch R, Asseff C, Podos SM, Becker B: Filtering valve implant surgery for eyes with neovascular glaucoma. *Am J Ophthalmol* 89:338–343, 1980.

24. Krupin T, Kaufman P, Mandell AI, Terry SA, Ritch R, Podos SM, Becker B: Long term results of valve implants in filtering surgery for eyes with neovascular glaucoma. *Am J Ophthalmol* 95:775–782, 1983.

25. Cairns JE: The Molteno long-tube implant. *Trans Ophthalmol Soc UK* 103:39–41, 1983.

26. O'Brien CS, Weih J: Cyclodialysis. *Arch Ophthalmol* 42:606, 1949.

27. Stark WJ, Worthen DM, Holladay JJ, Bath PE, Jacobs ME, Murray GC, McGhee ET, Talbott MW, Shipp MD, Thomas NE, Barnes RW, Brown DW, Buxton JN, Reinecke RD, Lao CS, Fisher S: The FDA report on intraocular lenses. *Ophthalmology* 90:311–317, 1983.

28. Stark WJ, Worthen DM, Holladay JJ, Murray G: Neodynium:YAG lasers. *Ophthalmology* 92:209–212, 1985.

29. Jaffe NS: *Cataract Surgery and its Complications,* ed 3. St. Louis, CV Mosby Co, 1981.

30. Brightbill FS: *Corneal Surgery: Theory, Technique, and Tissue.* St. Louis, CV Mosby, 1986.

31. Crawford GJ, Stulting RD, Waring GO III, Van Meter WS, Wilson LA: The triple procedure. Analysis of outcome, refraction, and intraocular lens power calculation. *Ophthalmology* 93:817–824, 1986.

32. Savage JA, Thomas JV, Belcher D, Simmons RJ: Extracapsular cataract extration and posterior chamber intraocular lens implantation in glaucomatous eyes. *Ophthalmology* 92:1506–1516, 1985.

33. Praeger DL: Combined procedure: sub-scleral trabeculectomy with cataract extraction. *Ophthalmic Surg* 14:130–134, 1983.

34. McDonald MB, Koenig SB, Safir A, Friedlander MH, Kaufman HE, Granet N: Epikeratophakia: the surgical correction of aphakia, update, 1982. *Ophthalmology* 90:668–672, 1983.

35. Michels RG: *Vitreous Surgery.* San Francisco, American Academy of Ophthalmology, 1982.

36. Tolentino FI, Freeman HM: Closed vitrectomy in the management of diabetes. *Ophthalomology,* 88:643–646, 1981.

37. Hilton GF, McLean EB, Norton EWD: *Retinal Detachment.* San Francisco, American Academy of Ophthalmology, 1981.

38. Gonin J: Treatment of detached retina. *Arch Ophthalmol* 4:621–625, 1930.

39. Michels RG, Rice TA, Pierce LH, Welch RB, Scott JD: Retinal surgery. In Michels RG, Rice TA, Stark WJ (eds): *Ophthalmic Surgery,* CV Mosby Company, St. Louis, 1984, pp 255–311.

40. *Vision Problems in the United States.* New York, International Society to Prevent Blindness, 1980.

41. Liebowitz HM, Drueger DE, Maunder LR: The Framingham Study Monograph. *Survey Ophthalmol* 24(suppl):335–610, 1980.

42. Hyman LG, Lilienfeld AM, Ferris FL: Macular degeneration: a case controlled study. *Am J Epidemiol* 118:213–227, 1983.

43. Ferris FL, Fine SL; Hyman L: Age related macular degeneration and blindness due to neovascular maculopathy. *Arch Ophthalmol* 102:1640–1642, 1984.

44. Sperduto RD, Seigel D: Senile lens and senile macular changes in a population based sample. *Am J Ophthalmol* 90:86–91, 1980.

45. Klein BE, Klein R: Cataracts and macular degeneration in older Americans. *Arch Ophthalmol* 100:571–573, 1982.

46. Macular Photocoagulation Study Group: Argon laser

photocoagulation for senile macular degeneration. *Arch Ophthalmol* 100:921–918, 1982.

47. Jakobiec SA, Levinson AW: *Choroidal Melanoma: Etiology and Diagnosis, Clinical Modules for Ophthalmologists.* San Francisco, American Academy of Ophthalmology, 1985.

48. Zimmerman LE, McLean IW: Evaluation of enucleation in the management of uveal melanomas. *Am J Ophthalmol* 87:741–760, 1979.

49. Gass JDM: Comparison of prognosis after enucleation versus cobalt-60 radiation of melanomas. *Arch Ophthalmol* 103:916–923, 1985.

50. Gragoudas ES, Goitin M, Verhey L: Proton beam radiation of uveal melanomas: results of 5 year study. *Arch Ophthalmol* 100:928–934, 1982.

Chapter 34

Neurosurgical Diseases in the Aging Patient

William F. Meacham, M.D., F.A.C.S.

Among the many significant changes that have taken place in clinical medicine in the past 20 years has been the altered concept of surgical management of the disorders of the elderly. Prior to this time, there was virtually a routine dismissal of major surgical options for those of advanced years as being "too old for surgery." Strangely enough, a similar conception was present for the very young as many premature infants as well as the elderly were deprived surgical attention by clinical decisions based on age alone without regard to the possibility of success. There is no question that this clinical philosophy was based on the concept that the aged cardiovascular and pulmonary systems could not support the anesthetic/surgical endeavor with predictable success (1).

Along with the other disciplines of surgery, neurologic surgery has gradually adopted a more progressive attitude toward intracranial and intraspinal operations on individuals in the period of life generally regarded as "elderly." Undoubtedly, this has come about as the result of the improved ability to ensure the maintenance of normal physiologic support during the operative procedure, improvement in anesthesia, control of vascular systems, ability to obtain adequate hemostasis, and the availability of impeccable postoperative care. It is also true that contemporary population changes show an increasing number of elders who require the clinical care once given principally to the younger age groups. The predictable life span of the healthy newborn is now 70 plus years, whereas 30 years ago, it was 40!

The neurosurgical disorders occurring in the older age groups differ very little from those in the mature age groups under the age of 65

although the frequency may change significantly as further aging takes place. For example, we see an increase in the problem of metastatic intracranial tumors in the elderly as compared with primary glial tumors and meningioma (2).

This chapter will present the author's philosophy and ideas concerning the clinical problems of the elderly that relate to the nervous system, especially those conditions that may be considered benefitted by a surgical therapeutic attack. It is obvious that there are many situations with the elderly that remain controversial and to which no "recipe" type therapeutic approach can be applied. This leaves many of the critical decisions of the central nervous system to the interest and motivation of the surgeon and to the clinical condition of the patient.

INFLAMMATORY DISEASES OF THE CENTRAL NERVOUS SYSTEM

Probably the most frequently occurring infectious disorder of the central nervous system (CNS) requiring surgical treatment is brain abscess; yet, in modern times this is not a very common lesion in the older age groups. In some measure, this is due to the universal use of antibiotics for all infections. The occasional brain abscess patient in the elderly group has the lesion develop as a contiguous infection from the paranasal sinuses into the frontal lobe area. Some are from a middle ear-mastoid infection and spread into the temporal lobe or the cerebellum. Rarely, multiple brain abscesses will occur as the result of a septic bacteremia. These are almost always fatal unless a prompt and specific response to antibiotic therapy is obtained. The solitary abscess should always be treated with an appropriate antibiotic, particularly in the early phase when meningitis and local cerebritis are present. However, this ideal may be very difficult to obtain in the confused, disoriented, and stuporous senile patient. The diagnosis of brain abscess, once difficult, is now very simple with the use of the computed tomographic (CT) scan, which should be employed in every instance of suspected intracranial pathology in the elderly.

The once popular treatment for brain abscess known as marsupialization is no longer employed because the simple technique of needle tapping and aspiration is generally conducive to cure. Abscesses of the cerebellum most often respond to one or two needle taps, and they do not refill. The frontal and temporal lobe lesions may do likewise, but they are often seen to refill and require numerous taps and occasionally must be totally excised by open craniotomy. We no longer use microbarium as a marker to show refilling of the abscess because the CT scan can give very accurate information, and it should be used repeatedly as necessary for this purpose (3). The purpose of this therapy is not simply to remove purulent material, but to relieve tension within the abscess cavity, which then enables the neo-vascular capsule to further its protective function and the antibiotic to gain access to the infectious wall. This relieves the tension that could lead to rupture into the ventricle or into the subarachnoid space, thereby creating a life-threatening complication.

The response of the elderly patient to successful brain abscess therapy is rewarding if the accompanying cerebritis has not produced a serious neurologic deficit, and full recovery may occur. All patients should be kept on protective antiseizure medication for long periods after the infection has cleared.

Subdural empyema, epidural abscess, and spinal epidural infection are all clinical problems that occur very rarely but that are serious because they threaten survival and are associated with great functional loss following recovery. The diagnosis is made by CT scanning and the appropriate treatment is obvious—surgical evacuation along with appropriate antibiotics systemically. Spinal epidural abscess, usually secondary to furunculosis, requires prompt evacuation

to avoid the permanent paralysis occasioned by ischemic compression of the spinal cord and cauda equina. It is important to remember that a lumbar puncture done for diagnostic or myelographic purposes is hazardous under these conditions; if the needle passes into the subarachnoid space after traversing the epidural abscess a meningitis is ensured. Slow advancement of the needle with constant aspiration during each stage may result in securing purulent material from the epidural space, confirming the diagnosis, and avoiding disastrous results. The scan currently is the fastest and most certain diagnostic maneuver for epidural abscess.

INTRACRANIAL NEOPLASMS

It is unfortunate that the diagnosis of intracranial neoplasm in the elderly is often made at autopsy. The almost habitual tendency to attribute the alterations of consciousness, personality changes, and focal neurologic deficits to cerebrovascular disease or senile dementia in elderly patients is a reflection on clinical practice of earlier times (4). The ease of diagnosis by the use of the enhanced CT scan now places the responsibility on every physician who "assumes" no neoplasm is present. The unpleasant aspects of ventriculopathy, pneumoencephalography, and arteriography are currently no longer valid reasons to delay diagnosis because these procedures have been abandoned in favor of CT scanning, which is painless, brief, and without predictable risk. It is also true that intracranial tumors are more common in the elderly than in the younger are group, although the types may very considerably; the glioblastoma, for instance, diminishing in frequency after age 65 and the meningioma increasing after that age (5). The most common neoplasms in the elderly in our experience have been the metastatic tumor, followed by the malignant primary glioma, and finally the meningioma. The acoustic neuroma and pituitary adenoma occur much less frequently than those listed as commonly occurring.

The aging individual with a metastatic intracranial tumor presents a therapeutic problem of considerable neurosurgical importance. To assume that the problem is hopeless is unwarranted. We have seen useful palliation extending for periods of several years in some patients with tumors, and in others, all therapy was of no value. It is the author's conviction that virtually all metastatic cerebral lesions have an associated area of edema and swelling and patients with these tumors are promptly benefitted by the oral (or subcutaneous) use of dexamethasone. Often, the improvement in symptoms is dramatic, and this gives the clinician and the patient time to consider the advisability of surgical removal of the lesion. If it is solitary and if it is situated in an area where its removal can be accomplished without predictable risk, and where the benefit will result in useful palliation, rather than crippling survival, then craniotomy should be strongly recommended. This attitude assumes that the patient's general systemic situation is appropriate for the surgical attempt and that the primary lesion is not an immediate hazard to survival. For lesions that are located deeply within the hemisphere or in the basal ganglia it is advisable to consider the continued use of steroids and appropriate radiation therapy if possible. The author has not employed the subtotal removal of deep cerebral metastatic lesions by stereotaxic means in the elderly. It is obvious that patients with multiple metastatic foci and those with neoplastic meningitis are treated symptomatically without hope for significant palliation.

The malignant astrocytoma of Grade III and Grade IV classification, although not as common as in the 40–65 year age group, is a frequent neoplasm in the geriatric group. We consider these two gliomas as glioblastoma. Patients of any age with these tumors are considered to be without the likelihood of anything but temporary palliation with the best of therapy. Patients harboring such neoplasms are benefitted with steroid administration and should be considered for resection of the tumor only if the lesion can be removed from the frontal lobe or temporal lobe area. This can usually be done with predictable success without introducing further neurologic deficit (6). Lesions in the corpus callosum, parietal motor area, and dominant hemisphere speech areas should be left alone unless the surgeon wishes to debulk the central tumor mass, leaving the surrounding functional cerebral tissue undisturbed. In our experience radiation therapy has not proven to be of real benefit, nor has the use of chemotherapeutic agents been successful in curing this obstinate tumor.

The meningioma is a benign tumor occupying areas within the calvarium where clusters of arachnoidal granulations occur—parasaggital, sphenoid ridge, olfactory groove, tuberculum sella, convexity, and torcular. In our experience the most common sites for this tumor in the older age groups are the sphenoid, parasagittal, and the pterional areas. Rarely, the meningioma may undergo a sarcomatous change and become highly invasive and virtually incurable. The meningioma is usually a very slow-growing tumor that allows the brain to adapt itself to the encroaching mass that is not invasive and therefore may produce no symptoms of intracranial pressure for a long period of time. Usually, headache and papilledema are not present, and only transient sensory motor symptoms may be described and then dismissed as a transient ischemic attack (7). Strangely, the meningioma often will invade and penetrate the dura, skull, and scalp, but not the underlying brain, which may be only compressed. The diagnosis of meningioma is simplified when one sees a protruding lump on the skull in the parasaggital, temporal, or convexity area. The CT scan study is now an essential study for this condition and should always be employed using the enhanced scanning technique.

In the older person, we no longer utilize the angiogram as a diagnostic tool because the objective is to remove the tumor, but not to endanger the associated major arteries or the dural sinuses. Small areas of tumor may be left if necessary. If this is done and if it is a slowly growing meningioma it will probably not show clinical signs of recurrence in the elderly patient's lifetime. If, however, the tumor can be removed totally without risk to the brain or to the vascular structures it should always be done (8). Convexity meningiomas routinely lend themselves to this endeavor, but the medially placed sphenoid ridge tumor or the tuberculum sella tumor are usually not so situated, and it is here that the surgeon must preserve the associated structures or the patient will suffer severely from crippling neurologic deficits.

In the elderly patient there is also some virture in only following the course of a meningioma. This is true for tumors that have produced few if any symptoms and if the patient is neurologically intact and is willing to cooperate in the frequent periodic follow-up (9). The author has now followed several patients for periods ranging from 4 to 8 years without their showing evidence of significant growth of the mass and without the development of new symptoms. In contradistinction, however, we have had patients with residual tumor show rapid recurrence within a period of 6 to 12 months. Such tumors are almost always of the fibro-angioblastic type. The psammomatous meningioma is virtually always slow and delinquent in its regrowth characteristics. It is appropriate to mention that radiation therapy may have a saluatory effect on meningioma growth activity.

Neoplasms of the posterior fossa are much less common in the elderly than in children and young adults although the acoustic neuroma or eighth nerve tumor is seen with increasing frequency in the older age groups. Beginning as a small tumor within the porous acoustica interna it may cause only annoying symptoms of tinnitus, hearing loss, and vertigo. However, as the tumor progressively enlarges it extends out into the cerebellopontine angle and may then impair the function of cranial nerves V, IX, X, and XI. Further enlargement compresses the lateral cerebellum and pons, and it may then cause obstructive hydrocephalus that jeopardizes survival. In recent years the use of the operating microscope and the use of microsurgical techniques have enabled surgeons to remove these tumors totally with preservation of the facial nerve, although the operative procedure may be lengthy. (See Chapter 12) In those older aged patients who have developed obstructive hydrocephalus from the growth of the acoustic neuroma it is advisable to carry out a ventriculo-peritoneal shunt and to delay the tumor operation until the patient has shown a favorable, stable response from the relief of the increased intracranial pressure. It has been the author's practice to carry out an intracapsular removal of this tumor, leaving the capsule and the seventh nerve intact but removing the capsule from the pontine and posterior surfaces as the tumor is ''gutted'' by piecemeal curettage and suction. This operation can be done easily and with reasonable safety, and it does not subject the elderly patient to a long operative procedure that may endanger facial nerve function. No attempt is made to remove the nodule of tumor within the internal canal of the ear. Similarly, those patients harboring only a small intracanalicular tumor are not subject to any operative procedure, but are followed periodically to determine by repeat scanning whether or not the tumor is enlarging enough to justify its surgical removal (10). This conservative approach to these tumors seems to be appropriate in the elderly. We have had no reason to alter our attitude concerning this approach. On only four occasions in the last 35 years have we had to carry out a secondary surgical tumor removal on older patients who were treated by subtotal excision.

Pituitary Tumors

Pituitary tumors have long been considered a rarity in the older age groups. However, autopsy studies have revealed the fact that pituitary adenomas are very common in the aged (11). A peculiar lack of symptoms in this age group is responsible for the frequent clinical failure to entertain this diagnosis. Most pituitary adenomas in older age groups remain as microadenomata and are probably prolactin producing, but otherwise, they usually cause no detectable hormonal or clinical changes. On rare occasions one may see an elderly person, male or female, with galactarrhea but with no other abnormal findings. Because pregnancy, menstrual regularity, and other growth features are not an issue in the elderly, there is little need for concern regarding the treatment of these tumors in the older age groups unless there has been enough enlargement of the tumor to cause impairment of vision. Unless there is rapid loss of vision beyond the bitemporal fields, radiation therapy may be adequate; otherwise surgical removal is mandatory. This is best performed by the currently popular transphenoidal approach. This procedure has revolutionized the safety and efficacy of pituitary tumor removal.

NEUROSURGICAL DISORDERS OF THE SPINE IN THE ELDERLY

Unfortunately, the most common intraspinal neoplasm in the aged individual is a metastatic tumor. These are usually in the thoracic area and are usually secondary to malignancies of the prostate, lung, and breast or from unknown primary sites (12). The progression of symptoms from spinal cord lesions is rapid and may begin as radicular pain, ataxia, and urinary incontinence. Plain x-rays are seldom of value as diagnostic tests for these extradural intraspinal masses, but CT scans and myelograms are usually diagnostic. Lumbar puncture for further diagnostic reasons should not be done unless it is for myelogram studies. Only if immediate neurosurgical assistance is available should this be done because the withdrawal of spinal fluid may precipitate additional cord compression by the sudden increased pressure from the mass lesion. If a complete block of spinal fluid flow is present only a small amount of dye is necessary to localize the lower limits of the tumors; otherwise a 12-cc dye injection is needed for a complete survey of the entire spinal canal. The CT scan or the magnetic resonance imaging study may make myelography unnecessary.

Clinically, the presence of a Brown-Sequard's syndrome (lateral cord compression) with ipsilateral motor loss and contralateral sensory loss is almost pathognomonic of intraspinal tumor. Likewise, progressive paraparesis is highly diagnostic of tumor.

The most common benign spinal cord tumor of the elderly is clearly the meningioma. It usually occupies the thoracic spine and produces slowly progressing symptoms that are often diagnosed as vascular disorders or spondylotic disease. The cervical area is next most often involved with either meningioma or neurofibroma, but the lumbar area is exceptionally free of meningioma in favor of neurofibroma.

The only effective therapy for all of these crippling tumors is to remove them surgically. Decompression of the spinal cord by tumor removal is well tolerated by the elderly patient, and excellent clinical recovery may be anticipated if the procedure is done carefully and before permanent capillary ischemia of the spinal cord has occurred. The subtotal removal of metastatic tumors may then require postoperative radiation therapy locally. If clinical recovery has occurred, this should be done; otherwise, there is little benefit to be gained if the patient remains paraplegic (13).

The disorder known as spondylosis results from spinal stenosis secondary to disc degeneration, osteophyte formation, facet hypertrophy, and enlargement of the ligamentum flavum (14).

This condition may occur at any spinal level, but is most common in the mid-cervical and low lumbar areas. The symptoms may be dramatically relieved if an adequate laminectomy is done in conjunction with the shaving of the facets to create a satisfactory enlargement of the canal. If pressure ischemia of the spinal cord, cauda equina, or nerve roots has progressed to an irreversible stage before the laminectomy is done, the degree of neurologic deficit may remain unchanged although its progression may be halted by the decompression.

Intramedullary tumors of the spinal cord are not common in the older age groups, although low grade astrocytoma and metastatic lesions are occasionally found. The removal of such tumors requires great caution and skill on the part of the surgeon; one must avoid operative damage to the cord parenchyma that would increase the neurologic deficit. In some cases a limited biopsy followed by radiation therapy constitutes the procedure of choice (15).

INTRACTABLE PAIN IN THE ELDERLY

The clinical entity known as tic douloureux or trigeminal neuralgia is almost totally confined to the older age group. There is no real sexual predominance for this condition in our experience. The cause of this disorder is not known precisely, although recent evidence suggests that it is due to vascular compression of the trigeminal posterior root. The diagnosis is made purely by history, there being no reliable objective test or findings of value. It should be emphasized that the painful attacks are brief and confined to the anatomic distribution of the trigeminal nerve and that the pain is never constant, although the attacks may be so frequent that the patient complains of "constant" pain. Unless the patient has typical trigeminal neuralgia no surgical procedures to relieve it should be done; otherwise the development of anesthesia dolorosa may ensue, which will defy all therapeutic attempts to control it.

Typically, the appropriate therapy for tic douloureux is the most conservative method that is successful. The use of Dilantin, Tegretol, and simple analgesics should be employed and maintained if effective. Unless the patient's systemic symptoms indicate a serious hazard to surgery, alcohol blocking of the peripheral nerve branches is useless except as a temporary measure. The same can be said for the section-avulsion of the peripheral branches. If, on the other hand, the conservative measures have failed and the patient's condition is favorable, a major surgical procedure may be employed, usually one that is the favorite of the surgeon. Currently, this usually means a radio-frequency procedure on the ganglion or a neurovascular decompression in the posterior fossa. Either of these may be successful, but the number of failures seen by this author after several attempts to obliterate the pain have been impressive, and it is virtually certain that a well-conducted, relatively safe, intracranial differential section of the posterior root will give permanent relief. It is a well-tolerated procedure, which is done with local anesthesia and spares the cornea and the first division of the fifth nerve. Unfortunately, it seems that this procedure is no longer taught in the neurosurgical training of residents, and its use has been relegated to the few older clinicians who can employ it with safety. In our community, the elderly patient with intractable tic pain desires one trip to the operating room for relief if conservative measures have been ineffective.

Glossopharyngeal neuralgia is much less common than trigeminal neuralgia, but is just as severe and cannot be tolerated when the attacks become frequent. The same medicinal controls should be tried, and if ineffective the rootlets of the ninth nerve can be severed in the posterior fossa.

Tic douloureux of the nervus intermedius is extremely rare, and may respond to Tegretol. If it does not, section of the nerve in the cerebello-pontine angle is successful, but this requires the very careful identification of the nerve by use of the microscope or magnifing loupe.

Intractable pain from metastatic lesion in older individuals should be tempered with the judicious use of narcotics in doses sufficient to control pain and to give a period of gratifying relief to the patient. It is foolhardy to insist on the use of such drugs on a 4-hour or 6-hour basis—the patient should have the drug when he or she needs it, not when the order requires or allows it. The concern about becoming an addict does not trou-

ble this author under these dismal and terminal circumstances. It should be noted that the use of the procedure known as spino-thalamic tractotomy (cordotomy) has little application in the elderly and is employed only rarely in the younger age groups. The percutaneous radio-frequency cordotomy performed under local anesthesia may be useful in the older person if the painful areas are local, unilateral, and intractable.

INTRACRANIAL ANEURYSMS

The appropriate therapy for unruptured aneurysms of the cerebral vascular system is a problem of great clinical importance, even though any approach lends itself to reasonable doubt. It is estimated that only 2% of all intact cerebral aneurysms will rupture in a year. This lends credence to the conservative philosophy of leaving such lesions undisturbed in favor of periodic observation to determine whether or not progressive enlargement has occurred (16). If there is evidence that this has happened within a short time period it is probably wise to recommend an operative approach to contain the aneurysm. If the aneurysm is located where there is a reasonable chance of success without serious neurologic deficit resulting, it should be clipped.

Subarachnoid hemorrhage resulting from a ruptured intracranial aneurysm is treated precisely the same as in the young patients with specific attention given to maintaining a normotensive blood pressure and the relief of cerebral edema by the use of steroids and osmotic agents if indicated. In the presence of cerebral angiospasm suffcient time must be allowed for the resumption of normal flow and the resumption of microvascular perfusion. If the older patient survives this critical period without a permanent major neurologic deficit and an alert mental state is present, the decision regarding surgical attack on the aneurysm must then be made. It is true that many clinicians favor a continued conservative approach in the older patient, but an aggressive surgical attack on the aneurysm may be surprisingly well tolerated in the systemically healthy senior patient. This author has consistently felt that aneurysms of the carotid artery at the level of the posterior communicating artery and those of the middle cerebral artery may be operated on with predictable success if damage to brain parenchyma has not already occurred (17). Those lesions of the anterior communicating artery and of the vertebral-basilar system may present technical difficulties that preclude an operative type of therapy. It should be understood that no recipe type of therapy can apply to these hazardous lesions and that each case must be individually appraised and its therapy decided upon (18).

Arterio-venous malformations are not a common problem in the older age groups. When such a lesion is disclosed by scan or by angiogram after a bleeding episode or after a convulsive seizure it is probably wise to avoid undertaking the excision of these lesions in the advanced age group. Useful survival usually occurs after such acute episodes, and although the potential for further trouble exists, it may be less than the risk of surgical removal. However, if some therapy is apparently essential, the deliberate embolization of the feeding arteries may be employed at less risk than total excision.

HYDROCEPHALUS IN THE ELDERLY

There are two forms of ventricular enlargement in the older patient that are frequently encountered, the pathophysiology of which is not completely understood. A frequently seen aspect of the aging process is atrophy of the brain parenchyma through loss of nerve cells and of the glia (principally, microglia). As a result, the subarachnoid pathways and the ventricles show a compensatory increase in size. This has been called *hydrocephalus et vacuo,* a term that is widely used, but is probably incorrect. At any rate the CT scan or more recently the magnetic resonance scan can easily disclose the enlargement of the fluid-filled areas and the atrophy of the cortex. The same picture may be seen in Alzheimer's disease but because there is no effective treatment for either of these disorders in the elderly there is no surgical consideration involved (1).

A possible treatable form of hydrocephalus in the elderly is normal pressure hydrocephalus. It is characterized by a triad of clinical problems consisting of dementia, gait disturbance, and urinary incontinence ("unwitting wetting"). This condition may be dramatically altered with ventricular decompression by performing a ventriculo-peritoneal shunt. At this time there is no reliable method of determining the ideal surgical candidate for this procedure. It has been shown that patients who have significant reflux of radioactive-labeled protein from lumbar subarachnoid space into the ventricles are probably good surgical candidates (19). In a review of our own series we found that the best results of surgical treatment occurred in those patients whose prime clinical problem was the gait disturbance. The poorest results were in those patients whose primary symptom was dementia. The operative procedure is easily done under light anesthesia and is well tolerated by the aging patient. Unfortunately, a good clinical result cannot be predicted preoperatively with any degree of certainty.

THE NEUROSURGICAL ASPECTS OF TRAUMA IN THE ELDERLY

Injuries to the head and spine are probably the most common cause of life-threatening disorders of the nervous system in older persons. Although such patients may survive the hazards of cerebral concussion quite well, they are materially handicapped from the more serious injuries. The older individual with arteriosclerosis and chronic chest disease may have little chance of surviving a closed head injury with associated cerebral contusion (20). The overall systemic stability and resiliency needed to combat such altered intracranial physiology are often lacking in the elderly, and the proneness of such patients to the complications of pneumonia and urinary tract infections, plus the impairment of cerebral autoregulation in the arteriosclerotic brain, may be overwhelming. Obviously, the important supportive care and attention required under these conditions necessitate a constant monitoring of such patients. Prompt attention must be paid to every possible complication, and because there is no specific therapy for the cerebral contusion itself the chances for a successful resolution are minimized.

As in the younger age groups fractures of the skull are well tolerated and require no treatment unless they are compound, in which case they must be debrided and closed. In the case of basal skull fractures resulting in cerebral spinal fluid otorrhea and/or rhinorrhea, recumbency with antibiotic coverage to negate the possibility of meningitis is appropriate and necessary. Depressed fractures of the convexity of the skull may be left alone unless the depressed fracture is greater than the combined thickness of all of the layers of the skull, in which case the underlying cerebral cortex may be lacerated or compressed. The elevation of or the actual removal of such an area of skull is thought by some to reduce the ultimate glial response and to minimize the likelihood of post-traumatic epilepsy. We suspect, however, that the result of this maneuver is principally one of cosmetic restoration, and this is usually not thought to be of prime importance in older patients.

There are three types of traumatic intracranial hematomas that are life threatening. Two of these conditions can be cured with reasonable ease if the diagnosis is made promptly. Probably, the most serious and the most ineffectually treated is the *acute subdural hematoma,* which is usually associated with a contused brain and which usually gives only minimal and temporary improvement when the hematoma is evaluated. The contused, edematous cerebral tissue then must be contended with by utilizing all the methods of cerebral decompression and by the maintenance of normal vascular perfusion to the brain tissue. The prognosis is grave, and total recovery is rare.

The *chronic subdural hematoma,* on the other hand, is a potentially curable condition and is easily diagnosed if the CT scan is employed. Failure to utilize this diagnostic tool because the clinical evidence suggests that the symptoms are from a vascular disorder or from a degenerative disease is inexcusable. The insidious development of the symptoms from the hematoma following a fall or a mild lump on the head, often forgotten by the elderly, may well simulate those symptoms seen with a stroke or with the altered cerebration of a degenerative disorder. Enlargement of the hematoma by microhemorrhages from the neo-vascular membrane may finally produce brain compression incompatible with consciousness, and stupor and coma will intervene. It is apparent that the virtually universal use of the computerized scanner will tend to eliminate the likelihood of overlooking this disorder, and we can help eliminate its tragic ef-

fect if effective treatment then follows. It has been traditional to treat all subdural hematomas by burr-openings, evaluation of fluid hematoma, and drainage of the space via closed system if brain re-expansion does not promptly occur. Otherwise, the subdural membranes will ultimately fill with spinal fluid and may then persist permanently as a form of "external hydrocephalus." To obviate this, re-expansion of the hemisphere has been accomplished in some case by the method of injection of normal saline via lumbar puncture until the subdural cavity was obliterated and the cortex was approximated back to the level of the dura (21). A mild Trendelenburg position has offered some gravitational help in accomplishing this effect. Craniotomy with removal of the hematoma membranes, once popular, is now seldom used, but should still be employed when failure has attended the other attempts to re-expand the cerebral hemisphere (22). The possibility of bilateral subdural hematoma is always present, and when this situation is disclosed the two sides should be treated simultaneously and identically. It is well known that some subdural hematomas are spontaneously absorbed and can be watched closely by repeated scanning, but only if the patient shows no progressive deterioration. It remains true that the surgical approach ensures the best outcome even today (23, 24).

The *acute epidural hematoma* constitutes the most dramatic of clinical conditions that may be rectified and a happy outcome achieved. Only if prompt action is taken to recognize and to decompress an acutely compromised brain is this possible. The classical history consists of a blow to the head with transient loss of consciousness, then a lucid interval that is followed by confusion, headache, and alterations of consciousness along with other neurologic sequelae. Obviously, the sequence of events in the history may vary, and there may be no report of a lucid interval, but anytime a history of rapid and progressive deterioration of the patient occurring after a head injury is obtained, everyone should be alerted to the possibility of a hemorrhage from the middle meningeal artery. Therapeutic delay in this situation can be fatal, and it is essential to realize that the time consuming and useless procedures of skull x-rays, diagnostic spinal taps, and detailed neurologic examinations may result in the patient's unnecessary demise. Currently, a hastily performed scan of the head may be permissible, but only if the patient's vital signs are stable and there is no indication of approaching respiratory paralysis. Emergency burr openings should be made in the emergency room if rapid neurologic changes and respiratory arrest occur. If clotted blood issues, success is possible, and the control of bleeding and wound closure can be accomplished in a timely manner in the operating room. A tragedy seen many times by the author is that of having a moribund patient arrive in the emergency room with dilated fixed pupils, profound coma, and decerebrate posturing and then to be handed a group of detailed x-ray films taken by a well-meaning clinician some 50 miles away from whom the patient was referred with the findings of an obvious epidural hematoma. Fortunately, some epidural arterial injuries clot before a large mass of hematoma is present. The pitfall here is that it may give false assurance to the physician regarding the patient's safety. This lesion when clotted is often guilty of several small rebleeding episodes (the stuttering epidural) that may ultimately produce the same havoc described above with untreated epidural hematoma.

Injuries to the bony spine in elderly patients are well tolerated if there is no associated injury to the neural elements. It is almost axiomatic that old patients with vertebral compression fractures or fracture dislocations without neural damage do well if they are not confined to bed in traction or in halo casts that will immobilize and confine them. It is well established that the elderly patient will tolerate this type of confinement very poorly, and it is almost a formal invitation to respiratory infection, confusion, and disorientation. Unless it is imperative that an operative procedure such as spinal fusion be performed the older patient will do well and usually better with simple braces and a short period of limited physical activities.

When damage to the spinal cord or cauda equina occurs the prognosis becomes infinitely worse. The old person who suffers an acute quadriplegic or paraplegic injury becomes at once a candidate for a series of complications. Pneumonia, urinary tract infection (indwelling catheter), pressure sores, and deep vein thrombosis all add to the usual picture of short period of survival for this unfortunate elderly victim.

Decompressive laminectomy has been of virtually no value to these elderly patients with acute traumatic transverse myelopathy.

Fractures of the odontoid are not uncommon in the elderly, but unless there is some neural damage (which is rare) it is wise not to employ tongs or halos, but to use a simple collar or a small brace because non-union is almost certain to ensue in any case (25).

It is hoped that the ideas expressed in this chapter will add weight to the fact that old people have a right to grow older and deserve the same neurosurgical care that would be offered a younger patient under similar conditions.

REFERENCES

1. Sammorajski, T: How the human responds to aging. *J Am Geriatr Soc* 24:4–11, 1976.
2. Long, DM: Aging in the nervous system. *Neurosurgery* 17:348–354, 1985.
3. Allen JH, Meacham WF: Colloidal barium sulfate as radiographic marker in surgical treatment of cauitary brain lesions. *Acta Radiologica* 9:15 1969.
4. Godfrey JB, Caird FJ: Intracranial tumours in the elderly. *Age Aging* 13:152–158, 1984
5. Holmes FF: Aging and cancer. *Cancer Res* 87:65–67, 1983.
6. Ransohoff J: Role of surgery in the treatment of malignant gliomas. *Cancer Treat Rep* 60:717–718, 1976.
7. Salcman M: Brain tumors in elderly patients. *Am Fam Phys* 27:137–143, 1983.
8. Salcman M: Brain tumors and the geriatrics patient. *J Am Geriatr Soc* 30:501–508, 1982.
9. Tomita T, Raimondi AJ: Brain tumors in the elderly. *JAMA* 246:53–55, 1981.
10. Silverstein H, McDaniel A, Norrell H, Wasen J: Conservative mangement of acoustic neuroma in the elderly patient. *Laryngoscope* 95:766–770, 1985.
11. Rovacs K, Ryan N, Horvath E, Singer W, Ezrin C: Pituitary adenomas in old age. *J Gerontol* 35:16–22, 1980.
12. Valenstein E: When to suspect spinal cord lesions in the elderly. *Geriatrics* 34:80–95, 1979.
13. Stewart J, Millac P, Shephard RH: Neurosurgery in the older patient. *Postgrad Med J* 51:453–456, 1975.
14. Fast A, Robin GC, Florman D: Surgical treatment of lumbar spinal stenosis in the elderly. *Arch Phys Med Rehab* 66:149–151, 1985.
15. Huang CY, Matheson J: Spinal cord tumours in the elderly. *Aust NZ J Med* 9:538–541, 1979.
16. Ducey RG, PitKethly D, Winn HR: Enlargement of an intracranial aneurysm in the eighth decade. *J Neurosurg* 62:600–602, 1985.
17. Meacham, WF: The surgical treatment of intracranial aneurysms. *Am Surg* 17:311–315, 1951.

18. Symon L, Vajda J: Surgical experiences with giant intracranial aneurysms. *J Neurosurg* 61:1009–1028, 1984.

19. Petersen R, Mokri B, Laws ER: Surgical treatment of idiopathic hydrocephalus in elderly patients. *Neurology* 35:307–311, 1985.

20. Kirkpatrick JB, Pearson J: Fatal cerebral injury in the elderly. *J Am Geriatr Soc* 26:489–497, 1978.

21. Markwalder TM, Seiler RW: Chronic subdural hematomas: to drain or not to drain. *Neurosurgery* 16:185–188, 1985.

22. So SC: Chronic subdural haematoma in the elderly. *Aust NZ J Surg* 46:166–169, 1976.

23. Robinson RG: Chronic subdural hematoma: surgical management in 133 patients. *J Neurosurg* 61:263–268, 1984.

24. Waga S, Sakakura M, Fujimoto K: Calcified subural hematoma in the elderly. *Surg Neurol* 11:51–52, 1979.

25. Pepin JW, Bourne RB, Hawkins RJ: Odontoid fractures, with special reference to the elderly patient. *Clin Orthop Rel Res* 193:178–183, 1985.

Chapter 35

Neuropsychiatric Aspects of Surgery in the Elderly

Richard A. Margolin, M.D., Charles E. Wells, M.D.

The psychiatric aspects of surgical treatment in the elderly include both the reactions of the mentally normal elderly patient when subjected to the stresses of surgical procedures and also those special problems posed for the surgeon by elderly patients with pre-existing psychiatric disease. Overall, the elderly probably tolerate operations mentally as well as younger individuals, but certain complications, such as delirium, occur more commonly in the aged patient. Psychiatric symptoms may be present preoperatively, or they may arise de nova in the perioperative or postoperative periods. These symptoms are important because they can be the first sign of physical complications and because they can also interfere with management and delay recovery (1). Awareness of the nature, causes, and treatment of psychiatric symptoms presenting in the surgical setting can help the surgeon avoid some of the usual pitfalls and ensure a more favorable outcome.

Psychopathology among the elderly is certainly not rare (2), and because it tends to coexist with physical illness (3), it is often encountered in the surgical setting. It must be remembered that it can equally well reflect organic brain disease or a functional (psychiatric) disorder. Those psychiatric symptoms and illnesses that are especially important and that are frequently seen in connection with surgical therapy will be stressed herein. Neurologic symptoms and diseases are also important when they coexist with the need for geriatric surgery, but they will not be covered here, however, because excellent reviews of geriatric neurology exist (4, 5). An understanding of the basis of psychopathology in the older surgical patient is best attained by a review of the relevant normal psychology and neurobiology of aging.

THE NORMAL AGING PROCESS

Normal aging involves change in both the mind and the brain. Unfortunately, there is yet to be developed a fully comprehensive or satisfying conception of either the healthy adult psychology or of the normal changes associated with the aging process. The same is true of the age-associated anatomic changes that occur in the brain. Nevertheless, it is necessary to explore these issues in order to have some framework for the consideration of the *pathologic* changes that are associated with psychiatric disease in later life.

The maintenance of good mental health in the senescent years clearly requires an intact neurologic function and the preservation of established normal psychological mechanisms. There is a complex and poorly understood interplay between microanatomic and physiologic changes of the brain, on the one hand, and the psychological variables in behavior, on the other. In healthy individuals, this neurologic/psychological relationship is basically stable. This stability allows relative retention and even enhancement of long-standing personality traits, cognitive skills, and affective style. The progressive development of insight, values, and perspective, even in the face of physical decline, can be said to represent "successful aging." Most elderly persons in the United States do in fact possess good general physical and mental health and never require institutionalization. In many elderly people, however, the impact of acute or chronic disease, significant losses (often the death of a spouse, relative, or close friend), or other stressful factors overwhelms their psychological stability and some psychiatric disease ensues.

504

Stereotypes, mostly of a negative sort, have long characterized society's perception of the elderly. Butler and Lewis (6) referred to these negative views generally as "ageism." Recent research has debunked many myths about the limitations of the elderly. An important finding is that variability is increased in the aged in many physiologic and psychological processes (7). Therefore, stereotypes and "ageism" are dangerous and often unfounded.

Certain questions and topics are beyond the scope of this chapter. For example, the various theories of aging and the relation between aging and disease (i.e., the distinction between normal and pathologic aging) are both important to the understanding of the psychobiology of the aged, but are thoroughly discussed elsewhere (8–10). Although age-related psychological changes and changes in the neuroanatomic and neurophysiologic substrate are actually inseparably intertwined, we will consider them separately herein.

Normal Psychology of Aging

The psychology of aging is best approached from a developmental perspective; that is, one that views senescence as representing a further stage of adult individualization. Whereas there is lively debate and several theories regarding psychic development and structure, it is generally agreed that adult psychological function comprises at least the basic components of *cognition* and related skills, such as memory and learning, *mood*, and *affect*. These building blocks are organized into the comprehensive and stable attributes of *intelligence, personality,* and *behavior.* It is possible to consider the psychology of aging from a biologic standpoint that stresses brain-behavior relationships and also from a psychosocial standpoint, stressing the relationship between an individual and the community. Both are important and revealing perspectives for the geriatric surgeon. The field of gerontologic psychology has grown rapidly; our review will be selective and targeted to those aspects of the field likely to be of importance to the surgeon. Thorough treatments of the topic can be found elsewhere (11).

Cognition

Cognition literally means knowing, particularly with regard to the outside world. It is a generic term, encompassing a set of discrete mental processes. Cognitive skills include perceiving, recognizing, reasoning, and judging. Memory and learning are closely related mental capabilities; intact consciousness and attention are also obvious prerequisites for successful cognition. Normal aging is associated with a mild decrement in cognitive abilities.

There are both motoric and non-motoric aspects of cognition. It is the motoric manifestations of cognition, measured for example by reaction time, that particularly decline with age. The importance of this motoric decrement in aging is readily apparent. Many tasks of modern life, such as driving a car, require speed, as well as dexterity. Response speed impairments interfere with the performance of such tasks by the elderly. Not all cognitive tasks of daily life require rapid response speed, however. Storandt (12) cites reading and gardening as examples of activities that the elderly may find enjoyable and at which they may excel, but for which time is not a critical factor.

Memory

Memory is a complex process, consisting of at least three subtypes: immediate, recent, and remote. There are age-related declines in memory, as documented by formal laboratory experiments (13). Visual and verbal memory demonstrate different patterns of change with aging; verbal and especially numerical retention are relatively well preserved (14). Predictably, the elderly perform most poorly on memory tasks that are time-constrained; their deficit is less apparent when response is not limited. Experiments have shown that mediators, such as mnemonic devices, can improve memory skills in the elderly. Such experiments have practical significance, and their results need to be translated into clinically useful techniques.

Learning

A depth of processing model (15) has been used to explain the relative impairment in learning noted in the elderly. This model states that information is learned more or less thoroughly depending on the "depth" at which it is processed. It is known that the elderly do not organize information into categories as well as the young and that their ability to form visual (mental) images is also inferior (12). Again, speed is an issue. Older people do learn, but more slowly (12).

The age-related decrement in cognitive and other intellectual capacities is routinely modified by educational, occupational and health status, and motivational factors (12). For example, an individual with a lifelong history of scholarly pursuit may preserve intellectual abilities quite intact into late life.

Mood and Affect

Mood refers to a feeling state that is stable over a reasonable period of time; affect is best thought of as the expressivity of mood. Little hard data exist about the emotional life of the elderly, but it is clear that wide variations in temperament exist. There is general consensus that the formerly widespread stereotypes of the elderly as cantankerous, crotchety, irritable, and stubborn are inaccurate and flawed. The variability of capacity and response among the elderly in other aspects of psychological function predicts similar variability with regard to mood and affect.

Intelligence

Although a universally accepted definition of intelligence is elusive, it is generally accepted to have verbal and perceptual-integrative qualities. Verbal skills, measured by tests of vocabulary and stored information, decline little with aging. Perceptual-integrative intelligence, however, measured by performance on objective tests, such as block design (object assembly), does decline progressively with age (12).

Personality

As stated above, normal psychological aging is associated with a relative preservation and even accentuation of long-standing personality traits. Personality is another elusive concept, but can best be understood as an amalgam of beliefs, attitudes, and patterns of behavior. Whereas there is now felt to be no characteristic "geriatric" personality, it is true that certain topics are frequently thought about and discussed by the elderly. Likewise, interviews with the elderly regularly reveal certain commonly held attitudes. Among these, attitudes about illness and longevity are especially relevant to this chapter. The will to live, for example, is certainly not directly related to chronologic age, but it is true that many very old individuals feel that life has passed them by or that they have lived long enough. Such views do not necessarily equate with depression.

Behavior

Changes in mental/emotional function are often translated into behavioral differences between the elderly and younger adults. Some evidence suggests that older individuals are more cautious. In psychological tests, for example, the elderly will more likely avoid making responses, whereas the young will more readily guess, even if they guess incorrectly. These stylistic differences have practical ramifications.

Stress and Coping

It has been alleged that the elderly have impaired coping skills, but this is not certain. On the one hand, aging often does involve being buffeted by more and more stressful circumstances (e.g., loss of independence, health, and social standing) while simultaneously having fewer and fewer resources to deal effectively with these stresses. On the other hand, the elderly are, by definition, "survivors" who must have at least a minimally adequate repertoire of coping strategies to have been able to attain advanced age.

Activity Level

Most elderly show a reduced level of physical and mental activity. There are both anatomic/physiologic and psychological reasons for this decline. Of interest is the fact that wide discrepancies between *actual* and *subjective* physical capabilities are frequently encountered. Long-established patterns are evidently important in determining how individuals adapt psychologically to declining physical capacities. Reduced physical and mental activity may be caused by depression or boredom. Conversely, inactivity can cause mood disturbances by increasing isolation. It is important to recognize that fatigue can also reflect underlying disorders, such as anemia and heart failure, or it may be an expression of the excessive use of sedative drugs.

Social and Economic Factors

The well-recognized increases in longevity in recent decades have been paralleled by not so well-appreciated changes in social structure. Whereas even 30 years ago most elderly lived as part of an extended family, today this is less likely the case. Changes in family structure, especially divorce, coupled with the remarkable physical mobility in American society, mean that more elderly are entirely alone and others have relatives living only at a great distance. Such social isolation can readily affect their attitudes toward illness and health care.

Economic considerations cannot be ignored by the elderly. Although the percentage of elderly living in poverty has recently declined, many if not most of these people live on fixed incomes. In the United States, most elderly patients rely on Medicare for reimbursement of medical costs. As has been widely appreciated—not least by the elderly!—the percentage of costs reimbursed by Medicare has decreased in recent years. Policy developments by the U.S. Department of Health and Human Services in the mid-1980s threaten to increase the elderly's costs for medical and surgical therapy.

Concurrent Medical Illness and Psychological Function in the Aged

The presence of concomitant chronic medical illness is important in surgical decision making. It has been estimated that 75% of surgical patients over age 70 have one or more associated diseases (16). The presence of these diseases often adversely affects the response to surgical care. Whereas there are surely many reasons for this adverse effect, the impact of chronic illness on the psyche may be one of the mechanisms involved. For example, chronic cardiac, pulmonary, or renal disease, as well as poor nutritional status, have been correlated with relatively impaired cognition in elderly populations. Recovery from illness and operations includes both subjective and objective aspects. It is frequently noted that the elderly take longer to recover fully. Again, psychological factors may mediate this finding.

In the very old or in those elderly who have overwhelming medical problems, the simplest and most basic capabilities may be extremely important, both for maintaining self-esteem and for preservation of a minimally adequate quality of life. Intact mental functioning and the ability to move are perhaps the most basic attributes necessary for a meaningful existence (17).

In summary, the mental health of the elderly is influenced by at least four factors—psychological, social, economic, and physical. When one or more of these factors become seriously disturbed, psychopathology is likely to ensue.

Normal Aging Changes in Structural and Physiologic Attributes of the Brain

Anatomic and physiologic changes of the brain associated with aging are important to geriatric surgery because the brain is the substrate for higher mental processes, such as cognition, memory, speech, etc. A comprehensive review of the anatomic and physiologic changes of the aging brain is beyond the scope of this chapter; excellent treatises on these topics exist (18, 19). Herein, therefore, those aspects of neuroanatomy and neurophysiology in which age-related changes have routine or critical importance in the surgical setting will be emphasized.

The past several decades have witnessed dramatic advances in our ability to determine parameters of human cerebral structure and function in vivo. Certain morphologic changes are now well documented in the aging human brain, both at the macroscopic and microscopic levels. Grossly, it is accepted that there is a progressive loss of brain weight associated with aging (19); up to 100 g of loss may be normal. The brain also shrinks in size with advancing age. Established neuroradiologic techniques, such as x-ray computed tomography (CT), have revealed progressive enlargement of the ventricles and sulcal space in normal aging (20). Microscopically, post-mortem histopathologic analyses have shown loss of neurons in most but not all brain regions (21). The cortex, which is most closely associated with higher mental processes, is particularly affected by cell loss, demonstrating up to 50% reduction in some regions (22).

There are also distinct age-related biochemical changes in the brain. Post-mortem neurochemical studies have shown age-related reductions in most neurotransmitter levels and in levels of their synthetic enzymes (23); an important exception is monoamine oxidase, which increases with age.

These structural and chemical changes are compensated for by the physiologic reserve capacity of the brain. Such mechanisms as redundant neural circuitry work to preserve the functional integrity of the brain. It is evident that the brain's reserve properties are substantial and that the higher mental functions are frequently preserved despite age-associated structural disruption of neuronal architecture. Only when damage is severe or focal does mental aberration result.

Newer imaging modalities, especially positron emission tomography, have shown age-related differences in a number of physiologic processes of the brain, such as cerebral blood flow (CBF), glucose and oxygen metabolism, and neurotransmitter function. Several groups have documented modestly declining CBF with advancing age (24, 25). It has also been shown that CBF and neuropsychological function are significantly correlated (26, 27).

Not all neurophysiologic processes necessarily deteriorate with age, however. Recent research suggests that the very healthy elderly have no significant decrements in the basal level of cerebral glucose metabolism (CMR glu) (28). This is important because under ordinary circumstances glucose is the sole fuel for oxidative metabolism in the brain. Thus, the ability of the brain to support higher mental processes should not be considered intrinsically impaired by the aging process. More typical elderly persons, such as those with chronic diseases, do show age-dependent decrement in CMR glu (29). CMR glu has likewise been shown to be significantly correlated with neuropsychological function (30).

In the area of neurotransmitter physiology, Wong and his associates (31) have elegantly identified in vivo the existence of age-related reductions in parameters of dopamine receptor binding, and analogous findings are suspected for the acetylcholine system.

Senile Sensory and Perceptual Changes

Vision Loss (Presbyopia) and Hearing Loss (Presbycusis)

Age-associated impairments in most sensory modalities are quite frequent; visual and auditory deficits are the most significant. Most elderly persons demonstrate presbyopia, the lengthening of the minimum focal point for accurate vision. The effect of this condition is to interfere with visual acuity for close objects, such as written text. Other common ophthalmologic and neuro-ophthalmologic disorders in the elderly include cataract, glaucoma, diabetic and other retinopathies, and strokes that involve visual pathways. Visual deficits are readily linked to behavioral changes, by promoting isolation and insecurity, and to depression. Partial or complete treatment exists for most senile visual disorders, and aggressive management is indicated when cure is possible.

Presbycusis, or senile hearing loss, is common. It is manifested by reduced acuity for high frequency sounds. Generally, perception of spoken words in conversation is not as impaired as perception of such sounds as music or a ticking watch. When voice perception is affected, female voices are more easily recognized. Also, voice perception is more often impaired in group conversation than in individual discourse. Most senile hearing loss is of the sensorineural type, and men are more commonly afflicted (32). Presbycusis can lead to many of the same changes in mood and behavior as are caused by visual disturbances. Sadly, the two are not mutually exclusive.

Pain Sensitivity

Evidence regarding age-related differences in pain sensitivity is incomplete and equivocal (33). Some studies suggest increased pain thresholds in the aged; others do not. Pain has both sensory/perceptual and affective aspects. Clinically, these are always intermixed. Negative response bias and personality factors may mitigate the reporting of pain by older individuals. Overall, the old are probably more like the young than not in their handling of pain.

Sleep Changes in Aging

Sleep laboratory and community epidemiologic studies clearly indicate that the elderly sleep less than younger individuals. Also, the nature of their sleep is different. The complex electrophysiologic architecture of sleep is now well appreciated. The elderly seem to have delayed rapid eye movement (REM) onset and less total REM time. Sleep-related complaints are certainly common among the elderly and may be particularly evident in the relatively inactive patient (32). Chronic administration of hypnotic drugs is counterproductive in the aged patient and can produce daytime sedation and even reversal of the sleep-wake cycle.

PATHOLOGIC BRAIN AGING

Because of the prevalence in the elderly of diseases that affect the brain and also for theoretical reasons, it is difficult to delineate a clear boundary between normal aging changes in brain structure and physiology and true pathologic changes. The differences encountered are usually quantitative and statistical, not qualitative or absolute. With regard to structure, it is clear that more cell loss and atrophy are present in dementia, for example, than in normal aging. Efforts to translate this fact into a reliable clinical tool (e.g., CT-based dementia diagnosis) have been impossible, however. Cell loss and degeneration are clearly linked to age-related brain disease in at least one case, namely that of the decreased volume of the nigrostriatal tract associated with Parkinson's disease.

Physiologically, substantially supranormal declines in CBF and CMRglu have been shown in dementia. Imaging of these processes may therefore become a useful clinical tool in the future.

Functional Status

A useful term that incorporates both psychological and neurologic components of age-related change is that of *functional status*. This term refers to the overall capacity of an elderly individual to act in the world as an independent agent. Both psychological and neurologic aspects of functional status become relevant in the setting of geriatric surgery.

An important distinction is that of the old versus the very old. Although no exact chronologic age boundary has biologic significance, the important point to understand is that the very old may be physiologically different from the "young old," who are more like middle-aged

persons. The age of 85 years is generally used to distinguish this very old group.

GERIATRIC PSYCHOLOGY IN RELATION TO SURGICAL THERAPY

Specific Normal Psychic Responses to Surgical Trauma

Beard (34) points out that an operation is a major traumatic life occurrence for anyone. He has described the prototypical sequence of reactions to a major surgical procedure by psychologically healthy elderly individuals so well that it is worth paraphrasing his description as a point of departure for our discussion:

An individual's surgical experience begins with a symptom that leads him to his physician. Fearing disability, he may procrastinate. The patient's family often becomes involved when the decision to operate is made. Upon hospitalization, he enters an unfamiliar world in which he has little to say about what happens to him. He feels powerless and is full of questions for which he has little information. Blind trust in the skill and knowledge of those he contacts is often required. His connection with his family and his once familiar world wanes. The operation itself is often preceded by several special examinations that can themselves be confusing or painful. He may hope that these studies will prove an operation to be unnecessary. Above all, if it is needed, he hopes that the surgical procedure will be curative.

The day of the operation itself is usually long and arduous. It includes exposure to mind-altering preoperative medications, the trip to the operating room, the induction of anesthesia, the operation itself, and then the beginning of recovery. In the immediate postoperative period, the patient is almost completely in the hands of strangers and he may see familiar faces very little. He is uncomfortable, and consciousness may be dimmed by metabolic disturbances and narcotic or sedative drugs. Time becomes elusive and disorientation frequently occurs.

As recovery proceeds the patient may be restless, irritable, and anxious. Again, there are many questions and doubts. On discharge from the hospital, he is required to make decisions without ready access to expert opinion. Adverse reactions to medications and behavioral abnormalities may first appear at this time.

Gradually, recovery becomes rehabilitation. Subtle changes in countenance, gait, and voice document the elderly patient's return to the preoperative level of control of his own life and the resumption of his accustomed activities.

As this account makes clear, even in the best

of circumstances, certain strong emotions are a natural part of the surgical experience for the elderly. Anxiety and fear in moderate degree, as well as feelings of isolation, are certainly common and need not be considered intrinsically pathologic. There are many reasons for fear and anxiety in the elderly surgical patient. Many older persons have known someone who has died during an operation. Some may be more afraid of dying during anesthesia than of the operation itself (35).

The distinction between fear and anxiety is subtle. Fear is defined as an unpleasant, often strong emotion caused by awareness of danger; anxiety adds an element of anticipatory apprehension. Although fear closely corresponds to a real danger, anxiety often is chronic and departs from the reality of a present danger. Anxiety is also associated with other mental processes, such as worry and rumination. Depressed mood and denial of illness are other frequently observed psychopathologic symptoms.

The boundary between the presence of such symptoms as normal reactions to a stressful experience and their occurrence as features of a more serious psychiatric illness may be subtle. The essential distinction is whether or not the symptoms interfere with normal functioning for an individual. Thus, to feel anxious or somewhat depressed when facing a surgical procedure or recovering from it may not be unusual or abnormal for many elderly patients; the addition of behavioral aberrations, such as anorexia or persistent insomnia, to these symptoms, however, may indicate the presence of a psychiatric disorder.

What is the incidence of psychopathology among the elderly in the surgical setting? Estimates have varied, but in a study of surgical patients of all ages, Titchener and colleagues (36) found a 15% incidence of postoperative psychosis. Furthermore, Heller and associates (37) found a 33% incidence of organic brain syndrome after open heart procedures. There is reason to believe that the elderly are a high risk group for the development of perioperative psychopathology. Millar (1) evaluated 100 consecutive elective general surgical cases in patients over age 65. He correlated a preoperative standardized psychiatric interview with postoperative nursing notes and a repetition of the standardized

interview. Thirteen of his patients showed preoperative psychiatric disturbance, and 21 demonstrated abnormalities postoperatively. Advanced age (over 80), a *major* surgical procedure, and polypharmacy all were significantly associated with increased psychiatric morbidity.

In further considering the psychological aspects of geriatric surgery, we will next discuss the preoperative psychiatric evaluation that a surgeon should perform and then some aspects of the doctor-patient relationship in this setting.

PSYCHOLOGICAL AND PSYCHIATRIC COMPONENTS OF THE PREOPERATIVE EVALUATION

Psychiatric aspects of the preoperative evaluation should include elements of history taking, a mental status examination, contact with the patient's family, and above all, thoughtful consideration of the impact of an operation on the totality of the patient's condition. Though necessarily brief, there is much evidence to suggest that this part of the evaluation is essential and of practical value to the surgeon. In addition, some data for psychiatric assessment will be obtained in other parts of the patient's evaluation and throughout it by the process of careful listening.

There are various parts to a preoperative psychiatric history. The process begins with identification of past or present psychiatric disease and clarification of whether it has any direct bearing on the current surgical problem. For example, surgical repair of wounds resulting from a self-inflicted injury sustained in a suicide attempt would be an obvious setting in which inquiry about mental and emotional symptoms would be germane. Depression, anxiety, and psychosis may be easily explored by direct or indirect questioning. A past history of major psychiatric disease is important to elicit because of its possible impact on the patient's behavior in the current setting and also because the stress of an operation can reactivate dormant illnesses.

A behavioral history is as important a part of the evaluation in the elderly as in any patient group. Occult alcohol or drug abuse is not rare in the aged, and it must be identified in order to prevent unexpected development of a postoperative withdrawal state, with its serious associated morbidity. A complete medication history is crucial for preventing adverse (allergic and otherwise) reactions and drug interactions. The elderly consume both prescribed and over-the-counter medications frequently. They also use psychotropic medications at a higher rate than the young.

Indications for including the family in the psychiatric assessment are more frequent for an elderly patient than for a younger one. This is so because a family member may have valuable historical data to offer that the patient might have forgotten or neglected to mention (38). The family can also provide information about the patient's overall situation, including his or her hopes and fears and his or her attitudes about terminal care. Social and economic factors can often be explored more easily in discussion with the family.

The mental status examination need not be a forbidding procedure for the surgeon. Key components to be assessed are orientation; mood and affect; cognitive skills, such as the ability to reason; memory (especially short-term memory); and the presence of symptoms of psychosis, such as hallucinations and delusions.

As an adjunct to the mental status examination, the use of brief quantitative cognitive function rating scales might be mentioned. These measures have the advantage of enhanced reproducibility. An excellent example of such scales is that developed by Folstein and colleagues, the Mini-Mental State Examination (39). It can be administered in approximately 5 minutes and has been validated by application to a large and diverse patient population.

Although the surgeon's mental status examination is necessarily brief, it can be argued that the assessment of preoperative mental function, especially cognitive function, is cost effective in terms of time expenditure, because it can provide a baseline for comparison in the event of postoperative psychopathologic complications.

However brief, the neuropsychiatric preoperative assessment should be comprehensive, including consideration of emotional well-being and sensory function (34). There are certain qualitative factors that must be included. One is the evaluation of the contribution of a surgical procedure not only to the extension of life but also to its qualitative improvement or preservation. The surgeon should reflect upon the com-

parative risk of an operation versus conservative treatment or no treatment. Weiss and Lesnick have pointed out that, although every patient deserves the maximum skill of which a surgeon is capable, the older surgical patient's limitations also require careful consideration (16). In their words, the surgeon "must know when to be more or less aggressive in order to achieve the optimal result." The timing and the magnitude of the procedure may also need to be modified by factors associated with mental or emotional illness (40).

Others involved in preoperative assessment can complement the surgeon's evaluation. The anesthesiologist is especially important in this regard, both as a backup for the completeness of data gathering and as another source of reassurance when discussing specific anesthesia-related issues with the patient. The patient's own wishes and opinions are germane and should be sought out preoperatively. The medical ethicist and/or psychiatrist can play a valuable role in assisting the surgeon in certain difficult cases.

Surgical Style and a Surgeon's Attitude toward the Elderly

Certain intangible aspects of the doctor-patient relationship are especially important in geriatric surgery. These include the style of communication, sensitivity to the values and wishes of the patient, and the creation of a real rapport. Beard, for example, has stressed the importance of unhurried and open communication with an elderly patient (34). Communication is a two-way street. The surgeon must be a sincere active listener to the patient's concerns, as well as a provider of facts and opinions for the elderly patient's considerations. The surgeon's explanations of the reasons for the surgical procedure, the process itself and its associated risks, some preliminary aspects of postoperative recovery, and the likely outcome must be done in a straightforward way and in common-sense, layman's language. Specific unfamiliar procedures that the patient is likely to encounter should be explained in advance. These might include cardiac catheterization, endotracheal intubation, artificial ventilation, central line placement, etc. Advance explanation can diminish anticipatory anxiety and surprise.

educational level than most younger individuals.

This fact, when added to sensory changes and the emotional stress of an impending operation, compels a measured, non-threatening conversation. Repetition and the use of diagrams (to incorporate another sensory modality) may be useful adjuncts in presenting factual information. In view of the frequent coexistence of cognitive impairment, sensory (particularly hearing) loss, and cautious behavior among the elderly, the value of patience and attention on the surgeon's part is obvious.

Similarly, communication with the family is crucial. The older patient may rely more often on concurrence by family members in the final assenting to clinical decisions. The surgeon's instructions and other points can also be reinforced by the family when an elderly patient's poor memory or lack of attention has caused such information not to be assimilated directly. Admittedly, communication with an elderly surgical patient and the family is not always possible and is seldom easy. Surgical emergencies are more common in the elderly, and under many of these circumstances no family or friend may be readily available (40).

Sensitivity to the patient's world view is invaluable. Despite the ravages of illnesses, most elderly patients, even those with cognitive impairment, tenaciously guard their right to self-determination (40). An individual's dignity and self-esteem are closely connected to this right. A surgeon will maximize his or her effectiveness if the patient is involved in the act of decision making as much as possible. In fact, the establishment of real rapport between the surgeon and the elderly patient enhances the chance of a favorable surgical outcome and ultimately is the absolutely best safeguard for the surgeon in the event of an unfavorable outcome.

A final point on this issue is the advisability of involving the patient's internist or other primary care physician during all phases of the surgical process. Such consultation is reasonable with compromised patients of any age, but there are specific reasons for it in the geriatric surgical situation. The patient will presumably have ready rapport with his or her own family physician. Elderly patients may more easily trust and have confidence in the surgeon if they know that their own physician is involved. The primary care physician who knows the patient well can also alert the surgeon to the patient's idiosyncrasies. Admittedly, such involvement of a primary care physician is not always possible.

As has been underscored elsewhere in this volume, the surgeon must discard ageism and other stereotypes. Progress in technique has steadily reduced the mortality rate that the elderly experience from major surgical procedures, and it is no longer clear that age per se is a specific surgical risk factor.

PSYCHIATRIC DISEASE IN THE ELDERLY IN THE SURGICAL SETTING

The surgeon may face psychopathology in the elderly age groups from patients with known psychiatric disease and also in the previously mentally healthy aged individual. Futhermore, psychopathology may present due to anxiety incurred preoperatively, in the hectic perioperative period, or during a prolonged postoperative course. The presence of a known psychiatric condition in an elderly patient is not in itself a contraindication to an operation; however, special care may be required for the proper management, and the involvement of a psychiatrist may be desirable. All the commonly occurring psychiatric disorders of adult life can be seen in the elderly; moreover, certain conditions are especially frequent in this phase of life. Table 35.1 summarizes the psychiatric illnesses that the geriatric surgeon is likely to encounter.

Delirium

Definition and Presentation

Delirium is a behavior state characterized by

Table 35.1 Common Psychiatric Disorders in the Elderly Surgical Patient

Organic mental syndromes
    Delirium
    Dementia
Affective disorders
    Unipolar depression
    Bipolar affective disorder (manic-depressive illness)
Psychosis (including schizophrenia and psychosis secondary to depression, mania, or organic brain disease)
Adjustment disorder
    With depressed mood
    With anxiety

a generalized alteration of mental function. Arousal, attention, perception, cognitive, and other intellectual skills, such as memory and speech, and the emotions may all be disturbed (41). The hallmark of delirium is the clouding of consciousness, which can wax and wane. Changes in arousal are variable in both degree and intensity, but there are two broad forms: a so-called quiet delirium and a florid, agitated form (loud delirium). Attention span is regularly disturbed; delirious patients are usually easily distractible and are also spontaneously distracted by internal and external stimuli of surprisingly low magnitude. Perceptual aberrations, such as illusions and auditory or visual hallucination, are common. Visual hallucinations are in fact more common in delirium than in many other psychiatric conditions. Disorientation to time and place is routine. A curious and relatively frequently occurring phenomenon is the mistaking of the unfamiliar for the familiar. Affective disturbances include irritability and especially lability.

Delirium usually has an acute onset, but rarely it can arise subacutely over several days. Postoperative delirium is most common 3–5 days after the operation, but it may be noted just after the effect of anesthesia has resolved (41). Frequently, delirium is associated with insomnia; this relationship can create a vicious cycle in which each problem contributes to the persistence of the other. Delirium is also referred to as an acute confusional state; the latter terminology is more commonly employed by neurologists.

Etiology

The list of factors that can produce peri- or postoperative delirium is long. (Table 35.2) Even anticipatory anxiety associated with the prospect of an operation may be involved (16). Often, two or more factors join to be causative for inducing delirium. Its occurrence in the immediate postoperative period suggests intraoperative hypoxia, cerebral emboli, or an anticholinergic syndrome (41).

Incidence and Significance

Delirium is the most common and arguably the most important psychiatric complication of sur-

Table 35.2 Common Causes of Postoperative Confusion in the Elderly

Environmental	Metabolic
Intensive care unit	Hypoxia
Intubation	Acid-based disturbances
Restraints	Hyponatremia
Isolation	Hyperosmolar coma
Traction devices	Acute renal failure
Sensory deprivation	Fever
Decreased auditory acuity	Dehydration
Decreased visual acuity	Infection
Bandages and dressings	Sepsis
Drug reactions	Pneumonia
Anticholinergic agents and	Urinary tract infection
anticholinergic side	Wound infection
effects of other drugs	Meningitis
Anesthetic agents	Miscellaneous
Narcotics	Trauma
Hypnotics	Unrelieved pain
Antiemetics	Anxiety
Tranquilizers	
Vascular	
Myocardial infarction	
Stroke, especially embolic	
Pulmonary embolism	
Hemorrhage	
Shock	
Heart failure	

gical therapy in the aged. In one study 14% of surgical patients had some degree of delirium (1). The significance of delirium becomes more important when it is realized that injuries (especially falls) and other accident-related causes of excess morbidity are much more likely to occur in the delirious patient.

Treatment

Delirium is usually reversible, often by time alone. However, in the surgical setting, an especially aggressive search for causes is always indicated. This is so because of the high probability that it is an iatrogenic event. Perhaps in no other area of medicine is the time-honored rule of *primum non noncere* more applicable. Treatment often consists only of support while removing the offending factor that initiated delirium. Other steps include close (even constant) observation of the delirious patient and the use of physical restraint, when necessary. Pharmacologic treatment is definitely of secondary value and quite often can be counterproductive in that the commonly employed drugs can themselves cause or exacerbate delirium. Drug treatment is, however, indicated when the patient's condition is likely to lead to injury to him- or herself or another. In such instances, antipsychotic drugs in low dosage may be helpful. (Table 35.3) These are preferable to the benzodiazepines or other related sedatives. A benzodiazepine, such as lorazepam, may, however, be valuable as a hypnotic for a brief period if insomnia is extreme or persistent.

Awareness of the reversibility of delirium can aid the surgeon in dealing with a patient's family by reassuring them of the prospect of the patient's ultimate return to his or her formal normal mental stats (16).

Dementia

Definition and Presentation

Dementia is characterized by a loss of intellectual ability in adult life of sufficient severity to interfere with social or occupational functioning (42). By definition, it presumes prior normal development of such ability. It presents along a continuum from mild deficits in specific cognitive capacities through global impairment of higher mental functions, to loss of control of even basic human bodily functions, e.g., bowel and bladder control and personal hygiene. In contrast to delirium, dementia is not an acute or subacute process, but rather a chronic one. Thus, it should always be identifiable preoperatively.

The demented patient, as can the delirious one, can display inappropriate behaviors or behaviors dangerous to him- or herself or to the caregiving staff. These activities can include cursing, kicking, scratching, spitting and attempting to loosen or remove restraints, to arise from a bed over (or through!) side rails, or to remove intravenous or other catheters. Urinary and/or fecal incontinence are especially challenging behaviors to manage. Elderly demented patients can easily become dehydrated or malnourished because of poor fluid and food intake. Although cognitive skills and memory are the most regularly affected mental functions, demented patients are often emotionally disturbed. A so-called catastrophic reaction has been identified in dementia in which a stressor that would be considered relatively minor by the non-demented person instead provokes a severe behavioral decompensation. Typical stressors capable of producing a catastrophic reaction include hos-

pitalization itself (i.e., change of environment), physical restraint, and separation from the family. Agitation, paranoia, and wandering are regularly encountered in advanced dementia. It should also be noted that dementia and delirium are not mutually exclusive.

Etiology

According to present-day knowledge, dementia is considered to be a clinical syndrome that can result from a number of distinct underlying pathophysiologic processes. In the United States, the most common cause of dementia today is Alzheimer's disease (primary degenerative dementia), and the second most common cause is multi-infarct dementia. A mixture of these two etiologies ranks next, and a multitude of rarer etiologies account for the remainder of cases: tumors, metabolic and endocrine disturbances, infections, etc.

Incidence and Significance

The incidence and prevalence of dementia increase steadily with advancing age. Although less than 7% of all people over age 65 are afflicted, as many as 20% of persons aged 85 and older may have significant dementia.

Operating on an elderly patient with dementia may be one of the most challenging tasks a surgeon can face. Issues that must be considered include those of a medicolegal nature (e.g., informed consent and competence) and postoperative management techniques. Although methodologically sound studies are lacking, it is widely believed that demented patients tolerate surgical procedures less well than non-demented patients of comparable age (40).

Treatment

Whereas there is currently no successful treatment for Alzheimer's disease, some other conditions that can cause dementia are remediable (43). Regardless of etiology the *symptoms* of dementia that can interfere with surgical therapy are relatively treatable acutely. Quite low doses of antipsychotic agents, such as haloperidol, can usually control agitation. Anticholinergic drugs, commonly used to control extrapyramidal and other side effects of the antipsychotics in the treatment of schizophrenia, are usually not needed in conjunction with the low doses of antipsychotics employed for behavioral control in dementia. Useful adjunctive steps include maximizing the patient's contact with the family while hospitalized, reassurance, and importation of familiar personal items into the hospital room.

Psychosis

Definition and Presentation

Psychosis is an acute or chronic mental state of faulty relation to reality. A psychotic person may have false perceptions and beliefs about himself or herself and the world outside that he or she holds despite contradictory evidence. Psychotic symptoms in the elderly include hallucinations and delusions, particularly of the paranoid type. It is important to recognize that psychotic symptoms appearing de novo postoperatively may actually reflect the existence of delirium, and a thorough search for organic causes must be undertaken before presuming these symptoms to be functional in nature.

Etiology

Preoperatively diagnosed psychosis may reflect a long-standing psychiatric disorder, such as schizophrenia. Psychosis can also be seen in major depression or mania. Postoperative psychosis is an entity long known to surgeons. Whether or not it reflects a distinct diagnostic entity, however, is controversial (1).

Incidence and Significance

Because schizophrenia has approximately a 0.8% prevalence worldwide and afflicted patients in industrialized societies are living longer, it is not rare to encounter such patients in late life. The new onset of psychosis in later life is also a recognized clinical entity (44). The significance of psychosis for the geriatric surgeon is primarily the need it occasions for diligent attention to the patient's behavior. Psychotic patients are frequently unpredictable behaviorally and may be uncooperative or noncompliant with instructions.

Treatment

The management of psychosis includes both pharmacologic and supportive components. Anti-

psychotic drugs are often necessary, but should be used in the lowest doses possible in order to prevent side effects to which the elderly are more susceptible. (Table 35.3) Useful supportive measures are substantially the same as those listed above for dementia.

Depression

Definition and Presentation

Depression is a vague term, referring both to a symptom and to specific clinical disorders. Feelings of loneliness, isolation, and sadness (depressed mood), as well as loss of energy, appetite, and interest in formerly enjoyable activities, are typical symptoms. Other symptoms include feelings of guilt and/or worthlessness, impaired ability to concentrate, recurrent unpleasant thoughts, especially of suicide, and reduction in sexual interest. Signs of depression include weight loss, sleep disturbance, and psychomotor agitation or retardation. A major depressive episode is diagnosable given the presence of four or more such signs and symptoms to a significant degree over a period longer than 2 weeks (42). Chronic depressed mood in the absence of severe functional impairment suggests a related diagnosis, dysthymic disorder. Exaggerated grief and bereavement reaction are also encountered in the elderly. Depression may be manifested preoperatively, or it may arise postoperatively.

Etiology

The etiology of geriatric depression is certainly multifactoral, with biochemical, psychodynamic, interpersonal, sociological, existential, and genetic factors contributing to different degrees

Table 35.3 Psychotropic Drug Recommendations for the Elderly Surgical Patient

Indication	Drug	Dose
Depression	Nortriptyline	10–25 mg HS/BID
	Desipramine	25–50 mg HS/BID
Psychosis, delirium and agitation	Haloperidol	0.5–5 mg HS/BID[a]
Anxiety	Lorazepam	0.5–1 mg BID/TID

[a]A concomitant anticholinergic agent, such as benztropine, 0.5 mg daily or may be needed to prevent extrapyramidal side effects, but usually only at higher antipsychotic doses.

in individual patients (45). In the elderly, depression may often be caused or aggravated by symptoms of medical illnesses.

Endocrinopathies, intracranial or abdominal masses, and neurologic disorders, such as Parkinson's disease and some strokes, are notoriously associated with depressive symptoms. Many medications are known to produce depressive symptoms in the elderly, but the antihypertensives should be mentioned in particular because of the frequency of this side effect and the frequency of their use in the elderly.

Incidence and Significance

Epidemiologic studies have shown a considerable prevalence of depression among the aged and have in fact identified it as the most common geropyschiatric disorder. Blazer and Williams (46) found an almost 15% rate of dysphoric symptoms in one representative group of elderly, but only 4% of the individuals they studied met criteria for diagnosis of a major depressive episode. Cheah and Beard (47) noted a much higher prevalence of depression, 31%, in hospitalized patients on a medical unit.

Although it varies considerably in severity, the presence of depression should be considered serious by the surgeon. Shuckit and associates (48) found a 60% 3-year mortality rate in a depressed geriatric group, but only a 32% mortality rate in a non-depressed elderly control group. The presence of depression during preoperative evaluation may interfere with a patient's participation in rational decision making concerning an operation. Depression developing postoperatively can interfere with compliance with recuperative instructions, including medication use. Anorexia and resulting weight loss can induce a catabolic state that can impair wound healing. A major aspect of the significance of depression is its association with suicide. A number of studies in Europe and North America have shown a progressively increasing incidence of suicide with advancing age, at least in men. Although sometimes suicide occurs in non-depressed psychotic patients, it usually results from severe depression.

Treatment

Transitory depressive symptoms do not necessarily warrant treatment; significant depression, however, should be treated with a combination of psychotherapy and antidepressant drugs. (Table 35.3) Electroconvulsive therapy is felt to be particularly helpful in refractory geriatric depression and may also be used when antidepressant medication is contraindicated. Psychiatric consultation is useful in moderate or severe depression; sometimes, delaying an operation in order to allow pharmacologic and psychotherapeutic treatment to work may be desirable.

Bipolar Disorder

Bipolar affective disorder (manic-depressive disorder) is also commonly encountered in the elderly. Mania is treated acutely with antipsychotic drugs and lithium salts. It is advisable to control mania preoperatively if possible.

Anxiety Disorders

As mentioned, some anxiety in the surgical setting is expected; in fact, its absence would be surprising! However, anxiety that interferes with rational behavior should be treated. The benzodiazepines are the preferred agents for anxiety (Table 35.3), and a scheduled dosage scheme is recommended. Fears of inducing drug dependence by prescription of these agents are usually unwarranted in geriatric surgery, and pharmacologic treatment of significant anxiety can promote compliance and recovery.

Miscellaneous Conditions

Many other psychiatric conditions may of course be encountered by the geriatric surgeon. Medical progress has enabled individuals with developmental disabilities, such as Down's syndrome, to survive into advanced age. Elderly patients with personality disorders, alcohol and substance abuse, and Munchausen's syndrome may also be seen. It is impossible to delineate here specific treatments or approaches for these and other conditions, but the general principles outlined above should be useful.

Psychopathology in Relation to Specific Surgical Procedures

Although no psychiatric syndromes occur exclusively in relation to specific surgical procedures, it is true that certain problems may more likely be encountered after certain operations. One of the most intriguing such associations is the development of cognitive deficits, affective disturbance, or personality changes after cardiac procedures and carotid endarterectomy (49). Micro-emboli and hypoxia have been postulated as causes.

Colostomy, amputation of an extremity, and oral, esophageal, or laryngeal procedures that result in speech or swallowing impairment all are difficult operations for the elderly physically and psychologically. Procedures resulting in cosmetic deformity may produce depression. This is particularly true with mastectomy, even for some women well past menopause.

SPECIAL TOPICS

The Impact of Anesthesia

Although specifically covered in another chapter, the effect of anesthesia on mental function in the elderly is worth brief comment here. Conflicting reports about the impact of different types of anesthesia have appeared in the literature. Some authors have suggested that general anesthesia has adverse effects on postoperative mental function when compared to local or regional techniques (50, 51). Others have not confirmed this effect in elective procedures (52, 53). Bigler and colleagues, in a study of emergency hip repair in the elderly, found no difference in postoperative mental function between general and epidural anesthesia (54). Some confusion in the literature undoubtedly results from lumping early and late (permanent) differences in postoperative mentation together, because most studies found some early differences. Those differences, even if transient, could negatively affect the course of recovery by interfering with compliance and increasing the risk of complications.

Pharmacologic Considerations

The importance of pharmacologic factors in geriatric surgery cannot be overemphasized. A comprehensive review of geriatric pharmacology is beyond our scope here, but excellent references exist for both geriatric pharmacology as a whole and psychopharmacology in particular (55–57). Pharmacologic concerns are relevant to geriatric surgery for many reasons. First, the elderly utilize many drugs in general, both those prescribed by physicians and those purchased over-the-counter. One group of researchers found that 78% of an elderly cohort were taking at least one prescribed drug, and another study revealed that 7% of an elderly population were consuming 12 or more drugs simultaneously (58)! The elderly are also among the most frequent users of psychotropic drugs (59).

Second, complications of drug use in the elderly are both frequent and serious. Hurwitz and Wade found a drug complication rate of 15% in a group of elderly inpatients versus a rate of only 6% in a younger group (60). Drugs are even important in the etiology of surgical problems themselves. In a very recent and important paper, Ray and associates reviewed the role of psychotropic drug consumption in the occurrence of hip fracture in elderly institutionalized patients (61). They found that use of several classes of such drugs increased the risk of hip fracture and that this risk was also dose-related.

In the surgical setting, many classes of psychoactive drugs are used. Preoperative preparation includes anticholinergics, sedative, and narcotics; the perioperative period involves the anesthetics; and the postoperative period sees the further use of sedatives, hypnotics, narcotics, and tranquilizers.

Both pharmacokinetic and pharmacodynamic factors are important in geriatric pharmacology in the surgical setting. *Pharmacokinetics* refers to the disposition of administered drugs, including such processes as absorption, distribution, metabolism, and excretion, whereas *pharmacodynamics* refers to the responsiveness of the body to drug action (55). Our discussion here will be confined to the psychopharmacologic domain and to factors likely to be significant in the surgical setting.

Absorption and First-Pass Effect

Although no age-related changes in absorption of psychotropic medications have been convincingly demonstrated, a number of orally administered drugs are affected by first-pass hepatic enzymatic activity. These include some commonly used antidepressants (desipramine and nortriptyline) and narcotic analgesics (meperidine, morphine, and propoxyphene) (55). Decrements in hepatic function can at least theoretically lead to increased blood levels of these agents.

Distribution

Most psychotropic drugs are quite lipid soluble. The age-associated decrease in lean body mass and water is coupled with a trend to increased lipid stores. Thus, fat-soluble drugs have a larger volume of distribution, a fact linked to their tendency to accumulate in the body during steady-state dosing periods. An important exception to the lipid-solubility of psychotropics is that of lithium; as an ion, it is water-soluble.

Metabolism

Specific differences in pathways of drug metabolism associated with aging are not clearly evident; however, the rate of metabolism of many drugs is diminished by age. Many psychotropics are metabolized by liver to other active compounds. When possible, drugs that are metabolized only to inactive compounds are therefore preferable.

Excretion

Most psychotropics are excreted by the liver; exceptions are lithium and oxazepam that are renally cleared. Because creatinine clearance decreases with age, a smaller margin of error exists before toxicity ensues for lithium. The final common pathway of these various pharmacokinetic processes is the blood level of drugs and their active metabolites. A secondary factor is their level of protein binding, because it is the unbound drug that is active. Blood levels are often higher in the elderly after a given dosing schedule. Thus, it is important in many cases to measure blood levels. Diazepam, for example, has a fourfold increased half-life in the aged.

Specific Indications for Psychotropic Medication

The use of psychotropics in the treatment of specific psychiatric disorders presenting in the context of geriatric surgery has been discussed above and is summarized in Table 35.3. Here, two other general uses of psychotropics are reviewed. Pain relief is one of the commonest indications for psychotropic medication in connection with surgical procedures. Postoperative pain is traditionally treated with narcotics. As with the use of benzodiazepines for anxiety, adequate dosages and a scheduled administration scheme represent optimal therapy. Fears of inducing drug dependence are usually unwarranted and should not prevent adequate analgesia. Recent research suggests that it might, however, be possible to minimize narcotic use through the use of regional anesthetic blockade in some cases (62).

Sleep disturbance is a frequent problem in the elderly before the operation and postoperatively. Although the indiscriminate use of hypnotics is to be deplored, the importance of sleep in promoting recovery from a procedure should not be ignored. Insomnia can be treated with chloral hydrate, antihistamines, or benzodiazepines. A short-acting benzodiazepine, such as lorazepam, is perhaps the most appropriate agent for inducing sleep postoperatively.

Adverse Reactions

Some specific frequently encountered adverse reactions to psychotropic agents merit attention. Long-acting benzodiazepines, such as diazepam and chlordiazepoxide, when given as anxiolytics or hypnotics, can produce daytime sedation. A number of antihypertensive agents have been linked to depression. The most notorious is reserpine, which is fortunately little used today. However, alphamethyldopa and the beta-adrenergic receptor blocking agent propranolol have also demonstrated this property. The newer beta-blocking agent atenolol can be substituted for propranolol in many cases. Cimetidine has been linked to delirium in the elderly; the newer analogue ranitidine may not share this property (63).

The cardiotoxicity of the tricyclic antidepressants in overdose is well appreciated. Their most important cardiac effects when given in therapeutic concentrations are prolongation of the PR and QRS intervals. Although use of these drugs in the elderly requires careful monitoring, it is usually possible to administer them. In particular, they can generally be used in patients with pre-existing cardiovascular disease (59). Important exceptions are patients in the first several months following myocardial infarction and patients with bundle branch blocks. The latter case is not an absolute contraindication, but extreme care is required.

A potentially serious adverse reaction to tricyclic antidepressants and antipsychotic agents is the anticholinergic syndrome. This syndrome includes a variety of symptoms, but especially common are dry mouth, constipation, blurred vision, and, in severe cases, delirium. This reaction is quite common in the elderly, probably because of reduced central cholinergic function. It should be recognized promptly; treatment by withdrawal of the offending drug is usually sufficient to reverse the process, although some hours or days may be required. More extreme treatment by use of physostigmine is generally unnecessary and even unwise. Ideally, the syndrome can and should be prevented, because there are drugs with relatively little anticholinergic action among the antidepressant and antipsychotic groups.

Orthostatic hypotension is another serious complication of the use of many or all of the tricyclic antidepressants. It can also occur with the low potency antipsychotics, such as chlorpromazine, but less commonly. Orthostatic hypotension is a serious concern because it is frequently associated with falls and their attendant morbidity. Although some tricyclics may be less prone to inducing orthostasis, this is not certain and the problem may be at least partly idiosyncratic. The safest course is the careful monitoring of the lying and standing blood pressure and pulse when introducing a tricyclic and maintenance of circulating blood volume and hydration. Discontinuation of as many other drugs as possible, use of the smallest doses possible, use of divided doses, cautious increases of doses, and the obtaining of serum levels when in doubt are other useful steps (59).

The elderly are quite sensitive to the actions and side effects of the antipsychotic agents. This is probably due to reduced central dopaminergic function (31). Many aspects of the use of these drugs in the aged have recently been reviewed by Peabody and colleagues (64). These agents are clearly indicated in management of specific psychotic symptoms and have also been widely used in controlling agitation and other nonspecific behavioral aberrations. However, their use in the latter context is somewhat controversial, and some argue that benzodiazepines should be used first. Acute adverse reactions include dystonia, akathisia, and other manifestations of extrapyramidal dysregulation. Such side effects can be controlled by anticholinergic agents, but these have their own complications, as discussed above.

Drug Interactions

Both psychotropic drugs and drugs usually considered non-psychotropic can affect mentation and/or mood in the elderly. Furthermore, interactions of non-psychoactive with psychoactive drugs occur in the elderly, but are poorly understood. Some specific interactions merit attention: Alcohol increases benzodiazepine levels and those of some antidepressants, and cimetidine increases diazepam levels. Tricyclic antidepressants antagonize the effect of guanethidine, alphamethyldopa, and clonidine. Certain psychotropic drugs commonly prescribed for the elderly, especially the tricyclic antidepressants and related compounds, are well known to interact significantly with anesthetics. The anticholinergic effect of tricyclic antidepressants may add to that of preoperative anticholinergic agents, producing tachycardia and anticholinergic delirium.

Several important interactions are associated with the monoamine oxidase (MAO) inhibitors. They are known to potentiate the central nervous system depression of anesthetics, barbiturates, and narcotics, as well as the action of vasopressors. Fatalities have occurred when they are combined with meperidine, although the mechanism is unclear. Duncalf and Kepes recommend that MAO inhibitors be discontinued at least a week before surgery (35). A final important interaction is that of lithium with muscle relaxants and succinylcholine; this combination should be used with great care.

Indication for Psychiatric Consultation

Turning from pharmacologic concerns to more general issues, it is useful to consider the role of the psychiatrist in geriatric surgery. Certain situations that a surgeon may face naturally suggest psychiatric consultation. These include the prospect of operating on a patient with known psychiatric disease who has symptomatic psychopathology or who uses more than the simplest regimen of psychotropic drugs. The unexpected development of significant mental or emotional symptoms in a surgical patient may also be an occasion for consultation, as may mediocolegal problems, such as the determination of competence to consent to or refuse proposed treatment. Finally, the question of surgical consideration in the terminally or chronically ill may be an indication for utilizing psychiatric expertise. Research indicates that psychiatric consultation on elderly inpatients is an underutilized service relative to the incidence of significant psychopathology (65). Yet the value of such consultation, when indicated, is substantial.

Medicolegal Considerations

Competence and Informed Consent

A number of psychiatric diagnoses, either intrinsically or in severe form, call into question a patient's competence to participate in surgical decision making. Competence is actually a legal term, and as such it must ultimately be determined by a court of appropriate jurisdiction. In practice, however, psychiatric evaluation, including a formal mental status examination, plays a key role in determining competence.

A particularly thorny area in geriatric surgery is that of informed consent. Cognitive, affective, and behavioral changes in the elderly may interfere with a patient's capacity to reason. The depressed or paranoid patient may refuse an operation when it is life saving. The demented patient may be unable to comprehend the nature of the surgical intervention proposed (66). In such cases, psychiatric evaluation to assist in determining competence to give informed consent is indicated. Family support at such time, if available, helps substantially to promote the chance of a favorable outcome. Legal steps are available to the caregiving team in cases in which a patient is not able to act independently or intends actions (or inaction) contrary to his or her best interest, as understood by the surgeon. Yet a patient's will should be respected if competence is determined to exist, even if the patient's intent is at odds with the surgeon's opinion (67).

Philosophy and Medical Ethics in Geriatric Surgery

Philosophical and ethical issues and questions of values often arise in geriatrics. The prospects of a surgical procedure, which has the quality of drama and force, is thus frequently the stage upon which conflicts in these areas are played out. It therefore behooves the geriatric surgeon to consider philosophical and ethical issues. In doing so twin perils greet him or her. On the one hand, ageism has long engendered a defeatist attitude in which valuable procedures were denied the elderly because of mistaken beliefs about their frailty. On the other hand, the rapid technological advances of recent decades have sometimes led to overly aggressive surgical approaches to medical problems. This has led to creation of perhaps surgically cured but nevertheless still chronically ill and disabled individuals.

Morrissey and Schein have argued that surgical procedures in the elderly should be oriented toward preservation of functional integrity. This seems a reasonable viewpoint. An operation should be considered not only for what it might achieve but also in the light of what harm complications might cause. Moreover, these authors also advocate its consideration in the light of the expected course of the surgical problem in the absence of surgical treatment or with medical treatment. It seems clear that there is less margin for error in the elderly. It is also true that a surgical problem can be the final episode in a series of medical problems of escalating severity (40).

The very old patients with one or more debilitating chronic medical illnesses, with cancer, or with prominent cerebral dysfunction, such as occurs in dementia or after a severe stroke, often pose particularly poignant ethical dilemmas to the surgeon. In such cases, the decision to operate or not must inevitably involve quality of life considerations. Does one prolong life at any cost? There is a general consensus that surgical care must not be spared in any case in which clear benefit from it is anticipated; conversely, heroic exercises with no overall contribution to preserving or improving the quality of life are unwise. Recognition of such concerns, together with knowledge of geriatric physiology and broad experience, will guide the thoughtful surgeon to an appreciation of the indications for aggressive or limited operations, or no surgical procedure at all, in any given case.

CONCLUSION

Various neuropsychiatric aspects of surgical

care in the elderly have been reviewed. Consideration of the normal aging process, both psychological and neurophysiologic, is the foundation for understanding the reactions of normal elderly individuals subjected to surgical treatment. Certain common pathologic reactions occur frequently; delirium is especially important. The surgeon faces special challenges when operating on patients with known psychiatric diseases, such as dementia, psychosis, and depression, as well as those of extremely advanced age with multiple system dysfunction. Psychopharmacologic expertise is essential because of its implications for patient management and recovery. Parapsychiatric topics, such as the questions of legal competence and informed consent, and the realm of ethics, are also real and important concerns for the geriatric surgeon.

REFERENCES

1. Millar HR: Psychiatric morbidity in elderly surgical patients. *Br J Psychiatry* 138:17–20, 1981.
2. Blazer D: Psychiatric disorders. In Rossman I (ed): *Clinical Geriatrics*, ed 3. Phildelphia, JB Lippincott, 1986, pp 593–605.
3. Knights EB, Folstein MF: Unsuspected emotional and cognitive disturbance in medical patients. *Ann Intern Med* 87:723–724.
4. Coull BM: Cerebrovascular disease. In Cassel CK, Walsh JR (eds): *Geriatric Medicine*. New York, Springer Verlag, 1984, vol 1, pp 25–35.
5. Carter AB: The neurologic aspects of aging. In Rossman I (ed): *Clinical Geriatrics*. Phildelphia, JB Lippincott, 1986, pp 326–351.
6. Butler RN, Lewis MI: *Aging and Mental Health*, ed 2. Saint Louis, CV Mosby, 1977.
7. Rowe JW: Physiological changes of aging and their clinical impact. *Psychosomatics* 25:6–11, 1984.
8. Meier DE: The cell biology of aging. In Cassell CK, Walsh JR (eds): *Geriatric Medicine*. New York, Springer Verlag, 1984, vol 1, pp 3–12.
9. Goldman R: Normal human aging: a theoretical context. In Cassel CK, Walsh JR (eds): *Geriatric Medicine*. New York, Springer Verlag, 1984, vol 1, pp 13–22.
10. Costa PT, Andres R: Patterns of age changes. In Rossman I (ed): *Clinical Geriatrics*. Philadelphia, JB Lippincott, 1986, pp 23–30.
11. Birren JE, Schaie KW: *Handbood of the Psychology of Aging*, ed 2. New York, Van Nostrand, 1985.
12. Storandt M: Psychological aspects of aging. In Rossman I (ed): *Clinical Geriatrics*. Phildelphia, JB Lippincott, 1986, pp 606–617.
13. Poon L: Differences in human memory with aging: nature, causes, and clinical implications. In Birren JE, Schaie KW: *Handbook of the Psychology of Aging*, ed 2. New York, Van Nostrand, 1985.
14. Arenberg D: Changes with age in problem solving. In Craik FIM, Trehub S (eds): *Aging and Cognitive Processes*. New York, Plenum, 1982, pp 221–235.
15. Crauk FIM, Simon E: Age differences in memory: the roles of attention and depth of processing. In Poon LW, Fozard JF, Cermak LS, Arenberg D, Thompson LW (eds): *New Directions in Memory and Aging*. Hillside, NJ, Lawrence Erlbaum Associates, 1980.
16. Weiss MF, Lesnick GJ: Surgery in the elderly: attitudes and facts. *Mt Sinai J Med (NY)* 47:208–214, 1980.
17. Haavisto MV, Heikinheimo RJ, Mattila KJ, Rajala SA: Living conditions and health of a population aged 85 years or over: a five year follow-up study. *Age Ageing* 14:202–208, 1985.
18. Maletta G, Pirozzolo F (eds): *The Aging Nervous System*, New York, Praeger, 1980.
19. Bondareff W: The neural basis of aging. In Birren JE, Schaie KW: *Handbook of the Psychology of Aging*, ed. 2. New York, Van Nostrand, 1985, pp 95–112.
20. Schwartz M, Creasey H, Grady CL, De Leo JM, Frederickson HA, Cutler NR, Raporport SI: Computed tomographic analysis of brain morphometrics in 30 healthy men, aged 21 to 81 years. *Ann Neurol* 17:146–157, 1985.
21. Brody H. Organization of cerebral cortex: III. A study of aging in human cerebral cortex. *J Comp Neurol* 102:511, 1955.
22. Henderson G, Tomlinson BE, Gibson PH: Cell counts in human cerebral cortex in normal adults throughout life using an image analyzing computer. *J Neurol Sci* 46:113, 1980.
23. Waller SB, London ED: Noninvasive diagnostic techniques to study age-related cerebral disorders. In Bergener M (ed): *Psychogeriatrics: an International Handbook*. New York, Springer, 1987, in press.
24. Naritomi H, Meyer JS, Sakai et al.: Effects of advancing age on regional cerebral blood flow in studies in normal subjects and subjects with risk factors for atherothrombotic stroke. *Arch Neurol* 36:410, 1979.
25. Obrist WD: Noninvasive studies of cerebral blood flow in aging and dementia. In Katzman R, Terry RD, Bick LK (eds): *Aging*. New York, Raven, 1978, vol 7, p 213.
26. Ingvar DH: Patterns of brain activity by measurements of regional cerebral blood flow. In Ingvar DH, Lassen NA (eds): *Brain Work: Alfred Benzon Symposium VIII*. Copenhagen, Munskgaard, 1975, p 397.
27. MacInnes WD, Golden CJ, Gillen RW, Sawicki RF, Quaife M, Uhl HSM, Greenhouse AJ: Aging, regional cerebral blood flow, and neuropsychological functioning. *J Am Geriatr Soc* 32:712–718, 1984.
28. Duara R, Margolin RA, Robertson-Tchabo EA, London ED, Schwartz M, Renfrew JW, Koziars BJ, Sundaram M, Grady C, Moore AM, Ingvar DH, Sokoloff L, Weingartner H, Kessler RM, Manning SI: Cerebral glucose utilization as measured with positron emission tomography in 21 healthy men between the ages of 21

and 83 years. *Brain* 106:761–755, 1983.

29. Kuhl DE, Metter EJ, Riege WH, Phelps ME: Effects of human aging on patterns of local cerebral glucose utilization determined by the F-18 fluro-deoxyglucose method. *J Cereb Blood Flow Metab* 2:163–171, 1982.

30. Reige WH, Metter EJ, Kuhl DE, Phelps ME: Brain glucose metabolism and memory functions: age decreases in factor scores. *J Gerontol* 40:459–467, 1985.

31. Wong DF, Wagner HN, Dannals RF, Links JM, Frost JJ, Ravert HT, Wilson AA, Rosenbaum AE, Gjedde A, Douglass KH, Petronis JD, Folstein MF, Toung JKT, Burns JD, Kuhar MJ. Effects of age on dopamine and serotonin receptors measured by positron tomography in the living human brain. *Science* 226:1393–1396, 1984.

32. Agate J: Common symptoms and complaints. In Rossman I (ed): *Clinical Geriatrics*. Phildelphia, JB Lippincott, 1986, pp 138–149.

33. Harkins SW, Price DD, Martelli M: Effects of age on pain perception: thermonociception. *J Gerontol* 41:58–63, 1986.

34. Beard BH: Management of psychiatric problems. In Greenfield LJ (ed): *Major Problems in Clinical Surgery*, ed 3. Phildelphia, WB Saunders, 1975, pp 124–138.

35. Duncalf D, Kepes ER: Geriatric anesthesia. In Rossman I (ed): *Clinical Geriatrics*. Phildelphia, JB Lippincott, 1986, pp 494–510.

36. Titchener JL, Zwerling I, Gottschalk L, Levine M, Culbertson W, Cohen S, Silver H: Psychosis in surgical patients. *Surg Gynecol Obstet* 102:59–65, 1956.

37. Heller SS, Frank KA, Malm JR, Bowman FO, Harris PD, Charlton MH, Kornfeld DS: Psychiatric complications of open-heart surgery: a re-examination. *N Engl J Med* 283:1015–1020.

38. Djokovic JL: Preoperative assessment of the elderly. *Wis Med J* 82:20–22, 1983.

39. Folstein MF, Folstein SE, McHugh PR: "Mini-mental state." A practical method for grading the cognitive state of patients for the clinician. *J Psychiatr Res* 12:189–198, 1975.

40. Morrissey K, Schein CJ: Surgical problems in the aged. In Rossman I (ed): *Clinical Geriatrics*. Phildelphia, JB Lippincott, 1986, pp 472–493.

41. Strub RL: Acute confusinal state. In Benson DF, Blumer D (eds): *Psychiatric Aspects of Neurologic Disease*. New York, Grune and Stratton, 1982, vol 2, pp 1–23.

42. American Psychiatric Association: *Diagnostic and Statistical Manual of Mental Disorders*, ed 3. Washington, DC, APA Press, 1980.

43. Wells CE: The differential diagnosis of psychiatric disorders in the elderly. In Cole JO, Barrett JE (eds): *Psychopathology in the Aged*. New York, Raven, 1980, pp 19–31.

44. Roth M: The natural history of mental disorder in old age. *J Ment Sci* 101:281–301, 1955.

45. Schmidt GL: Depression in the elderly. *Wis Med J* 82:25–28, 1983.

46. Blazer D, Williams CD: Epidemiology of dysphoria and depression in an elderly population. *Am J Psychiatry* 137:439–444, 1980.

47. Cheah KC, Beard OW: Psychiatric findings in the population of a geriatric evaluation unit: implications. *J Am Geriatr Soc* 28:153–156, 1980.

48. Shuckit MA, Miller PL, Berman J: The three-year course of psychiatric problems in a geriatric population. *J Clin Psychiatry* 41:27–32, 1980.

49. Folks DG, Franceschini J, Sokol RS, Freeman AM, Folks DM: Coronary artery bypass surgery in older patients: psychiatric morbidity. *South Med J* 79:303–306, 1986.

50. Blundell E: A psychological study of the effect of surgery on eighty-six elderly patients. *BR J Soc Clin Psychol* 6:297–303, 1967.

51. Hole A, Terjesen T, Breivik L: Epidural versus general anaesthesia for total hip arthroplasty in the elderly patients. *Acta Anaesthesiol Scand* 24:279–287, 1980.

52. Karhunen U, John G: A comparison of memory function following local and general anaesthesia for extraction of senile cataract. *Acta Anaesthesiol Scand* 26:291–296, 1982.

53. Riis J, Lomholt B, Haxholdt O, Kehlet H, Valentin N, Danielsen U, Durberg V: Immediate and long-term mental recovery from general versus epidural anesthesia in elderly patients. *Acta Anaesthesiol Scand* 27:44–49, 1983.

54. Bigler D, Adelhoj B, Petring OU, Pederson NO, Busch P, Kalhke P: Mental function and morbidity after acute hip surgery during spinal and general anaesthesia. *Anaesthesia* 40:672–676, 1985.

55. Carruthers SG: Principles of drug treatment in the aged. In Rossman I (ed): *Clinical Geraitrics*. Phildelphia, JB Lippincott, 1986, pp 114–124.

56. Salzman C: *Clinical Geriatric Psychopharmacology*. New York, McGraw-Hill, 1984.

57. Ban TA. *Psychopharmacology for the Aged*. Basel S. Karger, 1980.

58. Skoll SL, August RJ, Johnson G: Drug prescribing for the elderly in Saskatchewan during 1976. *Can Med Assoc J* 121:1074, 1979.

59. Richelson E: Psychotropics and the elderly: interaction to watch for. *Geriatrics* 39:30–42, 1984.

60. Hurwitz N, Wade OL: Intensive hospital monitoring of adverse reactions to drugs. *Br Med J* 1:531, 1969.

61. Ray WA, Griffin MR, Schaffner W, Baugh DK, Melton LJ: Psychotropic drug use and the risk of hip fracture. *N Engl J Med* 316:363–369.

62. Jones SF, White A: Analgesia following neck surgery. Lateral cutaneous nerve block as an alternative to narcotics in the elderly patients. *Anaesthesia* 40:682–685, 1985.

63. Jenike MA: Cimetidine in elderly patients: review of uses and risks. *J Am Geriatr Soc* 30:170–173, 1982.

64. Peabody Ca, Warner D, Whiteford HA, Hollister LE: Neuroleptics and the elderly. *J Am Geriatr Soc* 35:233–238, 1987.

65. Rabins P, Lucas MJ, Teitelbaum M, Mark SR, and Folstein M: Utilization of psychiatric consultation for elderly patients. *J Am Geriatr Soc* 31:581–585, 1983.

66. Hamerman D, Dubler NN, Kennedy GJ, Masdeu J: De-

cision making in response to an elderly woman with dementia who refused surgical repair of her fractured hip. *J Am Geriatr Soc* 34:234–239, 1986.

67. Abernathy V: Compassion, control, and decision about competency. *Am J Psychiatry* 141:53–60, 1984.

68. Koin D: Surgical concerns. In Cassel CK, Walsh JR (eds): *Geriatric Medicine*. New York, Springer Verlag, 1984, vol 2, pp. 275–288.

Chapter 36

Extended Care and Rehabilitation for the Elderly

Brian A. Bacon, R.R.A., Wanda G. McKnight, A.R.T.

The method of providing acute and extended medical care for this country's elders has been and will be a subject of major national interest for many years. As the population of older Americans grows larger, its members will become even more dependent upon the medical services and other services related to extended care. The purpose of this chapter is to examine the needs of the elderly in the extended care setting and to dwell somewhat on institutional options that are designed to maximize the rehabilitation, independence, and quality of life for the elderly.

EXTENDED CARE DELIVERY SYSTEMS NOW AVAILABLE TO THE ELDERLY

Many long term care delivery systems are now available for those elderly patients who need such services. Unfortunately, these current delivery systems are still loosely organized and are not very well coordinated with each other or with the acute health care system, resulting in potential for discontinuity of the care for the aged and disabled.

Ironically, it is at the time in their lives when they begin to have greater health care needs that many elderly people are least likely to have the financial means to pay for these services. Therefore, financial reimbursement for services is a major problem in the long term care setting. Although Medicare pays for most acute care hospital services and some physician services, it excludes most nursing home and long term care services. The Medicare program does offer limited financial coverage for skilled nursing and home health care, designed primarily for those

elderly patients who have good rehabilitation potential. Only medically related services are covered under the Medicare program. It will not pay for custodial, personal, or homemaking services. Medicaid is the primary payer of indigent nonskilled long term care in this country. It is not a widely appreciated fact, but about 90% of the Medicaid funds today are utilized for long term medical care. Only 2% of today's Medicaid funds are spent on non-institutional care (1). Fortunately, a large portion of the non-institutionalized elderly people are still being cared for by family and friends. Some, however, receive inadequate care because personal care, home health care, and housing needs for the indigent elderly cannot be met by community services. New and still unproven systems, such as Social Health Maintenance Organizations and various types of day care programs, are being created in an attempt to meet the needs of this segment of elderly patients.

PROBLEMS UNIQUE TO THE ELDERLY

Elderly patients face problems as individuals and as a part of our society that are uniquely theirs because of their increased dependence on medical services and their dependence on others to assist in the carrying out of their daily activities. As one ages, one tends to require more medical care. As other chapters have stressed, our vision and hearing become less acute with advanced age. These changes become more pronounced as we enter our sixties, seventies, and beyond. The senses of taste and smell are diminished, and our enjoyment of food is lessened. Muscle strength is reduced, and joints do not move as well. The ability to carry out the activities of daily living is therefore progressively diminished. These anatomic and physiologic effects of aging and the nursing and perisurgical aspects of these changes have been discussed in great detail in the preceding chapters.

Women generally live longer than men, and their health care needs are usually greater than for men. One of the major enemies of the elderly female is her increased likelihood of experiencing a fall. This may lead to a need for prolonged care and rehabilitative services. One study indicated a woman's chances of falling increases from 30% at age 65 to 50% at age 85 and over. Men's chances of falling increase from 13% at age 65 to a peak of 31%, which then declines at age 85. Tripping over objects that are hard to see and "drop attacks" (loss of postural control) are the major causes of these falls. In elderly women over the age of 85, the incidence of fractures from these falls increases. The study by Exton-Smith and Evans in 1977 showed 70% of patients who sustained fractures had a history of previous falls (2).

ATTITUDES TOWARD THE ELDERLY

Because of recent interest in and research into the subject, the "old age" stereotype has been defined, examined, and re-defined. Until recently, older people have generally been perceived as conservative, inflexible, withdrawn, passive, dependent, religious, and long suffering with various forms of physical and mental deterioration (3). Although some elderly people may fit this stereotype, the vast majority of the elderly of today are individuals very much like the rest of the current population, except that they have simply lived longer. Many are very alert, well-educated, intelligent, and physically active.

Evidence suggests that health care providers who work with many of these older patients have developed at least a neutral position and usually a much more positive attitude toward the elderly than those who have had little or no such contact with them. Evidence also shows that health care providers prefer working with those elderly patients who have disease-related problems and who have more potential for rehabilitation, rather than with those who require care strictly because of the effects of normal aging processes (4). Car-

ing for the elderly can be a rewarding experience for the care giver, and it usually fosters within the health care worker a greater appreciation for this group of people.

A very important aspect of providing appropriate and effective care for the elderly patient who may need long term care is the ability of the health care provider to achieve a compatible match of personalities with that of the patient. Particularly in the home setting, this bi-directional compatibility is important. The frequent one-on-one contact in the patient's home with the patient and with the other family members makes the compatible personality match very important. This aids in the patient's recovery, in his or her attitude, and it bolsters the sense of well-being. It also provides both the patient and the health care giver greater rewards from their relationship. A positive attitude and a sense of optimism on the part of the patient are paramount for a rapid and successful rehabilitation process.

REHABILITATION CONSIDERATIONS FOR COMMON DIAGNOSES

Rehabilitation of the Fractured Hip

The medical profession is now becoming more aggressive in the overall approach to the care of the aged. This attitude has created an environment that encourages other health care workers to treat elderly patients with the same attitude: Their opportunity for successful rehabilitation should be as good as are the opportunities available for the young. The result of this trend can be seen in the example so often seen today with the successful rehabilitation of elderly patients who have had repair of a fractured hip. The surgical and physical aspects of the success with this type of rehabilitation are also discussed in Chapter 30.

Patients with fractured hips sometimes become very confused when they are recovering from this injury, even if they have had no history of chronic mental impairment. The sudden injury and rapid hospitalization can cause disruption in the daily routine and result in considerable confusion in the elderly person. The rehabilitation process for this type of patient will be greatly enhanced if this temporary disorientation is treated as such and the patient is not arbitrarily categorized as "senile" or "crazy" (5). (See Chapter 35) Hip fracture patients recover best from their injury when they are able to be discharged from the hospital as early as possible after surgical repair. This should be recognized as the ultimate goal of the health care team from the time of hospital admission. (See Chapter 30)

Even with the medical profession's best efforts to speed the patient's recovery, the elderly patient may become emotionally distraught during part of the hospitalization. He or she will almost assuredly be worried about the other family members, spouse, or the home. If the older patient's spouse is living, it is not uncommon for him or her to fear for the other's well-being while the two are separated. The health care team should be conscious of this situation and make every effort to reassure the patient that all is well with things at home. Again, a return to the home environment as early as possible is the best and only remedy (5).

Although the recuperative rates for patients with fractured hips vary greatly, the successful rehabilitative process is always rewarding for all of the therapists involved. Education of the patient is critical. The older person must learn how to function at home in such as way as to prevent future injuries. This educational process must begin in the hospital and continue into post-hospital care. The physical therapy, which also begins in the hospital and is continued in the patient's home, is most effective when there is clear and frequent communication between the physical therapists, nurses, and others involved. All of this is best done under the direction of the orthopaedic surgeon.

Other Musculoskeletal Problems and the Elderly

Osteoarthritis or degenerative joint disease is the form of arthritis that most often plagues the elderly. These disorders are hereditary and age-related, but obesity can be a major contributing and complicating factor to this disability. Rehabilitative efforts for the aged patient with arthritis include weight control, if appropriate, and physical therapy. Protection of the knees and hips with balance and support, such as use of a cane or walker, may be helpful.

Rheumatoid arthritis is another common condition of the aged characterized by chronic and inflammatory peripheral polyarthritis, which is often symmetrical in its distribution. Swelling and proliferation of the synovial membrane eventually spread and cause destruction of the articulating cartilages. As the disease progresses, movement may be limited; deformity and muscle wasting become apparent. Tender nodules may also be present beneath the skin, and effusion of the joints may develop. Usually the disease begins in middle life and progresses throughout old age. Only in rare cases does the patient become totally incapacitated (6). When this condition exists, much effort must be given to its care and it must be recognized as a progressive situation. Often patients with these and other musculoskeletal disorders are more susceptible to fractures from falls.

The risk of orthopaedic trauma, mainly hip fractures, increases exponentially with age in patients who have Alzheimer's disease and other neurologic conditions. It has been observed that one in three women and one in six men over the age of 80 who have Alzheimer's will have fractured hips (7). Myra Levin's model for nursing indicates that the goal of nursing care for these patients is to maximize their potential and independence by integrating and maintaining the full use of any remaining abilities. The four patient elements addressed are the patient's energy (adequate rest to avoid fatigue), the structure of the patient's body (promotion of healing), the patient's personal self (recognition of individuality and self-worth), and the patient as a social being (inclusion of family and friends in care). Addressing these items may be difficult in the hospital acute care setting, but in the home care environment it is likely that the atmosphere will be conducive to this type of time-consuming nursing attention. The Alzheimer patient may be unable to absorb or remember much information that was received in the acute care setting because of memory loss, aphasia, and apraxia. A long term care environment, either in the patient's home or in other settings outside the hospital, may be the best environment for these patients to reach their full rehabilitative potential. (7) (See Chapter 35)

Neoplasms

The most common malignancies with which

the elderly are afflicted include malignant tumors of the lung, colon, and breast. The incidence of these particular cancers plateaus after age 70 or 80. Neoplasms that increase in incidence into the years from 80 to 100 include cancer of the prostate, leukemia, and lymphoma (8).

Elderly patients who have had surgical resection of intestinal or genitourinary neoplasms, and who have had the required ostomies, may be cured, often live a long time, and usually require long term care. Colostomy patients are especially in need of counseling and support from relatives and from members of the medical and nursing professions in order to maintain a good attitude and a reasonably good quality of life. Education in the care of the colostomy is essential for these patients and also for the family. Many of these elderly patients will have other medical problems that complicate the care of the colostomy. There are local ostomy associations that are eager to help the new ostomy patient adapt to the new way of life, but strong help and support from the family and good follow-up care in the home are also required. For those patients who require long term care, quality nursing care and extensive education of the family and patient can make life more pleasant and reduce future hospitalizations (9).

Circulatory Disorders

Atherosclerosis occurs in over 90% of elderly individuals. This disease in the elderly affects all vessels. The peak incidence of myocardial infarction occurs from age 50 to 70, and then it decreases in those over age 90 (8). Another major circulatory disorder, peripheral arterial occlusive disease, increases with age and is promoted by diabetes and smoking. This disease often leads to lower limb amputation in the elderly. Smokers with arterial occlusive disease tend to require amputation much earlier than non-smokers. Smoking of cigarettes positively correlates with a higher incidence of intermittent claudication, and heavy smokers are at three times the risk of non-smokers for needing all types of vascular operations. Patients who have quit smoking appear to show nearly the same low risk as non-smokers, because there is an apparent halting of these vascular changes after a period of smoking cessation (10).

The rehabilitation team can reinforce the edu-cation of the patient, especially about the ill effects of smoking. In the case of amputees who can be fitted with a prosthesis, the home care therapist plays an important role in monitoring the patient's progress and providing education and assistance when needed.

Visual Disorders

Other conditions frequently encountered that complicate the long term care of elderly patients are the many types of visual problems seen in that group. Although older patients may actually have correctable visions problems, they frequently fail to see the ophthalmologist regularly. The possibility of a correctable lesion should be investigated and ruled out before poor vision is accepted as a fact of life for the elderly patient. Recent technical advances that have been made in the field of ophthalmology can benefit many visually impaired elderly patients. These advances are discussed in detail in Chapter 33. Many eye problems, especially cataracts, respond dramatically to surgical interventions. Again the family members should be active participants in the analysis of the patient's visual problems. If the patient's vision is affected to the point that he or she is considered legally blind, the physician and the social worker can help the patient and family obtain available community services that will be of assistance in the home. Some communities have specific "low vision" services that provide excellent optical assistance for patients. If not, local ophthalmologists or optometrists often provide these services. There are many community organizations that are available to help patients obtain such items as talking books, large print material, electronic low vision aids, and braille books (11).

Mental Depression

Depression is the most widespread mental problem for the elderly. It is generally caused by lack of career and family, financial instability, sickness, infirmity, and death of the spouse. The problem of mental depression in older people will increase as the numbers of elderly people increase (8).

A recent study at the Boston City Hospital indicated that hospitalized elderly patients are at high risk for developing symptoms of depressed psycho/physiologic functioning. Four effects of psycho/physiologic dysfunction are confusion, anorexia, falling, and incontinence. The dysfunctions they identified can often be attributed to the patient's reaction to being hospitalized. Patients who are moved from their home environment to nursing homes, chronic care facilities, or housing projects for the elderly are also susceptible to increased morbidity and mortality in the year following their relocation (12).

Our society, led by the medical profession, can best address this problem in the elderly by adopting a more compassionate and inclusive attitude toward elderly people. This issue is discussed again later in this chapter and in Chapter 35.

Diabetes and Related Problems

Elderly diabetic patients usually have related complications that eventually will require medical or surgical treatment. Quality long term care can assist these patients by helping them to become less reliant on the acute care setting. Most of these patients can be managed by regular visits to their physician for adjustments in diet and medication. Ignorance, fear, and denial will result in a delay in treatment and lead to worsening of potential complications that may eventually require intensive medical or surgical attention. Some elderly patients will live with the complications of diabetes, such as foot ulcers, for years before they finally seek treatment. Education of the patient and family by the physician and the nurse can help prevent these problems. Home care nurses have extensive experience in dealing with these patients, and they can often help the physician prepare the patient for accepting surgical treatment, such as amputation, when it becomes necessary.

Unfortunately many elderly diabetic patients, like most others with life-long illness, are not financially independent and cannot afford extensive follow-up home care visits. Community services are often available to assist these people in obtaining proper access to the medical care system.

Safety Considerations

Health problems common to the elderly, such as hypertension, decreased vision, and dizziness, make the older person very susceptible to injury.

Joint stiffness and reduced coordination are major conditions that increase the likelihood of an accident occurring. Ninety-five percent of the elderly in this country live at home and are therefore reliant on themselves or their families to assure that adequate safety measures are taken in the home. The family can play an important role in this regard. Regular visits to the physician, especially for medication management, are important aspects of helping to maintain the patient's optimum health status and reduce the chance of injury. Simple practices for the older person, such as rising to an upright position slowly before standing, refraining from working with the arms above the heads, avoidance of the use of ladders or stools, and storage of foods, clothing, and medicines in low cupboards all can do much to prevent dangerous situations in their home. Obviously, the family members of the elderly can do much to encourage these safe practices. The family members should also develop a helpful attitude and should consciously identify hazards in the home that, when removed, will make life much easier and safer for the elderly. The feeling of being cared for, appreciated, wanted, and needed also contributes to the maintenance of total well-being and safety for the elderly. Elderly persons will usually develop a healthy attitude in response to a respectful, positive, safety-oriented approach from those health care workers and family members who care for them (13).

Nutritional Implications for the Rehabilitation of the Elderly

The nutritional needs of the post-operative elderly patient differ from those of a younger patient only to the degree that some slight changes in body composition occur with aging. A 6% decline in lean body mass is seen in aging individuals as each decade is spent (14), and between the ages of 25 and 75, approximately 45% of muscle protein content is lost. Occurring at the same time as the loss of lean body mass, the content of body fat increases and the total body water decreases. Diuresis, immobility, and infection can therefore more easily lead to dehydration in the postoperative elderly patient (15). Preoperative nutritional status is, to a considerable degree, predictive of the ability for good postoperative wound healing (16), and if the nutritional needs are assessed, they can alert the surgeon to the increased need for additional postoperative nutritional support. Involving a trained dietitian in the pre- and postoperative care and planning for the elderly surgical patient can help the patient understand his or her nutritional needs. This will result in a smoother, less complicated recovery and rehabilitation period. It is also important to keep the postdischarge plan of continued nutritional support in mind when assessing the patient's home environment, i.e., will he or she have access to the proper diet? A home health nurse can help the patient and family understand the nutritional needs and alert the physician if those needs are not being met.

Exercise in the Elderly

Not only does the elderly person who gets regular exercise sleep, eat, and feel better, it has been also shown that regular physical activity tends to slow the rate of the physical and mental decline, which has been known to show a gradual increase with aging (17). Regular exercise usually lowers levels of body fat, increases lean body mass, and increases muscle strength. Regular exercise and physical activity are especially beneficial, and they help to keep the elderly person independent and self-reliant for as long as possible. Exercise testing is often necessary for the elderly, especially if exercise has not been a regular activity in the recent past. Because prevention of injury is a major concern in the elderly, exercise instructions given to the patient are of great importance. The instructions and even the exercise testing may be given by a nurse, nurse technician, or physical therapist. Exercise testing and instruction regarding the extent of physical activity expected from the patient might easily become a part of the home-bound postoperative care if a physical therapist is available. An exercise program for the elderly person can be as important an aspect of preventing future surgical problems and complications as any medication.

DISCHARGE PLANNING

In no other group of patients is hospital discharge planning as important as it is when one is involved in providing complete medical and surgical care for elderly patients. The special needs of older patients are varied. Some will not have adequate family support to assist them with plans for rehabilitation. Some will be wealthy, some will have adequate financial resources, but many will lack adequate financial support. Some patients from all financial categories will need short or long term institutionalized care.

Early discharge planning is important for several reasons. First, acute care is more costly, and hospital days spent waiting for postdischarge arrangements to be made represent money and time wasted. In many instances third party payers, including Medicare, will refuse financial reimbursement for these "unnecessary" days. On the other hand, if the patient is discharged and readmitted within an arbitrarily determined time frame with the same principal diagnosis, payment may also be refused. Either situation places the financial obligation for the uncovered days upon the hospital. Some hospitals are in financial straits as a result of these denials.

Another equally important reason for early discharge planning is for the mental well-being of the patient. A smooth recovery and an immediate return to a familiar environment—be it home or the nursing home—ensures the patient that his or her "world has not ended" or changed drastically. If the patient's condition is such that return to home is not feasible, early planning for a new environment allows the patient and family time to adjust to the idea of living in a nursing home for a short while or in some cases permanently. Discharge planning is sometimes a lengthy process, especially when complicated skilled nursing care will be needed after hospital discharge.

Assessing Patient Needs for Extended Care

Home Care

Most elderly patients will strongly desire to return to a home environment. This often can be made possible in a supportive family environment by using the services of a home health care agency. Studies have shown that the long term care of a patient is greatly enhanced when individualized nursing care is available, rather than using the traditional method of task-oriented nursing care (18). Home health nurses are trained to care for patients who have dietary restrictions, who need appropriate medication administration, and who need wound care. The nurse is generally capable of assuring the physician that the patient's health needs are being met. Even if the elderly surgical patient is almost totally recovered from an operation, a home health care nurse may be helpful if strong, capable family support is not available. The best instructions given in the hospital may be easily forgotten or confused during the transition to the routine of being at home. If the patient has a chronic medical problem, medications or dietary restrictions may need to be re-established into his or her postdischarge routine. Other services or agencies that provide meals or assistance with shopping are available in many communities, and the discharge planner and home health nurse are usually very knowledgable about the availability of such services. Selection of a post-hospital discharge treatment modality will depend to a large extent upon the degree of support available in the home and family environment.

The Surgeon's Role in Appropriate Home Care Utilization

The vast majority of home care agencies work in concert with the surgeon to provide high quality medical services as ordered by him or her. These agencies are generally eager to communicate with the surgeon to ensure that he or she understands the care that is being provided and that they are providing only the care that has been ordered through proper channels. Without this input and constant reassessment, the home care agency cannot legally render care and receive reimbursement for services.

Appropriate referral channels include those available through the hospital's discharge planning or social services department and through the physician's office. This pathway provides the physician, the hospital, and the agency a documentation trail to ensure that the care is appropriate in quality and quantity. Most hospital personnel making referrals are aware of the agencies that will do the best job for the physician and patients.

Beyond these two types of referrals, the physician's control of the selection of a dependable home care agency may weaken. Appropriate referrals are sometimes suggested by family or friends, but it is inappropriate and, in fact, illegal for the agency to contact the patient or family without a physician's order.

Unfortunately, the competitiveness in the home care industry has forced some agencies to "find" patients because they do not receive adequate referrals from hospitals and physicians' offices. There are even situations in which the agency is willing to pay hospital personnel, physician office personnel, or physicians for these referrals. Some agencies obtain copies of discharge lists from hospitals and use this information to contact patients personally.

These practices are limited to a few agencies, and their reputations may be well known by other agencies and the hospital personnel who are making referrals. The physician is "the boss" for all home health care services, and as such can be very effective in ensuring that unnecessary services are not provided or billed. Generally speaking, if surgeons are asked to sign orders for patients for whom they are not sure they have requested home care, they should not sign them. The physician should contact the agency and ask for information explaining the referral, i.e., who contacted the agency making the referral? If he or she thinks the patient does not need home care or that the agency identified the patient illegally, the orders should not be signed.

If the physician finds the conduct or services of an agency to be unacceptable, he or she should discuss this with the Medicare intermediary in the area. By becoming more involved in the home care for his or her patients, the surgeon can play a vital role in helping those good home care agencies that are available to carry out the exact program as intended.

Frequent follow-up office or clinic visits and clear communication with the patient and family are the best avenues through which the surgeon can assess the effect of home health care. Altering, updating, and discontinuing physician orders as needed are important steps to maintaining appropriate home care.

Institutionalized Care

In some situations nursing home care after hospital discharge may be the most appropriate option for the elderly patient, although only about 5% of all persons aged 65 years and older live in nursing homes (1). It has been estimated that as many as one third of all nursing home place-ments are made hurridly (19), and consequently, it is not uncommon for the needs of the nursing home patient and the services offered by the nursing home to be incompatible (20). Wachetel and his co-workers have attempted (21) to analyze the predictors of post-hospital discharge care and have found considerable differences between the needs of men and women. For example, for a man the presence of a spouse reduced the likelihood of his need for nursing home placement, but for a woman, the presence of a spouse had no bearing on her chances of needing nursing home placement. The presence of a relative in the home had even less effect on the likelihood of nursing home placement than the presence of a spouse. Social and family support, then, appears to be more meaningful for the man needing postdischarge care than it is for the woman in a similar situation. The elderly patient's diagnosis, of course, had a significant bearing on the post-hospital needs and possibility of requiring nursing home placement. Patients of both sexes with mental disorders tended to be discharged more often to a nursing home. Nervous system disorders, such as strokes, and respiratory disorders in men and musculoskeletal disorders in women were highly predictive of nursing home placement in Wachtel's study. They suggest that these predictors may be helpful in "triaging" patients who will need assistance with nursing home placement. They stress, however, and we support their contention, that discharge planning for the elderly patient should begin the day of the admission to the hospital.

Choosing a nursing home. When the decision is made to utilize an extended care facility after the patient is discharged from the hospital, comprehensive information should be made available to the nursing home. This particular issue is discussed in Chapter 4.

When possible, the family should participate in selecting the nursing home. Visiting the nursing home can help the family decide which environment is best suited to the patient's needs. Contact with the state licensing agency might help identify those nursing homes in which substandard conditions have been reported. Only skilled nursing facility beds are paid for by Medicare and usually only for a short period of time. Often the elderly must pay for the nursing home

out of their own pockets until their funds are depleted to the point that they qualify for Medicaid. Medicaid also offers reimbursement for intermediate care.

Most elderly patients fear the prospect of institutionalization. With the assistance of the family who can help in evaluating the nursing home and in explaining the discharge process at the hospital, the patient's fears should be minimized. Problems relating to nursing home placement that generally concern the patient include the threat of loss of privacy, the impersonal atmosphere, the loss of family and social relationships, and the associated deterioration of morale. Considering that these and other drawbacks are real and objectionable disadvantages of institutionalization, it should be used as a last resort for the care of the aged and disabled (22).

The Congressional budget office estimates that 10% to 20% of patients in skilled nursing facilities and 20% to 40% of those in intermediate care facilities could be cared for outside of these facilities. Some estimates suggest that up to 50% of institutionalized patients could be cared for in less restrictive settings depending upon the criteria of need that are used (22). As more people in our society live longer and longer, these facts and their solutions will become critical in containing costs in our health care environment.

Adult Day Care

Community-based adult day care centers specifically designed for the impaired elderly are growing in numbers, and they provide yet another rehabilitation option for the elderly. The services provided through these centers vary, but they often include physical and psychosocial rehabilitation services, supervision of health maintenance, and respite care (23). Day *hospital* care in Britain has been developed to facilitate and prolong independent living for the elderly. The development of this category of care coincides with both the promotion of early discharge of elderly in-patients from hospitals and the prevention of unnecessary hospital admissions; however, there are no data to show that day hospital care is more cost effective than other alternatives to in-patient hospitalization (24).

Hospice Care

Hospice care is an alternative for the terminally ill elderly. Hospice care has been available in the United States for 13 years during which time the demand for this type of service has increased dramatically. This increased use is in part due to the funding by Medicare for hospice care. Preparing the patient and family for the inevitable death of the patient, pain control, pharmacologic management, psychosocial care, and cost containment are major features of a hospice program.

When properly coordinated, the benefits of hospice care to the terminally ill patient are many. In most cases, the patient is able to live in his or her own home until death. An often-voiced concern of physicians, however, is the fear of losing crucial continuity of care. They understandably find it difficult to relinquish the management of their cases to others after having seen their patients through many crises (25).

Improving Post-Hospital Adjustment

Today physicians and hospital personnel are more aware of the need for adequate patient education in preparation for a patient's post-hospital environment. Educational tools, such as pictorial information, pamphlets, or videotapes, seem to be effective. The overall goal of this strategy is to help the patient speedily attain an optimal level of functioning following an operation or an illness. To promote patient compliance, educational tools should be well organized, readable, repetitious, and specific. The more realistic or life-like the presentation, the greater probability there is for the patient to comprehend and retain the message (26).

PREVENTIVE CARE FOR THE ELDERLY

Because of the elderly person's lessened ability to survive emergency medical and surgical situations, preventive care in older patients is extremely important. The goals of preventive care are to maintain and improve, if possible, the quality of life, health, and vigor; to enhance the patient's independence; and to prevent conditions from reaching a crisis point before they are recognized and treated.

To meet these goals, a preventive care plan should include periodic and systematic assess-ment of the physical, mental, and social status of the elderly person (27). These objectives may be met by a support group of family, friends, and health care providers. In preventive care, it is important to remember several special characteristics peculiar to the elderly. Many times, older people are slow to ask for help. They are generally more accepting of unpleasant situations and tend not to complain. They understandably have a great fear of losing their independence, which is an attitude seldom seen in younger individuals. Some of the elderly of 1987 may have unpleasant memories of the institutions of the past and of the medical care of their youth. In addition, many of their peers will have died in institutions, and the elderly person may fear a similar fate for themselves. Indeed Branch and Nemeth found that 17% of 776 persons over age 70 whom they questioned had not seen a physician in the previous year, even though they thought that they should have done so. Twelve percent of that group specifically thought that all of their medical problems were all due only to their age (28).

Another important factor in preventive care for the elderly is a conscious awareness on the part of the care giver of the family "climate." Most families wish to care for their elders, but they often need advice, supportive assistance, and encouragement from time to time. A "holiday" that provides the other family members a time away from a stressful situation and constant responsibility can be an important contribution to the welfare of the elderly patient.

Most important to remember, however, is the fact that older people, like younger people, are individuals with different strengths, needs, and weaknesses. Each person requires an individual assessment and should not be stereotyped. As Holloway so aptly put it, "Age itself should not deny the right to be treated in a dignified and understanding way, even if time is needed to achieve this end" (29).

SOCIO-ECONOMIC CONSIDERATIONS

The current socio-economic and political atmosphere mandates that specific mention be made of the financial aspects of caring for the elderly. During the 1970s, the amount of federal and state funds that were used for the Medicaid and Medicare programs increased to an alarming degree. In fiscal year 1975, for example, 66% of the personal health care for persons 65 and older was funded through public programs, and this percentage has continued to grow (1). This alarming rate of growth has focused much attention on the rising costs of health care, especially that which is federally funded, and this has resulted in efforts to reduce the federal government's obligation to fund health care for the poor and old. These efforts which have been used by those employed for the review process are sometimes unbelievably callous.

The changing philosophy of the federally funded programs has led to a disturbing situation for all physicians, particularly those caring for a significant number of elderly patients, most of whom have only Medicare as a source of financing hospital services. This issue is mentioned in this chapter because of the harmful effect these changes may have on extended care by the cessation of payment for acute care before it is appropriate and, worse, by the denial of payment for hospital readmission. This is being done because of inadequate funds for the Medicare program. The rules for physician's participation in the Medicare program and the punitive measures employed by the federal government and those responsible for the management of the program for perceived noncompliance are designed to place extreme economic pressure upon the physicians and the hospitals. Physicians are expected, in fact they are demanded, to follow such stringent rules of admission, discharge, and readmission time frames that the potential for inadequate care is very great. The punitive action is then taken when it is perceived that the quality of care was substandard. Hospitals are denied payment for any hospitalization or action that is deemed inappropriate by the Medicare reviewer (professional review organization—PRO). the detrimental effect that these changes are having upon health care of the elderly is already apparent. (See case report)

L.B. is an 81-year-old obese woman with diabetes and hypertension. She had a previous history of adenomas of the colon. She had had a transanal resection of the large adenoma about 4 years ago. It had focal areas of atypia, but no formal bowel resection was performed. A recent colonoscopy done elsewhere had re-

vealed multiple colon polyps. Biopsies of some of these polyps in the splenic flexure also revealed areas of atypia.

Because of the patient's multiple medical problems, she was referred to the university hospital where a senior staff surgeon evaluated her closely on an outpatient basis. She was admitted to the hospital, and preparations were made for an exploratory laparotomy and a left hemicolectomy. The patient became nauseated the day of the scheduled operation and was unable to tolerate the bowel prep that was being used for cleansing and sterilizing of the colon prior to her laparotomy. The patient requested to be discharged from the hospital, rather than proceed with the operation. She agreed to reconsider the procedure at a later time. After she was feeling better, the patient was discharged from the hospital on the third hospital day.

Several days later, the patient agreed to be readmitted for the left hemicolectomy. In order to save time and hospital days, the patient agreed to have the bowel prep for several days at home. This was done, the patient was admitted to the hospital, and the following morning a left hemicolectomy was performed for six separate colonic polyps, two of which had atypical changes but none of which had become invasive. The patient developed a wound infection in the large obese abdominal wall. The diabetes was controlled carefully. The wound infection was treated aggressively, and the patient was discharged from the hospital after 3 weeks of hospitalization.

The PRO reviewed the patient's two hospitalizations and refused hospital payment for the second admission because the patient had had a "premature" discharge from her first hospitalization. Her hospital bill of $21,740.25 is non-recoverable and is the hospital's loss. The physician reviewer from the PRO program will now reconsider the recommendation for payment for the second hospitalization by the surgeon, the patient, and the university hospital.

As a result of a more competitive spirit in the health care industry coupled with decreased federal support for the Medicare and Medicaid programs as mentioned above, a larger variety of health care delivery options have recently become available. The number of home health care agencies has quadrupled in recent years. Health maintenance organizations have seen a similar growth. Unfortunately, the opportunity for fraud and abuse in these arenas has also grown. By the nature of their needs, the elderly are much more susceptible to less-than-honorable agencies than are other patient populations. Discharge planners and surgeons as well can help to some degree in the protection of their elderly patients from these evils. This issue was discussed earlier in this chapter. It is hoped that the competitive nature of the health care industry will result in "survival of the fittest" of the multitude of home health agencies and other alternative health care delivery and payment systems.

The hope that American citizens might continue to enjoy the finest medical care available anywhere in the world rests squarely and solely on the shoulders of the medical profession. Physicians must rely upon their own integrity and good judgement when caring for their patients, rather than willingly submit to capricious rules for which the stimulus is obviously purely economic. The Hippocratic Oath is older and more precious than the regulations of the Medicare program or those of any other third party payer. One cannot help but question the goals and ethics of a physician serving as a reviewing official who is willing to deny payment for obviously needed hospital care because of some minor technicalities pertaining to the hospitalization. The authors recognize that this present set of circumstances is most likely temporary. Nevertheless, the potential for the present situation to destroy many good things about health care in this country is sufficiently alarming to justify this discussion as part of this record.

HEALTH PLANNING FOR THE FUTURE

Whether many of these relatively new forms and methods of alternative health care delivery systems will endure and survive remains to be seen. The impact that they will have on the health care of this nation's elderly is also uncertain at this point. It seems clear, however, that our elders as a political and social group have gained sufficient attention and clout to ensure that their voice will be heard, and their needs will be addressed. The issue of long term care and its costs is receiving much attention now, and it is hoped that in the near future there will be a more suitable solution to this financial dilemma.

Currently, a few private insurers are experimenting with the concept of private insurance policies for long term care coverage. Planning for this is complex because of the difficulty in predicting the magnitude of the future needs and costs. Congress and the Health Care Financing Administration are also supporting research projects designed to find ways to provide long term care at a reasonable cost. One such program is the Social Health Maintenance Organization. This initiative provides long term care on a prepaid basis, emphasizing non-institutionalized care. Experiments such as these are under way across the country at the time of this writing (22). Our society must address the problem and should eventually find a way to offer individuals an opportunity to plan for their own future long term medical care needs. In the meantime, our elders will depend upon the compassionate health care system and intrepid physicians, whom they have come to know and trust in past years, to support them in their final years.

From a broader perspective, perhaps the greatest challenge facing our country in the near future pertaining to the elderly lies in the education of society as a whole about the needs of the elderly. The initial step in this regard is to integrate the elderly into our everyday lives, rather than considering them as a separate group. As Arie (30) points out, surely we will want our own children to have every opportunity to benefit from learning about aging and the elderly while they are young. This type of integration would foster a natural, continuous concern for the future elderly and would ensure that their needs will be addressed. After all, "they" are "us" a few years hence.

REFERENCES

1. *Fact Book on Aging: A Profile of America's Older Population*. Washington, The National Council on the Aging, Inc, 1978.
2. Exton-Smith AN, Evans JG: *Care of the Elderly: Meeting the Challenge of Dependency.* New York, Grune and Stratton, 1977.
3. Bassili JN, Reil JE: On the dominance of the old-age stereotype. *J Gerontol* 36:682–688, 1981.
4. Baker RR: Attitudes of health care providers toward elderly patients with normal aging and disease-related symptoms. *Gerontologist* 24:543–545, 1984.
5. Ceder K, Thorngren KG, Wallden B: Prognostic indicators and early home rehabilitation in elderly patients with hip fractures. *Clin Ortho Rel Res* 152:173–184, 1980.
6. Smith C: Orthopaedics and the elderly. *Nurs Times* 80:46–49, 1984.
7. Wells DL: The elderly orthopaedic patient with Alzheimer disease. *Ortho Nurs* 4:16–22, 1985.
8. Pushparaj N, O'Toole K, Hyland M, King DW: Diseases associated with aging. *Comp Ther* 9:7–16, 1983.
9. Jackson AS: Living with a colostomy. *Nurs Times* 75:70–75, 1979.

10. Liedberg E, Persson BM: Age, diabetes and smoking in lower limb amputation for arterial occlusive disease. *Acta Orthop Scand* 54:383–388, 1983.

11. Weinstock FJ: Managing geriatric vision disorders: where to get help. *Geriatrics* 38:96–102, 1983.

12. Gillick MR, Serrell NA, Gillick LS: Adverse consequences of hospitalization in the elderly. *Soc Sci Med* 16:1033–1038, 1982.

13. Mayo Clinic: Home safety for the elderly. *NCMJ* 44:379, 1983.

14. Forbes GB: The adult decline in lean body mass. *Human Biol* 48:161–173, 1976.

15. Beaumont DM, James OFW: Aspects of nutrition in the elderly. *Clin Gastroenterol* 14:811–827, 1985.

16. Dickhaut SC, DeLee JC, Page CP: Nutritional status: importance in predicting wound-healing after amputation. *J Bone Joint Surg* 66A:71–75, 1984.

17. Dustman RE, Ruhling RO, Russell EM, Shearer DE, Bonekat HW, Shigeoka JW, Wood JS, Bradford DC: Aerobic exercise training and improved neuropsychological function of older individuals. *Neurobiol Aging* 5:35–42, 1984.

18. Miller A: A study of the dependency of elderly patients in wards using different methods of nursing care. *Age Aging* 14:132–138, 1985.

19. Moss FE, Halamandaris JD: Too old, too sick, too bad. In: *Nursing Homes in America*. Germantown, MD, Aspen Systems Corp., 1977.

20. Kleh J: When to institutionalize the elderly. In: *The Geriatric Patient*. New York, HP Publishing Co, 1978.

21. Wachetel TJ, Derby C, Fulton JP: Predicting the outcome of hospitalization for elderly persons: home versus nursing home. *South Med J* 77:1283–1285, 1984.

22. Harrington C, Newcomer RJ: Social/health maintenance organizations: new policy options for the aged, blind, and disabled. *J Pub Health Policy* 6:204–222, 1985.

23. Szekais B: Adult day centers: geriatric day health services in the community. *J Fam Pract* 20:157–161, 1985.

24. Donaldson C, Wright K, Maynard A: Determining value for money in day hospital care for the elderly. *Age Aging* 15:1–7, 1986.

25. Gardner K: *Quality of Care for the Terminally Ill, An Examination of the Issues*. Chicago, Joint Commission of Accreditation of Hospitals, 1985.

26. Wong S, Wong J, Nolde T: Total hip replacements: improving post-hospital adjustment. *Nurs Manage* 15:34C–34G, 1984.

27. Carnes M: Preventive health care for the elderly. *Wisconsin Med J* 82:15–18, 1983.

28. Branch LG, Nemeth KT: When elders fail to visit physicians. *Med Care* 23:1265–1275, 1985.

29. Holloway E: Disability and the elderly. *Br Med J* 282:1533–1534, 1981.

30. Arie T: The future for the elderly. *J Am Geriatr Soc* 29:557–562, 1981.

Chapter 37

Projections for the Future

R. Neal Garrison, M.D., F.A.C.S., Phil J. Harbrecht, M.D., F.A.C.S.

Predictions for the future of surgical care of the elderly are akin to painting a picture from memory. Each artist in his or her own way would see different aspects of the scene and highlight certain views as determined by a personal perspective. Utilizing what current trends and avenues of surgical interest are in the forefront today, we will try in this chapter to mold a logical forecast of surgical practice in the 21st century. Our clairvoyance is hazy at best, but we have an optimistic vision for both the aggressive, enlightened surgeon of the future and for his or her elderly patients. We envision that both parties will benefit from a mutual respect for each other and a clear understanding of the accomplishments of surgical care. The aged patient will not necessarily live longer, but should have a more productive, vigorous existence in which to enjoy the fruits of his or her life's labors.

SOCIAL, ECONOMIC, AND POLITICAL TRENDS

As noted in several previous chapters, the geriatric population is growing faster than any other age group. The U.S. Census Bureau recorded that 26.3 million people, or 11.4% of the population, were 65 years of age and over in the United States in 1981. These numbers, when compared to previous decades, represent a steady increase in that portion of Americans aged 65 and over. This is due, in part, to a modest increase in longevity and, except for the post-World War II baby boom, a decline in the birthrate. By the year 2030, the elderly group is expected to be 17% to 20% of the entire population (1). The number of elderly people over 75 years of age is projected to grow even more rapidly, representing over 9% of the population in the same time frame. This trend toward a gradual

aging of the American population is not expected to crest in the foreseeable future; consequently, more elderly will require the expertise of the surgeon.

As a group, the geriatric population experiences a decline in overall health and an increased need for the use of health services. This need is reflected in the figures for fiscal year 1977 when the 11% of the population over 65 years of age accounted for 29% of the total health care dollars spent in the United States (2). At the same time, the elderly occupied approximately 30% of the beds listed for general surgery usage. Geriatric medicine has been recognized as an entity worthy of study and pursuit. Much socioeconomic planning for these much needed services has occurred at all levels in both the private and governmental sectors. Day care centers, nursing homes, and retirement communities for the elderly are commonly found today, and specific dedication of hospital beds strictly for the geriatric patient will become a necessity in the not-too-distant future.

THE ROLE OF SURGICAL TREATMENT FOR TODAY'S ELDERLY

In the wake of the needs of this expanding geriatric population, surgeons have become bolder in the treatment of old people even though the risk of anesthesia and of the operative procedure is greater than that reported for the younger age groups. The mortality from similar operations in similar groups of the elderly over three different time periods between 1951 and 1977 has been reported as essentially unchanged (3). However, mortality varies greatly for the various types of procedures performed in different body compartments on different organ systems, for emergency versus elective procedures, and for the very old versus the healthy sexagenarian. One study in 1979 listed a mortality rate of 6.2% in 500 patients over 80 years of age who underwent all types of surgical procedures (4). It has been forecast that in the foreseeable future more than 100,000 patients over the age of 65 will die each year during or following general anesthesia and a major operation (5).

The more aggressive approach to solving the surgical problems of old people stems not only from the surgeon's greater familiarity with and availability of elderly patients but also from the many improvements in the supportive care that can be provided by modern hospitals for their surgical practice. The ability to continue life by artificial means and the ethics and financial limitations of so doing are now matters of almost daily newspaper note and media discussion. Whatever may be the eventual level of ethical limitations established and dictated by political and public opinion, supportive care for the elderly and others should continue to improve. The availability of sophisticated surgical equipment and the gradual increase in knowledgeable surgical care should and will become more widespread and standardized throughout the country. All of these factors will allow greater freedom and safety for the careful surgeon and the elderly patient, and continued success should bolster his or her confidence in attacking remedial surgical problems in the risky geriatric patient.

The role of surgical therapy in the elderly is greatly influenced by the continual decline of many physiologic organ functions that occurs with the aging process. Similarly, there is an increased incidence of certain disease processes that lend themselves to surgical therapy as age progresses while at the same time factors arise that will complicate their anesthetic and surgical management. Of particular importance are the changes that occur in the heart, lungs, and kidneys. Atherosclerosis increases progressively in the industrialized societies over the entire adult life span. A point is usually reached, depending on hereditary, dietary, and environmental factors, at which cardiovascular function and clinical symptoms reach a critical stage. Over 60% of hearts examined at post mortem exhibit coronary arterial calcification in elderly patients. Even in the absence of specific arteriosclerotic

cardiovascular vessel narrowing, an age-related increase in blood pressure has been noted to occur in the elderly along with a marked reduction in cardiac output. These combined processes result in clinical disease (i.e., coronary heart disease, congestive heart failure, cerebral vascular disease, and peripheral vascular disease), a combination of which accounts for over half of the deaths in the aged population. Conversely in many instances there are various clinical manifestations of atherosclerosis that are amenable to surgical intervention.

There is a similar age-related decline in the function of respiratory and renal systems. After age 40, there is a steady decrease in the vital capacity with a concomitant rise in the residual volumes of the lungs. This is a direct result of the loss of elasticity within the alveolar walls. A dramatic fall in renal function has been noted so that, by age 65, even in the absence of a specific disease process, the creatinine clearance usually has fallen to one-half of the normal values for the younger age groups. These changes, and other age-related diseases, markedly alter the ability of the elderly to withstand the stress of a surgical procedure. Our crystal ball does not envision, for the near future, any significant medical progress in an understanding of the complex relationships between aging and the inevitable decline in organ function that occurs with it. Therefore, for the time being surgeons will need to adapt geriatric surgical care to accommodate these persistent risk factors.

Preoperative and intraoperative monitoring has become a science in and of itself. The overall assessment of the patient and his or her ability to withstand the contemplated surgical stress is especially important in the elderly and will remain so in the foreseeable future. The significance of the physiologic decline and associated diseases so measured by our monitoring techniques will be increasingly appreciated, and as the techniques become more sophisticated and reliable, the surgeon will become more comfortable in selecting and applying the indicated operative techniques needed for the care of an elderly elective surgical candidate. He or she will be able to minimize the risk in each individual patient by matching the risks of the operative insults with the abilities of the patient's declining organ function to tolerate the procedure.

Several physiologic score cards currently exist on a limited scale, and in the future, many more will be devised, aided by computer technology to weigh the significance of the multiple variables measured. (See Chapter 2) Noninvasive studies of the function of individual organ systems have become and will become more accurate and their use more commonplace. Cardiovascular and pulmonary blood flow distribution will be monitored routinely. The metabolic status, with liver function and nutritional assessment using amino acid profiles, glycogen stores, intraorgan blood flow, and immunologic status, will be routinely assessed for all surgical candidates. In the elderly patient, the measured inefficiency of these systems will be viewed in terms of their contribution to operative risk. It will continue to be the surgeon who ultimately balances the risk of the operative procedure and his or her ability to perform that procedure with the knowledge of how these various dysfunctions and physiologic variables will respond under stress. Judgement and risk assessment will remain a central and vital ingredient for the surgeon of the future.

Surgeons already recognize that extensive and lengthy surgical operations for peripheral vascular disease can be done quite safely and that the elderly will respond with only a slight increase in the mortality rate over that in the younger population. The increased mortality rate for this category of cases is primarily attributed to the increased cardiac risk in many elderly patients. There is even some evidence that the long term results of peripheral reconstructive vascular procedures are better than in younger patients. This phenomenen is probably reflective of the more virulent course that peripheral vascular disease runs in younger patients. However, even in such favorable cases as peripheral vascular procedures, a failed reconstruction or an operative complication adversely affects the ability of the elderly patient to survive. In the VA Hospital Cooperative Study of Amputation (6) there was a significantly higher mortality rate among patients in whom an amputation was done within 3 weeks of their vascular procedure. Advanced age was a definite factor in this elevated mortality. Thus, the limited physiologic reserve of the elderly can be strained even in favorable situations, such as with peripheral vascular

procedures where the stress would appear at first glance to be minimal.

Operations that involve the entrance into the major body cavities (i.e., laparotomy or thoracotomy) represent a great stress on the physiologic resources of any patient and thus are a greater threat to the elderly patient who usually has marginal reserves when compared to his or her younger counterpart. The ability of the elderly to withstand such major procedures is further impaired when even minor degrees of contamination or pre-existing infection exist. In a review of 255 laparotomy patients over the age of 65, 22 late deaths occurred with a predominant theme of sepsis and organ system failure (7). The inability of the elderly patient to avoid and/or recover from significant infection was the most common denominator in the increased mortality noted in these celiotomy patients. The nature of the surgical disease encountered and the impaired immunocompetence noted in most elderly patients mitigate against any major improvement in the results of celiotomy for these conditions in the near future. Advances in this area will hinge upon an improvement in our initial assessment and recognition of the immunologic and nutritional status of each individual patient and the development of techniques to augment and correct major defects in these systems.

The outcome for operations performed on the elderly is also unfavorably influenced by the severity of the disease process for which the treatment is being done and by the emergent nature of the procedure. Currently the increased mortality noted after emergency operations is more a function of the severity of the underlying disease that necessitated the emergency procedure than a lack of time devoted to preoperative assessment and preparation. With most emergency procedures, the predominant cause of death is shock from blood loss and the inability of the host to mount a sustained cardiovascular response or overwhelming infection from unrecognized or neglected disease. Many times these patients are not salvageable from the onset, and it seems that this emergent, desperately ill patient frequently is more and more likely to be in the most advanced patient age groups. Any major improvement to be seen in the outcome of these patients may possibly stem from the development of better techniques of care and resuscitation. Prevention of the situation, however, utilizing well-planned elective surgical and medical treatment plans—for example, the early diagnosis and elective resection of abdominal aortic aneurysms—offers the patient better hope of a satisfactory outcome. With the realization that the risk of a surgical procedure is multiplied many times over when such procedure is forced into an urgent time frame, more physicians and surgeons will be stimulated to recommend earlier and more extensive elective surgical procedures where a better result can be predicted.

To summarize the last few concepts, the elderly patient can usually withstand a clean operation of significant severity if done electively and without technical misadventure. The presence of very limited degrees of organ function does not seem to affect adversely the outcome of a well-done procedure provided overwhelming disease is not present and/or a complication of considerable magnitude does not occur. However, the existence of established infection, contamination, and the unfortunate situation of far advanced disease are seen as the factors most likely to affect the aged patient, and these are due, in part, to neglect and delay on the part of referring physicians, the patients, and their families. Preoperative infection and overwhelming septic disease will persist into the postoperative period and will usually foretell a dismal outcome. Both organ system failure and the frequency of the dreaded secondary operative procedures worsen an already dim chance for survival in the majority of these individuals. The present trend toward an early and a more aggressive surgical approach to the elderly patient on an elective basis should alleviate some of the risks associated with advanced disease states that have up until now unfairly influenced the perception of increased operative risk in even elective surgical situations. This attitude continues to exist and to be fostered by both primary care physicians and by public opinion.

THE ROLE OF SURGICAL TREATMENT FOR TOMORROW'S ELDERLY

The future, near term, for the surgical care of the elderly will be determined by the strong demographic and therapeutic trends that we have noted. These trends foretell of more well-planned surgical procedures on an ever-expanding population of old people. With a better understanding by surgeons of the physiologic barriers they must overcome and with the continued improvements in the systems available for the supportive care that they can provide, there should be a gradual acceptance of a more aggressive elective approach toward many operations. It is hoped that this attitude will diminish the number of forced emergency procedures, which are clearly a dangerous undertaking in the elderly. Even major and extensive operations will become more commonplace in the aged patient as the risks and benefits of such procedures are better interpreted, the surgical techniques refined, and the preoperative assessment simplified and better outlined. It is important that those particulars in an individual's physiologic makeup that would represent an absolute contraindication to a surgical procedure be identified. The older patient will have available a much improved surgeon with an armamentarium of sophisticated techniques and treatment options. It is anticipated, however, that some worsening in the morbidity and mortality associated with elective surgical procedures will be unavoidable as greater percentages of older, poorer risk patients with multiple associated diseases are added into the operative case-mix pool.

For the longer term, a description of our surgical future holds many possibilities, some of which approach the philosophical and many of which are speculative at best. There is always the possibility of a major natural disaster or a dramatic change in the environment in which we live as has occurred many times throughout recorded history. In recent times, mankind seems to be assisting in the likelihood of the premature occurrence of such a metamorphosis. From holes in the protective ozone layers to famine and deforestation of the great plains of Africa, the human species persist in an effort to better themselves for the present at the future expense of their fellow beings and of the environment. Perhaps a more urgent danger, considering the distrustful nature of the human animal, is a real possibility of a nuclear holocaust. Any one or any combination of these scenarios would obviously alter the need for surgical services and would affect how medical services are delivered.

However, none of these dismal possibilities can be predicted with any degree of confidence, and thus none can be prepared for to any significant degree. It seems therefore to be morbid and unsuitable that they be dwelled upon any further at this time.

The demographic trends, which promise an increased potential patient base, and the overall medical and technical trends toward increased surgical therapy in the elderly are indeed strong, promise to remain so, and will likely persist for many years. All such trends tend to level off, however, and there is the very real potential for other developments, in the absence of a major disaster, that would increase or diminish the role of the surgeon in the care of the elderly over a longer term.

Societal issues will dramatically influence the practice of the art of surgery in the elderly. Of major importance in this vein is the view that the current society holds of its elderly. The knowledge, wisdom, and judgement that this segment of the population brings to our collective experience are still held in high esteem, and they are thus sought out by the younger segments of many cultures and ethnic groups. In such a society, the surgical care offered to the elderly will flourish with new ideas and new types of investigations. The health care resources will be expended at a rate proportional to that esteem with which the elderly is held and proportional to that segment's needs. This position of honor and respect of the elderly, if inappropriately applied, could evolve into an intense preoccupation with a prolongation of life as an end in itself, with no consideration as to the quality or usefulness of that prolonged life. Or, a contrary position could develop that would view the elderly segment of the population as a drain on the needs of society as a whole. If the future should see a period of time of dwindling natural and financial resources, the working, young majority might tend to regard the elderly as competition, and thus it is conceivable that rationing of many of the more expensive and more vital procedures might occur. The limiting of overall health care services to the elderly would occur in such a situation. This phenomenon already exists in some countries where avant-garde surgical procedures, such as kidney and heart transplants, are reserved for the better physiologic candidates, i.e., the young with a longer potential survival. The view that the young have a right to vital medical services, and thus to life itself, to the exclusion of the elderly is a current theme in some populations even today and will probably persist.

The need for surgical services and the other expensive procedures done in the future may depend to a great extent on the progress of research made into the aging process itself. Proposed theories abound to solve this mystery of nature. If aging is due to a combination of environmental insults, which slowly inflict damage on organ systems incapable of self-repair or duplication, avoidance or mitigation of such insults may be possible. If these environmental insults are due to contact with transmitted virus particles, exposure to carcinogens, or the generation of free radicals released by polyunsaturated fats within our diets, appropriate prevention and early treatment may prolong the life span. Such preventive practices would place more elderly patients in the operative pool, and the physiologic deterioration usually associated with the aging process would not be as great; thus, overall operative risk in these aged patients would lessen.

If aging involves a pre-programmed genetic clock, and cells die after a species-specific number of doublings, as shown by Hayflick in tissue cultures, the human life span is essentially fixed as it has appeared to be for the extent of recorded history. Medical achievements made under this theory might then compress the period of predeath deterioration and senescence without actually increasing the life span to any significant degree. Control of the major lethal diseases, such as cancer and atherosclerosis, in the elderly would increase the average life span of mankind approximately 10%, but would not lengthen the maximum life span. The survival curve would still reflect the fact that only a small percentage of the population would survive to live more than 100 years (approximately 0.03%).

An autoimmune theory for aging is unique and deserves mention. It proposes that reactions between cells rather than within cells are the cause of aging. Antigens may be produced by the generation of defective proteins as naturally occurring genetic mistakes are made during the DNA and RNA replication phases of cellular growth and division. Clones of cells are thus formed in response to the "foreign antigen," and a series of prolonged histo-incompatibility reactions occur, damaging a variety of tissues. The frequency of such ''self-inflicted attacks'' increases with age as more antigens are formed and immune tolerance is lost. Key control organs with little ability for replication (i.e., the neuroendocrine system) undergo chronic malfunction as a result of this immunologic reaction, and thereby other organ systems are affected. Such a scenario would dictate that the maximum life span of a complex organism, just as the cell itself, is genetically fixed and cannot be altered.

Of the aforementioned theories, none is mutually exclusive of the others, and many other possible causes of aging have been proposed and are possible. Whether physicians can prolong the maximum life span, increase the average life span, or decrease the period of preterminal senescence, the role for the discipline of surgery in all of the scenarios remains undefined. Will there be a prolongation of the demographic trends of today, thus creating a larger and larger base of patients with more and more surgical problems? Or will there be a population of healthier oldsters with less need for the expertise of the surgeon? Perhaps healthier oldsters with only very specialized needs for surgical procedures should be the ideal situation that physicians and society should strive to achieve.

A gradual shift from the surgeon's role of today is likely to occur in any event. Transplantation of tissues and implants of artificial devices will become more commonplace. Unraveling of the mysteries of the immunologic system will permit us to use more of these major advances and will stimulate the development of an extensive knowledge base. A more efficient practice of organ procurement, preservation, and transplantation is now being implemented nationwide. The augmentation of immunologic competence prior to surgical therapy as opposed to the prophylactic antibiotic approach to infection prevention used today will improve the infectious limitations of surgical care of the elderly. This one development will improve all of surgical care, but is most important in the elderly patient who already has an impaired immunologic system. Major contributions in the fields of oncologic diagnosis and many treatment options await a clear understanding of how human beings identify immunologic self and cope with non-self.

Some areas of the practice of surgery seem potentially stable, whereas others are potentially expendable or are under threat of regression. Individuals will continue to require the services of the trauma surgeon to repair the damage they inflict upon themselves and others. The orthopaedic and urologic disciplines should expand in response to the increasing numbers of elderly; however, there will be more emphasis on the prevention of the degenerative processes, rather than on the repair of the damaged parts that result from trauma. There will be attempts and perhaps successes in expanding surgical treatment of diseases of the brain and neuroendocrine systems. The aging process is in many ways a failure of this system to maintain a friendly homeostatic environment for the other vital organs. An imbalance of neurotransmitters will be linked to many of the diseases that are associated with the aging process. In particular, the various forms of senile dementia so frequently encountered in the elderly will be recognized and corrected at an early stage, thus preserving a vigorous and useful existence for many. Surgeons will develop techniques for the repair of injured neuropathways, and precise diagnosis and correction will be possible, thus averting neurologic disability.

Advances in therapeutic techniques may expand or diminish the areas now recognized as the surgical arena. The present trend toward less invasive methods will persist and in some instances diminish the number of opportunities and indications for invasive surgical procedures. For example, the current approach toward the biliary tract through an endoscope is a valuable technique for the surgeon and in the risky elderly patient may become a replacement for the classical surgical approach. Similarly, balloon angioplasty, angioscopy, and optically directed laser angioplasty have the potential to lessen the need for formal surgical intervention both in peripheral vascular and coronary atherosclerosis. Development of these treatment plans will require the surgeon to be on the forefront of their development because only he or she can truly assess their impact upon risk in comparison to the alternative surgical approach. Certainly with the elderly, the least risky procedure that will be effective will be the one that will be accepted by both physicians and the public. Anesthetic procedures will shift toward regional block techniques, and the depressive effects of the general anesthetics will be avoided. New drugs and anesthetic techniques will allow more extensive surgical procedures to be performed on poorer risk patients and will significantly shorten the hospitalization and recovery time for these procedures.

SUMMARY AND CONCLUSIONS

The ideas expressed in this chapter may appear in many ways to be projections for an uneasy and unpredictable surgical future. However, barring a major natural or man-made disaster, present demographic trends for the elderly population and technological advances are so strong that in the near future, we can see nothing other than an increasing demand for surgical procedures of an ever-increasing level of technologic difficulty. The political and economic demands will support an aggressive approach toward surgical disease with inherent assumption of cure or at least improvement. The medical resources necessary to provide this level of support for elderly illness and disease in the near future will be available as the political clout of the elderly becomes stronger.

For the longer term, we foresee a persistence of near term trends with gradual leveling off but not cessation of the trends. There will be a proliferation of new approaches with the development of new surgical procedures and anesthetic techniques that are less invasive and therefore better tolerated by the elderly. There will be gradual success in controlling some of the degenerative processes and infirmities associated with aging and gradual improvement in the average life span. Most of this improvement will be in the productive years of life. It is doubtful that any significant prolongation of maximum life span will become a reality; however, the period of preterminal morbidity can and will be shortened. Surgical developments should and will be in the forefront in lengthening the vigorous lifetime of the elderly. Finally, there are foreseen many socio-economic stresses and disturbances for all of mankind; however, an overall gain in multiple areas will allow society and surgical progress to flourish together. Surgical care for the elderly offers a challenging vista most ensured and foreseeable in the near future and with hints of potential achievement in the more distant future. This must be exciting to most surgeons, who so frequently even today must combine the visionary with the practical.

REFERENCES

1. Panneton PE, Wesolowski EF: Current and future needs in geriatric education. *Pub Health Rep* 94:73–79, 1979.
2. Kovar MG: Health of the elderly and the use of health services. *Pub Health Rep* 92:9–19, 1977.
3. Ziffren SE: Comparison of mortality rates for various surgical operations according to age groups. *J Am Geriatr Soc* 27:433–438, 1979.
4. Djokovic JL, Hedley-Whyte J: Prediction of outcome of surgery and anesthesia in patients over 80. *JAMA* 242:2301–2306, 1979.
5. DelGuercio LRM, Cohn JD: Monitoring operative risk in the elderly. *JAMA* 243:1350–1355, 1980.
6. Kihn RB, Warren R, Bube GW: The "geriatric" amputee. *Ann Surg* 176:305, 1972.
7. Harbrecht PJ, Garrison RN, Fry DE: Role of infection in increased mortality associated with age in laparotomy. *Am Surg* 49:173–178, 1983.
8. Hayflick L: Aging under glass. *Exp Gerontol* 5:291–303, 1970.

Index

Page numbers in *italics* denote figures; those followed by "t" denote tables.